THE POPULAR MEDICAL ENCYCLOPEDIA

The Popular Medical Encyclopedia

BY

Morris Fishbein, M.D.

DOUBLEDAY & COMPANY, INC.
GARDEN CITY, NEW YORK

Library of Congress Catalog Card Number 56–9054

Revised Edition

W

PREFACE

THIS VOLUME discusses in simple language the diseases that affect mankind, some of the more important symptoms that occur in disease, some of the methods that are employed in the treatment of disease, and the methods by which disease is spread and prevented.

For facility in use, the book has been arranged in alphabetical order. Some of the sections, for completeness, are rather long, notably those dealing with child care, prenatal care, and similar subjects. In the majority of instances, however, information given has been made as concise as possible.

This book is not intended to substitute in any way for care by a physician. When remedies are mentioned, dosages and methods of use are not supplied simply because any remedy that is capable of accomplishing an effect is just as likely to be harmful if given in wrong dosage. Self-diagnosis is dangerous. The purpose of this book is, therefore, to be helpful to the physician, for it has long been established that an informed patient is more co-operative and better than one who is left in complete doubt as to what is going on.

The physicians of America decided officially that proper education of the public regarding health is a responsibility of the medical profession. *Hygeia, the Health Magazine,* now called *Today's Health,* published by the American Medical Association, of which I was editor for some twenty-five years, was planned for such education of people who want to know about health and disease.

The best advice that can be given to anyone who is ill is to consult a competent physician at the earliest possible moment and to be guided by his advice.

This book is regularly revised to keep it up to date with new discoveries in the field of disease prevention and medical care.

MORRIS FISHBEIN, M.D.

THE POPULAR MEDICAL ENCYCLOPEDIA

ABDOMEN The portion of the body below the chest and diaphragm and above the legs; the abdomen contains the stomach, intestines, liver, gall bladder, spleen, kidneys, bladder, and other organs.

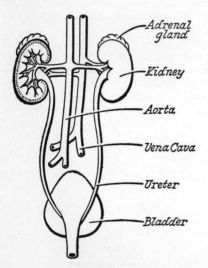

The lower abdomen contains among other important structures the adrenal glands, which lie above the kidneys; the large blood vessels, which carry blood from the heart to the smaller arteries of the body and return the blood from the veins to the heart; the ureters, which carry urine from the kidneys to the bladder; and the bladder, which holds the urine until it is released from the body

ABDOMINAL PAIN (See also *Stomach Ulcers, Appendicitis, Gall Bladder, Peritonitis, Hernia, Kidneys*, and *Intestines*) Nothing is quite so alarming or disturbing to the average person as a sudden severe pain in the abdomen. The diagnosis of the cause of such a pain is one of the most delicate and difficult of medical tasks. Colic or a griping pain may come from overeating or from eating foods that are particularly irritating. Abdominal pain is sometimes due to inflammation of the lungs, which is reflected to the abdomen along the nerves. In the early stages of pneumonia and pleurisy children sometimes suffer most with abdominal pain.

A pain in a localized spot in the abdomen is most often due to an acute inflammation of the appendix. In a grown person the gall bladder may be the chief cause of the pain; the outlet or gall

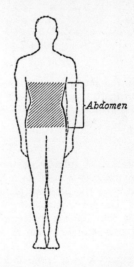

ducts may have been blocked by a stone or the gall bladder itself may be infected or swollen. The attempt to pass a stone from the gall bladder or the kidney down the tubes that carry the secretions away from these organs will produce a serious pain.

A sudden obstruction of the bowels by worms or irritations may be the cause of a severe abdominal pain. In children sometimes one part of the bowel will be drawn into another part, causing what is called an intussusception. The child with this condition will suddenly scream and may even partially collapse. The child may lie quietly between attacks but each attack of pain is so severe that the first reaction is repeated. Any time a child has a severe abdominal pain with such a reaction, the doctor should be called immediately, because delay may be serious if not fatal.

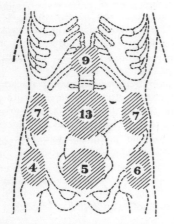

This drawing shows the number of different structures in each part of the abdominal area that may be the cause of pain there

A sensation of fullness or weight in the abdomen may be due to a nervous condition or to the presence of an ulcer or tumor. The development of gas in the bowels or the stomach is frequently a cause of pain and irritation as well as nausea.

Occasionally a pain in the abdomen is due to inflammation of the bones of the spine. Rheumatism or arthritis affecting the spine will reflect themselves with pain in front, although sooner or later the pain is related back to the spine. Therefore a persistent pain in the abdomen should never be neglected. Most of these conditions can be treated if a proper diagnosis is made early. A pain that comes and goes should never be neglected.

One of the most serious sudden pains is the result of perforation of an ulcer of the stomach or of the duodenum. This pain comes on suddenly and severely and is unlike anything the person ever suffered before. At such times the slightest movement will add to the sharpness of the pain.

The most common cause of pain in the abdomen is ordinary stomach-ache —less elegantly called a "belly-ache." The average person who has a stomach-ache suffers a rather well-defined pain somewhere along the middle of the abdomen and occasionally on the left or right.

Too many people when they get a pain try to remove it by taking a large dose of castor oil, epsom salts, or some other laxative or cathartic. This acts about the same way dynamite would act

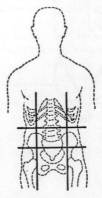

The precise location of pain in the abdomen is important in determining the possible cause or causes. This is the way doctors divide the area: Upper section reading from left to right: right hypochondriac region—epigastric—left hypochondriac
Center section reading from left to right: right lumbar—umbilical—left lumbar
Lower section reading from left to right: right inguinal—hypogastric—left inguinal

in a small closed place. If it cannot break out at one point, it will break out at another.

Therefore the best advice when abdominal pain occurs is to find the cause as soon as possible and then to treat it accordingly. Second, never take any powerful remedy until the cause has been determined.

ABORTION Almost half the married women of the United States have had a miscarriage before they are thirty-five years of age. Estimates indicate one abortion to every two and one half childbirths in cities and one in five in rural areas. About one third of the 700,000 abortions in the United States each year are spontaneous, the others induced.

Abortions occur most frequently in the eighth to the twelfth week of pregnancy. "Immature labor" is interruption of pregnancy from the sixteenth to the twenty-eighth week; "premature labor" is interruption from then to the thirty-seventh week.

Spontaneous abortion occurs from any cause that brings about death of the unborn child. Infection, high fever, or asphyxiation of the mother may induce abortion. Syphilis, malformations, or injuries may stimulate expulsion of the fetus. Changes in the action of the glands and wrong nutrition may have this effect.

The chief signs of a threatened spontaneous abortion are pain in the womb or uterus; bleeding; and expulsion of all or parts of the unborn child from the mother's organs. Severe pain and bleeding of a pregnant woman should be considered a threatening sign. She should go to bed immediately; the physician should be secured as soon as possible.

ABORTUS FEVER See *Undulant Fever.*

ABRASION A spot rubbed bare of skin or mucous membrane. Usually serum or blood flows from this spot. The best treatment is thorough washing with soap and water and the application of a clean sterile bandage.

ABSCESS Whenever an area of the body becomes infected with accumulation of pus, the condition is called an abscess. A large collection of pus in the chest cavity is called empyema. The abscess forms because pus-forming germs like the staphylococci or streptococci, or less often others form poisons which destroy the cells. Inflammation occurs and the white blood cells or leukocytes come into the area and help to take up and liquefy the material. The white blood cells give the pus a creamy appearance. Eventually the wall of inflammation around the abscess thins out so that the pus may burst through. Thus a boil, which is a form of abscess, "points" or "comes to a head." Physicians consider it safest to open the abscess with a sterilized knife after cleaning the area, so that the pus may be cleanly and wholly removed without damaging tissue unnecessarily. Should the abscess break into the abdominal cavity, it might set up general infection or peritonitis. If an abscess breaks into a large blood vessel, the infection may be quickly spread through the whole body, causing sepsis. In control of the infected area antiseptics may be applied or there may be injections of the sulfonamide drugs or penicillin or other suitable antibiotics.

ACCIDENTS (See also *Hemorrhage, Poisoning, Shock,* etc.) Fourth in the list of causes of death in the United States are accidents. A good knowledge of first aid and of resuscitation would save some of the lives lost by accidents. The *Red Cross First Aid Book* should be studied by everyone. Some people have more accidents than do others for a variety of psychologic reasons. These people are accident-prone.

ACETANILID This drug is a derivative of aniline combined with acetic acid. It has also been called antifebrin because it acts to bring down a fever. Its chief effect is to relieve pain. Thus acetanilid is a constituent of many common headache remedies. Nevertheless, because it is derived from aniline, acetanilid is a poison and should never be taken except when prescribed by a doctor. An overdose of acetanilid depresses the action of the heart; it also interferes with the ability of the red blood cells to carry oxygen so that the person affected becomes blue and short of breath.

ACETIC ACID   The sour substance of which vinegar is characteristic. Glacial acetic acid and trichloracetic acid are used as caustic substances to destroy warts, corns, or other horny tissue growths.

ACHLORHYDRIA   Changes in the wall of the stomach sometimes reduce the total amount of hydrochloric acid in the gastric juice. Complete absence is exceedingly rare, occurring in about 10 per cent of people with disturbances of the stomach. Cases of decreased acid are, however, fairly frequent. In most cases the digestion carried on in the intestines takes care of the absence of digestion in the stomach. With insufficient acid the stomach empties more rapidly than when acid is present. The treatment is to give small doses of dilute hydrochloric acid in a whole glass of water before each meal, as prescribed by the doctor. However, the giving of plain water or any inert substance called a "placebo" often has the same effect, so that the result is probably more psychologic than actual. The functions of the stomach, including its secretions, are greatly susceptible to influences from the nervous system.

ACHONDROPLASIA   Also called "dwarfism." Sometimes there occurs before birth a disturbance of the growth of bones so that the child is born with a large head, a small face, approximately a normal trunk, and very short limbs. Such dwarfs have been known for thousands of years and were court jesters in the Middle Ages. One sees them often nowadays on the stage. There is usually one with each troupe of Minnevitch's harmonica players. The cause of the failure to grow is not known.

The mental condition is usually nor-mal, but these little people often become spoiled by their parents. Seldom do they reach more than four feet in height.

The achondroplastic dwarf differs from the cretin type of dwarf because of the abnormal proportions and because the mentality of the achondroplastic dwarf is normal.

ACHYLIA   The complete absence of all secretions of gastric juice by the stomach. A condition exceedingly rare. More common are achlorhydria and anacidity, which refer to a lack of sufficient hydrochloric acid in the juices secreted by the stomach.

ACIDOSIS   A true acid state of the blood never actually occurs during life. Acidosis is, therefore, merely the tendency toward production of overacidity that may arise in certain diseases. Acid is always developing in the body but is usually carried away in excretions from the body.

There are some conditions affecting digestion in which acidosis develops, either because of increased production of acid or because the alkaline substances are lost by way of the bowels. This happens when there is much loss of fluid from vomiting or diarrhea. The treatment is to replace the loss of fluid and to hinder the production of acid substances by giving water, salts, and glucose. If these cannot be taken by mouth, the doctor will inject what is needed into the tissues or veins.

The most obvious symptoms of acidosis are headache, weakness, rapid breathing, and a sort of fruity odor to the breath. The most certain tests are made in the laboratory. Such tests of the blood and urine will show the amount of the alkali reserve and the acid state.

Certain foods are definitely associated with the formation of acid. These include lean beef, white bread, chicken, egg yolk, oysters, veal, wheat, pork, fish. Other foods tend to yield alkaline reactions. The alkaline-forming products include tomatoes, prunes, carrots, lima beans, oranges, lemons, cantaloupe, lettuce, peaches, potatoes, and dried peas.

Sodium bicarbonate is frequently taken to overcome an acid condition. The symptoms of excess acidity are signals of trouble, which should be investigated carefully. Sometimes the trouble is constipation; sometimes the difficulty is in the gall bladder. When a fire bell rings the fireman does not pour water on the fire bell; he recognizes the signal and goes to the fire. When acid eructations occur, the difficulty is not always with the acid.

Diabetes is the chief disease in which acidosis occurs. In diabetes the body is unable to use sugar, so that fats are incompletely burned in the body and acid substances are produced. The acid substances accumulate, and the body must develop alkaline susbtances to neutralize them.

Acidosis also develops in some diseases of the kidney, but it is never so severe in these conditions as when it is associated with diabetes.

Usually excess acid in the secretions of the stomach is associated with excessive work, worry, indulgence in alcohol or tobacco, or imperfect utilization of fluid. It is sometimes associated also with ulcer in the stomach. Before doing anything about excess acid in the stomach, however, find out the extent of the excess and whether or not anything needs to be done about it.

Citrus fruits have been offered as a means of overcoming acidosis; if the body is really acid, it will take six quarts of orange juice to get it over on the alkaline side. But oranges may well constitute a part of an alkalinizing diet. Some people warn against eating meat for fear it will have an acid tendency. Chemists have estimated that it would require four and one half pounds of lean beef in a single meal to produce a slight shift toward the acid side.

ACNE Acne is the scientific name for a chronic inflammatory disease of the oil glands and hair follicles of the skin. This condition is called by most people merely pimples and blackheads.

Acne occurs most often in boys and girls between the ages of twelve and twenty-five. The pimples and blackheads occur mostly on the face but can be found on other parts of the body, especially the back. In many cases the skin is excessively oily, so that there is much dandruff in the scalp and much itching, redness, and scaling behind the ears.

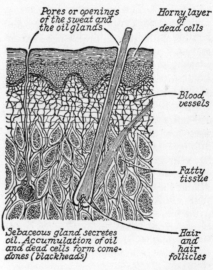

A cross section of the skin showing the tissues that secrete perspiration and the relationship of the hair to the skin

Acne is not caused by uncleanliness alone. Many people who are excessively active in caring for the skin and wash it constantly still have acne. The most recent view is that acne is related in some way to wrong action of parts of the glandular system of the body.

Often acne is associated with difficulties related to digestion; in many instances it seems to be related to excessive indulgence in stimulants and sugar. Drugs like bromides or iodides, to which many people are sensitive, will increase the number of pimples.

Doctors differentiate various kinds of acne, such as acne vulgaris. Cleanliness is important in preventing infection with pus-forming germs and secondary abscesses and scarring. Blackheads should be squeezed out under careful conditions of cleanliness. The face should be washed thoroughly with hot water. The skin may be soaked in hot boric-acid solution containing about three heaping tablespoonfuls of powdered boric acid to three quarts of hot water. The face may be soaked for ten to fifteen minutes with towels wrung out in a hot solution of this kind. This will remove the grease and loose skin from the face. After this heating process the blackheads may be squeezed out properly with a special blackhead extractor. Then the skin may be treated with successive applications of cold water to contract the pores.

Specialists in diseases of the skin provide various ointments, salves, and pastes for irritated and infected skins. Ointment made with sulfonamide drugs or antibiotics like penicillin and terramycin are useful in preventing secondary pus infections but should be used only when prescribed by the doctor.

The X ray has been found to be one of the most effective treatments. X ray must be given by someone who has specialized in its use. Improperly used, there are great dangers.

Much has been said about controlling the diets of people with acne. Sugar seems to be harmful in many cases. Since there appears to be some sensitivity in the skin of such patients, many specialists insist that those with acne be restricted in their fat, chocolate, alcohol, and iodine. These substances seem sometimes to be especially important in bringing about reduced ability of the skin to resist infection.

Many skin specialists insist also on the avoidance of spicy and peppery foods. Recent research emphasizes the glandular relationship more than previous studies. In many lesions treatment with ointments of hydrocortisone has resulted in prompt improvement, a method which is still experimental.

ACONITE An alkaloid drug derived from a plant formerly much used in medicine in ointments to relieve pain. In an overdose it is a dangerous poison. Once it was used in fevers. Whenever poisoning occurs, as shown by vomiting, motor weakness, burning in the abdomen, and a fall in the pulse and breathing rates, the stomach is washed by encouraging vomiting and by using a stomach tube. Atropine and digitalis are antidotes.

ACRIFLAVINE A brownish-red crystalline dye substance which is used in the treatment of various infections. This group includes also proflavine.

ACRODYNIA A disease of infancy with increased sensitivity of the soles and palms, rheumatoid pains, and a brilliant red eruption. The condition is usually associated with a deficiency of vitamins A and B complex in the diet.

ACROMEGALY "Giantism." When the anterior portion of the pituitary gland becomes excessive in its action, there is enlargement of the hands, feet, jaws, lips, nose, and tongue, to which the general name "acromegaly" is given. Closely related is gigantism, in which all the body is affected uniformly with overgrowth.

The person who develops acromegaly first notices thickening of the soft tissues, accompanied particularly by changes in the bones. The jawbones are enlarged, and the lower jaw sticks out. The nose is thickened, the lips become coarse and protruding, and the ears become large. The hands and feet look like paws. The voice becomes deepened, due to thickening of the vocal cords. The hair grows thicker, and it appears most profusely over the whole body, both in women and in men who are affected. Soon the sex glands are found to be disturbed, and these giants fail to have the sexual power that is often associated with them. Hardly any cases are known in which women with acromegaly have had children.

Usually the great size of the person

is associated with an inordinate appetite; these people eat a vast amount of food. Sometimes the disease reaches a point at which its advance ceases, so that the person will experience no further changes and will be enabled to live almost a normal existence. In other cases one portion of the body may suddenly develop a giant character, such as the great toe, or the thumb, or one or two fingers. In most cases, however, the condition proceeds gradually to the point where great weakness develops, and eventually death.

No method is known by which the growth of the gland or its excessive secretion can be stopped by remedies given internally. Sometimes it is controlled by the use of the X ray or by surgical operation.

Giants are far more frequent among men than among women. In those cases also it is the pituitary gland that is primarily responsible. Seldom do giants reach a height greater than seven feet with a varying number of inches, although rare instances are recorded of men who reached eight feet in height. Robert Wadlow, the Alton giant, was well over eight feet tall. There are certain cases in which large size may be reached without any determinable evidence that there is anything wrong in the glandular system. Conceivably certain portions of the nervous system may be associated with the processes of growth, and the changes in the nervous system may be primarily responsible.

The one hope in a severe case of this type seems to lie in removal of the excess portions of the gland or in some effort to control the condition by attacks on other glands which may be related to the pituitary.

ACTINOMYCOSIS This serious disease of men and animals is caused by fungus growths, which grow in extended chains. The actinomyces grows like a star. When the condition affects cattle it is called lumpy jaw. Cattle are attacked by the disease more frequently than men.

When a human being is affected with actinomycosis, it is usually from chewing grass or straw or grain which has been infected with the organisms. Therefore the condition is more frequently seen in laborers and farmers than in other classes of people.

When the fungus gets into the body, it enters usually through decayed teeth or diseased tonsils, following the chewing of a straw. The first sign is usually a hard lumpy swelling at the lower edge of the jaw or in front of the ears, such as occurs in mumps. After the skin becomes elevated and lumpy, pus forms, and soon there is an open running growth. The material from this growth is also infected, and it is necessary to observe sanitary precautions around such people.

The treatment of actinomycosis involves surgical removal of the infected material. Sometimes the X ray is used. Antibiotics and sulfonamide drugs are also employed to control the infection. The patient must be kept clean and everything possible done to avoid contamination of other people or of materials with the pus from the infected area.

Meat from animals with actinomycosis is condemned and infected animals are destroyed.

ADAM'S APPLE The prominent cartilages of the larynx which are seen in the front of the throat in men.

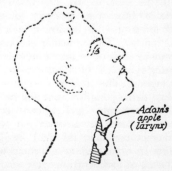

The Adam's apple is a cartilage in the neck

ADDICTION, DRUG See *Narcotic Addiction*.

ADDISON'S DISEASE Above the kidneys lie two small bodies known as the adrenal glands. One portion of these glands secretes a substance now generally called adrenalin, which has the power of constricting the blood vessels and raising the blood pressure. Another portion of the glands, known as the cortex, which is the outer portion, secretes a different substance, generally called cortin.

The adrenal glands are necessary to life. If they are removed from the body of an animal, the animal dies. When the glands become infected with any organism which destroys their tissue, the destruction of the glands is followed by death.

More than seventy-five years ago a British doctor named Addison described the condition which is now known as Addison's disease. Since 1927 extracts of the cortex of the adrenal glands of cattle have been prepared and are taken as a substitute for the cortex of the adrenal glands of the human being.

When the adrenal glands are removed either surgically or by disease, a number of changes take place in the functions of the body. There is a progressive loss of salt and of water, which leads to a lessening of the amount of fluid circulating in the blood and of the amount of fluid in the cells of the body. The result of such a decrease in fluid is the appearance of shock. Associated, there will be a loss of weight, vomiting, muscle weakness, a lowering of the blood pressure and, finally, a lack of flow of urine. The muscular weakness is probably the most important manifestation of a lack of adrenal material in the body. This is the symptom of which patients complain first and most. Another symptom which attracts considerable attention, however, is the bronzing of the skin; this may involve not only the skin but also the mucous membranes of the body.

The discovery of cortin is now recognized as one of the greatest discoveries of modern medical science, since it makes possible the saving of life in cases which were formerly invariably fatal.

Each year not more than three to four hundred cases of this disease are reported in the United States. There are, however, instances in which there may be a depression of the function of the gland rather than a complete disappearance of its secretion. Under such circumstances the use of the preparation cortin or one of its substitutes may be helpful in controlling the symptoms.

An extract of the adrenal glands is now available under the name of desoxycorticosterone acetate. A more recent discovery—aldosterone—is much more powerful. The pure cortin is exceedingly expensive and difficult to secure. Usually Cortisone or the more potent Meticorten or prednisone is given.

There is a definite relationship of vitamin C to the function of the cortex of the adrenal gland, so that extra amounts of vitamin C are given also.

Finally the elimination of sodium from the body in this disease is an important factor in developing the weakness and the other symptoms, so that a high intake of sodium chloride and a low intake of potassium are also considered to be essential.

ADENOIDS In the throat and back of the nose lies a considerable amount of tissue which doctors call lymphoid tissue. Lymphoid tissue picks up infectious germs and helps the body to get rid of them. Occasionally, however, this tissue itself becomes infected and inflamed. The lymphoid tissue enlarges. Then it becomes more dangerous than helpful to the body and requires removal.

The adenoids, which lie back of the nose and which may be reached through the throat, are lymphoid tissue. When a doctor wants to see whether or not a child has enlarged adenoids, he passes a throat mirror down into the throat. This enables him to look up into the back of the nose and to see the size and character of the adenoid tissue. In the case of a small child the doctor may reach into the throat and pass his fingers up and back of the nose; then he can actually feel the size of the adenoid tissue.

Usually, if the adenoids are infected or inflamed, the tonsils and the other lymphoid tissue in the throat will be inflamed and vice versa. A child with infected and inflamed adenoids may be quite sick with a fever, have difficulty in breathing, and sometimes also a chronic cough. When the adenoids have been repeatedly infected, they may remain permanently enlarged; in fact so large as actually to interfere with breathing. Moreover, the child with chronically infected adenoids catches frequent colds. Usually the child will breathe through its mouth because of the trouble in breathing through its nose.

The presence of inflamed and enlarged adenoids leads to frequent disturbances of the Eustachian tubes and trouble with hearing. Children with enlarged adenoids were once considered stupid; probably such children seldom heard and were, therefore, slower in their reactions. This made them seem stupid. The enlargement of adenoids tends to give the child an expression which is known as an "adenoid face." The mouth is open all the time, the eyes staring and a little dull. The lines leading from the sides of the nose to the mouth are smooth, exaggerating the narrowness of the face and thinness of the nose, and thus tending to enhance the stupid appearance. Moreover, the constant breathing through the mouth tends to make the palate high and pointed, and this interferes with proper growth of the teeth.

Definitely enlarged or inflamed adenoids ought to be removed. Since this condition is usually associated with enlarged and inflamed tonsils as well, the tonsils and adenoids are removed at one operation. The removal of the adenoids is not a difficult operation in a child. It involves a simple cutting procedure with a special apparatus and is carried out under an anesthetic. It does not require a long time.

Parents frequently ask whether or not it is possible to treat the adenoids with various drugs which might be applied directly, or with vapors which can be inhaled, or by the X ray, or by some other method which would not involve an operative procedure. Unfortunately none of these methods has any certainty in its application.

The operation is not a serious or difficult procedure and results in complete removal of the adenoid tissue, with a wide opening for breathing space through the nose. Occasionally, however, even a small portion of the adenoid tissue which is left may again become infected and enlarged.

ADENOMA A glandular tumor, diagnosed and treated according to the organ involved.

ADHESIONS When tissues heal, fibrous scars are formed which cause the portions to adhere to each other. Following operations within the abdomen, adhesions are said to cause pains on pulling or stretching because fibrous tissue is not elastic.

ADOLESCENCE Adolescence is the period between childhood and full-grown adulthood.

In girls this period begins at about twelve years of age and lasts ten years. In boys it begins at about fourteen years of age and lasts for a varying period, from seven to ten years. During this period important changes take place in the body and mind of the child. These changes are the characteristics that distinguish the grown man or woman from the child. During the period of adolescence growth is more rapid than at any other time except during the first two years of life. The rapid growth may bring special stresses which need to be met by considerate understanding and wise information.

The muscles develop somewhat more slowly than do the bones in this period. For a while it was thought that this was responsible for "growing pains." Now it is recognized that these pains are usually associated with rheumatic conditions. The appearance of so-called "growing pains" is an indication for the doctor to look for signs of rheumatic disease and especially for rheumatic fever.

Once girls during the period of adolescence became pale, thin, and anemic. The condition was called chlorosis and was believed to be a part of the change from childhood to womanhood. Now it is recognized that the habit of putting the girl at the time of adolescence under control, so that she did not get out of doors much, wore heavy garments, and was otherwise deprived of sunlight, exercise, and proper food, produced in her a secondary anemia. Thus with the coming of the modern attitude toward women there has been practically a disappearance of the condition called chlorosis.

There are four critical periods in the lives of women—birth, adolescence, marriage, and the climacteric. In each of these critical periods the woman needs the best advice that medical science can give as to the changes that are taking place in her body. The adjustment of the body of the growing girl to the manifestations of her sex that become apparent at this time is especially difficult. The first few years may be marked by irregularities and severe symptoms. Any departure from the normal demands special study.

Especially important is a recognition of the extent to which the changes that come at this time in the growing girl may affect her mental life. Extraordinary unhappiness, distress, or inability to sleep should have special consideration from the mother and may necessitate consultation with a doctor. The normal girl sleeps well, eats well, enjoys companionship, and is happy. The manifestation of a desire for seclusiveness is an indication that something is wrong. It is not natural for young girls to be constantly by themselves.

Such symptoms as undue sensitiveness or negativism, which most parents would call pure cussedness, are signifi-

cant. Whenever a growing child is refractory and opposes every possible suggestion, the situation needs study.

The growing boy in adolescence also needs advice as to the problems that confront him. The appearance of interest in sex, the changes in the voice which sometimes arouse ridicule, and the mental attitudes developed at this time may mark the child's entire life.

ADOPTION In most instances people pick out a child because he is dark or fair, fat or lean, because his hair is curly or straight, blond or brunette. The wise couple will realize from the first that the health of the child is much more important than the tilt or turnup of his nose.

An extremely cute baby may be just the opposite when he reaches eight years of age. The fat babies get thin and the thin ones get fat; the curly-headed blond six months of age may be a straight-haired raven at fifteen.

The child with a positive Wassermann test has a condition which demands a great deal of attention before he is suitable for adoption.

The child who has come from a family with tuberculosis may pass through a long period of invalidism before he is healthful.

Mental deficiency can be recognized after three or four months of age, but some mental taints do not appear until later in life. Some conception of the amount of mental defect in the ancestry of the child being considered for adoption is desirable.

Some hereditary defects can be controlled to a certain extent through environment, but it is far safer to be sure of the heredity of the child and not to take chances.

Most people who want to adopt a baby want an extremely young one so that he will not know that the parents are not his own. It is undesirable to adopt a baby during the first few days of his life. At least several months should be given to observation of his physical and mental state before he is taken by the family for rearing.

Most of the children available for adoption are either illegitimate, those abandoned by their parents, or those taken away from disorderly or vicious parents by legal authorities.

The demand for children for adoption far exceeds the supply. Girls are requested more often than boys.

Sometimes parents want a child to replace an infant who has been lost, in which case they endeavor to duplicate the physical and superficial characteristics without giving sufficient attention to the mentality and the heredity.

One woman suddenly decided to adopt a baby because she thought he would look sweet in a coat which she could make from some leftover pieces of white fur.

Parents usually ask for golden-haired, blue-eyed girls with sweet dispositions. It is merely necessary to take the prospective parents through the nursery in order to cause them to take the first child who may happen to hold his arms out to them.

The child is not only the direct descendant of his parents but the sum of all of the ancestry of both for hundreds of years back. Moreover, nature has extraordinary ways in that it suddenly projects a black sheep into a thoroughly good family, and raises great statesmen, multimillionaires, and intellectual giants out of mud heaps. At least 70 per cent of weight can be placed on the immediate parents in the selecting of an infant with a view to getting a clean history from the point of view of mentality and 30 per cent on the influence of the more remote ancestors.

Pick out a child with as good an ancestry as possible, pick the child young, and take the child only on trial. Most institutions having children available for adoption now have definite procedures which prospective parents follow in order to be assured that satisfactory results will be secured.

AEROPHOBIA A morbid fear of drafts of air, also a morbid fear of being up in the air.

AFTERBIRTH The structure, consisting of the placenta and the membranes, which comes from the uterus or womb of the woman following the birth of a child—the placenta being that portion by which nutrition and oxygen are brought to the child by way of the mother's body previous to birth.

AGALACTIA A lack or failure of the secretion of milk by the mother following the birth of a child.

AGAR A form of seaweed which is used in medicine as a means of providing bulk in the material excreted from the bowel. Sometimes drugs are added to the agar; sometimes mineral oil or petrolatum.

AGE See *Senescence.*

AGRANULOCYTOSIS See *Granulocytopenia.*

AGUE The name formerly given to malaria; also used for describing chills associated with various other conditions.

AINHUM A rare disease, seen chiefly in Africa, in which the little toes, and sometimes the other toes, drop off. The course of the disease is slow and the cause is unknown, although it is believed to be some special form of parasitic infestation.

AIR CONDITIONING The human being is sensitive to the atmosphere in which he lives. Air is the most necessary of all substances needed for life. A human being can live about forty days without food, about four days without water, but only about four minutes without air.

Air is a mixture containing approximately 21 per cent oxygen, 78 per cent nitrogen, and a fraction of 1 per cent of a number of other gases. The air of our large cities is contaminated by the gases that come from the bodies of man and from industry, by dust and germs of various kinds, and even by droplets of fluid.

The air that surrounds the human body is used, first, for breathing, second, to help control the temperature of the body. There is a heat-regulating center in the brain. When the body gets cool, the amount of blood circulating through the skin is increased and radiation takes place from the surface of the body.

All air contains a certain amount of moisture. The moisture increases with the temperature. The moisture in the air is reflected by the measurement of the humidity. The effects of bad air are due to high temperature, the high relative humidity, and the lack of motion. When the air is in motion, it tends to evaporate water from the surface of the body more rapidly than when it is not in motion. This produces a cooling effect.

The best temperature for a room is from 65 to 68 degrees, with sufficient water vapor in the air to produce a relative humidity of from 30 to 60 per cent.

Once it was thought that only the chemical constituents of the air were important in distinguishing good air from bad air. More recently it has been recognized that the physical qualities of the air are also important. Dusts and pollens may be primarily responsible for symptoms like those of hay fever and asthma from which many people suffer.

When a room contains a great many people without arrangements for free ventilation they begin to feel drowsy and fatigued. This sensation results from a combination of the warmth and the accumulation of a certain amount of dioxide which is exhaled in the air from the lungs.

Once all sorts of diseases were believed to be due to bad ventilation and to gases coming from marshes and sewers. Now it is known that these diseases are actually due to germs which are transferred from one person to another. Moreover, the marshes were breeding places of mosquitoes and other insects which carried diseases.

Once it was thought night air was unhealthy. Night air is just as healthy as day air, provided it is not contaminated by germs or infested with insects which carry germs. Everyone knows now that the wind comes up and the mosquitoes fly toward nightfall.

In cold weather there is a tendency to overcrowding and lack of ventilation. This means a greater likelihood of infections being transferred from one person to another. Unsatisfactory ventilation may be a factor in the increase of coughs, colds, and other respiratory diseases during the winter.

With the coming of modern air conditioning, there is more and more tendency toward proper ventilation. The average home, however, can easily be ventilated by opening the windows occasionally and allowing a brisk circulation of air through the rooms. Indeed the ordinary home as now built contains enough chinks, cracks, and space under doors and windows to permit a good deal of fresh air to circulate constantly.

Mechanical systems of air conditioning have value in crowded places, like factories, workrooms, motion-picture theaters, and public halls. Frequently such systems constitute the only means by which a sufficient amount of good pure air can be secured.

Unfortunately most air-conditioning apparatus is operated without any recognition of the functioning of the human body. The human body adapts itself to a good many extraordinary conditions. Sudden changes in temperature from cold to warm or from warm to cold place considerable stress on the physiology of the human body.

Most experts believe that the difference in temperature between the inside and outside air should not be more than from ten to fifteen degrees in warm weather. When the temperature outside is exceedingly cool, people should wear plenty of warm clothing in order to maintain the body temperature at reasonably stable level.

In maintaining the cleanliness of air all sorts of useful devices have been developed. Air-conditioning and air-filtering apparatus help to remove pollen and dust.

Few housewives understand how to clean a room without filling it with dust. The modern vacuum cleaner takes dust out of the air and out of furnishings in a room without stirring it up. The old-fashioned carpet sweeper is better than a broom. The obsolete feather duster scatters dust in the air, whereas a moist or oiled cloth removes it without disturbing it.

Good ventilation is particularly important during sleep. Sleep occupies or should occupy approximately one third of the twenty-four hours. Good ventilation during the hours of sleep helps take the place of bad ventilation which may be likely during hours of work indoors. During sleep the temperature of the body may be controlled by suitable covering. Thus the temperature of the room may be somewhat lower during sleep than is permissible during the day.

Old people and invalids usually require a higher temperature for comfort because their bodies produce less heat than do the bodies of younger people.

Because air is so universal, characteristics of the air such as odor, moisture, or movement are likely to be much more emphasized than their importance in relation to health merits. Apparently much of our belief in the importance of fresh air is based on the will to believe.

The story is told of a man who could not sleep one night because the air seemed to be stagnant. He got up and tried to open a window but had no luck with it. Finally he picked up a shoe and broke the glass. Then he went to bed and slept comfortably. The next morning when he looked around he found that he had broken the glass door of his bookcase.

AIRSICKNESS See *Seasickness.*

ALBINOS Some people are born with the absence of pigment in the skin. The condition is called albinism and the people who have it are called albinos. When there is a complete absence of pigment from the body, the pupil of the eye appears red and the iris of the eye pink or bluish. The hair is white or a very pale yellow and silky in texture. The skin is white or pink and does not tan on exposure to sunlight. In certain areas of the world a considerable number of people have this condition, as it is inherited, although it tends to breed out of the family rather than to intensify.

The white person who is an albino is more likely to have a complete absence of pigment than any one of the colored races. These are likely to have pigmented spots mixed with the areas in which there is an absence of pigment. Incidentally, it is believed that albinos do not grow as tall, as strong, or as lusty as other people of the same race. Sometimes the lack of pigment material in the eye tends to interfere seriously with vision and to cause imperfect development of the eye.

Albinos have been found in practically every part of the world and in most races. However, they are not frequent. They had been reported to occur about once in 100,000 births in Russia and in France but once in 30,000 in Italy, once in 20,000 in Scotland and once in 10,000 in general in North America. However, among Zuñi and Hopi Indians albinos have been found in the percentage of 4 or 5 for each 1000 births.

Among some of the Indian tribes in which albinism is frequent marriages between two albinos are not permitted. However, there are instances in which persons with an albino strain have married, thus intensifying the condition. Two brothers married their first cousins, all representing an albino strain. One marriage produced ten albinos (nine boys and one girl) out of fifteen children, and the other marriage produced three albinos (one boy and two girls) out of eight children. Moreover, seven pairs of boy and three pairs of girl albino twins have been recorded.

There is not much that can be done about this condition once it occurs. It must be recognized that such conditions are inherited and everything possible should be done to prevent intensification of the breeding of the albino types by discouraging intermarriage between persons with albino strains.

ALBUMINURIA (See also *Kidneys*) The appearance of albumin in the urine, found usually by adding strong acid or by heating the urine. An early sign of disturbance of the kidneys, which permit the albumin of the blood to pass into the urine.

ALCOHOL The use by man of alcoholic drinks dates back to a time long before the beginnings of written history. Fermented liquors contain not only ethyl alcohol but also higher alcohols of the type of methyl, propyl, butyl, and amyl alcohol. So important is the drinking of alcoholic liquors in the economy of every nation that vast sums have been spent on the study of the effects of such drinks on the human body.

Alcoholic drinks include whisky, gin, beer, ale, stout, wines, and malt liquors.

The excessive use of alcohol cannot be defended successfully by anyone. Used in excess, alcoholic liquors produce serious damage to the human body, destroy the co-ordination of the nerves and the muscles, render the user susceptible to accident and exposure to the elements, resulting in disease. There is plenty of evidence that alcohol taken in excess actually injures the germ plasm of the body. The children of chronic alcoholics are notoriously likely to be both physically and mentally affected. The person who has taken alcohol excessively loses command of his judgment, his inhibitions disappear, and he may become a menace to society.

Many people who use alcohol with great moderation derive pleasure from it. The vast majority of people do not incline to be drunkards. There is no scientific evidence that moderate doses of alcohol, even if taken daily by a normal person, are deleterious either to him or to his children. Most medical evidence does not indicate that an occasional drink taken in this manner by a normal person will lead to chronic alcoholism.

Medical evidence inclines to the view that the person who drinks to excess is like the one who takes drugs to excess —a psychologically inferior person who finds in the drugs or in the alcohol an escape from social situations to which he cannot adjust himself.

What does alcohol do when it gets into the human body? When the alcohol is taken up by the blood from the digestive tract, it goes to the various organs of the body. A small part is eliminated through the lungs, kidneys, and skin. Alcohol has even been found in the milk of nursing mothers. The alcohol taken up by the body is oxidized and thereafter can be used as a source of energy. Small doses of alcohol may cause a slight rise in the rate of the heart; large doses always lower the blood pressure and weaken the pulse.

When a person takes a dose of alcohol, he feels a warmth and reddening of the face due to the fact that the blood vessels of the skin are dilated. On the brain alcohol has, in the end, a depressing effect. Its early effects are to make the drinker less keenly aware of his environment. This helps him to escape to some extent from his worries, anxiety, and self-criticism. However, it interferes with his judgment and his mental alertness.

Alcohol is still a great problem socially, scientifically, and medically. One of the most serious problems created by alcohol is the danger that arises when a person with lessened judgment and mental alertness, brought about by alcohol, endeavors to drive a motorcar.

The drinker difficult to cure is the person who drinks to escape from his troubles. The normal man meets his problems squarely. The abnormal man escapes sometimes by developing a disease, sometimes by overeating, oversmoking, occasionally by taking narcotic drugs, and even more frequently by indulging in alcohol to excess.

The slowing action of alcohol on the

brain has been proved by tests with the electric encephalogram. The signs of slowing are manifested further in slurring speech, staggering gait, emotional changes, and failure in co-operative action.

Finally, it has been proved that some of the serious effects of alcohol, such as alcoholic neuritis, delirium tremens, hallucinations, and even hardening of the liver, result from deficiencies of nutrition associated with the taking of alcohol. People who drink do not eat the foods they should have, in either the amount or the quality. In some instances such symptoms as alcoholic neuritis, alcoholic pellagra, and alcoholic delirium tremens are due to deficiencies of thiamine, nicotinic acid, and other portions of the vitamin B complex. Finally, the effects of alcohol on the brain frequently result in unnecessary crime. This makes it a psychiatric as well as a medical problem.

In a recent study of the mental aspects of illness it is pointed out that every alcoholic has some form of neurotic character disturbance. He has social anxiety, and indeed, it is urged that the alcoholic is a narcissistic person —which means that his self-love is such that he finds little satisfaction in social relationships. When under the influence of alcohol his self-esteem is raised to a level of tolerance. Then he can be friendly but because of his unusual sensitivity the alcoholic person is likely to be irritable on the slightest provocation.

Some persons have periodic drinking bouts between which they are said to be trustworthy and, in fact, most of the time quite remorseful about their previous intoxication. They represent a special problem because there is an individual psychological difficulty in each case.

Means have been sought for conditioning alcoholics against alcohol by various drugs which make the product distasteful or which produce nausea and vomiting. Many psychologists believe that such methods of treatment produce depression which may be worse than the original symptoms. In any event it is clear that the approach to every case of alcoholism is psychological and that it is necessary to help these people to make a realistic approach to their problems.

The alcoholic drinks include, as I have pointed out, malt, liqueurs, wines, and distilled liquors. Malt liquors usually have less alcohol than do wines or distilled liquors but they have a higher amount of carbohydrate and protein.

In most foreign countries beers and ales, which are malt liquors, are taken as part of a meal and help to provide the total number of calories that may be required by the individual for the day. In this country malt liquors are frequently taken between meals. They add a considerable amount of calories to the diet and thus help to put on weight. Light beer contains less carbohydrate and more alcohol than dark beer. Bock beer is made with more malt and hops per barrel and therefore contains more alcohol and carbohydrates than ordinary beer. Ale, porter, and stout differ from ordinary beer by using a different type of yeast in the brewing. In general a cup or half pint of beer provides 150 calories or 300 calories per pint. Wines vary, providing, in the case of muscatel, port, or sherry, about 150 calories to the glass. Champagne provides around 100 calories to a glass. Some wines are artificially sweetened.

Whisky is proportionately much stronger in alcohol and provides about 150 calories per ounce. Cocktails vary according to the amount and the nature of the materials that are put in them. There are no other food values of alcohol beyond the energy value in calories that has already been mentioned.

The average man who attends a banquet has already had his breakfast and luncheon, which usually give him enough calories for the energy output of the day. At a banquet he gets about 2500 calories in the form of food and another 700 in the form of drinks. To use up these extra 3200 calories a person would have to play a fast game of handball or squash racquets for five and a half hours, walk sixty miles, or run thirty miles.

Studies of the social effects of alcohol show that women are likely to be less judicious in their drinking than men, exactly as they are less judicious in their smoking of cigarettes.

All this information leads to the conclusion that alcohol and alcoholic drinks have a certain definite place in our economy and in our social existence but that, like other drugs—and alcohol is a drug—they must be used with the greatest of care and intelligence.

It must always be remembered that the action of alcohol is essentially depressing, that its chief effects are to dull the perception of unpleasant feelings and surroundings, to diminish self-criticism, and to diminish the fear of taking any action which might excite remark or be regarded by other people as not appropriate or polite or civilized.

Thus under the influence of alcohol people become more communicative, talk more freely, and have their emotions easily aroused. Alcohol is therefore unsuitable for the highest mental efforts or for the performance of any feat requiring skill, fine control, alertness, or prolonged muscular action.

The adult who is presumed to be responsible for himself will soon realize if he is a normal individual the harm that it does him when he drinks to excess and he will confine his use of alcohol to those convivial, social occasions which long usage has come to recognize as warranted.

In 1949 a drug called antabuse was found capable of killing the appetite for an enjoyment of alcoholic drinks. Since the drug must be repeatedly used, psychologic treatment must accompany its use to get a more permanent result.

ALEXIA A scientific word that describes inability to read because of word blindness. Various forms depend on inability to comprehend the significance of what is seen; inability to read aloud although the person understands what he reads; or, as in musical alexia, the inability to read music.

ALIMENTATION The act of giving or receiving nutriment.

ALKALOSIS The opposite of acidosis, meaning an increased amount of alkali in the blood over what is normal.

ALLERGY (See also *Asthma, Hay Fever, Hives,* et cetera) Allergy was first described more than fifty years ago under the name "hypersensitiveness." It referred to the fact that people sometimes reacted with disturbances when substances to which they were sensitive got into their bodies. Now a wide variety of terms is used to describe this condition, including hypersensitiveness, idiosyncrasy, atopy, anaphylaxis, and allergy—but allergy is the one most frequently used. There are no doubt differences in sensitivity to various substances like metals and proteins but for the average person these conditions are exceedingly complex.

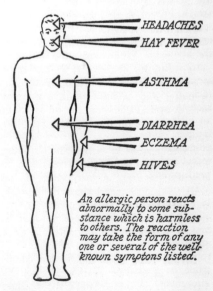

An allergic person reacts abnormally to some substance which is harmless to others. The reaction may take the form of any one or several of the well-known symptons listed.

Allergy gives rise to many symptoms besides those of hay fever and asthma. Some of the areas where allergic symptoms occur are indicated

The exact mechanism of excessive sensitivity to various substances is unknown. The view is now generally accepted that the mechanism of allergy is a reaction taking place in the cells or tissues of the body against the substance to which the person is sensitive. In producing this state there may be hereditary or various other factors which predispose to producing sensitivity. Some have thought that the sensitivity was due to the production in the cells of certain toxic substances which were released in the blood. People who have a tendency to develop asthma, unusual eruptions on the skin with itching, running of the nose, or swelling of the tissues often have also symptoms which indicate that there has been a special reaction of the nervous system at the same time. Quite possibly the allergic response releases substances which act on the glands and the nervous system. Incidentally, the effects of the substance to which the person is sensitive may be felt at some other portion of the body than that at which the substance is introduced. In other words, the person with asthma may have the attack following the eating of a substance, the inhalation of the substance, or the injection of the substance into the blood.

In addition to the factors already mentioned that induce an allergic attack, it is now recognized that psychic factors may predispose or precipitate an allergic condition. Tension, conflict, fatigue, exhaustion, overwork, disappointment, anxiety, fear, or grief may sometimes be the precipitating factor in predisposing to an allergic attack.

In some cases it has not been possible to desensitize or cure a person with allergy until the mental elements have first been eliminated. For instance such an attack will sometimes clear up when the person is in the hospital and return when he goes back to the original environment. It is believed that the psychic factors predispose to allergic attacks by altering the excitability of the nervous system, which in turn brings about a change in the blood supply to the tissues involved in the allergic attack.

The number of persons in the United States who have allergy is now believed to be in the millions, and the definite increase that has taken place is not wholly due to the fact that doctors and people generally have become allergy-conscious. Indeed it is believed that at least 3 per cent of the entire population have allergic symptoms related to the nose, throat, and lungs and this does not include the many millions who have only very mild hay fever and asthma and therefore do not come to medical attention.

Most recent in the treatment of allergies are the antihistaminic drugs like pyribenzamine, benadryl, neo-antergan, chlor-trimeton, neohetramine, and thephorin.

ALOES A cathartic substance derived from a plant of the same name.

ALOPECIA See *Baldness* under *Hair*.

ALTITUDE SICKNESS (See also *Seasickness*) The average person is adapted to living at altitudes under 5000 feet. When you go higher than 12,000 feet above sea level, you are likely to develop much discomfort. Changes take place in the body which result in symptoms. One American investigator who climbed the Andes in Peru in 1922 asserts that the following changes occurred as he went to a higher altitude. First there was an increase in the rate and depth of breathing as the oxygen pressure decreased. Next the number of red blood cells and red coloring matter of the blood increased. This is in response to the demand for oxygen. Third, the red coloring matter of the blood known as hemoglobin took up more oxygen.

The symptoms which result at a high altitude include those that represent a shortage of oxygen, such as dizziness, mental dullness, occasionally headache, vomiting, sometimes difficulty in hearing and seeing. At great heights there is slight fever. Sometimes there is bleeding of the nose. In other cases there may be weakness of the limbs sufficient to make walking difficult. The pulse becomes more rapid in the effort to supply the tissues with more oxygen. If efforts are made slowly, one becomes gradually accustomed to the higher altitude. For severe symptoms the breathing of a mixture of oxygen with air gives relief.

Altitude has become particularly a problem in aviation. Altitude sickness differs from mountain sickness in the fact that the latter is continuous, so that the body becomes more or less accustomed to the lack of oxygen. The lack of oxygen in airplane flying is temporary and one does not become accustomed to it.

At 18,000 feet altitude about 25 per cent of normal people collapse in a period of one half to one hour unless they are provided with extra oxygen. Associated with this may be changes in mental function and emotional control which lead to disturbed judgment. One of the most common aftereffects of prolonged lack of oxygen in aviators is a state of fatigue which makes a long rest period necessary to overcome the condition. In some cases, as the result of repeated periods with lack of oxygen, nervous symptoms develop which have been called aeroneurosis. In this condition there are fatigue of the mind and body, nervousness, irritability, and sometimes gastric disturbances. Army fliers suggest that oxygen always be given on reaching 8000 feet when climbing and that when coming down oxygen be continued until 1000 feet altitude is reached.

The condition called airsickness resembles seasickness and is due to repeated oscillations of the body in a ship or an airplane. The chief symptoms are dizziness, nausea, vomiting, pallor, and sweating.

ALUMINUM When aluminum is taken into the body a small amount of the substance remains, chiefly in the liver and the spleen. Most of the aluminum is promptly passed from the body in the urine and in the bile. The body easily takes care of any insignificant amounts of this metal that may be taken into the body as a result of eating food cooked in aluminum cooking utensils. There is no evidence that aluminum absorbed as a result of using aluminum cooking utensils has any harmful effect on the ordinary consumer. The claim has been made that aluminum in foods or the use of aluminum cooking utensils in some manner may promote the growth of cancer in the human body. There is not the slightest scientific evidence to support this claim.

Aluminum is used in medicine in the form of an aluminum hydroxide gel which is prescribed chiefly as an antacid substance in the treatment of ulcer of the stomach and duodenum or whenever there seems to be excessive acid in the stomach. It has a slight astringent effect and serves also to coat the affected area and thus to protect it against the action of acid. Furthermore, such gels of aluminum hydroxide tend to increase the mucin secretion, which is also favorable to the treatment of ulcer. Many different preparations of this type are now available and are frequently prescribed by physicians. They should not, of course, be taken unless prescribed by the doctor for the specific case and in the amounts which he thinks desirable in that case. One such preparation is official in the United States Pharmacopoeia. It contains about 4 per cent of aluminum hydroxide.

Another preparation of aluminum which is used in medicine is called aluminum subacetate. This is used as a mild astringent and an antiseptic substance in dermatology. Many of the preparations used for sunburn and also those used to prevent underarm perspiration contain substances of this type. Since the substance may be irritating in high concentration, it is customary for the doctor to prescribe it sufficiently diluted with water to make it harmless.

AMAUROSIS Blindness that occurs without any apparent lesion of the eye itself but from disease of the optic nerve, the retina, the spine, or the brain, which are concerned in vision.

AMBLYOPIA (See *Eye*) Absence of vision.

AMEBIASIS (See also *Dysentery*) A form of dysentery due to infection with a parasite called *Endamoeba histolytica*. The disease is diagnosed by finding the organisms in material from the bowel. It is treated with drugs like emetin and chiniofon, which are specific against amebae; also terramycin and Milibis.

AMENORRHEA (See *Menstruation*) Absence or abnormal stoppage of the menstruation.

AMINO ACIDS Research by Dr. W. C. Rose, leading authority on proteins, indicates that only eight of more than twenty amino acids are necessary to maintain the nitrogen required for health and growth of the human body. When the proper amount of nitrogen is being taken in and used up, the condition is called "nitrogen balance." The protein in the diet is considered adequate when the nitrogen balance is maintained. The eight amino acids now considered essential for the health of the human being are isoleucine, leucine, lysine, methionine, phenylalanine, threonine (first discovered by Dr. Rose), tryptophane, and valine.

Quite possibly other of the amino acids are necessary for the growth of children, for pregnant women or mothers nursing babies, or even for adults under exceptional circumstances. These protein foods are just as necessary for the health of the human body as any of the vitamins. The amount of protein in the ordinary diet of the active adult cannot safely be reduced under fifty grams a day, of which as little as five grams may be in the form of animal protein.

Amino acids are now prepared in pure form and used to treat starvation or malnutrition. They are given before and after surgical operations when needed.

AMINOPHYLLINE A drug used particularly in conditions affecting the heart, including angina pectoris.

AMMONIA This product, used in households, will burn the tissues if applied in concentrated solution. Weak vinegar acts as an antidote.

AMNESIA Lack or loss of memory, especially inability to remember the proper words, frequently associated with changes in the tissue of the brain.

"AMOG" This is a term derived from the Malay language similar to the English "amuck." The term "running amuck" refers to a condition of hysterical excitement which follows an infectious disease such as malaria or brooding on personal relationships. Among Malay women there is a condition called "latah" which begins with a shriek, after which the woman is likely to imitate everything that is said and done in her presence and to shriek at her employer.

AMYOTROPHIC LATERAL SCLEROSIS Degeneration and hardening of portions of the spinal cord which is promptly reflected in the muscles of the body is called amyotrophic lateral sclerosis. This is the disease that killed Lew Gehrig, famous ball player.

The spinal cord is only eighteen inches long in a full-grown man and weighs less than one ounce. It is, therefore, much shorter than the spinal or vertebral column in which it lies. The tissue of the spinal cord is divided into parts which are anterior, meaning the front; lateral, meaning on the side; and posterior, meaning the back.

Obviously whenever there is a change of any kind in these tissues, the effects on the human body are far-reaching and serious. When something happens to the nervous tissues, the muscles which are controlled by this nervous tissue are likewise affected. The cause of amyotrophic lateral sclerosis is unknown. It is apparently not due to any well-established condition affecting the blood, and certainly there has been shown to be no infectious cause. It has been suggested that there are conditions within the body at birth which ultimately reveal themselves in this disease. The condition is seen mostly in mature age, usually between forty-five and sixty years of age, and affects men more often than it does women.

The chief symptoms are a progressive twitching of the muscles with increasing weakness and wasting away. The symptoms of the condition seem to be occasionally foreshadowed by vague feelings of exhaustion, occasional cramps, numbness, and a burning sensation. Usually, however, the patient comes to the doctor because he has noticed a gradual wasting of the muscles of one or both hands with twitching. From this point on progressive weakness and wasting are the most important symptoms.

The condition is seldom painful, although in some instances there may be severe pains. Unfortunately the condition does not tend to improve; the progressive wasting of the muscles and, associated therewith, inability of motion or action continue. Treatment helps to maintain the tone of the muscles and to alleviate worry.

ANALGESIA Absence of sensibility to pain, such as may be brought about by the use of drugs, anesthetics, or nerve blocking.

ANCYLOSTOMIASIS (See *Hookworm* under *Worms*) The scientific name for hookworm disease.

ANEMIA When the concentration of red coloring matter in the blood falls below normal, there is anemia—regardless of the number of red blood cells, the condition is anemia. Sometimes anemia is due to the fact that the loss of blood or the destruction of blood cells takes place more rapidly than new blood cells can be produced. In other instances the production of cells falls below the normal rate of destruction of red blood cells.

To understand these causes it is necessary to know the present view of the manner of production of blood cells and also the manner in which they are lost from the body. If there is a severe hemorrhage due to any kind of injury, a great amount of blood cells can be lost. Most of the blood cells are produced in the bone marrow. In the presence of disease of the bone marrow the production of red blood cells is less. There are certain poisonous substances which can damage the bone marrow seriously and in that way reduce the formation of red blood cells.

The first and most simple cause of anemia is the loss of blood. Usually the fluid and the red blood cells as well as the red coloring matter will return to normal within two months provided the patient lives. The loss of blood may result from tearing of a blood vessel, rupture of an internal organ of the body, bleeding from an ulcer in the stomach or intestines or from an ulcer in the bowel, occasionally from childbirth or tuberculosis. In some conditions there is a constant loss of a small amount of blood, so that the total becomes serious. This happens from persistent bleeding from piles, ulcers of the stomach and duodenum, conditions of the female organs related to childbirth, and varicose veins in the throat and stomach.

With a large, severe hemorrhage the person concerned feels weak and faint, becomes dizzy and thirsty. The pulse becomes rapid because of the necessity to get the blood around the body and weak because the volume of the blood is low. The skin is pale, cold, and slightly bluish. Breathing, at first deep and rapid, becomes weak and shallow. The person who loses much blood is restless, as if anticipating a serious event. Cold perspiration is another sign of blood loss. With continued loss of blood the pressure falls steadily and may finally reach a point at which shock occurs. Most of the symptoms are due to the diminution in the volume of the blood and the failure of the body cells to receive the oxygen that they require. Obviously it is important in cases of loss of blood in this way to stop the hemorrhage as soon as possible, since the ultimate outcome depends entirely on the amount and rapidity of loss of blood, the promptness with which treatment is begun, and the ability of the body to restore the blood to normal volume and red-cell content.

If one third of all the blood is lost suddenly, death may follow immediately unless the condition is corrected by putting in blood plasma. Over a period of time two thirds of the blood in the body might be lost, as within a period of twenty-four hours, and still the patient might recover.

When there is much loss of blood, the blood pressure should be recorded every half hour and emergency treatment should be instituted if it falls as low as 75 to 95 millimeters of mercury at the time when the heart is contracted. As much as a pint to a quart of blood from a donor may be given, or plasma or serum from a blood bank can be given. In the absence of these materials a salt or glucose solution can be used to help keep up the volume. Certainly anyone who has had such a hemorrhage should be kept quite warm, but not too hot. As recovery occurs, a good diet with plenty of protein, minerals and vitamins, and extra iron may be supplied to stimulate the formation of red blood cells.

Anemia frequently results from defective formation of blood. This may be due to some deficiency in nutrition as, for example, the lack of iron and protein or the special substance derived from the stomach or liver which is important for the formation of red blood cells. Apparently there are cases in which the thyroid gland is not sufficiently active to stimulate the mechanism involved. Copper and cobalt are important in the formation of red blood cells. As has been mentioned already, there are some cases in which chemicals like benzene, arsenic, gold, and the sulfa drugs can damage the bone marrow so that it cannot produce cells adequately. There may also be damage by X ray and radium or the growth of tumors in the bone marrow.

A lack of iron is important in relationship to anemia. Iron may be deficient in amount when there is a considerable loss of blood, when iron is not taken into the body in sufficient amounts, or when it is not properly absorbed from the bowel. The growing infant may deprive its prospective mother of iron. There are also cases in which infestation of the bowel with worms like the hookworm produces a deficiency of iron and of blood.

Many years ago young girls used to suffer frequently with the condition called chlorosis. This in turn was the result of bad nutrition and bad hygiene, overwork, constipation, and menstrual disturbances. Now the anemia of young girls has given way to an anemia which appears more often in women between the ages of thirty and fifty and is associated with excessive menstrual flow and sometimes with lack of sufficient hydrochloric acid in the stomach.

The anemia that is due to increased destruction of blood may be due to poisonous materials which may damage the red blood cells or to some condition in the formation of the cells which makes them too easy to damage.

In any event, with either of these types of anemia the person concerned feels weak and tires easily. He becomes short of breath on exertion and is likely to complain of faintness, dizziness, and palpitation. Occasionally there is swelling of the legs. If the anemia develops gradually, the number of red blood cells may fall from a normal of 6,000,000 to as low as 1,000,000 and the red coloring matter may be only 20 per cent. The hemoglobin, or red coloring matter of the blood, is measured by various technics—the simplest being colored charts in which the color of a certain percentage of red coloring matter is said to be normal, the next 90 per cent, and so on down. By actual weight 15 grams (or ½ ounce of hemoglobin) for every 100 c.c. (or one-fifth of a pint) of blood is said to be normal. However, accurate measurement is exceedingly difficult, so that the usual color scales would probably register anything above 13½ grams as representing 100 per cent.

Obviously patients with such a drop in the number of red blood cells are seriously sick. In any anemia of this kind the doctor will examine the blood regularly in order to determine the extent of the damage to the red blood cells and to determine also whether the condition has been reversed as shown by continued improvement. If improvement fails to occur, it may be necessary to undertake more radical measures like surgical operations or transfusion of blood.

Once the cause of bleeding is removed, the patients usually improve rapidly if they are given abundant fresh air, sunlight, and a nourishing diet containing spinach, meat, liver, eggs, apricots, peaches, foods rich in vitamins and proteins. Iron is usually considered necessary to produce more hemoglobin and red coloring matter and more red blood cells by speeding up the function of the bone marrow that builds the cells. The doctor prescribes iron in the form he considers best suited to the patient concerned.

In cases in which the formation of red blood cells is inadequate the condition can be approached only by attacking the cause. Causes of blood destruction must be removed as rapidly as possible.

ANEMIA, PERNICIOUS Since 1822 it has been known that there is a condition in which the body fails to produce a sufficient number of red blood cells of a quality and character capable of supporting the health of the body. In that year a doctor named James S. Combe, of Edinburgh, described accurately a case of pernicious anemia. Then another doctor whose name is now famous, Thomas Addison, gave a well-nigh perfect description of the condition in 1849. The disease was considered to be incurable until 1926, when Drs. George Minot and William Murphy, of Boston, found that the taking of a half pound of liver daily would control the condition.

Pernicious anemia rarely occurs before the age of thirty. Most of the cases develop in people past forty or fifty years of age.

Early it was recognized that some disturbance of the digestive system of the body is associated with pernicious anemia. For instance an absence of hydrochloric acid in the secretion of the stomach may appear years before the pernicious anemia and may continue even when treatment with liver has been carried on. A doctor named Castle found that the normal person has in the secretion of his stomach a certain substance called an intrinsic factor—that is, developed within the cells—which reacts with food to produce a substance that is necessary in maintaining the normal formation of blood. This substance is absorbed from the bowel and stored in the liver and other tissues. In pernicious anemia the substance is not present in the liver. The exact nature of this substance is not known but its absence will interfere with the formation of normal red blood cells.

The discovery of the method for saving the lives of people with pernicious anemia was most important because the death rate from that disease had been rising steadily, moving up from 12 for each 100,000 of our population in 1921 to about 18 for each 100,000 in 1926. Today, as a result of the discovery of the treatment of pernicious anemia with liver extract, the death rate has dropped to 5 for each 100,000—a decline of almost 70 per cent.

The person with pernicious anemia is pale and his skin develops a lemon-yellow color; the tongue gets sore at the edges. The condition comes on gradually with an increasing sense of fatigue and tiredness, weakness, shortness of breath, headaches, and disturbances of digestion. If the condition persists without control, the nervous system becomes affected. There is numbness and tingling of the arms and legs, eventually difficulty in walking and lack of control of the usual functions of the body. The liver and the spleen become enlarged.

The red bone marrow becomes soft and of a deep red color. In describing the condition Dr. Thomas Addison wrote: "It makes its approach in so slow and insidious a manner that the patient can hardly fix a date to his earliest feeling of that languor which is shortly to become so extreme."

When the doctor examines the blood, he frequently finds that there is a greater reduction of the red cells than of the red coloring matter. Because of the insidious approach of the disease the red cells may drop to 2,500,000 before the person begins to realize that something is wrong.

Only since the discovery of the microscope and the use of the laboratory for studying the composition and character of the blood has it been possible for physicians to make the kind of studies that are necessary in differentiating various blood diseases from each other. Now we know that there are many different forms of disturbances of the blood which may affect the fluid matter, the chemicals dissolved in the fluid, the red blood cells, the white blood cells of various types, the blood platelets or materials involved in causing the blood to clot.

In the most serious cases the doctor not only uses all these technics to examine blood taken from a puncture of the ear or finger but he may actually take a sample of the bone marrow from the breastbone in order to determine whether or not any important changes have taken place in that blood-forming tissue. The doctor will not diagnose anemia from the blood alone because, as has already been shown, there are so many different kinds of anemia and because the treatment must be definitely related to the peculiar variety. Then again, the doctor is enabled to determine the nature of the anemia by studying the blood before and after the use of various forms of treatment. The giving of iron will bring about stimulation of the formation of red blood cells and of red coloring matter in the blood. The giving of liver extract will have a definite effect on the bone marrow when that substance is absent from the tissues of the body. Obviously the patient who is completely at rest while undergoing treatment is likely to recover much more rapidly than the one who tries to work or engage in other activities which may interfere with the forces of the body while treatment is going on. Then again the doctor who treats the patient with liver extract, iron, or both must determine exactly how much of each of these substances is necessary in an individual case. He must also determine the manner in which the material is to be given. We know from the results of experience that liver extract is sixty times as effective when given by injection into the body as when given by mouth. The injection may be made directly into the muscles and thus the action is prompt. It is known that a unit of liver extract injected daily into the muscles in a person whose red blood cells have fallen to 1,500,000 for each cubic millimeter of blood will cause an increase to about 2,500,000 red blood cells in each cubic millimeter of blood a month.

One of the most amazing sights in modern medicine is the rapidity with which patients improve once the diagnosis has been made and the treatment given by the doctor.

Associated with the administration of the liver extract there should be improvement in the diet by including liberal amounts of liver, green vegetables, and fruit. Occasionally doses of hydrochloric acid may be given to take the place of the hydrochloric acid that is absent from the stomach. If the condition is diagnosed early and proper treatment given soon, the majority of patients recover promptly. However, there is a tendency toward relapse, so that these patients should be seen regularly by the doctor over a considerable period of time.

Folic acid and the more recently discovered vitamin B_{12} have the power to stimulate formation of red blood cells far more powerfully than liver extract. With vitamin B_{12} the intrinsic factor of the stomach wall may be given.

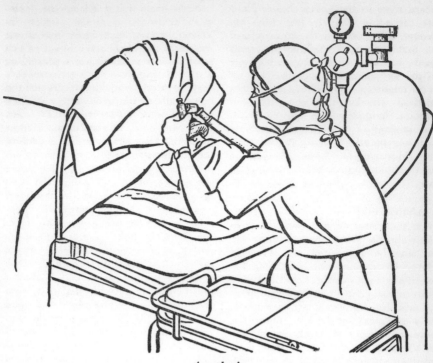

Anesthesia

ANESTHESIA Only a little more than a hundred years have passed since the boon of anesthesia was first conferred on mankind. Before anesthesia the operating room was a place of terror. Today fear of pain associated with surgery has been removed. Anesthesia now includes the use not only of nitrous oxide oxygen gas, ether, and occasionally chloroform but new gases such as ethylene and cyclopropane.

Anesthetic substances can now be injected into the spine so as to block sensations away from portions of the body without interfering with consciousness. In addition to such block anesthesia there is also a technic in obstetrics known as continous caudal analgesia in which very small amounts of the anesthetic are placed around the nerve roots after they have come out from the spinal cord. This is used to produce childbirth without pain.

For operations on the arms or legs or other portions of the body anesthetic solutions may be injected around the nerves that affect the area concerned. A single section is thus blocked off from the rest of the body. A typical example is the way in which teeth may be pulled and tonsils removed without pain when a local anesthetic is injected around the tooth or the tonsils or when the anesthetic is injected into the nerve area somewhat removed from the place where the operation is going to be done but in an area which gives rise to the nerves that carry the sense of pain from that area.

Another interesting development is the injection of sedative drugs directly into the blood so that unconsciousness is produced for a definite period of time. For longer operations the needle is left in place and the anesthetic is continued in small amounts. Operations done on board ships in the United States Navy are carried out largely with this procedure, using particularly drugs related to barbituric acid. Among the drugs used in intravenous anesthesia are evipal and pentothal sodium.

So important is anesthesia in modern medical practice that the American Medical Association has created a special section for hearing new contributions on the subject at its annual meetings. Moreover, anesthesia is recognized as a definite specialty in medical practice.

ANEURISM An aneurism arises from the stretching of a weak place in the wall of a blood vessel. In the walls of blood vessels there are layers of elastic tissue. They enable the vessels to dilate and contract. Sometimes a thick-walled rubber balloon when blown up will develop an extra pouching out at some point where the rubber has been thinned out. This can also happen to a rubber tire which has been weakened by either a physical or chemical injury.

The most frequent cause of the thinning out of the wall of a blood vessel is an infection which destroys a part of the elastic tissue. Sometimes, however, a physical injury may cause it. I have seen an aneurism result from a bullet which scraped the wall of a large blood vessel. Sometimes an aneurism may develop immediately after birth because a portion of the blood vessel may not have grown properly.

Of course if an infection in the body is attacking the walls of the blood vessels, that is a serious matter and should have attention. However, even curing the infection will not restore the tissue that has been destroyed.

A person with an aneurism must be exceedingly careful not to injure the thin sac filled with blood, because a breaking of the sac may result in a serious hemorrhage. Sometimes it is possible by use of surgery to open the tissues down to the point where the aneurism exists and then to tie off the blood vessels or to remove the aneurism.

Some years ago a distinguished surgeon developed a technic which involved the insertion of coiled wire inside the aneurism, causing the blood to clot inside the aneurism and thus preventing a rupture. Advances in surgery now save many lives by removing the thinned-out blood-vessel wall and substituting new material from blood-vessel banks which are maintained in hospitals. Plastics have also been developed to substitute for blood-vessel wall.

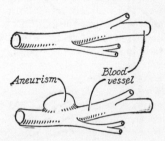

An aneurism is a weak spot in the side of a blood vessel which puffs out like a balloon

ANGINA, VINCENT'S See *Vincent's Angina.*

ANGINA PECTORIS The very name "angina pectoris" means pain in the chest. Interference with the blood supply to the heart muscle is the cause. In coronary thrombosis the interference with the blood supply is prolonged and brings about serious damage to the tissues. In the case of angina pectoris the interference may be momentary and may not result in permanent damage.

The heart is not nourished chiefly by the blood which passes through it and which it pumps to the utmost ends of the body. It is nourished by its own blood vessels, which come to it as blood vessels come to other tissues and organs of the body. These blood vessels originate in the largest blood vessel which comes off from the heart. Obviously, therefore, any changes which occur in this large blood vessel may interfere with the flow of blood through these vessels into the heart. Occasionally also, as people get older, the blood vessels thicken and harden. In association with this process they also become narrower. When they become narrower, they cannot furnish as much blood as when they were wider and more elastic. When there is a general change of this type, affecting the other blood vessels of the body, those which supply the heart with blood are also affected.

A muscle at work requires a certain amount of blood-carrying oxygen in order to do its work satisfactorily. The tissue of the heart is muscular tissue. If a muscle does not have enough blood and oxygen, it manifests this disturbance by a pain in the heart. The heart reveals its inability to get sufficient blood for its use by a similar pain.

When pain occurs in angina pectoris, the symptom usually does not last long because the blood supply is diminished only briefly. Sometimes the pain comes on because the heart is trying to do too much work. If the work is lessened, the blood supply is sufficient and the pains disappear. Occasionally a sudden fall in the blood pressure will bring about a lessened flow of blood into all of the vessels. A drop in blood pressure usually occurs during sleep. The pain of angina pectoris may come on in old people at such times.

The pain of angina pectoris is a most significant symptom. If we know the nature of the pain and the kind of circumstance that brings it on, we can avoid it. The pain in angina pectoris is usually under the breastbone just to the left of the upper portion. It is the kind of pain, however, that may radiate to the shoulder or down the arm, sometimes to the left side of the neck or to the pit of the stomach. Most important of all, it is a short pain. If the pain lasts for long, there is something else wrong besides angina pectoris.

The attacks of pain in the heart may come on from overwork, from exertion, and particularly from exertion soon after one has eaten a heavy meal. A man who may be able to walk rapidly without distress at a time when he has no food in his stomach may be unable to walk even a hundred feet after he has had a heavy meal. The attack of angina pectoris is likely to occur following a meal which is eaten too hastily, in which case considerable air is taken in with the food. It may also follow a meal which is indigestible or eaten when one is too tired. The best advice that can be given to anyone who has angina pectoris is not to eat when tired, not to eat heavily at any time, not to take any exercise within half an hour after a meal, and always to eat slowly. The food selected should be soft and easily digestible.

While exertion does not always bring on an attack of angina pectoris, it frequently does so. Therefore people with this condition should not walk facing strong or cold wind. They should be exceedingly careful about walking upstairs and up inclines, and should not permit themselves to be hurried.

Finally, it is known that an attack of anger may precipitate an attack of angina pectoris. Any emotion may, therefore, precipitate an attack, but especially anger, grief, or worry. Many a businessman has his first attack of angina pectoris after he has suffered severe reverses in the stock market or in his own business.

Angina pectoris may occur in people in any business or occupation, but it is more likely to occur in those who work under strain or who are forced to put out a good deal of energy. For this reason cases of angina pectoris occur more frequently in people who live in the city than in those who live in the country. Cases are seen more often in the cold or temperate zones than in the tropical areas.

From what has been said, it should be obvious that the person with angina pectoris need not despair. It is quite possible for him to live a fairly normal existence, provided he takes care of himself. Here are ten commandments which are especially applicable to the person with angina pectoris:

1. Do not subject your heart to sudden, strenuous, or prolonged physical activity.

2. Eat regularly, slowly, and temperately.

3. If you are excessively overweight, seek sound counsel as to how best to dispense with this form of heart handicap.

4. Try to avoid physical activity for at least thirty minutes after eating, particularly after the heaviest meal of the day.

5. Avoid emotional stress and strain. Worry is an important factor in its relation to heart strain.

6. By appropriate measures, keep your body as free as possible from so-called foci of infection.

7. Regular intestinal elimination is highly important.

8. Average not less than eight hours of sleep in a room abundantly supplied with fresh air.

9. Perennial health demands a proper balance between work, play, and rest.

10. A periodic examination may often reveal defects of which you are unaware.

Recently two specialists in diseases of the heart made the following interesting statement about angina pectoris: "Persisting in golf after angina is perhaps comparable to persisting in eating candy after diabetes appears." In eight out of one hundred cases of deaths from angina pectoris the patient died while playing golf. Every golfer knows the frequent temptation to violent exercise. There is the danger of bad weather and strong wind, there is the possibility of short but stiff climbs, there is the necessary exertion in getting out of the rough, of climbing out of a trap, and the hurry necessary to keep pace with more rapid golfers.

In thirty-three out of one hundred fatal cases of angina pectoris long journeys had been taken just before the final disaster. There is always associated with a long journey unusual activity in getting ready, loss of sleep, overeating, emotional stress, and the trip may include as well overindulgence in smoking and alcohol.

If there is one disease above all others in which moderation must be preached, that disease is angina pectoris.

In three cases of death from angina pectoris the fatality followed a violent loss of temper during a business argument. In two cases patients became overexcited at football games. In two others the attack came on when the persons were called on suddenly to make speeches for which they were not prepared. A person with angina pectoris should never put himself into a position, once he has learned that he has this condition, in which he may be suddenly submitted to an extraordinary stress.

Scientific medicine has developed a method of relief for the acute attack. Small ampules filled with a drug called amyl nitrite are prescribed by doctors for people with this disease. In the majority of cases the inhaling of this drug will bring about prompt relief. Some of the patients do well with treatment involving the use of nitroglycerine. Peritrate is a long-acting dilator of coronary vessels. These drugs are potent and should never be taken except with the advice of a doctor who will determine the true cause of the pain.

Relief of the acute attack is not the chief matter of importance. The doctor who is responsible for the patient with angina pectoris will regulate the entire life of the patient according to the suggestions that have already been mentioned, in order to minimize the number of attacks. This regulation will also be helpful in overcoming various disorders in the body which are responsible for the onset of the attacks.

The pain of coronary thrombosis, as has already been mentioned, is like that of angina pectoris and occurs for the same reason. Some part of the heart muscle is deprived of its necessary blood supply. However, in coronary thrombosis the blood supply is cut off because a clot or some other obstruction forms in one of the branches of these blood vessels. Thus a portion of the heart muscle has to do without any blood, and pain results. Moreover, the obstruction, once established, is sufficiently long in its duration to permit a good deal of damage to be done to the part of the heart concerned.

ANISEIKONIA There are many strange Latin names that describe disturbances of vision due to changes from the normal in the shape of either the eyeball or the mechanism that brings the image through to the brain. For instance astigmatism is a condition in which parallel rays are focused at different points and is usually due to a change in the curvature of the cornea, or outside of the eye.

There is another condition in which there is marked inequality in the refraction of the two eyes. This occurs in a person who is farsighted in one eye and nearsighted in the other eye. Sometimes either farsightedness or nearsightedness is combined with astigmatism.

One of the most recently discovered conditions is one in which the images which fall on the retina in back of the eye are unequal in either size or shape. This condition is called aniseikonia. There are apparently instances in which such inequality in the retinal images is responsible for eyestrain and in which correction of the refraction or the wearing of suitable glasses does not bring complete relief.

Instruments have been developed to test the ability of a person to see images equally with either eye. A person with aniseikonia will think that a table is level when it is actually tipped or vice versa. If a table is level and looks tipped, the person can be asked to tip the table until it seems level to him. The amount of tipping necessary to make the table seem level will give an idea of the amount of distortion present.

Eye specialists say that about 2 per cent of people have aniseikonia that can be corrected. About one third of all the people who are given glasses to correct this condition report that they are entirely relieved of the symptoms; another one third say that they have partial relief.

While the correction of aniseikonia will not clear up headaches, which may be the result of many different causes, there are instances of headache in which correction of this solution will bring about some relief.

To a person who has aniseikonia to a large degree the world looks as it did in the motion picture called *The Cabinet of Dr. Caligari* or in some of the other modernistic pictures that one sees in which everything seems to be leaning in the wrong direction. For such people it means a great deal to have the world put back on the level.

ANKLE, SPRAINED A sudden turning of the foot may stretch or pull a ligament so that bleeding and inflammation follow. Heat, as by soaking in hot water, helps to relieve inflammation. Strapping with adhesive keeps pull and pressure off the injured tissues. Latest treatment includes injection of a local anesthetic which relieves pain and permits earlier use of foot.

ANOREXIA (See *Appetite*) Loss of appetite.

ANTHRAX The anthrax germ was first described by Pasteur. It is found in the hair, hides, and the fresh excretions of human beings and animals. On the outside of the body it forms infections which are called malignant pustules or boils. Inside the body the germ usually gets into the lungs of wool sorters or persons working with hides, so that anthrax of the lungs has been called "wool sorters' disease." An epidemic of anthrax of the face once occurred in the United States due to the use of infected shaving brushes imported from Japan. Following this epidemic, laws were passed which controlled the importing of such shaving brushes.

The anthrax germ usually gets into the body from contact of a wound or scratch with material containing the germ, from inhaling the spores of the germ, or occasionally by transmission from some infected animal to man by the medium of the fly or mosquito. Several days after the germs get into the body the symptoms appear.

The prevention of infection with anthrax in human beings involves the prevention of the disease in animals and the prevention of the spread of the disease from animals to man. The workers most likely to be affected by anthrax include agricultural workers, butchers, veterinary surgeons, and workers with hides.

In preventing the spread of the disease workers should always wear overalls or rubber aprons when working with suspected animals, wash and disinfect the hands thoroughly, and avoid contact with any person who has a sore or an abrasion. The preventive measures common to all industries include general cleanliness, the avoidance of dust, the wearing of overalls, caps, and gloves, and warning workers to report any lesion of the skin to the physician so that he may examine it. All waste water or sewage from factories where the possibility of anthrax exists should be thoroughly disinfected before it is permitted outside the plant. Tanneries and woolen mills should have proper ventilation apparatus, including exhaust fans to take care of dangerous dusts.

The presence of anthrax is marked by painful itching, which is followed in a few hours by the appearance of a red spot. This swells and pus appears at the center. The malignant boils spread rapidly and the tissue becomes gangrenous. Naturally when such an infection gets into the lung, the condition is exceedingly serious with all of the symptoms of a most serious infection and the difficulty in breathing likely to follow any serious infection in the lungs.

Because anthrax is a rare disease the diagnosis is not made usually until rather late, sometimes only at post-mortem examination. Fortunately serums which are effective against anthrax have been discovered; the sulfonamides are also useful in this condition to control secondary infections.

ANTITOXINS Antitoxins are substances which react against poisons or toxins. They are usually made by injecting the toxin or poison of a disease into an animal (such as the horse) which then develops the antitoxin in its blood. The blood is taken from the animal after a sufficient amount of time has elapsed. The serum or fluid material which contains the antitoxin is removed from the blood and then injected into a person who is suffering with infection.

The value of antitoxin in diphtheria is now so well established that it is considered one of the greatest discoveries of all time. Diphtheria antitoxin neutralizes poisons of diphtheria and is employed both as a curative agent and also to prevent diphtheria. However, in the prevention of diphtheria several other methods which are considered more desirable are employed. For instance diphtheria toxoid is a preparation of the actual toxin of diphtheria modified by the addition of materials which cause it to lose its ability to produce the toxic effects. Diphtheria toxoid is a detoxified toxin.

The antitoxins which are recognized as among the most useful in medicine include those against botulism, snake bite, diphtheria, scarlet fever, lockjaw, and staphylococcus infections. Other antitoxins have been used in erysipelas, epidemic sore throat, and meningitis. However, the sulfonamide drugs and penicillin are so effective against some of these infections that the use of the antitoxin or antiserum has been abandoned in most instances in favor of the chemical remedy.

When a human being has in his blood enough antibodies or antitoxins to overcome an infection, he is said to be immune to that infection. However, immunity to infection is divided into two kinds—natural and acquired —and acquired immunity is divided into passive and active immunity. In active immunity the antisubstances are created in the body. In passive immunity the antisubstances are introduced from outside the body. Antitoxins are, therefore, substances which produce passive immunity in the body by supplying the antibodies which promptly antagonize the poisons of the germs. Therefore passive immunity is much prompter than active immunity because it puts in the antipoison directly, whereas the injection of a substance like diphtheria toxoid causes the body to develop its own antisubstances.

Perhaps next most important after the diphtheria antitoxin is that for tetanus, or lockjaw. This antitoxin is useful not only in the prevention of tetanus but also in its treatment. Once lockjaw has occurred, exceedingly large doses of the tetanus antitoxin must be given to overcome the effects of the poison. In the United States Army and Navy all troops are now injected with the tetanus toxoid, which causes the soldier or sailor to develop in his own blood substances capable of preventing an infection with lockjaw.

The scarlet fever antitoxin is likely to be used only in times when an epidemic of this condition prevails in the community, and the staphylococcus antitoxin only in cases of severe infection in which the staphylococcus has gained entrance into the blood. Again the effects of penicillin in staphylococcus infections are so adequate that this substance is likely to be given a trial in serious cases before resorting to the use of the staphylococcus antitoxin.

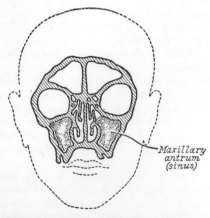

The large sinuses at the sides of the nose in the jaws are called maxillary sinuses. They are located in a bone known as the maxilla, which is the upper jawbone

ANTRUM (See *Sinuses*) A cavity or space, usually within a bone, most frequently used in referring to the maxillary antrum or maxillary sinus.

ANUS The scientific name for the outlet of the rectum, or lower end of the bowel.

AORTA The largest blood vessel, coming from the heart, from which the entire system of arteries proceeds.

APHRODISIAC Any thought, substance, or drug that arouses the sexual instincts. Medicine knows of no true aphrodisiac drugs capable of use without harm, but the mind exerts considerable control.

APOPLEXY Brain hemorrhage, commonly called apoplexy or stroke, is coming to be one of the most frequent causes of death because of the increasing age of our population. In 1890 less than 3 per cent of the people in the United States were over sixty-five years of age; today about 9 per cent of people are over sixty-five years of age.

A stroke usually affects a person who has high blood pressure and hardening of the arteries or other serious changes in the blood vessels of the brain. The stroke often comes on in the midst of excitement or any other condition that raises the blood pressure. For instance a man at work suddenly falls as though struck down and is thereafter unable to move the muscles of his face, his arms, or his legs. In a typical instance an elderly person goes to sleep and awakens during the night with a sharp cry to find that some part of the body has become paralyzed.

There are all sorts of superstitions and notions about a stroke. One of these insists that a third stroke is always fatal. There is no basis for this belief except that a person who has had repeated strokes and whose body has been worn down as a result is more likely to die after the second stroke than the first and after the third stroke than the second.

When a stroke occurs in a young person, it is often due to the fact that a small clot has broken loose from a wound or tissues elsewhere in the body and has lodged in one of the small blood vessels in the brain. Any sudden blocking of the blood to the brain produces symptoms like those of hemorrhage into the brain, which presses on the blood vessels and thus prevents the passing of blood to the tissues of the brain.

Whenever a stroke occurs, the first step should be to put the affected person to bed, allowing him to lie flat on his side while he is unconscious. This will help to prevent the tongue from falling back and producing choking and strangulation. Everything possible must be done to maintain the strength of the heart and the flow of blood to the brain. Of course a doctor should be called immediately so that he may control the administration of food, water, and other activities necessary to keep the patient alive.

On recovery from the first attack of unconsciousness following a stroke the person affected will find that certain parts of the body have been paralyzed. This may be due to actual destruction of certain nerves or just to the inflammation and pressure. The inflammation will tend to lessen with the passing of time and often just good care and rest permit recovery to go on, so that eventually the paralysis disappears as new blood vessels grow into the area concerned.

After the hemorrhage has stopped it becomes possible to determine the extent of the paralysis and to see what can be done to take care of the patient, who is no longer able to take care of himself. The future of such a patient is, in many instances, not hopeless. After the hemorrhage is absorbed, there may be gradual recovery of portions of the body that have been paralyzed.

Sometimes it is difficult to move a heavy man or woman who has had a stroke. Such persons should not, however, be pulled or jerked. They should be lifted or rolled gradually into a new position. If the patient has use of his arms, it may be possible to fix a bolt in the ceiling and to suspend from this a rope or tape by which the patient may raise himself and thus aid in movement.

Persons who become unconscious usually are deprived of fluids. They are unable to drink or swallow. It is therefore absolutely necessary to see that fluids are put into the body either by injection with a tube or by injection under the skin. The feeding of such patients may be exceedingly difficult, requiring in many instances the use of a tube passed directly into the stomach or occasionally feeding directly into the bowel or even into a vein.

In the daily care of the patient who has been paralyzed after brain hemorrhage it is especially important to give proper attention to the skin. A daily bath with soap and water is necessary for cleanliness and for the avoidance of secondary infections. Such patients should be moved at frequent intervals —at least every two or three hours— so that there will not be continuous pressure on any portion of the body where the bones are next to the surface, resulting in the possible formation of a bed sore or an ulcer on the skin.

APPENDICITIS In 1886 a Boston surgeon named Reginald H. Fitz definitely described the condition now called appendicitis. Almost immediately thereafter another surgeon recommended prompt operation once the diagnosis of appendicitis was made.

Many animals do not have an appendix. These include the skunk, the raccoon, the bear, the walrus, and the baboon. Other animals, including the gibbon, the chimpanzee, the dog, the cat, the sheep, and the tiger, do have an appendix like that of man.

The appendix is a small fingerlike projection from the large bowel varying in length from one to six inches. It comes from that portion of the large bowel called the cecum, which is in the lower right side of the abdomen. Because it lies near the bladder and the rectum, inflammation or infection of the appendix may cause symptoms which are related to these two organs.

For a long time it was thought that appendicitis resulted always from food which lodged in the appendix and blocked it. Occasionally such materials as stones, seeds, hairs, pins, small bones, or even lead shot have been found in the appendix when it was removed in a surgical operation; occasionally worms are found in the appendix. However, there are innumerable cases of appendicitis in which no such materials have been found. In such cases it seems likely that there is an infection caused by germs which have lodged in the appendix and set up an inflammation and a reaction.

When the wall of the appendix becomes infected, it swells. This interferes with emptying of the organ and leads to the formation of an abscess. The pressure of material that cannot get out produces pain. Eventually, also, the swelling may become so great that the appendix bursts. Bursting of the appendix is an exceedingly serious accident because the infection is then spread throughout the abdominal cavity, producing an inflammation of the lining of the abdominal cavity called the peritoneum. Inflammation of the peritoneum is called peritonitis.

Some faddists have argued that appendicitis is a disease of civilized people only and that it does not occur among savages or primitive peoples. They insist that appendicitis results from the sort of diet that civilized man eats. Careful studies among savages and uncivilized people by medical scientists now indicate that appendicitis occurs in Java, India, and the Philippine Islands. Differences have not been found between appendicitis in Americans, English, Japanese, Chinese, or Malayans. In fact some of our Army and Navy officers in the South Pacific area already report a considerable number of operations for appendicitis among the Japanese and the Malayans. Some faddists have argued that the Chinese do not have as much appendicitis as persons in the United States because they live on a special type of diet. However, surgeons of long experience in China say that appendicitis is far more common among the Chinese than we are led to believe. Indeed they believe that the difficulty has been, instead, a lack of scientific medical attention and a failure to diagnose the condition properly—a failure which, incidentally, was frequent among civilized men be-

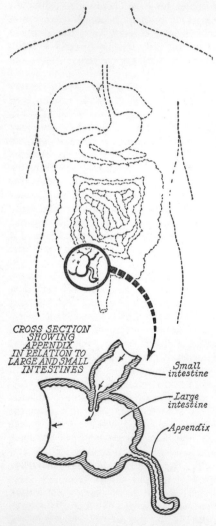

CROSS SECTION
SHOWING
APPENDIX
IN RELATION TO
LARGE AND SMALL
INTESTINES

Small
intestine

Large
intestine

Appendix

The appendix is a small sac attached to the bowel which seems to cause trouble out of all proportion to its size

fore Dr. Reginald Fitz, of Boston, called attention to the exact nature of the disease.

In the United States about sixteen thousand people die every year from appendicitis, so that it is about fifteenth among the causes of death. If children are eliminated from the statistics and only persons above the age of fifteen are taken into consideration, appendicitis would be eighth or ninth in the list of causes of death.

In most cases when death occurs in appendicitis the person concerned has delayed in securing a diagnosis and an immediate operation necessary to save life. In most cases also the person concerned has tried to cure a pain in the abdomen, or what he calls a gastrointestinal upset, by taking a large dose of some cathartic. The best possible advice is to avoid the use of any cathartic or even a laxative for a pain in the abdomen until the cause of the pain is definitely known.

When appendicitis begins, the person usually says that he feels ill with nausea and loss of appetite and that he has a soreness over the abdomen. Sometimes he vomits. Usually he blames it on something that he recently ate. Soon the pain in the abdomen becomes constant and localizes on the right side rather low down. The area becomes tender to touch; the pulse becomes rapid, and the temperature rises to well over 100. Sometimes there is difficulty in moving the bowels or in urinating. This is explained by the fact that the appendix is close to the bladder and rectum, as has already been mentioned.

May people have been led to believe that appendicitis is always accompanied by severe or projectile vomiting and exceedingly serious pain in exactly one spot. We know now, however, that there are many cases of appendicitis in which the symptoms are not so definite. The physician promptly takes a specimen of blood and counts the white blood cells. A large increase in the number of white blood cells indicates to the doctor that there is a serious infection and that the blood is reacting against it. The trained finger and brain of the doctor can determine the exact spot of the pain and thus make certain of the diagnosis. Particularly in winter months the doctor finds the diagnosis somewhat difficult because signs like those of appendicitis sometimes occur in beginning pneumonia. Pneumonia in the lower part of the lungs sets up an inflammation along the diaphragm, the large muscle for breathing which separates the chest cavity from the abdomen. This causes pain, which is felt over the area where the appendix lies, and rigidity when the doctor tries to press on the abdomen.

The modern surgical operation for appendicitis is so well standardized that any competent surgeon who works in an accredited hospital can give reasonable assurance of a prompt recovery if the operation is done before the appendix bursts. If, however, the appendix has become gangrenous, or if there has been rupture of the appendix with the extension of the infected material into the abdominal cavity, recovery may be delayed for several weeks. In the majority of cases, when the diagnosis is made early and the treatment promptly administered, the doctor may get the patient up after two or three days and out of the hospital after seven to ten days.

Penicillin, terramycin, aureomycin, and other antibiotics prevent peritonitis so that death from secondary infection has become rare.

APPETITE When hunger occurs, there are contractions of the stomach. There is a difference between hunger and appetite. People who eat regularly and in fair amounts seldom feel hunger. They do, however, have appetite at regular intervals of eating.

Eating is a habit. Sometimes eating becomes a habit indulged to excess. Appetite is a longing for something that we want. We have excessive appetite when we are too frequently hungry. Appetite may follow excessive exercise, particularly in the open air. Ordinarily a good appetite is considered to be an indication that the person who has it is healthy.

Sometimes children develop excessive cravings for food in response to psychologic conditions in their environment. The eating of food may be a substitute for some serious disappointment or a means of getting attention. One child developed an excessive craving for food after its favorite nurse was discharged. Another child developed such an excessive craving following the birth of a new baby into the family.

There have been many arguments as to whether or not wine, beer, or cocktails increase or decrease the appetite. The majority of experience indicates that the taking of small amounts of such drinks will awaken or increase the appetite. However, these substances eliminate the contractions that are associated with hunger.

New drugs recently discovered called benzedrine and dexedrine have the power of diminishing appetite and are now prescribed in weight reduction.

Complete loss of appetite and failure to eat is called anorexia nervosa. It is usually associated with some emotional instability. It occurs more frequently among women than among men.

ARACHNODACTYLY This is a condition in which the fingers and toes are long and thin. The term comes from a Latin word meaning "spider" and it means that the fingers are spiderlike. Apparently there is a tendency to hereditary transmission of a condition of this type.

ARCHES, FALLEN (See discussion under *Feet*) The arch of the foot is under constant pressure from standing on the feet. Breakdown of the arch results in flatfoot.

ARCTIC HEALTH (See also *Frostbite*) The development of aviation greatly increased travel into Arctic regions. Emergency landings may cause people to be exposed without preparation to the unusual climate. These hints may be most helpful in saving life.

The peculiar hazards of the Arctic area relate primarily to cold and snow. Snow blindness is the result of the effects of glare on the eyes. Special goggles are supplied to keep off the glare. The Eskimo makes a snow shield from a scrap of wood; he takes a rectangular piece of thin wood, about six inches long and one inch wide, and burns holes or slits through it at about the width of the eyes. This shield can be placed across the bridge of the nose and held by a piece of string passing around over the ears and in back of the head. Vision is possible through the slits, which serve at the same time to bar the glare of the sun. Another help is the blackening of the cheeks and the bridge of the nose with soot, charcoal, or dirty engine oil. This blackening helps to cut down reflections from the sun.

Tight shoes encourage freezing and damage to the feet. The shoes worn in the Arctic regions must be big enough to allow the person to wear at least two pairs of heavy socks. If the shoes are not sufficiently large for this purpose, it is well to remove the shoes entirely and to wrap the feet in improvised coverings made of canvas or similar materials.

The hands and feet must be kept constantly warm and dry. For keeping the hands warm heavy woolen inner mitts with canvas or other windproof outer mitts are recommended.

Many a serious accident has occurred from touching cold metal with a bare hand. The metal will freeze to the skin. In the first reaction the tendency is to tear the hand away from the metal; this will destroy the skin. The metal should be thawed loose from the skin.

The Eskimo diet has been planned in relation to the cold. Fat is the basis of this diet, since it is a heat-producing food. The Arctic soldier obtains his food from animals and fish. A government agency warns against the eating of polar-bear livers, which are said to be poisonous. Warning is also given against living exclusively on the meat of the rabbit, just because it happens to be plentiful. A continued diet of rabbit produces a condition called rabbit starvation, with diarrhea beginning about a week after the rabbit diet has been established. Practically all fish have enough fat to make them good Arctic food. The liver of the cod, which is the basis of cod-liver oil, is an especially good food and can be eaten boiled.

Among the most important of the recommendations are those having to do with the avoidance of frostbite. Frostbite often comes without the victim's knowledge. If the skin becomes stiff and grayish or whitish in color, frostbite is under way. Under such circumstances never apply snow or ice. This used to be the recommended treatment. Now we know that it is much better to warm the affected part gradually, avoiding even the gentlest of rubbing or massage, since this may destroy human tissue. Frozen feet are especially serious. If the feet are frostbitten, shoes, and coverings should be removed immediately; when possible, a warmer type of footgear should be employed. The feet should be wrapped in cloth or fur until they thaw. Thawing is accompanied by a burning sensation and may be an extremely painful condition. After frostbite the skin blisters and peels exactly as it does in sunburn.

ARGYROSIS Use of silver solutions like silver nitrate or argyrol may result in deposit of silver in the skin called argyrosis. The result is a gray-blue appearance which has to wear off gradually.

ARTERIOSCLEROSIS When the blood vessels become less elastic, thickened, and hardened, many changes related to the changes in the blood vessels occur in the body. Such hardening of the arteries causes the death of many people who live past middle age. Nevertheless the body can accommodate itself to hardening of the arteries

so that people who pass sixty-five or seventy years of age without any type of accident may go on to live for a good many years.

A blood vessel is a tube like a water hose that contains elastic tissue in its walls. The wall will stretch and, after it stretches, will come back to its original size. If the walls stretch to accommodate an increased amount of blood flowing through them, the blood pressure will not change. However, if the walls will not stretch, the increased amount of blood puts extra pressure on the walls and high blood pressure develops.

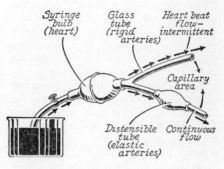

Mechanism showing how hardened blood vessels increase blood pressure

Hardening of the walls of the arteries, or arteriosclerosis, is frequently associated with high blood pressure. It is not, however, the cause of high blood pressure. The exact causes of arteriosclerosis are not known. Sometimes the condition occurs more frequently in some families than in others. It has been associated with excesses in drinking alcohol and smoking. However, people have died from delirium tremens after a long career of heavy drinking without having hardening of the arteries. Some have believed that overeating, particularly the overeating of fats, may be responsible for hardening of the arteries. The evidence in support of this contention is also insufficient to give complete acceptance. Modern research on animals indicates that a high fat diet may have some relationship to hardening of the arteries. In most cases the changes in the walls of the blood vessels take place after the fourth decade of life.

We know of no specific treatment for hardening of the arteries. Doctors generally recommend good hygiene and the avoidance of excesses of all kinds, and graceful mental and physical adjustment to getting old seems to be helpful when hardening of the arteries sets in. The drugs that are administered to people with hardening of the arteries are usually given with a view to causing these people to rest more frequently and to reduce the mental stresses from which they may suffer. One of the reasons for such treatment is the fact that the high blood pressure associated with the artery whose wall is not elastic may produce an accident like a hemorrhage if there is too much pressure.

Since there is no specific treatment that will restore the elasticity to the hardened blood vessels, everything possible should be done that will take off the extra stress. People with hardened arteries usually feel better after warm baths, hot-air baths, and similar physical therapy. Most of the symptoms of hardening of the arteries are related to the high blood pressure and the difficulty of maintaining good circulation. Transient attacks of dizziness, drowziness, and ringing in the ears are the symptoms most frequently complained of. Sometimes these clear up without any treatment except the rest and hygiene that have been mentioned, particularly after the person concerned has gotten used to the symptom. In some cases, however, the changes in the blood vessels of legs and the interference with circulation produce cramping, blueness of the tissues, and other signs of a lack of sufficient circulation.

When the arteries of the heart or brain happen to be involved, the situation is much more serious because of the importance of these tissues in the maintenance of life itself. Hardening of the arteries of the heart is responsible for from 25 to 40 per cent of cases with chronic heart disease.

ARTHRITIS A survey indicates that there are at least 7,000,000 people in the United States with rheumatism. This disease is responsible for more days lost from work than any other chronic disability except the nervous and mental diseases. Rheumatism includes arthritis, gout, neuralgia, neuritis, lumbago, and other conditions.

Arthritis is an inflammation of the joints which occurs in many different forms. For instance there is the arthritis due to infection of many different types, that due to degeneration of the tissues of the joints, of which the cause is unknown but which sometimes follows injury, arthritis associated with gout and other disturbances of the digestion and metabolism of food, inflammation of the joints associated with nervous disorders like locomotor ataxia, inflammations following the growth of tumors, and many inflammations of the joints associated with sensitivity to foods and drugs. Then there are disturbances of the joints related to the bones that are involved in the joints.

When the cause of the arthritis can be definitely determined as an infection, with the germs that cause gonorrhea or tuberculosis or syphilis or scarlet fever or typhoid fever, the condition can be treated with much more satisfaction than when the inflammation in the joint is simply a degenerative and inflammatory change of which the cause is unknown.

In one great clinic 7 per cent of all the patients treated suffered from chronic rheumatism. People with rheumatism are likely to feel better on nice warm days and worse on cold rainy days. When they feel better, they credit the last treatment that they tried for the improvement. For this reason there are innumerable remedies for rheumatism sold to the public. Most of these contain some product of salicylic acid or some sedative drug. The worst danger in their use is the fact that they make the person feel better temporarily, so that he is likely to depend on the product and not do what can be done to stop the progress of the disease.

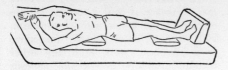

THE SUPINE POSITION

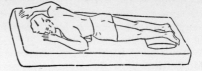

THE PRONE POSITION

Positions assumed in bed by the arthritic patient to obtain physiological rest

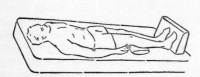

GOOD POSITION

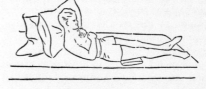

POOR POSITION

The recumbent position assumed in bed by the arthritic patient to prevent deformity and to improve general circulation

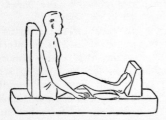

GOOD POSITION

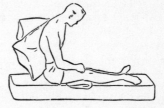

POOR POSITION

The functional position assumed by the arthritic patient sitting up in bed for occupational therapy

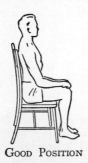

GOOD POSITION

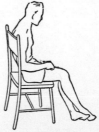

POOR POSITION

The sitting position assumed in a suitable chair by the arthritic patient

There are cases of arthritis in women which are related to the activities of the sex glands. This form of arthritis, called menopausal arthritis, is frequently controllable by treatment directed to the general condition.

The condition called rheumatoid arthritis is far more frequent than the form due to infection with some definite germ. Certain factors are known to be definitely related to this type of arthritis. Fatigue, shock, injury, exposure to dampness, rain, and cold have all been mentioned as factors which contribute to this type of inflammation. In many cases the person who is affected definitely relates his disturbance to some such exposure, to a surgical operation, an emotional strain or fatigue. In this condition there are pain and swelling of the joints, often associated with chills and fever and signs of acute infection.

When the onset is gradual, the symptoms appear usually first in just one joint. There may be pain and stiffness in this joint for weeks and months before any other joint is affected. Eventually the condition becomes chronic, however, and other joints, particularly those of the fingers, hands, and knees, are involved simultaneously on both sides of the body. The amount of pain in the joints varies and is not always proportionate to the amount of swelling. In many instances there is relatively little pain except when the joint is exercised or involved in intensive motion. The arthritis that affects the hips and the spine is more painful than that affecting other portions of the body.

The hands of the person with this kind of arthritis are rather typical of the condition. The fingers develop an appearance which has been called "sausage finger," in which there is a pod-shaped swelling of the joint of the finger nearest to the wrist. The joints farthest removed from the wrist are not so likely to be involved. Eventually, however, all of the fingers may be involved and the swelling will appear in the knuckles and the wrist. The knees are generally affected and usually early in the disease.

The toes seem to be little involved, apparently because the toes are seldom moved individually.

Another common appearance in this condition is the nodules which occur under the skin in about 10 per cent of all cases. These nodes are usually found around the elbows, wrists, fingers, and occasionally at the ankles. They vary in size from a small pea to a large walnut. They come and go but in general tend to persist for months.

As has been mentioned, this type of arthritis is a chronic condition. There are periods when the patients seem to be entirely free from disturbances even for months but gradually the condition tends to become more and more pronounced and the involvement more extensive. In the worst cases the patients become confined to bed because of permanent deformity.

Rheumatoid arthritis differs considerably from the degenerative type. Usually rheumatoid arthritis comes on before forty years of age, while the degenerative type comes on between fifty and seventy. Persons with degenerative arthritis are likely to be overweight, whereas those with rheumatoid arthritis are underweight. The rheumatoid condition may involve any joint in the body, while the degenerative type usually affects the knees, the spine, and the fingers. The little nodules under the skin which are present in 10 per cent of rheumatoid cases are not seen in degenerative arthritis. Whereas the rheumatoid inflammation tends to produce permanent deformity of the joints, degenerative arthritis does not usually have that effect.

In addition to the typical arthritis that has been described this condition may have many modifications, depending on environmental factors.

Unfortunately there is no specific form of treatment which will definitely prevent the advancement of rheumatoid arthritis. However, everything possible is done to increase the patient's resistance and to put him in the best possible health. Furthermore, special attention is given to every one of the inflamed joints to prevent any type of permanent deformity.

All observers are agreed that rest is important even though the patient feels that he can go on working. The doctor is likely to demand, however, at least one to two hours rest in bed every day after lunch and a real rest cure in the worst cases. In difficult cases the use of a hospital or sanitarium is desirable so that the different methods of treatment that are used may be applied under controlled conditions.

We do not know of any diet that is especially valuable in this kind of arthritis. Most of the patients are undernourished and underweight. In order to bring them back to health a diet with at least 50 grams of protein daily and with all the necessary vitamins and mineral salts is desirable. Such a diet will be rich in vegetables and fruits.

Vaccines have been developed which are supposed to be useful. They are usually made out of bacteria that are isolated from the body of the person concerned, particularly from the nose, throat, and bowel. Their use seems to be still experimental. A number of patients are reported to have been benefited by such treatment. Many, however, feel that the effect of these vaccines is the same as comes from using a nonspecific protein to stimulate the reaction of the body of the patient against any kind of infection.

The use of the heat cabinet, which produces artificial fever, has been reported to benefit some patients but there seems to be no evidence that it is routinely helpful. Such relief as occurs seems to be just temporary.

Drugs, particularly derivatives of the salicylates such as aspirin and sodium salicylate, seem to be valuable in controlling the pain of rheumatoid arthritis.

Frequently used remedies are salts of gold. There are several preparations of gold salts which are now tried and apparently anywhere from 20 to 40 per cent of patients report improvement when this treatment is given by a physician who has thorough knowledge of the technic of use of these preparations.

Of recent years particular reliance has been placed on treatment with dry heat, diathermy, massage, and exercises. The chief function of these procedures is to increase the circulation of the blood in the area of the joints and to keep the muscles around the joints in the best possible physical condition. The application of heat is most important. Some prefer moist heat with packs wrung out of hot water such as are used in the Kenny method. The use of electrical diathermy, which conveys the heat directly into the joint, is felt by some to be less beneficial than the packs or the hot tub bath.

Some years have passed since investigators first observed that women in pregnancy and people generally during jaundice were relieved of rheumatic symptoms. The investigators decided that some substance circulating in the blood under such circumstances must be responsible. Dr. E. C. Kendall of the Mayo Clinic therefore attempted to find in the bile salts a product that could bring about these effects. Earlier it was determined that the substance concerned was one of the many hormones secreted by the adrenal gland. From the cortex of the adrenal gland Kendall found a substance called Cortisone. Several different forms of Cortisone which should be taken only as prescribed by the doctor are now available. A new, more potent form is prednisone or Meticorten or Sertane or Deltra. The results thus far reported on patients with rheumatoid arthritis are excellent. Patients are relieved in a short time from pain and from their serious crippling. However, the investigators find also that, while the substance has therapeutic value, the use of the material daily is necessary in order to supply the missing hormone from their bodies. Investigators found also that the pituitary gland develops a hormone which has the function of stimulating the adrenal gland to action, thus causing the adrenal to develop more Cortisone. This substance is called adrenocorticotropic hormone; it is known by its abbreviation ACTH, or by the name Corticotropin. It has been found efficient against rheumatoid arthritis. Nevertheless this substance also must be taken daily.

Some people with rheumatic conditions do very well with a change of climate, particularly to warm, dry areas such as those of Arizona and New Mexico. However, a week's stay will not accomplish much. Proper treatment means anywhere from six months to a year in the improved climate.

The orthopedic surgeons do a great deal to improve the control of the deformed joints and bones and muscles. Proper orthopedic care does a great deal for the functioning of these tissues.

Finally, people with rheumatic conditions are likely to suffer with mental depression. Attention must be given to their psychology. Army surgeons have reported many instances in which the rheumatic conditions were definitely made worse by nerve strains associated with the war.

ASBESTOSIS A condition occurring among workers who inhale dust and other materials from asbestos. The inhaling of asbestos fibers produces fibrous changes in the lungs which represent an attempt of the tissue of the lung to wall off the foreign substance. Asbestos contains about 41 per cent of silica and 2½ per cent of iron oxide. The lungs react particularly to silica, producing a condition that is called silicosis. Workers with asbestos also develop warty growths on the skin which are called asbestos corns.

ASCHHEIM-ZONDEK TEST See *Pregnancy*.

ASCORBIC ACID (See discussion under *Vitamins*) Vitamin C.

ASPHYXIA Most times when a person becomes asphyxiated, a doctor is not easily available. This applies particularly to babies who are suffocated in their cribs, to persons shocked by electricity, or to those asphyxiated by illuminating gas. During the past ten years American industry has organized to take care of patients who have been asphyxiated. Many a large industry has a first-aid team which knows just what to do when such an accident occurs. The first step is resuscitation. Many different machines have been developed to aid resuscitation. Many fire departments and hospitals have such devices easily available. However, it is not desirable to wait until someone finds the device and brings it to the spot where the asphyxiated person lies.

Let us assume that the person has been drowned. He should be put immediately in a horizontal position with the back upward and the abdomen down on a clean place on the ground. The head should be turned to one side and can rest on the victim's hand so as to keep his mouth out of the water or out of the sand. If the body can lie slightly inclined downward on a slope of 20 or 30 degrees, elimination of fluid from the throat and the breathing tubes will be facilitated. With the person in this position resuscitation is begun by what is called the prone-pressure technic, which involves alternate pressure and release on the chest so as to force air in and out of the chest. People who do not know this technic should receive instruction so as to be able to practice it successfully when an emergency arises. Everything possible must be done at the same time to keep the asphyxiated person warm, because failure to do so may result in shock which in turn may be responsible for death.

So frequently do linesmen working on electric wires become shocked and asphyxiated that the light companies have developed a special technic which they call "pole-top" resuscitation. The shocked linesman will probably be found hanging by his safety belt. The rescuer is taught to push the victim's head forward, encircling the waistline with the arms, placing one open hand on the abdomen and grasping the first hand with the fingers of the other to insure a firm grip. The rescuer then applies pressure on the abdomen in an inward and upward direction, then completely releases the pressure, making about eighteen or twenty pressures per minute.

The figures seem to show that nobody can live whose lungs have been without a change of air for over twelve minutes. In fact there are few, if any, records which show that anyone has lived after being submerged under water for more than four minutes. Nevertheless, resuscitation may be attempted for long periods of time with the hope that the period during which the individual has been without air is less than has been originally estimated.

The idea of blowing air into the lungs and sucking it out again by the use of a machine evidently was first developed around 1909. Some of the first machines that were developed were dangerous because they could blow up the lungs so large as to damage the tissues. Practically all modern machines are equipped with stop valves which prevent this hazard. In many large cities ambulances have been especially equipped with resuscitation apparatus with the view to giving the injured individual the aid of the machine at the earliest possible moment and also during the time when he is being transferred to the hospital.

ASTHENIA See *Exhaustion* and *Fatigue*.

ASTHMA Of all the diseases that are due to excessive sensitivity to various substances, bronchial asthma is the most important. It has existed since early times because the very name of the disease comes from a Greek word that means panting or gasping for breath of a fairly severe degree. A slight degree of difficulty in breathing was called dyspnea, which merely means shortness of breath.

There are many different types of asthma. They have been classified rather arbitrarily into the asthma that is due to allergy, that due to irritation of the bronchial tubes, that which is largely mental in its cause, that related to diseases like infections, tuberculosis, or other changed conditions of the body,

and, finally, all of the asthma that cannot be related to any definite cause.

People of any age can have asthma but at least half the cases appear between the ages of twenty and forty. The condition seems to be twice as common among boys as among girls. Men who are in occupations in which they are especially exposed to the inhalation of various dusts more frequently have asthma than do others. This includes, for instance, bakers, furriers, cotton spinners, upholsterers, barbers, druggists, dentists, poultry dealers, and workers with various flours and dried beans.

A person with asthma may be sensitive to several different dusts. For instance a woman who had her asthma only when she began working in a beauty shop was found to be sensitive to orris root. When the orris root was replaced by buckwheat flour, the symptoms disappeared, but after ten months she became sensitive to the buckwheat flour. When removed from this contact, the asthma disappeared but at a later date she became sensitive to rye flour.

The tendency to sensitivity resulting in asthma is more frequent in some families than in others. As a part of the asthmatic constitution there may be glandular conditions, conditions of the nervous system, psychological factors, and chemical changes in the body which need to be studied by the doctor because of their relationship to the asthma. In many instances asthma first appears following an infection of the nose, throat, or lungs with various germs including that of tuberculosis. Various chemical or metallic irritating dusts may be a factor in producing the first attack of asthma. Indeed hypersensitiveness to dusts, particularly house dusts, is one of the most frequent causes of an asthmatic attack. House dust is composed of a great variety of molds, fungi, and similar materials.

Among the most common causes of asthma in children are sensitivities to foods, whereas these are responsible for only a small percentage of cases among adults.

In an asthmatic attack the person finds it increasingly difficult to breathe until he struggles for air and thinks he is suffocating. As a result he breathes more rapidly and his pulse becomes more rapid. Because plugs of mucous secretion get into the bronchial tubes, the blood does not get an adequate amount of oxygen. Therefore the person seems blue and the heart beats more rapidly. The constriction of the bronchial tubes makes the air come and go with a high-pitched sound. Because the breathing is difficult the muscles of the chest are strained.

Frequently the attack of asthma will come with a strong desire to sneeze, followed by a lot of secretion coming from the nose and lungs. Often there will be frequent yawning before the attack, sometimes itching of the skin or an eruption. All of these are symptoms of the sensitivity. Because of the constriction of the tubes and the flowing of secretion coughing is not infrequent in the effort of the asthmatic person to clear the chest and throat. Most alarming, however, is the sense of suffocation that is not relieved by strenuous efforts to breathe, by increasing the flow of air, opening the window, or by remaining absolutely quiet. However, patients soon learn that they can best combat the shortness of breath by remaining quiet and motionless. They are likely to bend the body so as to increase the breathing space in the chest and throat. When the attack passes, the breathing becomes easier and the anxiety disappears.

Often the asthmatic attack occurs at night. The reason for this is not known, although there are many theories having to do with the sensitivity of the nervous system and the accumulation of the irritating secretions. Some people have attacks almost every night, whereas others may be free from asthmatic attacks for weeks or months.

Eventually the asthma may become chronic. In the chronic asthmatic the severity of the attacks is less and the shortness of breath is likely to be less disturbing. However, the constancy of the symptoms may eventually produce changes in the appearance of the chest. There is also likely to be loss of weight due to difficulty in eating, and occasionally there may be secondary effects on the heart, the lungs, the digestion, and other parts of the body.

Obviously the prevention of asthma depends on detecting the substances to which the person is sensitive and eliminating these items from his surroundings. This is not, however, as simple as it may sound. It involves numerous tests, including skin tests, and may need the services of specialists in many different fields. Frequently the best recommendation is to have the patient with asthma that is difficult to diagnose go to a hospital so that the allergy tests may be made along with X-ray studies, heart studies, examination of the sinuses, laboratory studies of the blood and the sputum, and a complete study, during the patient's absence, of the environment in which the patient lives.

When a person has an acute attack of asthma, the doctor may administer immediate relief by an injection of a substance called epinephrine, or adrenalin, which will relieve the bronchial spasm. The amount of the epinephrine to be given and the manner in which it is to be injected are, of course, to be determined by the doctor for the individual patient. Many patients who have had asthma for a long time learn how to inject themselves. In some instances members of the family learn how to give the injections so that immediate relief is obtained when an attack comes on at night. There are also other devices which can be used to relieve asthmatic attacks such as vaporized epinephrine or adrenalin that can be taken by inhalation. Sometimes drugs like ephedrine are taken internally to produce relief. The antihistaminic drugs as mentioned under *Allergy* are often useful in cases of asthma. ACTH and Cortisone are powerful in asthma otherwise uncontrollable and the physician can inject them as needed.

Many a person with severe asthma

has obtained relief by wearing a mask which protects him against dusts and vapors to which he is sensitive.

The problem of avoiding exposure is one that varies with every case. A farmer may be sensitive to the dandruff from animals yet the nature of his occupation makes it impossible for him to avoid contact. People become sensitive to the dusts from horsehair in upholstered furniture or to down or feathers in pillows or mattresses. It is now possible to purchase pillows and mattresses made with other than the sensitizing substances. It is also possible to cover pillows and mattresses with airtight coverings that are fastened with zippers and thus protect the person against contact with the dusts. A person who is asthmatic should avoid any occupation in which he comes frequently in contact with hairs, feathers, dye substances, or similar materials.

Usually it is recommended that a person with asthma sleep alone in a well-aired room in which the temperature and the humidity are under control. Such patients do better if the air of the room is reasonably moist. All upholstered furniture, rugs, and other dust catchers should be removed from the bedrooms. The walls should be painted rather than papered because papered walls may yield dust and dye substances. Such rooms are best cleaned with an electric vacuum cleaner. Usually it is best for a sensitive person to be out of the house when any serious cleaning is to be undertaken. Animals should not be permitted in the house, since the coat of the animal may not only yield its own dandruff but also dusts that the animal may pick up. Indeed the sensitivities may be so serious that people coming to visit a person who is sensitive to dust should avoid, if possible, bringing in dust on their shoes or clothing.

The person with asthma should eat little at night, since a full stomach makes breathing more difficult. Excessive indulgence in alcohol has been known to bring on an attack. In general damp localities are unfavorable for

people with asthma. Other substances known to incite an attack of asthma are changes in temperature, cold winds, tobacco smoke, gas fumes, insect powders, or strong odors from any source.

In some cases the doctor is able to desensitize the patient against the asthma.

ASTIGMATISM (See also discussion under *Eye*) The human eye can be farsighted or nearsighted, in which case the rays of light are focused either in front of the retina, the seeing tissue at the back of the eye, or behind it. When the eye is at rest and parallel rays are focused exactly on the retina of the eye, it is said to be normal. When parallel rays of light coming into the eye are focused at different meridians or angles, the eye has astigmatism.

Astigmatism is usually due to a change in the curvature of the cornea, or outside membrane of the eye, with or without some shortening or lengthening of the diameter of the whole eyeball.

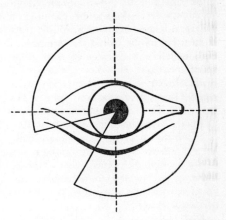

A chart of the mechanism of astigmatism showing the four planes of distortion because of curving of the eyeball

Occasionally astigmatism is also caused by defects in the curvature of the lens of the eye.

The exact causes of these anatomical differences are not known, beyond the fact that the shape of the eyeball differs in various people, so that there is a tendency for astigmatism to appear in members of the same family. The shape of the eyeball itself is inherited. There are, however, cases in which injury, inflammation, or operative procedure on the cornea of the eye will change the curves and thus produce astigmatism. There are also instances in which, apparently, pressure on the eyelids may distort the eyeball and thus produce astigmatism.

Probably every eye has some astigmatism. However, many people do not have enough disturbance of this type to make any attention necessary. In other cases, however, the blurring of vision brought about by the astigmatism makes it necessary to wear corrective eyeglasses for properly focusing the rays of light on the retina. Whenever there is a considerable degree of astigmatism, the acuteness of vision diminishes for both distant and near objects.

The specialist who examines the eyes is likely to suspect there is some astigmatism when the eye cannot be brought to see the line of letters numbered 20 at twenty feet distance by the use of spherical lenses. One of the simple tests is to use what is called the astigmatic dial, which is a clock with lines radiating to each of the hours. If the person is unable to see all of the rays with equal clearness, the astigmatism is responsible. The lines that are seen more distinctly and the lines seen least distinctly indicate the principal meridians. By the amount of blurring or the place of the blurring, the expert who examines the eyes is enabled to determine the areas in which the curvature of the lens needs correction.

ATABRINE See discussion under *Quinine.*

ATAXIA The word "ataxia" is a medical term which means that people are disorganized. Actually there are many ataxias known to the doctors. The ones most commonly known to the public are locomotor ataxia, sometimes called tabes dorsalis, which is a disease of the nervous system now known to be related to infection with syphilis; chorea, which is usually called St. Vitus' dance; multiple sclerosis, of which the cause is not known; and Parkinson's disease, also called paralysis agitans and the shaking palsy. In addition there are a half-dozen other ataxias which have associated with them the names of physicians who first recognized the particular disease, which in each case represented a disturbance of some certain portion of the nervous system from the brain down to the spinal cord. Some of these highly specialized forms of ataxia are known to run in families and represent inheritance of failure to develop in certain portions of the nervous system. Since the nervous system is concerned not only with motion but also with sensation, many of these conditions are associated with disturbances to the sense of taste, sense of touch, sense of smell, the ability to see, and other special senses.

Whenever anyone develops symptoms of disorganization of the relationship between the nervous system and the other parts of the body sufficient to interfere with co-ordination of movements, to bring about inability to walk, or to cause the making of motions which have no purpose, the person should have immediate and careful attention from a doctor, including an examination directly related to the nervous system, preferably by someone who has specialized in the study of such disturbances. Physicians who do such special examinations are called neurologists. The neurologist by studying the functional state of the nerves in different portions of the body can determine the portion of the central nervous system that is disturbed and damaged. He can find out whether or not a degenerative disease might have a relationship to the symptoms. In many of these difficult conditions, proper care may slow and often stop the progress of the disease. Surely it is folly not to take advantage of the specialized knowledge that medical science has developed in these fields.

ATELECTASIS A condition in which the air is lost from the small aveoli, or air chambers, in the lungs, giving the lung a contracted, solid appearance when viewed with the X ray.

ATHLETE'S FOOT See *Ringworm*.

ATOMIC ENERGY The observations made at Hiroshima and Nagasaki established facts about what happens when a city is subjected to the explosion of an atomic bomb. According to a group of experts who have had extensive experience in this field, it can be assumed that the amount of induced radioactivity or contamination with radioactivity in the vicinity of the explosion is negligible. Teams of medical workers can enter the area immediately.

The first problem is the treatment of external injuries resulting from radiation burns, the effects of blast, and penetrating injuries. The authorities say that a third of the population of the bombed city will be killed outright or will die in days to weeks no matter how soon they are given medical care. The next third of the population will live if they get medical care quickly and if it is adequate. The remaining third can survive without medical aid unless they happen to be subjected to an epidemic or the destructive results of the disruption of transportation, sewage system, water supplies, and similar facilities.

Experience with the burns resulting from atomic bombs indicates that most of these patients ought to be taken immediately to a hospital, where they are given the modern treatment of burns. These burns are manifested by swelling, redness, and the formation of blisters. The burns resulting from irradiation are much more serious.

Scientists are now investigating the problem of how much irradiation a human being can stand. Irradiation is usually measured in units which are called roentgens and which are designated by the symbol r. From 50 to 200 reproduce nausea and a lessening of the white blood cells and a thrombocyto-

penia in the blood, followed usually by bleeding. From 200 to 400 r produce the same symptoms, including also anemia, severe nausea, vomiting, diarrhea, and hemorrhage. While death occurs to a small number of such patients, the majority recover. Exposure to 400 to 600 r makes the person seriously ill. He has all of the symptoms that have been mentioned, but much worse. Less than half the people exposed to such doses recover. When people are exposed to as much as 600 r, the chance of survival is slight. Only a few people can survive that kind of exposure even with the best of medical care.

What treatment can be given to people who have been exposed to the effects of the atomic bomb? All of the blood disturbances that have been mentioned are best treated with daily transfusions of whole blood. Large doses of the antibiotic drugs like penicillin are given to control the infections. When there is a severe destruction of the white blood cells, these are needed particularly because the body has no defense against infection. The physician must treat the severe inflammations of the bowels, the accumulation of water in the body, and the diarrheas. Frequently it becomes necessary to give nourishment by injection. Since the patients are apprehensive, frightened, and mentally disturbed, sedatives are needed to restore their balance. In radiation burns the pain persists for days and drugs may be needed to control this pain.

We are just beginning to understand the serious problems associated with atomic warfare. What disturbs the experts particularly is the possibility that water and food supplies could be contaminated by radioactive isotopes which would themselves be taken into the body and which localize in bone and destroy human beings. Whole cities could be made uninhabitable and water supplies could be hopelessly contaminated by this method. Protection of communities against atomic bombs constitutes one of the major problems of modern medicine.

ATROPHY The death and degeneration of tissue of the body.

AUSCULTATION The act of listening for signs within the body for determining changes that have taken place in the lungs, the heart, or other organs, sometimes done with the ear but usually employing a listening device called a stethoscope.

maturely or small is no greater now than formerly; it is, in fact, much smaller because of the advances of modern obstetrical science. We hear much more about such babies because newspapers discuss such subjects now while formerly they did not do so. It is now possible to save the lives of such babies in far greater number than was formerly possible.

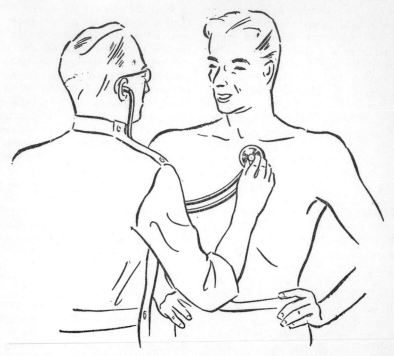

The doctor uses a stethoscope to hear sounds of the opening and closing of the heart valves and the breath sounds in the lungs

AUTONOMIC NERVOUS SYSTEM See *Sympathetic Nervous System.*

BABIES, PREMATURE Babies rarely survive if they weigh less than 2.2 pounds, or 1000 grams, at birth.

Not long ago a newspaperman inquired whether it is true that more tiny babies are being born now than in the past. The number of babies born pre-

There are records of the survival of large numbers of babies who weighed less than 2.2 pounds at the time they were born. Since these records show that such babies catch up with normal babies by the time they are six months to a year old, every possible effort is made to save their lives. Use of the baby incubator, breathing oxygen mixed with carbon dioxide, feeding of mothers' milk, and application of other developments of modern medical science let these babies survive to become healthful children and adults.

The birth is reported of a baby weighing only 1.6 pounds, or 735 grams. By the time this baby was one year old it weighed 17 pounds and 5 ounces.

According to statistics of the Children's Bureau, 5 per cent, or one twentieth, of 23,000 babies born alive recently in this country were prematurely born. In the city of Chicago 4 per cent of 97,000 babies born alive in 1936 and 1937 were reported prematurely born. This indicates that about 85,000 babies are born every year in the United States in advance of the time when they should arrive. They are underweight and undersized and demand special medical attention if they are to survive.

The first step in the survival of such a baby is to regulate the body heat. Old-fashioned incubators have been replaced by modern, electrically heated beds in which the temperature is regulated by a thermostat. Portable incubators have been developed, so that the baby can be put almost immediately after birth into such a device and then be taken to a hospital.

Authorities are agreed that mother's milk is the best possible food for premature babies. In most cities arrangements are now made to obtain this type for all premature babies.

The question is constantly raised as to whether babies born prematurely have mentalities as high as those of infants born after the usual time. In a recent review of the subject Dr. Arnold Gesell points out that the normal time before birth is about forty weeks, but that cases are on record of birth with survival after twenty-four weeks.

In order to find out whether babies born after six, seven, or eight months develop mentally as well as those born after nine months, examinations were made regularly on a number of such babies. Two children born prematurely were studied regularly for a period of two years. One child at the age of five months resembled in behavior equipment a child of three months, but many of the difficulties might have been due merely to the fact that it was seriously underweight.

One physician investigated the mental equipment of almost four hundred premature infants and found that in general they do not develop as well as infants born after the normal time. Their mentality is likely to develop a little later.

However, the majority of premature infants born after eight months without injuries at birth undergo normal mental development but progress more slowly than full-term infants during the first year. They usually walk and talk about six months later than do infants born after nine months and are somewhat slower in learning to co-ordinate.

There are, of course, many hazards associated with being born prematurely but Nature seems to do her best to enable such children to catch up, so that eventually they do become equal to children born after a normal time.

It is interesting, in this connection, to realize that some of the greatest men of history were born prematurely, including Charles Darwin, the French philosopher Renan, the great military leader Napoleon, Isaac Newton, and Voltaire.

BACKACHE Modern man has been described as a mechanical misfit. A small boy, asked to describe the spine, said that it was a long bone in the back of the body. "You sit on one end and your head sits on the other." There are many kinds of animals that have backbones which, because of their flexibility, adjust themselves to the needs of the animal concerned. The backbone of the boa constrictor has four hundred different bones; that of man is shorter. Four-footed animals walk with the backbone horizontal; man walks with the backbone in the vertical position.

The flexibility of the backbone makes it possible to perform a number of activities which otherwise could not be done. The human spine is like a spring, curved like the letter S. The top bulge of the letter S makes up the round shoulders, which occur in many human beings. The bottom of the letter S is the hollow of the back. As the human being gets older, the shoulders become stooped; the hollow in the back becomes less and then hollows the wrong way. As man gets older, the backbone tends to form an arch instead of a spring.

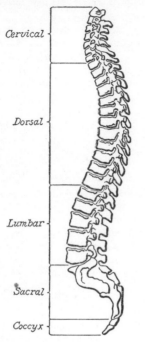

Cervical

Dorsal

Lumbar

Sacral

Coccyx

The bones of the spine are classified in groups

The spinal column or backbone is composed of small bones between which are cushions known as disks. Inside this column is a tube which contains the spinal cord. The nerves come out in little notches between the bones. The bones are bound together by strong tissues called ligaments. The disks are made of cartilage.

Obviously an inflammation, irritation, or infection of any portion of these tissues may result in pain in the back. A sudden overstrain or a long continued strain may throw one of these many joints into a wrong position. A disease may weaken some portion so that other parts of the spine will have to carry extra strain and stress.

Pain in the lower portion of the back is common among people of certain occupations, which submit the back to extra strain. This includes those who do heavy lifting or who stand long on their feet. It has been estimated that a traffic policeman who stands on his feet all day may be an inch shorter at night. After he has had eight hours of rest in bed, his tissues resume their elasticity and he is ready to begin another day.

The back is actually one of the strongest and most important parts of the body. If it could be given the same kind of personal consideration and attention that we give regularly to our teeth, skin, and other portions of the body that are easily visible, the human body would be a more efficient working mechanism and would probably last longer without breaking down.

The terms most commonly used to describe a painful back are lumbago, low back pain, and backache. There are so many different causes of such pain that it is desirable to determine the exact cause in every instance. Sometimes this can be done only with great difficulty and after long study. Such study will include the making of a number of tests which are familiar to physicians in general and particularly to orthopedic surgeons. X-ray pictures are helpful because they show whether or not the parts lie in proper relationship to each other. Especially important is a careful record of the conditions under which the patient works, the story of the time when the pains began, and the record of their development. For instance the tissues of the back may be abnormal at birth. There may have been a severe injury or many minor injuries to the bones, the ligaments, muscles, nerves, or other portions of the spine. The job may cause the person to stand in a bad position for a long period of time. Sometimes an inequality in the length of the legs forces an abnormal position of the spine. An infection which causes inflammation of the joints will result in overgrowth of tissue and pain.

Tumors may occur in the spine as in other portions of the body. Serious changes in the bones are known to be associated with excessive or deficient activities of various glands, particularly the parathyroid glands, which are definitely related to the deposit of calcium in the body. Interference with the circulation of the blood to the tissues will cause disturbances in the spine as elsewhere and this applies also to changes in the nervous system.

Finally, there are many cases of backache which are incidental to other diseases like gout, gall-bladder disease, ulcers of the stomach, childbirth, pulling on the tissues which support the uterus and other tissues within the abdomen.

Pain in the lower portion of the back appears often in women after childbirth, sometimes associated definitely with the organs of childbirth and at other times with disturbances of the intestines and kidneys. Some cases of backache—by no means the majority—seem to be largely mental rather than physical in their causation.

Occasionally backaches begin after operations in the abdomen and the pain is definitely associated with the healing and the formation of scar tissue.

Both the doctor and the patient are fortunate if a definite relationship can be found between the appearance of the backache and some special strain associated with the occupation or with daily life, since the treatment in such cases is clear.

SLIPPED DISCS—The discs which act as cushions between the bones of the spine may be squeezed or twisted out of place during a lifting injury or some similar movement. Special examinations determine whether or not such a disc is out of place. The treatment may be long rest, wearing of a brace, and, if these methods fail, surgery.

Often people with backache may obtain great relief by wearing proper braces or supports, which give the inflamed tissues a chance to rest and recover. The application of warmth and,

after sufficient healing has occurred, of massage and controlled movements may be helpful.

If constant pain of the back is associated with overweight, flat feet, or some similar condition, the treatment must be directed to that cause.

Physicians know of many drugs which are useful in relieving pain. It is better, if possible, to determine the cause of the backache and to bring about permanent relief rather than to try to get along over the years with pain-relieving medicines.

BACTERIA Bacteria is a term commonly used by people who do not say "germs." The term "germ" is commonly used to describe a microbe or a bacillus or any other infective agent. Usually bacteria means minute living organisms that can be seen only with the aid of a microscope and which multiply by dividing themselves into individual portions, growing separately, and again dividing. Many different forms of bacteria are described, depending on the shape and size, the poisons that they produce, their method of growth, and many similar factors.

Generally the famous French scientist Pasteur is credited with having discovered the germ causation of disease. He showed that the cause of chicken cholera was cholera germs. He proved that anthrax, which affected sheep, was due to the anthrax germ. He showed, finally, the possibility of inoculation against rabies, or hydrophobia, with the virus of that condition. We recognize today, however, a definite distinction between viruses and germs, or bacteria.

The famous bacteriologist Robert Koch worked out some rules for determining whether or not a germ is the specific cause of a disease. Among the criteria that he established were the following: (1) The germ must be taken from the body of an animal or a human being that has died of the disease. (2) It must be possible to grow the germ outside the human body, as is done on various substances like blood mixed with agar or beef broth mixed with gelatin. (3) It must be possible to reproduce the disease in an animal by injecting the germs into the animal. In the science of bacteriology all of these methods are used constantly.

The whole concept that cleanliness is next to godliness is the very basis of the science of the prevention of disease by the removal of germs. The modern sanitary experts insist that food, clothing, or any of the surroundings of man are not clean when they are free from visible dirt but only when they are also free from germs, or bacteria. In the control of infection sanitarians have found that repeated washing with soap and hot water and drying in the sun constitute perhaps the best method we have for eliminating bacteria from bed linens, clothing, rugs, furniture, and all of the other accessories of modern civilization.

In an experiment carried out at the University of Nebraska it was discovered that after underwear is worn one day the average count of bacteria per square inch is 400,000. If a shirt is worn six days consecutively without washing, the number of germs increases to nearly 10,000,000 bacteria per square inch. When the shirt is laundered and dried, the number of bacteria is reduced to 1000 per square inch or less. Washing alone is effective, but even better results are accomplished by drying thoroughly and particularly by drying in the sun.

BAKING SODA See *Sodium Bicarbonate.*

BARBER'S ITCH Often following some accidental infection of the skin of the face, the irritation of an ingrown hair, or the use of infected razors, shaving brushes, or towels, a germ called the staphylococcus, one of the most common pus-forming germs, will get into a hair follicle and set up a spreading infection. This occurs most often in people who have oily skins with excess secretion from the oil glands and excessive perspiration. The combination of a thick, wiry beard and a tender skin helps to make irritation of the skin easy. Occasionally the trouble will begin on the upper lip following a cold in which there has been constant secretion of mucus from the nose and rubbing and scratching of the skin below the nose. Sometimes the trouble begins at the point where the side of the nose is in contact with the cheek. Occasionally the trouble begins on the back of the neck, due to rubbing by a rough collar or scratching of the skin at the hairline

The scientific name for barber's itch, or barber's rash, is sycosis, which is not at all related to the term "psychosis," which refers to a mental disturbance.

Eventually the infection may cause bleeding and crusting, with falling of the hair and even secondary abscesses.

Because of the infectious character of this condition it is foolish for anyone to try to treat himself. Indeed the cure is difficult, so that the care of the skin should be regulated by the doctor until healing has occurred. In difficult cases there must be repeated application of hot, wet dressings of antiseptic solutions, the use of dusting powders to produce dryness, remedies taken internally to control the infection, perhaps the removal of hair by the use of tweezers, or in some instances the X ray. Most recent is the application of ointments containing penicillin or other antibiotics called tyrothrycin and bacitracin, with which cases have been cured in a few days. The disease is curable and will under proper treatment disappear in the majority of cases, but the personal supervision by the doctor and strict attention to details such as those that have been described are necessary to bring about prompt healing before there is permanent damage to the skin.

The possibility of the spread of barber's rash has caused most states to regulate the sanitation of barbershops. Some states insist that the barber wash his hands with soap and water before attending to each customer. They require placing brushes, combs, clippers, razors, and similar apparatus in boiling water before being used on each customer. They demand a new clean towel for each customer and that the headrest be covered with a clean towel or the paper changed after each customer. Towels known as steamers must be fresh and used only once without reboiling. Sanitary laws forbid the use of a styptic pencil and require instead a styptic powder used fresh for each bleeding spot. Barbers can help by refusing to give service to any person whose skin is badly infected or who has an eruption, unless the customer brings his own shaving brush, lather cup, and razor.

BASAL METABOLISM The normal human being produces heat at the rate of one calory for each kilogram of weight per hour. The average basal metabolic rate for normal men between the ages of twenty and fifty years is from 38 to 40 calories per square meter of body surface per hour. This value is the same for all normal men, whether they are tall or short, thin or stout, large or small.

The basal metabolic rate is a measure of the speed of chemical changes going on in the body. A low basal metabolism means that the heat produced by the development of energy from materials taken into the body is less than the average of most normal people.

The basal metabolism is determined by putting the person at rest on arising in the morning, without any breakfast. Then the gaseous interchange in the lungs is measured. By means of tables a standard figure is reached that is called the basal metabolism. The ordinary variation is from a figure of minus 7 to plus 7. Occasionally a person who is quite healthful will have a figure as low as minus 16 to minus 25. The basal metabolism is also determined by giving radioactive iodine and measuring with a Geiger counter the rate with which the thyroid takes up the iodine.

The basal metabolism is usually higher in childhood because children are active and growing. In certain diseases the basal metabolism is much greater than normal. Anger and fear will temporarily speed up the activities of the body and raise the basal metabolic rate. During sleep the basal metabolism is less than during waking hours. Undernutrition is associated with a lowered basal metabolic rate. A lowered rate is found also in occasional cases of anemia and in nervous disorders of the psychasthenic type or nervous breakdown. In cases in which the thyroid gland does not act sufficiently the basal metabolism is likely to be low. This might apply also to a deficiency of the pituitary gland and the adrenal gland. However, an excessive activity of any of these glands may increase the basal metabolic rate. The basal metabolic rate of the pregnant woman shows little change until the sixth or seventh month, when the weight of the mother increases. From that time on the rate is the sum of the metabolism of the mother and that of the unborn child. Mental effort causes an almost negligible increase in metabolism. Benedict, who was an authority on the subject, said that the extra calories needed for one hour of intense mental effort would be completely met by eating one oyster cracker or one half of a salted peanut.

BATHING (See also *Skin* and *Hygiene, Personal*) Water is one of the most valuable substances, internally and externally, for the health care of the human body. Its value has been established by thousands of years of experience and practice. Internally, water is absolutely essential for the health of the human body, since it takes part in every chemical reaction in the cells. It is absolutely necessary to aid digestion and the passage of waste material from the body. Externally, water is used for cleanliness and also in the treatment of disease.

Bathing habits vary among human beings according to their living conditions. However, the so-called "best people" bathe at least once a day. From this percentage the habit of bathing may vary up to once a season or as long as friends and neighbors can stand it.

The routine use of soap for cleansing is quite recent. In ancient times people oiled the skin; sometimes they cleansed themselves with a sweat bath. The famous courts of the King of France had no bathtubs, as anyone will discover by a visit to Versailles. This was no doubt responsible for the rise of the perfume industry in France.

Soap cleanses the skin by breaking up or emulsifying the oily secretions and dissolving this material. This makes it easy to remove the layer of grease and the accumulated dirt and debris along with it.

The ordinary bathroom contains a tub, but there may be a shower, or both a tub and shower. A shower bath is more stimulating, due to the sting of the spray and the quicker regulation of the temperature. The tub bath is useful because the water surrounds the body at an even temperature and pressure.

Many hygiene authorities recommend a freshening bath just before dinner in addition to the cleansing bath that is taken at night, or the freshening bath that is taken on arising in the morning.

A person who is tired after a day's work will find a warm shower relaxing, and a short cold splash immediately afterward stimulating. For cleansing the human body, a moderately warm bath with soap is best. Particularly important is thorough washing of portions of the body likely to acquire perspiration and, therefore, odor.

Since some people are sensitive to soap, it is desirable to wash the soap away thoroughly from the body with plenty of water after the soap has been applied.

The temperature of the water most effective and agreeable for the normal skin is from 95 to 100 degrees Fahrenheit. For most people the best cleansing soap is the ordinary white soap which is rubbed into a lather. A soft washcloth is helpful in making certain that the parts of the body that are hard to reach are properly cleaned. If the skin is easily irritated, drying is best accomplished by patting, rather than rubbing, with clean, soft towels. Brisk rubbing with a towel stimulates the circulation and will not injure the ordinary skin.

Baths can be harmful as well as beneficial. Among people with exceedingly dry skin, such as occurs in old age and among those who itch greatly, the skin may be made more sensitive by excessive use of hot baths and soap. In such cases the skin may need mild cleansing and oiling.

Cool baths are valuable for conducting heat away from the body. Frequently such baths are recommended to lower the temperature in fever. The chief value of the warm bath is to relax the human body. Hot water causes dilation of the superficial blood vessels. This excess stimulation causes profuse sweating. For that reason, hot-water baths are used in rheumatism. In taking a hot-water bath it is best to begin with the temperature around 98 degrees and then increase it up to 115 degrees Fahrenheit. One should not remain too long in a hot bath, since it may produce exhaustion and even collapse.

The so-called tonic bath has a stimulating effect. It usually means a quick cold shower or plunge used in the morning. Sudden changes in temperature produce sudden contractions of the blood vessels, after which there is a reaction. Each one must determine for himself how much of a bath and how much of a reaction is wanted.

After the quick cold tonic bath in the morning, particularly the cold shower, the skin should be rubbed vigorously with a rough towel. This adds to the stimulation.

Many people cannot take a cold bath in the morning. There is no evidence that a cold bath taken regularly every morning will harden the body against catching cold. Neither is there reason to believe that they are particularly healthful for the majority of people.

Scientists have made investigations on the effect of plunging a warm body suddenly into a cold bath. Some reports show that the immediate aftereffect is a lessened resistance to infection. The experiments have hardly been sufficient to make certain of this effect. However, there is evidence that people who are strong enough to stand persistent indulgence in a cold bath every morning are strong enough to resist almost anything else as well. Nevertheless there is no evidence that any weak person or a chronic invalid ever increased his resistance by this performance.

BED SORES People who are chronic invalids and those who have certain disturbances of the nervous system are likely to develop as a result of prolonged pressure on the skin over certain areas breakdown and degeneration of the tissue leading to what is known as a bed sore. The surface area of the body of an average man five feet eight inches tall and weighing about a hundred and fifty pounds is about 2800 square inches. However, not all of the skin is ever pressed upon. There are certain spots which carry the weight either standing or lying down. These include the heels, the buttocks, the lower portion of the spinal column, the tops of the large bones of the hip and thigh, the elbows, and the backs of the shoulders. These portions of the body may be under considerable pressure for long periods of time and the pressure is far greater than the $1\frac{1}{2}$ or 2 pounds of pressure to the square inch that is necessary to cause a breakdown in the tissue if for any reason it is not in the best of health.

Shifting of the weight or the redistribution of the pressure by changed position or posture is one of the best methods known for preventing excessive pressure at any one spot. It has been shown by taking motion pictures of sleeping people that even the sleeping person is likely to change his position slightly or even grossly every five or ten minutes. When a person is, however, paralyzed or unable to shift the position of the body, it is necessary for a nurse or attendant to see to it that movement occurs. In shifting the position of the body various devices are helpful, including soft pillows, inflated air cushions, rings made from wool, blankets and similar materials which will help to hold the patient in a different position.

Since the skin is so tender, it is important to make certain that the undersheets and clothing are not wrinkled. Clothing must not be too tight. In the case of very sensitive patients even a crumb of bread on which the patient rested for a few hours has produced a bed sore. Some laundries use starches and chemicals which make the sheets too hard. Soft, pliable sheets are less likely to cause bed sores.

If the skin is moist, it macerates more easily than when it is kept properly dried and powdered. People who cannot control the excretions of the body are likely to suffer from soiling and wetness. This applies also to cases of excessive sweating.

Among the most important procedures for prevention of bed sores is proper nursing. The nurse will wash the skin, dry it properly, treat it with alcohol rubs, massage tenderly, and use powder to decrease the possibility of maceration and irritation. Because a bed sore may be so serious, particularly in a person who is paralyzed or very old, the attendants must watch carefully for the first sign of such a condition. A threatened bed sore is shown by redness of the skin which disappears on gentle pressure. Unless the condition is promptly controlled, it may proceed to ulceration. Such ulcers demand the best and the most careful attention that can be given by the doctor so that death of the tissues may not occur. Strong antiseptics may injure the weakened tissue. Nevertheless many people are likely to try these first for the control of ulcers due to bed sores.

BED-WETTING (See discussion under *Child Care*) Scientifically known as enuresis.

BEE STINGS The sting of a bee is a form of injury familiar to many people. The mechanism by which a bee stings is the insertion of a sharp, fine, horny needle in which there are two barbs. When the bee puts the needle with the barbs into the skin, it anchors itself, and in its effort to get away it presses on the sac that contains the bee poison or venom. This pressure empties the venom into the skin. The injection of a very small amount of bee poison into the skin of a human being is followed by immediate reddening, with the development of a blister and a surrounding area of redness. Usually all signs of the sting will disappear in twenty-four hours. In about 2 per cent of people, however, there is sensitivity to the venom of the honeybee, and the symptoms may be so serious that even life itself will be threatened. There is a record of a person who died ten minutes after being stung by a honeybee.

Some research has been done on the effects of bee venom on animals and on the human body. For instance all the venom was taken from eight honeybees and injected into a rabbit. The heart of the rabbit was affected noticeably, and at the end of fifteen minutes the rabbit's heartbeats were too feeble to make a record. The effects of large quantities of bee poison on the blood of a dog were like those of rattlesnake poison. The red blood cells were broken down, so that the coloring matter escaped, the blood pressure fell, and the smooth muscles of the body, such as those of the intestines and heart, were forced to contract.

A chemical analysis of the poison of the bee shows that it contains both acid and alkaline materials and a substance which is like histamine. Histamine is a chemical that is released in the blood in cases of allergy. It is possible to desensitize people who are especially sensitive to honeybee venom by injecting them over a period of time with small doses of the venom, so that they build up a resistance to it. In the ordinary case of bee sting, however, it is merely necessary to apply some soothing lotion to the spot. Usually any of the lotions that will bring relief from itching will do for the purpose.

A person who has had multiple bee stings should be put promptly to rest. The action of his heart and kidneys should be watched carefully by the doctor, so that he can be given supporting treatment if his blood pressure falls rapidly. Some of the drugs that are used in severe asthmatic attacks may be injected under the skin by the doctor and bring about a promptly favorable reaction. These include the antihistaminic drugs such as benadryl, pyribenzamine, and neo-antergan.

For years there has been a belief that the sting of the bee or its poison may be of special value in the treatment of rheumatism, including inflammations of the muscles and joints. There are cases in which the use of bee or rattlesnake venom has produced reactions that have seemed to be favorable. However, the method has not yet had general medical support.

BEHAVIOR Since 1900 much has been said and written about behavior, and there are psychologists who are known as behaviorists because they believe that the study of the conduct of human beings in a purely objective manner will reveal much that is important for both mental and physical health.

The average parent is likely to say that the child behaves if the child conforms to what the parent thinks is right. Specialists in the care of children say that over half of the children that they see in a city practice have behavior problems. About 10 per cent of children will be brought to the doctor just because of behavior problems, but the remainder are discovered in the course of examination.

Some of the behavior problems that particularly concern parents have to do with the fact that a child will not eat, that he is unfriendly, that he wets the bed or shakes his head and rolls. Sometimes a child is unnecessarily destructive. It is hard enough for the average parent to deal with a child who has reached the age of reason; much harder is the attempt to discover in an exceedingly young child, like a preschool child, why he develops such extraordinary reactions. For instance one child twenty months of age refused for over ten months to keep down her food. Immediately after eating, the child would announce, "I am going to be sick," after which she usually was. Careful investigation showed that there was nothing physically wrong with her. She was the only child of parents in their late forties who were married after an engagement of twelve years. The father was himself neurotic and given to taking all sorts of medicine for vague complaints. He felt that his poor health was responsible for the troubles of the child. The mother was a schoolteacher who knew that this would be the only child and was apprehensive about her survival. Both parents had concentrated on the child, who naturally expected always to be the center of attention. The child was used to having anything she wished. When refused, she announced that she would be sick. In the hospital a three-year-old boy refused to give her a toy and called the rest of the children to watch her be sick. She was unable to produce. Association with other children who treated her in this manner brought about her cure. The whole basis of this child's refusal to co-operate in eating was the oversolicitude of her parents.

Another interesting example was that of a three-year-old daughter of a doctor who had married a graduate nurse. This child also learned that she could dominate her family by refusing to eat. Every meal was a battleground, with coaxing, wheedling, and promises. This child was placed in a school with other children and informed that nobody could leave the table until all had finished. She played with her food while the other children waited. One boy then said that she would have to sit at another table because "we do not want her with us because she is too slow and spoils our fun." This discipline was sufficient to cause her to co-operate. She began by eating a small amount of food; each day her plate was filled a

little fuller, and finally she was eating all the food necessary to keep her well. When she was taken home, it was found that she would not eat at home, although she ate well in the nursery school. Complete information to the parents as to how the results had been accomplished in the nursery school brought about a change in the procedures at home with eventual cure.

Obviously, therefore, the most important step in a behavior problem is a complete investigation of all the factors involved, including the onset of the condition, the changes of residence and schools, the child's emotional reactions to various situations, the example set at home and, as has been pointed out, something of the history of the parents. In most instances interviews with parents should be held in the absence of the child and interviews with the child in the absence of the parents. It is necessary to know the attitudes and feelings of the child toward other members of the family, his teacher, his playmates, and his authorities.

Children have certain mental as well as physical needs. They need not only food and water and clothing but also affection and self-expression. The child who does not have these needs satisfied is likely to respond with signs that show he is not well adjusted to his environment. Babies need a certain amount of cuddling. When they are deprived of emotional satisfactions, they respond in unsatisfactory ways. Dr. L. Emmett Holt points out that babies with restlessness, irritability, and vomiting quiet down when a calm, soothing nurse is substituted for an overwrought, tense, and agitated mother.

The growing child must feel that he is wanted, that he belongs in the home in which he is growing. Sometimes parents make the mistake of threatening a child with withdrawal of affection as a means of getting the child to do what the parent thinks is right. The usual response is to create in the child a vindictive behavior or a desire to hurt the parent.

Children do not like to be smothered with affection or unduly pampered. The parent creates a vicious circle by pampering the child, so that what the parent gives comes to be demanded.

Much has been said about security from the cradle to the grave. It is true that children need to be well fed and clothed and housed, but they also need to feel reasonably secure in their lives from the mental point of view. Children frequently insist that the stories that they learn to like be told always in exactly the same way. A change in the story makes the child think it is not being told correctly. His desire for security causes him to insist on a verbatim statement.

Incidentally, children are individuals exactly as are grownups. They have to grow and develop at individual rates of speed and not according to anybody's exact standard of what is thought right for the child. This does not mean, however, lack of discipline. Demands on the child should be reasonable. Unwise discipline creates anxieties, and the results of anxiety or fear are confusion and resentment. Dr. William S. Langford of the Columbia University College of Physicians and Surgeons has emphasized that the oversolicitous mother is one of the most frequent causes of bad behavior in a child. She may be aware of her difficulties but be unable to do much about them. Sometimes she is oversolicitous because she is trying to make up to the child for some earlier rejection of the child. Perhaps the child was unwanted. Perhaps the mother blames herself for some illness of the child and as a result develops an overprotective attitude. Perhaps the mother in her childhood was deprived of many things, so that she overwhelms the child with the things of which she herself was deprived. Indeed Dr. Langford cites a few typical remarks made in his office by oversolicitous mothers which represent the difficulties inherent in this situation. For instance: "He was a delicate baby at birth, and I have always given in to him until his brother came." "If I know he is physically fit, then I can punish him." "He has got to move his bowels for me or he won't have room in his stomach for food." "His bones are weak; it's my fault; I didn't give him enough viosterol." "I have to wash him but he would do it himself." The result of these reactions of parents to their children may be refusal to eat or lack of appetite, the eating of dirt and plaster, unnecessary vomiting, and either diarrhea or constipation. They may be associated with disturbances of sleep, disorders of speech, anti-social behavior, or strange emotional reactions.

BELCHING Eructation of sour material including acid of the stomach, or of air or gas, is called belching, which may or may not be audible. People who eat too fast swallow air and then belch it back. Some people get a peculiar pleasure out of loud frequent belching, and psychiatrists trace a connection with sexual motivations.

BELL'S PALSY Bell's palsy or Bell's paralysis is the name given by medicine to a paralysis of the muscles of the face, usually only on one side at a time, which occurs in most cases without any cause except exposure to cold. Long exposure of one side of the face to cold, such as occurs when one has been driving next to an open window or sleeping in the draft from a ventilator on a train or under similar circumstances, may produce this condition. Some physicians believe that an infection in the throat or ear or a specific virus may also be responsible.

The nerve affected is one of the large nerves of the head which controls the movements of the muscles of the face. A disturbance at any point on this nerve may be responsible, but in many instances it is believed that the nerve swells in an area where it passes through a tight bony canal, so that pressure produced by the swelling stops the passage of impulses along the nerve with the resulting failure of movement. The condition is called Bell's palsy because it was first described and analyzed by a British doctor named Bell.

This form of paralysis of the face comes on suddenly. Often the person affected is first aware of the condition when he awakens in the morning and finds one side of the face completely paralyzed. He usually feels all right otherwise, being without fever or pain. However, occasionally there is some pain in the side of the face around and above the ear.

When this condition occurs, the side of the face that is affected is motionless and without any expression. The mouth is drawn over to the sound side because the healthy muscles will pull on those that are paralyzed. The eye on the side that is paralyzed seems to be more widely open than usual, and tears may run down the cheeks. It may be difficult to chew or swallow and impossible to close the eye tightly on the side that is paralyzed. The inability to shut the eye may allow dust or cinders to get in with the chance of secondary infection.

In mild cases recovery may occur in two or three weeks or even less, but serious cases may go on for months and occasionally there may be a permanent weakness which leaves distortion of the mouth on the affected side.

Simultaneous infection of both sides of the face is so rare that there is some doubt as to the cause of the condition when it occurs. However, cases are known in which both sides have been affected at the same time.

Doctors usually recommend the application of heat to the side of the face that is involved and complete rest for the patient. After the acute stage of the condition is passed and pain and tenderness have disappeared, electric stimulation of the nerve and muscles may be begun and discontinued when voluntary movements of the muscles become possible. Electrical treatment gains nothing when it is prolonged unduly in the absence of improvement.

Since the strong muscles pull on the paralyzed or weakened ones, various devices have been developed to support the weakened side to prevent over-stretching of the paralyzed muscles. Such devices are applied by the physician who is familiar with the muscles of the face and knows how to splint them in proper position.

Occasionally, if the condition goes on, the sense of taste is involved, so that there is a loss of this sense on the front two thirds of the tongue on the side involved.

In the majority of cases there is almost complete return of function. In a small percentage, however, the mouth remains permanently drawn over to the opposite side and the eye cannot be closed. In such cases the surgeons perform plastic operations, transplanting tissues, including nerve transplants, with a view to restoring the function of the nerve to the paralyzed parts and to restoring the symmetry of the face.

Cortisone or prednisone, given promptly, has been found useful in controlling inflammation and in securing more prompt and more complete recovery.

BENADRYL A new antihistaminic drug used in allergic conditions like hay fever, asthma, urticaria, and other manifestations of sensitivity.

BENZEDRINE A stimulant drug which can also contract mucous membranes. Used in an inhaler to control symptoms of congestion in the nose. Also called amphetamine. The drug can help to control appetite in the obese.

BERIBERI Among the dietary deficiencies which affect human beings one of the first to be clearly understood was beriberi. In 1897 a Dutch physician named Eijkman in Java observed that chickens fed on polished rice developed forms of neuritis and a paralysis which did not affect chickens fed on whole rice. This observation led to a study of the composition of polished rice as compared with that of whole rice.

Rice is not, however, the cause of beriberi. The cause is the lack in the diet of a portion of the vitamin B complex known as thiamine. When the rice is polished, the outer portions are removed. With the outer portion go the protein, the fat, and the thiamine.

Beriberi is most prevalent among people who live largely on rice. It occurs, however, also on sailing ships which travel on long voyages and in populations which live largely on restricted diets for other reasons. Beriberi was formerly quite prevalent in the Far East and parts of Brazil, Newfoundland, and Labrador.

Since the cause of the condition has been determined, it is now rarely seen. Medical scientists are interested, however, in the possibility that a relative deficiency of thiamine in the diet may produce symptoms which do not go on to complete beriberi but which, nevertheless, constitute a part of that disease. For instance during World War I troops in Palestine developed neuritis which was due to dietary deficiency. That is one reason why so much effort was given in World War II to provide proper feeding for American troops all over the world.

Among the symptoms of thiamine deficiency which in beriberi go on to serious damage to the tissues of the body are inflammations of the nerves, collection of fluid in the legs and in the tissues of the heart, congestions elsewhere in the body, including the lower parts of the legs, and changes even in the adrenal glands. The symptoms would include tingling and numbness of the portions of the body reached by the nerves that are affected, tenderness of the muscles, wasting of the tissues due to secondary infections, fever, and general disability.

Occasionally invalids who are on greatly restricted diets will suffer from deficiency of thiamine. After surgical operations on the bowel, chronic diarrhea, ulcers of the stomach, chronic alcoholism, or long infectious diseases, there may be signs of thiamine deficiency. Food faddists who like to live on strangely restricted diets sometimes show signs of thiamine deficiency or moderate beriberi. A man who was a

chronic alcoholic and who always stopped eating during alcoholic bouts developed swelling of the legs and arms, shortness of breath, and some enlargement of the heart. When his alcohol was stopped and he was given enough thiamine directly by injection into his body so that it would certainly be absorbed, he began to eliminate the extra fluid, utilized oxygen to better advantage, and promptly recovered. A number of young women who volunteered for the purpose were given a diet deficient in thiamine for twenty-one weeks. They had loss of appetite and weight, severe fatigue, tenderness of the calf muscles, constipation, and apparent slight swelling in the heart muscle. After twelve days of a large dosage of thiamine all the defects disappeared.

BILHARZIASIS A parasite called *Schistosoma haematobium* gets into the human body principally when people swim in contaminated waters. The intermediary host of this worm is the fresh-water snail. The condition has previously been a tropical disease and apparently originated in the Nile Valley thousands of years ago. When the parasite gets into the skin, it produces an inflammation. Then the eggs get into the human bladder and other hollow organs of the body where ulcers and inflammations occur. Certain specific drugs like emetine and drugs of antimony will eliminate this parasite from the human body. Repeated infections in the intestine will cause ulcers and bleeding. The worst form, which is severe and which may lead eventually to death, is the Asiatic form.

BILIOUSNESS (See also *Cholecystitis, Hepatitis, Jaundice*)   From a strictly scientific point of view there is no such condition as being bilious or liverish. The term goes back to the time when people were thought to suffer with various humors of which the bile or bilious form was the worst. To the physician the term "bilious" indicates that the liver is not functioning quite as well as it should, so that there is an accumulation of waste products in the body. Sir Arthur F. Hurst, an eminent British physician, points out that biliousness occurs more commonly in men than in women but it is being seen more frequently of late in women and girls who frequent cocktail parties and who drink a great deal of alcoholic liquors without food at dances several nights a week.

An epidemic of jaundice may occur due to an inflammation of the liver following infection with an easily transmitted virus.

There are, of course, other instances in which infections of various types, such as with the amoebae or malaria or infections due to toxins or poisons, may cause insufficiency of the liver. Serious infections or inflammations of the liver go on to a condition called hepatitis, which merely means an inflammation of the liver. This will produce destruction of liver cells and ultimately jaundice. Habitual irritation of the liver by alcohol or other poisons may produce damage which progresses and leads to hardening of the liver as well as an obstruction. Fortunately the human being is constructed with about seven times as much liver as is needed to carry on the ordinary functions of the body. However, even this amount of liver may be incapacitated by persistently bad habits related to eating and drinking. The person who drinks a great deal does not eat as much as he should. Failure to eat results in vitamin deficiencies and deficiencies of essential proteins for rebuilding the tissues of the body. The person who is bilious feels worse in the morning. After a night of fitful, restless sleep he wakes with a headache, an unpleasant taste in the mouth, and a thick tongue. The lack of appetite results in still further depletion of necessary substances from the food intake.

The condition is not usually painful but there is a feeling of discomfort and a lack of well-being. The fatigue results in a disinclination to work either mentally or physically. The symptoms are likely to disappear toward noon, at which time the person is often hungry and is ready for plenty of lunch. Such people work better in the afternoon than in the morning and they also have more confidence in the afternoon.

Certain substances in the diet tend to make people with biliousness less comfortable than others. Chocolates, cream cakes, cream, the yolks of eggs, a great deal of fat, and fried food of all kinds will make these people less comfortable than diets high in protein. Alcohol must be avoided, and any substances likely to irritate the liver, such as an anesthetic, must be handled with great caution. In many cases the use of glucose, either taken in water, with orange juice, or by injection, is helpful. This, however, must be prescribed by the physician after he has determined the nature of the condition. The doctor can also promote elimination from the body of bile by the use of suitably prescribed laxative salts and similar preparations.

BIRTH CERTIFICATES Will Rogers, a few years before he died, needed a record of his birth in order to obtain a passport for traveling in foreign countries. He found that he had never had a birth certificate. As a result, even with the reputation he had, it was difficult for him to arrange to meet the requirements of the passport division of the Department of State. At that time Will Rogers wrote, "I now see that the purpose of a birth certificate is not to prove that you have been born, as I had thought at first. The purpose is to show when you were born, where at, and who to."

Occasions constantly arise in which people are unable to produce their birth certificates and as a result have difficulty in meeting requirements of the government. A birth certificate is especially valuable because it establishes citizenship, makes it possible to secure a passport when traveling, and to vote as a citizen after registration.

As soon as a child is born, due note should be made of the fact by the attending physician. He should arrange promptly to notify the health department and the department of vital statistics in his community that a new arrival is present and in good health. If a child dies during birth, an immediate certificate is demanded. On this certificate there must be not only a statement as to the cause of death but also any secondary causes which may have been noted. The birth certificate, when it is received from the health department, should be as carefully guarded as any other valuable paper such as a marriage license or a tax receipt.

If you do not have a birth certificate and if you know where and when you were born, you can write to the city clerk in the place concerned and on payment of a small fee get a copy of your birth certificate.

If a baby is expected in the family, it is desirable to pick out a suitable name even before the child is born.

Obviously a name for both a boy and a girl should be selected so as to have the right one, or both, available. Then when the baby is born the doctor can file a record of its birth, including the name of the father and mother and also the name to be given to the child. This will permit the health department to supply the parents with a suitable birth certificate when the record of the birth is received.

BIRTH CONTROL See *Contraception.*

BIRTHMARKS There are few people without birthmarks or other skin blemishes of one type or another. These blemishes have been studied by the experts with a view to determining their true character.

The so-called strawberry birthmark is a mass of blood vessels collected in a knot near the surface. Sometimes they are flat, but in other cases they are elevated. According to the distance from the surface, they are either brilliant scarlet in color or blue. Those very near the surface are brilliant scarlet. The deeper ones are blue. When you press on a strawberry birthmark, the color

disappears because the blood is in this manner forced out of the blood vessels.

Another type of birthmark contains more cellular tissue and less fluid. This type appears to be pale blue or gray in color and is not as spongy as the strawberry birthmark. When pressed upon, it does not lose all of its color because it contains fewer blood vessels than the former type of growth.

Usually immediately after birth these spots may seem insignificant and small. Thereafter they may grow, reaching a fairly good size by the time the child is three weeks or several months old. Then they may stop growing and, in fact, may sometimes disappear without further attention, although there is no certain way of knowing which ones will disappear and which will cause symptoms.

Another type of skin growth is called the port-wine birthmark. These marks are collections of small blood vessels with various amounts of pigment deposited from the blood into the skin. They seldom get larger and there is not much that can be done for them, although occasionally they disappear after suitable medical treatment with ultraviolet rays. If they are very large and unsightly, it is possible nowadays to obtain cosmetic preparations with which to cover them and to make them almost unnoticeable.

In the past it has been customary to treat skin lesions of this type with the electric needle, to freeze them with carbon-dioxide snow, to cauterize them with heat or various chemicals like carbolic acid or nitric acid, to cut them out, or to treat them with radium. All of these methods are useful in the right kind of cases when properly employed.

A more recent method is to inject the blood vessels in such growths with various chemical substances that cause a slight inflammatory reaction inside the blood vessels, eventually resulting in scarring with obliteration or disappearance of the birthmark. Such methods are exceedingly delicate, but when carried out under proper conditions by a physician who has been suitably trained in the method, the results are in most instances excellent.

A survey made by a surgeon in 1955 proved that ordinary strawberry birthmarks disappeared or became inconspicuous as children grew older without surgical or other treatment such as freezing or cauterization.

BIRTHS, MULTIPLE The average human mother has one baby at a time. When two or more babies show up at a single birth, the process is abnormal. It may also be inconvenient. Most mothers plan for only one baby. Of course modern methods of diagnosis and the use of the X ray make it possible for a physician to tell well in advance that two or three or even four babies are to be expected. Since there is only one authenticated record in all the history of medicine of five babies being born at one time and living longer than one hour, it is doubtful that any doctor has ever diagnosed the expectation of quintuplets. There is no authentic record of sextuplets—six babies at one time. Recently a picture has been shown of what are alleged to be sextuplets born years ago in Africa but there is no authentication for this story.

Twins occur once in 87 births, triplets once in 7100 births, quadruplets once in 757,000 births, and the chance of quintuplets is one in many millions. There is evidence that in some families and in some countries twins occur more frequently than in others.

As I have already indicated, quadruplets are rare but there are a good many records now available of the birth of quadruplets and their survival to a fairly advanced age. Although obstetricians report that one set of quadruplets occurs in about 512,000 births, Professor H. H. Newman asserts that the ratio is about one in 6,000,000. There is even a scientific law which insists twins occur once in 88 births, triplets once in 88×88 births, and quadruplets once in 88×88×88 births. If this law, known as Hellin's law, is true, then quintuplets occur once in 88×88× 88×88 births. This would make the chance of quintuplets one in 500,000,000 births.

It has been claimed that the only quadruplets ever to reacn maturity are the famous Mary, Mona, Leota, and Roberta Keys, of Hollis, Oklahoma. The bunch of Keys graduated from high school in 1933.

Pictures are available of the quadruplets known as the Morlocks, of Lansing, Michigan. Their names are Edna, Sarah, Wilma, and Helen and they were well-grown children in 1945.

Not infrequently two sets of twins born close together are advertised as quadruplets and featured in theatrical performances. So far as is known, none of the sets of quadruplets now touring the vaudeville stages is authentic.

Beaumont, Texas, incidentally, boasts the presence of the Perricone quadruplets. On October 31, 1935, they were six years old. These boys, named Bernard, Vincent, Anthony, and Donald, were born within one hour of each other. Bernard, the shortest, is three inches shorter than Donald, the tallest. One boy is left-handed, one can use both hands equally well, and the other two are right-handed. One eats corn bread but another won't touch it.

In New Haven, Connecticut, the Salzo quadruplets prove that quaduplets can be made to survive under modern scientific conditions. Their names are James, Michael, Salvatore, and Angelena. They were born on May 9, 1921, to Michael and Guiseppina Salzo. Finally Aberdeen, South Dakota, provides us with the Schense quadruplets, who were born on January 13, 1931, and who at the end of 1935 were all still alive.

Apparently some thirty-five cases of the birth of quintuplets have been recorded in the history of medicine but not even all of these are certain. There are, however, records which indicate that in one instance all five infants lived about an hour; in another instance one of the five lived for fifty days. Then in 1934 appeared the Dionne quintuplets. Their birth and growth have been a constant source of interest to all the world. For the first time in history quintuplets have all grown to the age of fifteen years and continue to offer promise of development to maturity. Moreover, they have grown and developed in a small town, far away from any medical center. The population of Callander, Ontario, Canada, where they were born and live, is about six hundred people. It is a French Canadian settlement, a small village on the east shore of Lake Nipissing, two hundred miles north of Lake Ontario. The people are of Norman descent and for over three hundred years have lived in Canada.

On May 28, at 4:00 A.M., Dr. Allan Roy Dafoe was called to the home of Mrs. Elzire Dionne, where an emergency, associated with childbirth, was occurring. Mrs. Dionne had married at the age of sixteen and had had six fulltime pregnancies, all of the children living except one. She had reached twenty-four years in age. All of her babies had been born within five hours of time and usually she was out of bed carrying on her home work by the fifth day after the birth. On the occasion of this pregnancy she had suffered considerably with symptoms which indicated some intoxication from the childbirth, including swelling of her legs, blurring of her vision, and a blood pressure over two hundred. After some rest in bed her symptoms lessened greatly.

When the doctor arrived on May 28, he found two babies already born under the ministrations of a local midwife, and a third was just being born. Two neighbors were helping and the father had disappeared. The last two were born inside the sacs in which babies lie before childbirth. The doctor released all the babies and tied the cord which joined them to the tissues which unite them to the mother and which carry the blood supply and nutrition to them. Then he baptized the babies, wrapped them in some remnants of cotton sheeting and napkins, and covered them with a heated blanket. Since the mother was not in good condition he next turned his attention to her, carrying out the necessary procedures to stop bleeding,

relieving her of the afterbirth. Finally she seemed about to die and the doctor hurried away to get a priest, two and a half miles distant, because the husband was gone and no one else was available for the purpose. When, however, the doctor returned, the mother was much improved, and the attentions of the priest were unnecessary. The mother then proceeded gradually and uneventfully to a complete recovery.

Thereafter by constant attention to the infants they were brought safely to their present age. They have had the finest of modern nursing and feeding care. Baby specialists throughout the world recognize the achievement of bringing these babies successfully to their present age as one of the greatest accomplishments in the history of medicine, since never anywhere previously had anyone been able to keep alive five successive babies weighing as little as these babies weighed at birth, regardless of whether or not they were quintuplets or were born one at a time from five different mothers.

BLACKHEADS (See discussion under *Acne*) A common name for the comedo.

BLADDER CONDITIONS From the kidneys there pass two tubes, called ureters, about a foot long and one fifth of an inch wide, which carry the fluid excretion from the human body, called urine, to the bladder. The bladder is a storage receptacle which is emptied from time to time. Ordinarily about thirty drops a minute come from the ureters into the bladder. The human bladder has an average capacity of something less than a pint but can stretch to contain as much as one and a half pints. The lower part of the bladder contains a good deal of muscle tissue, including certain round muscles that control this emptying. The upper of these muscles is automatic; the lower one can be controlled by the will of the individual. The upper part of the bladder is thicker than the lower part and here is where the stretching can occur.

When the tension in the bladder reaches a certain amount—about a quarter of a pound per square inch—the automatic muscle will open up. There also comes the desire to empty the bladder which produces the act of urination.

Since the bladder represents a tissue of the human body, it is susceptible to many of the conditions that may affect other tissues, including infection or inflammation, bruising, rupture or breaking, the growth of extra tissue in the form of tumors, and also the possibility of damage from foreign bodies that should not be in the bladder or from the formation of stones.

A tumor of the bladder may be exceedingly serious in causing bleeding, difficulties of urination, or other disturbances. One of the greatest inventions of medicine is the cystoscope, which enables the doctor to look directly inside the bladder. The cystoscope is essentially a long tube which is passed into the bladder. At the end of this tube is a light. Fluid is injected into the bladder through the tube so as to stretch the walls, the tube is turned from side to side, and the light is thrown on the bladder at various angles. By a system of reflecting mirrors the doctor is able to see any tumors or other growths that have occurred in the wall of the bladder. It is also possible to pass various wires, which can be heated at the end, or cutting instruments directly into the bladder by the use of this tube and in this way to remove excess growths of tissue. Treatment can be applied directly to irritated areas of the bladder wall.

In earlier days it was necessary to open the abdominal cavity in order to get at the bladder. That type of procedure is still necessary when growths occur of such great size as to make impossible removal by other methods, as well as when the damage to the bladder wall is such that repair is necessary.

Another method of treating tumors or other growths in the bladder is to use the X ray or radium. X ray is in general not so much used as radium because of the possibility of irritation of the wall of the bladder by the X ray. Radium is applied preferably by the use of the emanation of radium sealed in little tubes which are known as radon seeds, or else by radium needles. These have the advantage of being directly applicable into the tumor itself when a growth occurs inside the bladder.

INFLAMMATION OF THE BLADDER— Various germs may infect the walls of the bladder as they can infect other tissues of the human body, although an infection in the bladder alone, which does not concern the kidneys or other portions of the genitourinary tract, is rather rare. The germs get into the bladder either by extension from the urinary passages below or above or occasionally by way of the blood or the lymph channels. Naturally any abnormality that produces obstruction to the flow of the urine, with accumulation in the bladder, injuring the bladder wall, is likely to increase the possibility of infection and inflammation. This condition is called scientifically cystitis, which merely means inflammation of the bladder. Old people, those who are seriously run down because of chronic illness, or those who have to remain in bed practically all the time are more likely to develop such conditions than are others. An enlargement of the prostate gland which obstructs the flow of urine from the bladder will sometimes help to initiate infection and inflammation.

The typical symptoms of crystitis or infection of the bladder are frequent urination accompanied by burning and occasionally also by the appearance of blood. Whenever a person has to get up frequently at night to empty the bladder, there should be a careful investigation of the condition of the urine and the whole urinary tract. An inflammation of the bladder is not necessarily accompanied by fever, although an infection in the kidneys is likely to produce a fever.

Before the doctor makes a diagnosis of inflammation of the bladder, he is likely to want a good many important tests. These tests will include examination of the urine at various times, in various portions, as well as examples over a twenty-four-hour period. In serious cases he will want to use the cystoscope to look directly into the bladder to find out whether or not there has been a change in the wall of the bladder. The doctor will examine the prostate gland to see if it is enlarged or inflamed and to determine whether or not it is causing any obstruction to the flow of the urine. Studies may be made of the ability of the kidneys to excrete a dye substance called phenolsulfonephthalein or there may be other tests of the ability to excrete fluid from the body. Studies may be made to determine whether or not there is pus or gravel or bacteria in the urine.

Inflammation of the bladder is almost always secondary to obstruction or infection in the urinary tract either above or below the bladder, so that again it should be emphasized that such cases demand the most complete study.

Fortunately modern science has developed a number of technics for treating such inflammations, far superior to anything previously possessed by medical science. The sulfa drugs, penicillin, mandelamine, furadantin, or other drugs are now used, either taken by mouth so that they get into the urine or by way of the blood. Various drugs can be made up into solutions and injected directly into the bladder so that they are applied to the spot where the inflammation or infection exists.

Most serious of all infections of the bladder is probably tuberculosis, which in the bladder is secondary to tuberculosis in the kidneys in most instances. Isoniazid is a new drug which attacks the tubercle bacillus.

BLADDER STONES—A stone in the urinary bladder may get there from the kidney or may be formed within the bladder itself. The majority of stones in the urinary bladder form when there is obstruction to the flow of the urine and stagnation of the fluid and secondary infection. Stones in the bladder are much less common now than they were in previous generations. Nowadays doctors are able to determine the presence of a stone much earlier by the use of the X ray and by use of the cystoscope, which enables the doctor to look directly into the bladder. Before the discovery of these instruments it was necessary for the doctor to diagnose the presence of stones either by the symptoms alone or by the actual passing of portions of the stone from the body in the urine.

Incidentally stones in the bladder occur about twenty times as often among men as among women because men are much more likely than women to suffer from bladder conditions as they get older. This is due to infections of the prostate gland and to general infections that occur in the genitourinary tract. Obviously any man who suffers frequently with attacks of serious pain associated with the attempt to get rid of portions of kidney stones is likely also to show occasionally the signs of stones in the urinary bladder.

The kidney stones form in the kidney where the ureter, or tube, which carries the urine from the kidney to the bladder begins. The ureter is a tube about a foot long and a fifth of an inch wide. It carries the urine from the kidney to the bladder. Since the stone may be larger than the ureter, the passing of the stone from the kidney to the bladder may be exceedingly painful. Among the signs of stone in the bladder are frequent urination and almost constant desire to urinate. Even after urination has occurred, there is a feeling of discomfort or pain. The urination may be accompanied by some slight bleeding. If there is secondary infection, there is also likely to be burning.

A rather extraordinary phenomenon is sudden stopping of the flow due to the fact that the stone acts like a valve and blocks the exit. At such times, if the person will lie down, he will discover after he gets up again that the stone has come away from the opening as would a ball valve, so that it is again possible to pass fluid in the upright position.

The X ray has been the most important medium for diagnosing the presence of a stone in the urinary tract. Certain substances have been discovered which make the entire urinary tract opaque to the X ray, so that not only may the stone be discovered but the actual spot in which it lies may be determined. Moreover, it is possible by the use of the cystoscope to look directly into the urinary bladder and to pass additional tubes through the urinary bladder up into the ureters. Devices have been invented which can be passed into the bladder by way of the ordinary passages to break up the stone in position so that it may be removed piecemeal through the tube.

The decision as to what is to be done in such cases must be made by the doctor who is taking care of the patient. In most instances the methods that have been described are carried out much better in a hospital than in the doctor's office.

BLINDNESS See *Eye*.

BLOOD Most important of the organs, tissues, and fluids in the human body is the blood. Only fifty years have passed since some of the formed elements about which we talk glibly—the red and white blood cells and the platelets—were first identified. The manufacture of blood goes on constantly in the human body. In some diseases, such as pernicious anemia, the destruction of the cells may go on rapidly, or they may fail to be formed as they are needed. In some diseases the blood becomes too thick; in others, too thin. White blood cells are increased when there is infection, and greatly decreased in certain diseases.

The blood of man contains, when he is normal, from 4,900,000 red blood cells up to 6,050,000 in each cubic millimeter. The blood of woman contains from 4,400,000 up to 5,350,000 in each cubic millimeter. The body of a woman is smaller and demands less in the way of red cells in the circulation than does the body of a man. Each red blood cell is only three ten-thousandths (0.0003) of an inch in diameter. Those red blood cells grow in the bone marrow, especially in the ribs, the back bones, and the flat bones. In babies, however, the marrow of all of the bones takes part in building blood.

After the blood cells have been developed, they go from the bone marrow into the blood stream, being picked up by the veins. They are then carried to the lungs, where they take up oxygen. The oxygen is carried by the red coloring matter of the red blood cells, which is called hemoglobin. Hemoglobin is a complex substance containing some iron. If the number of red blood corpuscles falls below normal, or if the amount of hemoglobin in the blood corpuscles is deficient, the person has anemia.

Nowadays an examination of the blood is a vital part of any complete physical examination. The doctor punctures the ear lobe or a finger tip and withdraws a small amount of blood. Usually he will take a little more than a drop of blood for each of several pipettes, or tiny calibrated tubes, which are used for measuring and counting the number of red blood cells, white blood cells, and blood platelets. He will also spread some of the blood on a slide, which blood is then stained so that he may determine the different varieties of white blood cells and the relative numbers of each variety.

He may also take a small amount of blood to find out the total amount of hemoglobin or red coloring matter. Whenever any of these methods is used, the doctor is able to say that the blood is 80 per cent normal, or 60, or whatever the case may be. Small differences, as, for example, from 70 to 75 per cent, or from 80 to 90, are not significant.

BLOOD PRESSURE, HIGH Scientifically blood pressure above the normal is known as hypertensive disease. Since medicine has overcome the acute infectious diseases of childhood, the number of people who die from high blood pressure and associated conditions is much greater. We have always

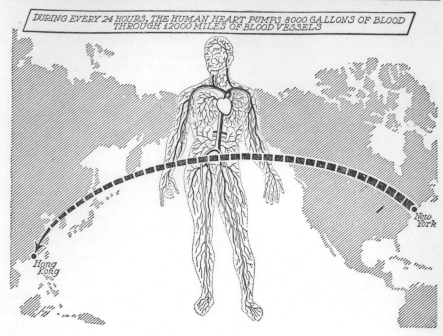

DURING EVERY 24 HOURS, THE HUMAN HEART PUMPS 8000 GALLONS OF BLOOD THROUGH 12000 MILES OF BLOOD VESSELS

Hong Kong

New York

The human circulatory system

known that rest and relaxation would help in the control of high blood pressure but never have they brought about permanent relief. Moreover, there have been persons in whose families high blood pressure was the rule rather than the exception. There have also been families in which the blood pressure of all of the members began to rise when they were young, bringing about death from brain hemorrhage, heart disease, or some associated condition in the middle thirties.

More than one hundred years ago the famous Richard Bright, whose name is associated with Bright's disease, suggested that there was some relationship between the kidneys and the occurrence of high blood pressure. However, this relationship has been definitely established only in recent years. The fact that high blood pressure may not appear until the age of thirty or forty has made difficult the study of the changes that take place in the tissues, since these come on insidiously and are hard to determine until after

death. These studies do show, however, that people who have high blood pressure belong to families in which the amount of disturbance of the blood vessels is much greater than in normal families.

Among certain types of people, as for example the natives of Africa, high blood pressure occurs rarely. However, among the descendants of these same people in our own country the condition is not unusual. The Chinese suffer relatively little in their own country from high blood pressure. It has been customary to state that those races which are not easily excited and which do not develop much nerve strain suffer much less with high blood pressure than do native Americans. However, such people also live in different climates and eat entirely different diets, so that there have been attempts to explain high blood pressure from the point of view of both climate and diet. For many years it has been thought that a high protein diet, particularly the eating of large quantities of meat, was associated with high blood pressure. Nowadays little of the real cause of high blood pressure is assigned to this source.

Not long ago a medical investigator proved that clamping of the blood vessels to the kidneys would result in raising the blood pressure of animals on which this experiment was performed. This led to the view that there was some substance in the kidney which got into the blood system and produced rise in the blood pressure. Operations performed on people with various diseases of the kidney resulting in lowered blood flow revealed that such disease was frequently associated with high blood pressure.

TREATMENT OF HIGH BLOOD PRESSURE—According to Drs. Irvine H. Page and A. C. Corcoran, treatment of high blood pressure involves first an evaluation of the patient's status. Young people need to be told methods of prevention. People with mild conditions of high blood pressure may not require any active treatment with drugs. Older women who have mild hypertension require reassurance, mild sedation, and a program of living that will not disturb their blood pressure.

DRUGS—Many new drugs are available, among which is hexamethonium. Thiocyanate is used for those who suffer from headache. Some doctors use a combination of thiocyanates and phenobarbital, a sedative, both of which must always be prescribed by the doctor. Other new drugs which depress blood pressure are Priscoline and Dibenzoline, which act by depressing the sympathetic nervous action. Mixtures of the alkaloids of ergot have recently come into use; one preparation is called Hydergine. Veratrum viride has been popularized. The derivatives of tetraethylammonium most used are hexamethonium, already mentioned, and pentomethonium, which act on the autonomic ganglia of the nervous system, making what is called a chemical sympathectomy. The patient who is going to be put under one of these drugs should be for a period in the hospital where the doctor can determine the effects. Usually a low sodium diet is given with these drugs since that helps to improve and prolong the action. Another new drug is Apresoline, tried under controlled conditions and frequently accompanied in older cases with a low sodium diet and with drugs to help the heart. Some of these drugs have toxic side effects; the doctors may give antihistaminics to control the side effects. The combined use of Apresoline and hexamethonium seems to act on both the nervous system and the kidney.

Among the newest drugs is a product called "Rauwolfia" which has been known in India since 1776. This drug is included in a variety of mixtures with various barbiturates. The drug acts as a tranquilizer. Recently introduced also is a tranquilizer which is a mepobromate called Miltown and Equanil.

In modern treatment the physician may prescribe any of the forms of the drugs mentioned.

SURGERY—For patients with uncontrollable high blood pressure, doctors may operate on the sympathetic nervous system to stop its function in relationship to the blood vessels. Operation is undertaken in selected patients only after failure with other less intensive and less disabling methods of treatment.

One of the most serious complications in high blood pressure is rupture of the blood vessels in the brain. This may possibly be prevented by the withdrawing of blood, which will tend to lower the blood pressure and which will tend also to keep the red blood cells and the red blood coloring matter, called hemoglobin, in proper amounts.

DIET—Many people with high blood pressure are seriously overweight. This tendency should be controlled by the use of proper diets. It should be emphasized that these diets include particularly the right amounts of vitamins and mineral salts. Frequently persons with high blood pressure have difficulty with the action of the bowel. It is quite possible to produce proper regulation here by the use of suitable foods and suitable remedies. A person with high blood pressure should not indulge in exercises like running or lifting of heavy weights or any type of activity which produces shortness of breath. However, mild exercises and mild massages tend to produce relaxation and aid physical health.

Based on experimental evidence, cautious experiments are now being made with diets low in fat and low in cholesterol. Experiments with animals indicate that these are important in hardening of the arteries.

The person with high blood pressure should avoid excitement. Many physicians prescribe suitable sedative drugs which tend to avoid overexcitement and produce sufficient amounts of rest and sleep.

As stated previously, the development of tranquilizing drugs has led to new and successful approaches to the problem of high blood pressure.

Thus it becomes clear that the treatment of this condition means complete physical and mental control and that with such treatment many a person with high blood pressure may be given added years of life.

The blood pressure of the average person depends on his age, sex, body weight, and constitution. The constitution includes the condition of the blood vessels. Up to the age of fifty the blood pressure rises slowly from 120 with the heart contracted and 80 with the heart relaxed to 130 with the heart contracted and 85 with the heart relaxed. After fifty the blood pressure needs to be studied perhaps more often than previously. The blood pressure of a fat man may be 15 millimeters higher than that of a lean man, whose blood pressure will be 10 millimeters of mercury lower than that for a person of normal weight.

Many factors influence our blood pressure. If we are mentally disturbed, if we are worrying a great deal, or if we are frightened, the blood pressure may rise. The blood pressure with the heart contracted is likely to rise more than that with the heart relaxed. This has been observed particularly among soldiers coming for examination in whom it was found that the fear of the examination itself may be sufficient to raise the blood pressure to a point which makes it impossible to pass the candidate.

Pain will cause a rise in the blood pressure, as will also irritation of the abdominal surface of the diaphragm, which is the large muscle that separates the chest cavity from the abdominal cavity.

Inflation of the stomach or overeating can cause pressure and thus raise the blood pressure. Cooling of the skin and chilling help to cause an increase in the blood pressure. It is believed that poor circulation of the blood and chilling cause the tissues of the body to release a substance called histamine, which in turn brings about a narrowing of the small blood vessels and thus a rise in the blood pressure.

Frequently when a fat person becomes undernourished, there is a fall in the blood pressure. This was seen particularly during World War II with the blockading of the Central Powers of Europe.

There have been all sorts of beliefs about the relationship of various foods to the blood pressure. We know, for instance, that people who have a tendency toward low blood pressure frequently are improved by taking large amounts of salt with the diet, but conversely a restriction of salt will not lower an abnormally high blood pressure. Dr. Leopold Lichtwitz says:

As food and diet greatly influence body and mind, it would be well to consider what happens to a man with a chronic ailment, such as arterial hypertension, when his diet is restricted in protein, salt, eggs and spices, and he is forbidden to smoke or to drink alcoholic beverages.

For a short time such limitations are more or less well tolerated, but over an indefinite period such a regime tends to make the man a social outcast and causes him to develop the psychology of invalidism. A few individuals refuse to accept the sentence and follow their own inclinations.

But there remain the great majority, poor devils whose life and activity center around their blood pressure, who become hypochondriacs, and who bore the doctors at every possible opportunity with the perennial topic of blood pressure.

Considering the lack of certainty as to a relationship between food constituents and hypertension, the long duration of the disorder, and the influence of the therapeutic management on the patient's mind and conduct of life, it seems wiser and more effective to regulate the diet principally with regard to quantity, to the amount of calories as well as to gross volume, restricting protein and salt only moderately and with regard to the individual requirement.

Blood pressure rises steadily with age. In one group of almost three thousand men over forty, the blood pressure was 150 in 16 per cent; in those over fifty, in 28.6 per cent, and in those over sixty, in 51.2 per cent. Another analysis included 42,000 instances in which it was shown that a blood pressure of 150 with the heart contracted, and 90 with the heart dilated, rose from 5 per cent at the age of twenty-five to 45 per cent above sixty-five years. Thus many people actually do have high blood pressure, and it might be considered for some types of constitution almost normal to have a blood pressure somewhat higher than 135 or 140.

Recently Drs. A. M. Master and S. Dack made a study of almost six thousand workers employed by the New York Telephone Company and many of the large department stores. They believe that a blood pressure over 150 can be classed as abnormal. The figures from many large life insurance companies indicate that a blood pressure over 145 is probably abnormal. However, the figures altogether seem to show that one fourth of men and two fifths of women workers over forty have a blood pressure around 150. Therefore it would be wrong to say that such a blood pressure is serious in relationship to the length of life.

Actually the exact relationship of high blood pressure to the length of life and to the aging process has not been fully established. The matter becomes especially important when it concerns the possibility of employing a man or a woman of advanced years, since some companies will not employ a person with blood pressure above 145. Indeed the New York experts say that it may well be that, after the age of forty, the old and now discarded dictum that the blood pressure should be 100 plus the man's age is not entirely wrong.

BLOOD PRESSURE, LOW

(*Hypotension*) The average blood pressure of men at twenty years of age is 120; at sixty years of age, about 135. In people who are overweight this pressure is likely to be higher. A variation of 5 millimeters of mercury above or below these figures may be considered within the average. Variations of more than 5 millimeters above or below are conditions for study.

There are many reasons why the blood pressure may fall below the average. This occurs whenever a person is nauseated, faints, or has a severe hemorrhage. There are, however, other conditions of general weakness in which the blood pressure is low and in which the physician needs to concern himself with building the person back into a good condition. For instance, following influenza, people are frequently weak, perspire freely on exertion, and appear weary, depressed, and tired without any apparent cause. When the infection is cleared up and the appetite returns, when the person begins to resume his daily physical activities, the pressure may rise promptly.

A similar condition may develop following any long-continued infection, and the method of taking care of the condition is obvious. Rest is necessary. If everyone who had a severe cold, even without a fever, would stay in bed in the acute stage and if every person who had a fever would stay in bed from one to three days after the temperature became normal, a vast amount of degenerative disease, of low blood pressure, and of general weakness would be avoided.

There are certain diseases which attack the glands of internal secretion which are concerned with keeping the blood pressure normal through maintaining proper elasticity in the blood vessels. Obviously any disease affecting these glands and interfering with their function may bring about low blood pressure. Since the blood pressure is a reflection of the power of the heart to push the blood through the arteries and veins and of the condition of the blood vessels through which the blood passes, any factor that greatly influences these two basic features of the circulation may bring about either a high or low blood pressure.

Dr. Wingate M. Johnson, after a survey of the available knowledge, feels that low blood pressure favors long life, but that it is not likely to be associated with physical vigor. There is a tendency to encounter low blood pressures more frequently than high ones.

BLOOD TYPES Modern investigations have shown that human beings can be divided into groups according to certain factors that are present in the blood and that the bloods of some groups may be mixed without danger, whereas the bloods of other groups will not mix satisfactorily. This classification of the bloods of various human beings is based on the fact that the fluid matter of the blood contains a substance called agglutinin, which, when it comes in contact with the red blood cells of certain other bloods, will cause them to clump together or agglutinate. The red blood cells apparently contain some substance which may be called agglutinogen, which enables them to be clumped together when they are acted on by the right kind of agglutinin from the fluid material of another blood.

By testing the blood of one person with that of another in many thousands of people it was discovered that human beings may be divided into groups according to the agglutinins and agglutinogens which they have in their blood. It is obviously impossible for a person to have in his own blood an agglutinin which would act on his own agglutinogen, because then his own blood would immediately clot.

Further studies made on these blood groups have shown that they are inherited and that various types of animals and various races of human beings have special arrangements of their blood groups. A person can transfer only one of these factors to his child. If the blood group is known to which a child and one parent belong, it can be definitely said that the other parent must belong to one of certain other groups and therefore could not possibly belong to some other groups. Today the courts in many states have recognized the scientific character of these observations. Evidence has been introduced in legal cases to show, for instance, that a certain man could not possibly be the father of a certain child, although it is not yet possible to show by this evidence that a certain man is quite certainly the father of a certain child.

Recently attention has centered particularly on the Rh factor. If an Rh positive marries an Rh negative a child born to the parents may have a dangerous disease of the blood called erythroblastosis.

In about one marriage in eight the wife is Rh negative and the husband Rh positive. In a marriage of this type there is the possibility that the reactions of the blood will be such that a disease will occur in the infant, causing its blood cells to change.

When a person who is Rh negative receives a blood transfusion of Rh positive blood, that person is likely to become immunized against the agglutination reaction. A Boston investigator found that nearly half of all the men who had an Rh negative factor and who were transfused during the war have become immunized and developed substances in their blood against the Rh factor. If an Rh negative person is immunized as a result of a blood transfusion, further transfusions of Rh positive blood may produce severe and possibly fatal reactions. The transfused blood is destroyed very rapidly. Later transfusions bring about reactions with fever and jaundice. When an Rh negative woman becomes pregnant and has an Rh positive child, she may become immunized and produce a substance which can agglutinate the red blood cells of all Rh positive people including those of her own children. Once the antibody is produced it may pass through the blood of the mother to the blood of the child and damage the child's red cells. When the child is born it will have a blood disease and some deaths have occurred as a result of this situation. Since Rh negative blood is necessary for the transfusion of all Rh negative persons and all children with diseases of the blood who may be born to Rh negative mothers, it becomes necessary for blood banks to have available Rh negative blood. Because of the importance of this situation the suggestion has been made that all prospective parents have tests made of the blood as to the presence of Rh negative or Rh positive factors. The test is technical but not too difficult and many laboratories already make the test available.

BODY ODOR The scientific name for this condition is bromidrosis. Those who suffer from it ought to pay great attention to personal cleanliness—in fact even more than ordinary people do. Of course a bath should be taken every day, or twice daily, because bathing is not likely to do any harm. A good soap should be used, preferably not one with an offensive odor of its own. Various special soaps are offered for the purpose, but it is not certain that they are any more beneficial than any good ordinary soap.

Certainly parts of the body in which perspiration is likely to be excessive may be treated with some of the preparations used to check this condition. Many of these are available in drug-stores. They are not likely to be harmful, because checking perspiration under the arms or on other parts of the body where it is excessive will not interfere with health. After the lotion has been applied and the perspiration effectively checked, an antiseptic dusting powder or talcum powder may be put on the skin.

If there is excessive perspiration of the feet, the doctor usually will prescribe a regular bathing with a 1 per cent solution of a substance called formalin, or liquor formaldehyde. Since, however, this is an exceedingly active chemical substance, it would not be advisable to undertake its use unless your doctor thought such use warranted. Some persons are sensitive to this substance and get eruptions when it is applied to their skin.

Chlorophyll preparations, introduced as capable of controlling body odors, have been disappointing. Combined with other substances, they may mask odors.

Usually it is just certain regions of the body from which the sweat with the offensive odor is excreted. This applies particularly to the areas under the arms, the feet, and occasionally more intimate parts of the body. Sometimes the extra secretion of sweat is associated with nervousness, and proper treatment applied to allay this nervousness will help to control the sweat.

In a few instances the application of mild doses of the X ray by competent specialists in diseases of the skin has been sufficient to control the condition completely.

BOILS A boil is an infection of the skin. Usually it follows a breaking of the skin, such as occurs when the back of the neck is constantly rubbed by a collar which has not been laundered smoothly. Boils occur particularly on those parts of the skin that are covered by hair follicles; the hair follicles offer increased opportunity for irritation and for the entrance of germs beneath the surface of the skin.

In some diseases, such as diabetes,

the skin reacts seriously to infection; boils occur with greater frequency in diabetics.

Repeated infections of the skin, such as pimples and boils, result from a generally lowered resistance of the body to disease. Such a lowering may come with increased fatigue and with bad diet, constipation, insufficient sleep or fresh air, and a general deficiency in all of the health habits that are associated with good hygiene.

Persons who have boils frequently should try to keep the body in the best physical state by establishing good health habits. All infections of the ears, teeth, throat, nose, or other portions of the body should be attended to, since frequently the germs coming from these portions of the body may localize elsewhere and set up secondary infections.

A boil is actually a deep-seated inflammation of the skin. Usually the germs causing the boils are the pusforming germs which are ever ready to attack when the resistance of the skin is broken down by any continued irritation or other disturbances.

There are innumerable methods for treating boils. Heat is frequently applied because it brings a good supply of blood. The blood aids in destroying germs. The blood also brings to the area where the boil is located the necessary white blood cells which wall off the boil from the rest of the body. The opening of a boil is a serious surgical operation. Not everyone is competent to do this. The idea that anyone who can see blood without fainting is competent to do minor surgery has long since been exploded by the deaths of people who have been seriously infected generally through careless handling of small infections. If a boil is opened improperly, the infectious material may spread to other parts of the skin and may even be forced through the wall that separates it from the rest of the body, in which case the infection may spread through the system and cause death.

In some instances X ray and ultraviolet ray have been applied when boils are long persistent. This, however, is a procedure which only a competent physician should attempt. The use of yeast for boils is certainly of no established merit. Vaccines or preparations of the killed germs taken from the boil sometimes seem to help in building up resistance.

A carbuncle is actually a group of boils and is simply more serious because it represents a more extensive infection. When carbuncles occur in aged people or in those who are recovering from illness, they are naturally much more serious than when they occur in the young. Nowadays the X ray is frequently used in the treatment of carbuncles. In serious cases the attention of an expert surgeon is required.

BONES Bones are the solid elements of structure that sustain the body, regulate its form and its position. The most important attribute of bones is their rigidity.

The number of separate bones in a man forty years old is 206. At every age up to twenty-two the number of bones in boys is different from that in girls because of the changes that take place in the joining together of small bones to make large ones.

The word "skeleton" is a Greek word that means a dried-up mummy. Nowadays the term "skeleton" means the bones and the joints.

Bones are made of a gelatinous material, which is the elastic tissue of the body, infiltrated with a great deal of calcium. Tricalcium phosphate makes up more than one half the weight of bone and gives it its stony hardness, its rigidity, and its strength. Tricalcium phosphate is not soluble in fluid. The calcium is brought to the area where the bone is going to be formed by the blood in other calcium salts, which are then changed over into tricalcium phosphate in the bone.

The exposure of a child to sunlight or ultraviolet rays and the action of these rays on a substance called ergosterol in the human skin create vitamin D, which in turn results in the depositing of calcium salts as the insoluble calcium phosphate. For that reason plenty of milk containing calcium and phosphorus and enough vitamin D or sunlight are necessary for proper growth of bones and teeth.

Everyone knows that the individual bones vary in their shape and size. The large bone of the thigh is quite different from the flat bone of the chest.

The center of the bones contains tissue which forms blood cells.

The breaking of a bone is known as a fracture. When a fracture occurs and the fragments are replaced in proper position, lime salts are deposited in the blood in the area where the fracture occurred. Gradually the scar tissue is transformed into new bone, so that the broken ends become firmly united.

Following World War I, 65 per cent of American soldiers who returned with various disabilities were found to require the attention of the orthopedic surgeon. These are the specialists in medicine who deal particularly with malformations and crippling injuries of the bones, muscles, and joints. The studies of many years have shown the possibility of making bone grafts to replace damaged areas, of transplanting bony tissue, and of creating new sockets for the heads of bones which have been destroyed. Pins or nails may be used to hold broken bones in place until healing has occurred. By their work the orthopedic specialists have done much to free human beings from pain and suffering; they have repaired the crippled and restored to useful activity people who would otherwise be permanently disabled.

BOTULISM Most dangerous of all of the forms of food poisoning is botulism, which is due to contamination of food by a specific germ known as the *Bacillus botulinus*. This germ is found in soil throughout the world. Naturally, therefore, it becomes possible for the germ of botulism to contaminate food that is grown in such soil. If this food is packed or preserved under conditions that are not quite safe with the germs still alive, the toxin or poison of the germ is formed and produces the form of food poisoning called botulism. Sometimes the toxin of the botulinus is so strong that as little as one part in ten million will kill a mouse. Many factors can modify the amount of toxin that is present. For instance the nature of the food, whether acid or alkaline, the amount of sugar that is present, or the extent to which the food has been heated before preserving will have a definite effect on the amount of botulinus present and the amount of toxin that develops.

In the record of various outbreaks of botulism that have occurred in the United States the foods that have been most often involved are string beans, corn, spinach leaves, asparagus, beets, and apricots. In the outbreaks which have occurred in Europe most of the foods involved have been sausages, meat and fish pastes.

Commercially canned foods are now so standardized in the methods of packing and handling that outbreaks of botulism from commercially canned foods have not occurred for a long time. Home-preserved vegetables and fruits served cold as salads have, however, been several times incriminated. Home canning that is done without sterilizing the containers and the food under pressure permits the spores of the botulinus to survive. It has been shown that some spores can survive boiling for six hours and can live under fifteen pounds of steam pressure for six minutes. Fortunately six minutes of boiling will destroy the toxin of the botulinus even if it will not destroy the spore. Therefore all home-preserved foods should be boiled for six minutes before they are tasted or served. It is known that the preservation of foods in a 10 per cent brine solution will make home-canned foods reasonably safe.

The principal symptoms of botulism are weakness and paralysis because this toxin seriously affects the nerves. Among the earliest symptoms are those affecting the eyesight. People who have been poisoned with botulinus toxin have difficulty in talking and swallowing and occasionally see double. The chief step in first aid for anyone who has been poisoned with botulinus toxin is to keep the patient alive and to secure as soon as possible the aid of a physician who may try the effects, if not too long delayed, of the anti-botulism serum.

BRAIN The brain is a tissue which, in the average man, weighs between three and four pounds. The size of the brain is not an index of intellect. Sometimes large brains are found in idiots. The accumulation of fluid in the brain will increase its weight.

The chief distinguishing feature between man and the lower animals is man's brain. It gives the human being the power to think and to reason, to speak and to create. There is a great deal of difference between the brain of a fishworm and that of a dog or a horse. Indeed there are differences between the brains of various dogs and various horses, exactly as there are differences between the brains of various men. One of the distinguishing factors between the mammals, for example, and lower animals is the fact that the mammals nurse their young and take care of them. Of course birds and even some snakes develop care of the young for brief periods, but the mammals have greater capacities than animals of a lower order.

A dog gets along much better than a snake. He can adapt himself to many conditions. In fact a dog's learning ability is far beyond that of lower animals. It is interesting that the seal, which is also a mammal, can be trained to performances which would be impossible for fish, which are not mammals.

The nearest brain to that of man is the brain of what are called the anthropoid apes—the monkeys that are like men. These monkeys, including the chimpanzee, orangutan, lemur, and the gorilla, have hands that grasp and a brain structure much like that of man. There are some experts who insist that these monkeys even have limited powers of reasoning. Intelligence tests made on the orangutan show that it is slow but

that it actually tries to get insight into every test situation. In fact it has been urged that the brain of this monkey can obtain the development necessary for the production of an idea.

The chimpanzees have attained great reputations as performers and as comedians. They have learned to use implements like spoons and straws. They develop marksmanship with sticks and stones, and they get great fun out of dressing up and masquerading as human beings.

Gorillas, too, develop remarkably. The one which is attracting great attention in a circus was raised in a home, as have been other gorillas in the past. The gorilla's brain is larger and weighs more than that of any other ape, and in many other ways is nearest that of man.

In the brain reside the centers for the special functions of the body such as seeing, hearing, and smelling, also the center for putting into action those tissues of the body that are under voluntary control.

The head end of all animals is the dominating end. Not only are the special centers that have been mentioned located in this area but also the nerve centers for sensation, combinations of sensations, memory, judgment, and the control and co-ordination of various activities. Here also is the center for consciousness. Because of the importance of all of these activities in relation to life the brain is protected by a vault of bone and by membranes and fluids which keep it from damage under any except extraordinary circumstances.

The brain is composed of various portions in which have been located the centers for certain activities. Obviously damage to these centers is reflected in the portion of the body for which the special center functions.

The outer portion of the brain is called the cortex. Experts believe that the higher intelligence and workings of the mind are functions of the cortex. Mind, thought, and their conversion into action are the functions of the brain, just as digestion is a function of the stomach. When any tissue works, it gets tired. The cells of the brain may get tired exactly as the cells of a muscle get tired from overuse. The people who think, therefore, that the mind is something quite apart from the body do not realize that the modern trend of medicine tends to consider the mind more and more in relationship to changes in the body and the occurrence of disease.

The gray matter comprises about 40 per cent of the front of the brain. Usually the left side of the brain is a little heavier than the right. We know today that one side of the brain may be dominant over the other. The activities of the right side of the body are dominated by the left side of the brain. That portion of the brain which is not in the cortex is like a vast telephone system where impulses come in, are rerouted, and go out.

The back portion of the brain, called the occipital, is primarily concerned with visual functions.

Examples of failure of the brain to function are aphasia (in which there may be a defect in the formation of words), loss of writing ability and verbal memory. In difficulties with words there is usually something wrong in the front part of the brain. Sometimes people have difficulties in understanding what is said to them. They cannot remember complex phrases. They are what is called "word deaf." In this condition the trouble is usually found toward the side of the brain, about halfway back.

There are cases in which people have difficulty in designating objects by name. When speaking, they stop because they cannot remember the name of some object that they want to mention. They may describe the use of objects. They read with difficulty but usually can spell out words. The trouble in this type of aphasia is found still farther back on the side of the brain.

These conditions are mentioned as examples, indicating how the doctor goes about determining the spot at which some trouble may lie when such difficulties occur. Occasionally there may be a softening of the tissue of the brain, a tumor, an injury from a blow, or a hemorrhage. Knowledge of the functions of the special areas of the brain gives the doctor evidence as to where to perform a surgical operation if that is necessary.

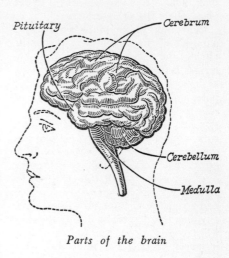

Parts of the brain

BRAIN CONCUSSION What happens when a human being suddenly becomes unconscious after a bump on the head? When the brain is examined after an injury to the head, there are sometimes signs of hemorrhage or loss of blood from the coverings around the brain. In other instances there will be disturbances in the way in which the spinal fluid circulates through the brain. Occasionally there will be crushing of some of the soft white material of the brain. In still other instances the fibers which act as the connection cords between different portions of the brain will be damaged or destroyed.

The important factor whenever there is a blow or an injury to the head is the amount of damage done to the brain. Even a slight crack of the skull is not so important as the pressure that may result from the bleeding inside the skull that occurs when the crack takes place. The visual evidence that the skull is cracked is some indication of the amount of the damage, because it takes a great amount of force to crack the skull. If the brain itself is being pressed on by fragments of bone or if the tissue of the brain is torn in an accident, the condition is serious. There is also danger of pressure on the tissue of the brain by blood that may get loose under the skull. The effects vary according to the place where the pressure occurs.

Concussion of the brain is actually a paralysis of the functions of the brain. Usually the person who has had a concussion is unconscious. He breathes with a shallow respiration; he has a rapid pulse and a low blood pressure, and the skin feels cold and clammy. A concussion may be so brief that recovery occurs almost immediately. Sometimes the damage after the concussion is so great that recovery of consciousness does not occur at all. Often after regaining his senses the person who has had a concussion is unable to remember anything that happened during the time when consciousness was lost. In many instances he does not remember what happened for an hour or two before unconsciousness occurred.

When a prize fighter is knocked out in the ring there is a short period in which the blood vessels in the head contract so that the supply of blood to the brain is reduced. This produces a condition called cerebral anemia, which merely means a lack of blood in the brain. The lack of a supply of oxygen to the cells of the brain prevents them from carrying on their functions. When a fighter gets "punch drunk" he has large portions of his brain put out of service by the pressure of small hemorrhages.

BRAIN HEMORRHAGE See *Apoplexy.*

BRAIN TUMOR Among the commonest of all of the disturbances of the nervous system are tumors of the brain. Once such conditions were considered hopeless as far as their control and treatment were concerned. Now it is recognized that early diagnosis may permit operations that will save life and restore people to useful activities. In one series of operations, including 400 consecutive cases of tumor of the brain, which were operated on, there were 224 cases in which the tumor could be removed completely and permanently. The diagnosis of a tumor of the brain in the final stages is not difficult but at the same time is not so helpful or important as the recognition of such tumors in people at an early date.

Certain signs of tumor of the brain are easily recognized, as, for instance, the changes at the back of the eye which indicate a high degree of pressure inside the skull, the pain which is continuous and does not yield to any kind of treatment, and the vomiting that cannot be controlled. These symptoms may result from other conditions. The one true symptom of a tumor inside the brain is the gradual and progressive loss of functions of the portion of the brain that is involved. So important is the occurrence of a brain tumor in relationship to life that it would be folly for anyone to attempt even to hint at the diagnosis of such a condition for himself.

Disturbances of function of the body which develop in relationship to a tumor of the brain are so serious in the vast majority of cases that few people would be likely to neglect these symptoms. When those portions of the brain concerned with thought happen to be involved, the difficulties with speech and writing and thinking become apparent rather promptly, although instances are known in which even such symptoms are neglected for months. When the portions of the brain concerned with movement happen to be involved, the difficulty is likely to be recognized somewhat earlier. When there is involvement of a combination of the powers of thought and the powers of movement, the disorder is quickly apparent.

At the very back and buttom of the brain is the portion called the cerebellum, in contrast to the front portion, which is known as the cerebrum. Involvements of the cerebellum produce disorganization of motion and action that is exceedingly serious. Sometimes there is at first merely unsteadiness or tremor. Later, awkwardness, lack of coordination, staggering, and dizziness may appear. Sometimes these people stand with the feet wide apart so as to be able to maintain their balance, and they tend to sway and fall toward the side where the tumor exists. As they walk they tend to sway about and deviate toward the side on which the tumor lies.

If a tumor in the brain presses on near-by structures, it may involve actions of the eyes or ears or of the other special senses which are controlled by nerves coming from that area.

In the modern diagnosis of tumors of the brain the physician may be helped by new methods including dye substances and radioactive isotopes which localize in such tumors. It is possible to inject air into the cavity of the skull and then to take a picture which may show changes in the shape of the brain or consolidation of tissue that has been pressed together or other changes which will be familiar to the trained eye. In other instances the doctor makes tracings of the activities of the brain, which are called brain waves, and thus finds differences from the normal pattern. There is likely to be an examination of the spinal fluid. In this procedure a needle is placed into the spine to determine whether or not the fluid comes out under pressure, whether or not it is stained with blood or modified in other ways.

BREATHING Breathing is a function of the lungs. When we breathe, oxygen in the air is taken into the lungs and carbon dioxide with some additional moisture is breathed out. The lungs are constructed like a sponge. Small spaces are surrounded by tissues which contain tiny blood vessels. When air comes into these spaces, the tiny blood vessels take up oxygen. When we exhale, the carbon dioxide is passed out of the blood and into the air spaces, then into larger tubes, known as bron-

chial tubes, and then into the trachea, or windpipe, and out of the body. The air changes take place at about the rate of four quarts per minute.

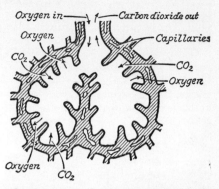

The lungs take in oxygen from the air and give off carbon dioxide from the blood

When we breathe normally during sleep, we breathe from twelve to fifteen times per minute. We breathe more rapidly when we stand up and when we exercise than when we are at rest. We breathe more rapidly also when we are excited.

In various people the capacity of the chest differs. The amount of air which passes in and out of the chest is known as the vital air. All of the extra air that can be breathed in above this amount is called complemental air. All of the extra air that can be breathed out after the lungs are emptied in the normal manner is called supplemental air. The vital capacity of the human being is the total of the three amounts.

Some people can stop breathing for from twenty seconds to a minute. If you breathe deeply or normally for about one minute and then take a deep breath, you can hold your breath about three times as long as you could if all of the air were expelled just before attempting to do without breathing. The factor that controls this is the amount of carbon dioxide in the lungs at the time when you begin to hold your breath.

Shortness of breath is a serious symptom. In many instances it is related to heart disease but in others to a different factor. People who are too fat are frequently short of breath simply from the extra load that they carry. Sometimes shortness of breath is associated with nervous exhaustion.

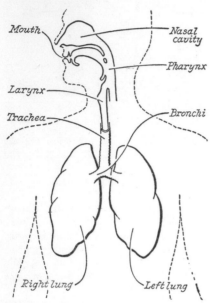

The swallowing and breathing paths

BRIGHT'S DISEASE (See *Nephritis*) Chronic inflammation of the kidneys.

BROMIDROSIS See *Body Odor*.

BRONCHIECTASIS When the lung around the breathing tubes becomes infected and the sections dilate, the condition is called bronchiectasis. Usually it affects just the lower lobes of the lungs, and in most instances the left side more than the right. There are all stages of the condition, depending on the amount of tube and lung material involved.

The chief symptom of bronchiectasis is a chronic cough with the expectoration of a great deal of purulent material.

It is necessary in every such case to make certain that other conditions like tuberculosis and silicosis are not present. The cough in bronchiectasis comes on at regular intervals and frequently gets worse if the affected person stoops over. The amount of sputum expectorated may vary from a quart in twenty-four hours to one tenth of that amount.

Naturally the breathing is difficult. Associated with the difficulties in breathing there may be blueness of the skin. The extra pressure put on the heart by the lung condition is also reflected in the blue color and the shortness of breath. If the condition is severe, there may be fever, loss of weight, night sweats, and even bleeding from the lung.

When an abscess or collection of purulent material occurs in any portion of the body, the best treatment, frequently, is to open the abscess to let the infected material blow out. Then direct treatment of the infected area can effect a cure.

Obviously the opening of a lung with a great many small compartments is not so simple as opening an abscess anywhere else in the body. If there happens to be a tuberculous infection in the lung, the treatment quite frequently involves the use of the system called pneumothorax. In that method air is injected into the area around the lung, causing the lung to be compressed and thus to be rested. The method, at first opposed by many, is now rather generally accepted as a useful technic in bronchiectasis.

Other technics for resting the lung, including operations on the phrenic nerve and actual removal of several ribs, have been tried in severe cases. Indeed bronchiectasis may become so severe that complete removal of the entire lung is necessary. This is an exceedingly serious problem. In a total of sixty-two cases of complete removal of a lung, according to many different surgeons, one half the patients died after the operation. The operation for removal of just one lobe of a lung is now done frequently with success.

Besides the surgical treatment, people with bronchiectasis are often helped by plenty of rest, nourishing food, plenty of fresh air and sunshine. The drainage of material from the lung is frequently helped by allowing the head to hang over the bed or by bending over a chair or in other ways facilitating gravity in pouring out the fluid material.

Sometimes specific germs can be found in the secretions from the lung and methods of attacking these germs by special remedies directed at the character of the germs may be helpful. This means, of course, the attention of a competent doctor who can have suitable laboratory studies made. The doctor can also provide for the drainage of material from the lung and direct the use of that procedure. New technics have been developed for inhalation of penicillin and other antibiotic drugs.

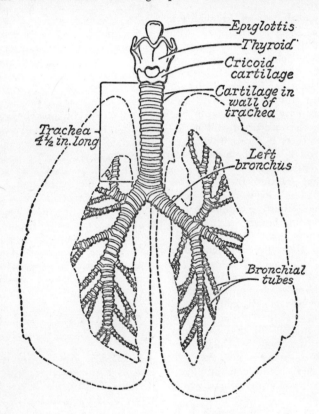

The anatomy of the breathing tract

BRONCHITIS The bronchial tubes are the large tubes that carry air from the trachea, or windpipe, to the final branches which go to the smaller cells of the lung. When these tubes become infected or inflamed, the condition is called bronchitis. Usually, however, the windpipe and the voice box, or larynx, are involved first; occasionally also the tonsils and throat.

Usually bronchitis follows an infection in the throat or a cold. It comes often after measles, whooping cough, or influenza. The chief danger of bronchitis is the possibility of pneumonia after the bronchitis. Almost any of the germs that infect the throat or lungs can infect these tubes. There are also cases in which the viruses which cause colds or influenza may infect the bronchial tubes. Sometimes the infection will pass from one person to another and infect the whole family.

Bronchitis comes on most often in the spring and fall when the weather is cold and changeable and is likely to affect small children more than those of adult age. Many people seem to be especially susceptible to bronchitis. This applies particularly to those who are sensitive to various pollens or dusts.

In the typical case of bronchitis a cough or a cold is associated with chilliness, tiredness, and soreness in muscles. As the infection spreads down the tubes, there is a feeling of tightness in the chest, a fever begins which will go to 101 or 102 degrees. With this comes an increase in the rate of the pulse and in the rate of breathing. Almost at once there is a cough which at first is dry, rough, and ringing but later soft and accompanied by the production of mucus and sputum. In most cases prompt attention will stop the condition. This means putting a child to bed at once, keeping the air in the room fairly moist, and using the usual measures that go with the treatment of a severe cold.

The remedies administered by physicians are those which tend to produce rest, lessening the cough, and preventing irritation in the throat. If the breathing is so difficult that the child appears blue, the doctor will make certain that air or oxygen gets into the lungs. The diet should contain plenty of milk, water, and citrus drinks, which provide alkali.

In order to loosen the cough it is customary to provide inhalations of steam by any simple device which will permit the child to inhale the steam. Great care must be taken, however, not to burn the patient by tipping over kettles or basins of boiling water. The purpose of the steam is to loosen the infected material so that it may be expectorated. In cases in which the bronchial tubes are especially sensitive, it is sometimes necessary to remove the child to a warm, dry climate to permit complete recovery so that chronic bronchitis will not follow.

The chief danger of bronchitis is, of course, the possibility of secondary pneumonia. In cold, changeable weather children should be carefully guarded against too much exposure of the body without adequate protection by warm clothing. They should be guarded also against sudden changes and extremes in temperature, passing too rapidly from a hot room to the outside cold. There is also danger from wet clothing. When the child comes indoors, the wet clothing should be promptly removed, the skin dried, and dry clothing substituted.

If an infection persists so that it seems to be tending toward becoming chronic, special attention must be given to the use of remedies that will overcome the infection. It is necessary to avoid exposure to dusts. Rest, fresh air, sunshine, and nutritious food tend to build in the body sufficient resistance to produce healing. A persistent cough means that there is continuing infection, inflammation, and irritation. Chronic bronchitis produces constant coughing, particularly during the night. The constant coughing tends to produce fatigue and depression, so that the whole condition leads to a vicious circle.

BRUCELLOSIS See *Undulant Fever*.

BRUISES Any injury to the surface of the body that does not break the skin, if sufficiently severe, will cause a bruise. If the skin breaks and bleeds, the condition is called a laceration. Most bruises result from actual blows with blunt objects such as clubs, rubber hose, or whips. Bruises also result from bumping into corners of chairs and tables, from falls, or from being struck by falling objects.

Occasionally bruises require more than merely passing attention because there may be a serious complication under the black-and-blue mark that is under the skin. For instance there are cases in which a bladder filled with fluid has been ruptured following a blow which seemed to cause only a bruise on the surface. Cases are known in which patients have passed into serious conditions, including peritonitis, because they neglected that kind of an injury. A bruise of the scalp is particularly important because there may be a fracture of the skull under it. Cases are on record of slight ruptures of the liver following a bruise which seemed merely to injure the surface of the body. Continuous bleeding from the broken part of the liver eventually resulted in so much loss of blood that the person became unconscious and died.

Some people bruise much more easily than others. This may be due to the fact that their blood vessels are more permeable, permitting blood to escape easily. In other instances it may be due to the fact that the blood itself does not contain enough of the materials necessary to produce prompt clotting. Some women bruise easily around the time of their periodic functions and do not bruise easily at other times. Fat people and those who are anemic are likely to bruise more easily than people in good health.

The changes in color of the bruised skin are due to the changes that take place in the blood that has escaped from the blood vessels. When the bruise occurs, the small blood vessels in the skin are broken, so that the blood gets out into the tissues. This blood at first is changed by the formation of the clot into a black mass. Gradually as the pigment material is absorbed it will change to blue, then to brown, and finally to yellow.

When a severe bruise occurs, it may be necessary to rest the part affected. If there is much swelling in an arm or a leg, the limb may need to be elevated to aid absorption of the blood. The application of heat will also aid the absorption of the blood.

A secondary infection in a blood clot may be a most serious complication.

Rarely indeed does blood collected in a mass under the skin have to be let out. Usually it is absorbed from within. In some instances, however, when the pressure of a clot may be menacing to neighboring portions of the body, the doctor may have to open the area in order to remove the accumulated material.

BUBONIC PLAGUE See discussion under *Plague*.

BUERGER'S DISEASE Buerger's disease is named after a physician named Buerger who first wrote a description of the condition, establishing it as a special disease. The scientific name for Buerger's disease is thromboangiitis obliterans.

This name describes a condition of the blood vessels in which the linings are inflamed so that blood clots form and passage of the blood is slowed. Usually Buerger's disease starts with pain in one leg and later appears in the other. The legs get cold. There may be spasms of the blood vessels in the legs. With the interference that occurs in the blood supply, there may be swelling and even ulceration and gangrene. Naturally the severity of the symptoms depends on the extent to which the condition has progressed.

While Buerger's disease involves the legs more often than any other part of the body, it may occasionally involve the arms and sometimes both the arms and legs. In still other cases it may affect blood vessels elsewhere in the body.

Buerger's disease mostly affects men between the ages of twenty and fifty. At one time it was thought that it affected particularly the Jewish people. Now it is known that it may affect people of any race or religion and that women are frequently affected as well as men. Out of 1000 patients with Buerger's disease seen in a large clinic, only one fourth were Jewish.

One of the most important aspects of Buerger's disease is its relationship to excessive smoking. A classification of patients made as to the number of cigarettes that they smoked varied from five a day in the first group to

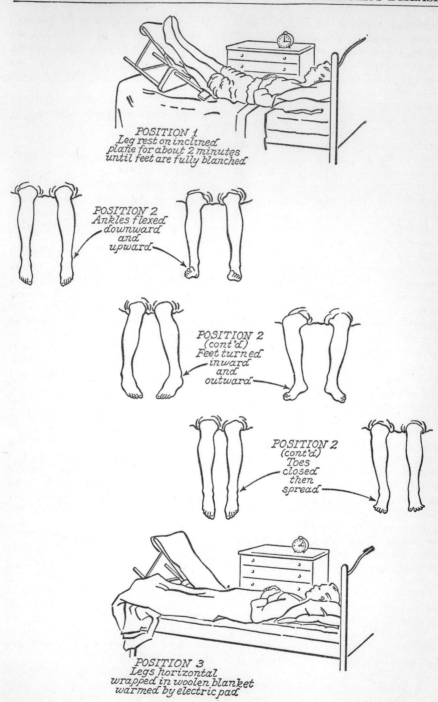

POSITION 1
Leg rest on inclined
plane for about 2 minutes
until feet are fully blanched

POSITION 2
Ankles flexed
downward
and
upward

POSITION 2
(cont'd)
Feet turned
inward
and
outward

POSITION 2
(cont'd)
Toes
closed
then
spread

POSITION 3
Legs horizontal
wrapped in woolen blanket
warmed by electric pad

*Exercises to encourage circulation of blood in the feet and improve elimination of
fluid which causes swelling*

twenty or more a day in the fourth group. Some of the patients in the fourth group smoked as many as sixty cigarettes a day. One patient smoked twenty cigarettes daily before breakfast. Ninety per cent of these patients were cigarette smokers; 66 per cent smoked excessively. Since smoking to excess has definitely been shown to have deleterious effects on the blood vessels and on the circulation of the blood, most physicians are convinced that there is a definite relationship between excessive smoking and Buerger's disease.

Because of the danger of gangrene as a result of Buerger's disease and the necessity for amputation to control the gangrene, people with this condition are urged particularly to watch carefully the care of the feet. Here are sixteen simple directions that are known to be helpful:

1. Wash feet each night with neutral (face) soap and warm water.

2. Dry feet with a clean soft rag *without* rubbing the skin.

3. Apply rubbing alcohol (70 per cent) and allow the feet to dry thoroughly. Then apply a liberal amount of vaseline or toilet lanolin and gently massage the skin of the feet.

4. *Always* keep your feet *warm*. Wear woolen socks or wool-lined shoes in the winter and white cotton socks in warm weather. Wear a clean pair of socks each day.

5. Use loose-fitting bedsocks instead of hot-water bottles, electric heaters, or any other form of mechanical heating devices.

6. Wear properly fitted shoes and be particularly careful that they are not too tight. Use shoes made of soft leather and without box toes.

7. Cut your toenails only in very good light and only after your feet have been cleansed thoroughly. Cut the toenails straight across.

8. Do not cut your corns or calluses.

9. Do not wear circular garters.

10. Do not sit with your legs crossed.

11. Do not use strong antiseptic drugs on your feet.

12. Go to your doctor at the first signs of a blister, infection of the toes, ingrowing toenail, or trouble with bunions, corns, or calluses.

13. Drink at least four quarts of water each day.

14. Eat plenty of green vegetables and fruit in an otherwise well-balanced, liberal diet, unless you have been ordered to follow some special diet.

15. Do not use tobacco in any form.

16. Have some member of your family examine your feet at least once each week.

Finally the doctor can make recommendations relative to the care of the legs, the improvement of the circulation, and other methods that will be helpful in controlling this condition.

BUNIONS See discussion under *Feet*.

BURNS Burns of the skin are among the most frequent of all injuries. In World War II they constituted approximately one third of the injuries suffered by men in the United States Navy.

In any exceedingly serious burn the first attention is given to shock. Eighty per cent of the total deaths from burns result from secondary shock. When the body is burned, plasma—the fluid material—is lost from the burned surface. Plasma also leaves the blood vessels and passes into the tissues, so that the circulating blood becomes concentrated. That is the reason why plasma is given and not whole blood.

Cases of extensive burns of the body sometimes result in death. Seldom is there recovery for anyone who has as much as one half of the surface of the body burned. Children die in many instances when even less than one half of the skin is burned.

Each year approximately 6000 fatal burns and scalds occur in the United States, and 40 per cent of the deaths concern children under fifteen years of age. The number of deaths is much smaller in the five months from May through September because children spend more time out of doors. The rate is higher in winter when the home fires are burning and the children are exposed to accidents. Stoves, grates, hot water, and matches account for about 60 per cent of the deaths from burns. In early childhood hot water is the leading cause of accidental burns. Electric burns are in their ultimate effects about the same as burns by direct heat. To prevent such burns as have been mentioned, babies and young children should be kept away from contact with boiling water, hot radiators, and similar sources of burns. Kettles, teapots, and cups of tea and coffee should be placed only where they will be inaccessible to children.

In various industries and in the Army and Navy where there are burn hazards, the use of asbestos gloves, helmets, and linings is being adopted. Also, as one of the discoveries of this war, there is the possibility of the use of burnproof or flameproof clothing.

Doctors classify burns into first-degree, second-degree, and third-degree burns. The classification concerns the extent of the surface burned and the depth of the burn.

For an ordinary burn it is customary in first aid to cover the area that is burned with a sterile or clean cloth at once and to sustain the patient by giving fluids. A doctor can give a narcotic by injection to relieve pain.

In a technic recently developed in the Navy the burned area is cleansed with soap and water, if this is not too seriously damaging to tissue, then treated with a mixture of blood plasma, to which have been added sulfonamides and enough tragacanth to make a fairly thick ointment. The area is then covered with layers of gauze soaked in warm normal salt solution, and over this is placed some wax paper, held in position by adhesive tape around the edges attached to good skin.

For ordinary home treatment the simple application of sterile gauze, soaked in warm normal salt solution, will do for most burns until they can have medical attention. In the case of serious burns, which are best treated in the hospital, it is customary to inject blood plasma and to relieve pain by the use of narcotic drugs. Pieces of skin that have become loosened are cut away with sterile instruments; then the protective dressings are applied.

Many different applications have been suggested to relieve pain and prevent infection in burns. Boric-acid ointment is applied to simple burns. In the British Army and Navy a triple dye ointment is used. Sometimes melted paraffin of light consistency is applied by the use of a spray mechanism. Most important is the prevention of contact with any germs from the nose and throat of the person who is caring for the one who has been burned. Generally a gauze mask can be worn to prevent germs from the nose and throat getting on to the burned area.

One of the most serious effects of burns is the possibility of scarring. That is the reason such careful attention is required by the surgeon in a case of severe burning of the skin. Sometimes scarring is so severe as to require plastic surgery with transplantation of skin from other parts of the body to take care of the defects that occur.

BURSITIS In certain portions of the body where there is likely to be much rubbing or pressure, there are little sacs of fluid which serve to minimize the effects of irritation. A bursa is a sort of shock-absorbing sac of fluid which helps to lubricate friction points in various portions of the body. Some of these are found at the top of the shoulder, some of them in back of the shoulder blades, some of them over the hips, and others in other places. Sometimes a bursa will form where there is repeated friction or irritation, as for example over a bunion.

When a bursa is bruised, irritated, or infected, it responds with an excess amount of fluid. If the injury is serious, blood will be mixed with the fluid. Bursas near the surface of the body can be felt with the fingers. When they are deep in the tissues, they make their presence known by pain which is worse on motion.

Housemaid's knee is a form of bursitis which results from chronic pressure on the kneecap associated with kneeling on the floor. Miner's elbow is a similar condition which affects the elbows of miners. Sometimes there is a bursa at the hip joint, sometimes under the buttocks, and occasionally at the back of the leg where the long tendon comes up from the heel. One of the most frequently irritated bursas is that under the big muscle over the shoulder. When such bursas become inflamed and when calcium gets deposited in them, they can cause disability and sometimes become so constantly painful as to interfere with sleep. The prevention of irritation or inflammation of a bursa depends on avoiding the source of irritation.

Cortisone can be injected directly into bursas to give relief in many cases of bursitis.

Surgeons treat bursas by placing a needle in the sac and removing the excess fluid. Continuous application of heat and rest will permit absorption of the excess fluid, if the original cause of irritation or inflammation is removed. The application of the X ray has been helpful in many cases. Sometimes surgery is necessary to remove the bursa completely.

CAESAREAN OPERATION

Whenever it becomes necessary to open the abdomen and then the uterus to aid the birth of a child, the procedure is called a caesarean operation. The term comes from the name of Julius Caesar who is said to have been born by this route. Formerly such an operation was an exceedingly dangerous performance. Nowadays with the development of new forms of anesthesia, new technics for controlling hemorrhage and new methods for determining the state and position of the child before it is born, the operation has much less risk. When the operation is performed by a competent obstetrician in a good hospital, the results are usually favorable. Frequently the operation saves life of both mother and child.

CAISSON DISEASE

This condition, also called compressed-air illness, the bends, and divers' palsy, develops in people, particularly in divers and those working in tunnels, who have been working under high atmospheric pressure and then been subjected to rapid reduction of air pressure. Under these conditions the nitrogen from the air dissolved in the body gets loose in the blood as nitrogen bubbles which obstruct the circulation.

The chief symptoms of caisson disease are pain in the legs or abdomen, dizziness or staggers, itching of the skin, asphyxia, and nervous symptoms.

Experience has shown that recompression of the worker and then slow decompression overcomes the symptoms of caisson disease. If the symptoms are not promptly relieved, the worker is placed in the high-pressure chamber or tunnel and is allowed to remain for a long time (overnight soak), thereafter receiving gradual decompression.

CALAMINE

A pink powder of zinc oxide with a small amount of ferric oxide used as a base for lotions and ointments for protecting injured skin.

CALCIUM

Calcium is a chemical element out of which bones, teeth, and similar hard structures of the body are composed. Calcium is prescribed, therefore, to aid the growth of bones and teeth. It also has definite effects in regulating the activities of the nervous system. The use of calcium in the body is dependent on adequate amounts of vitamins A, D, and C and also on effective action of the parathyroid gland. All of these are concerned in the mechanisms by which calcium is used in the body.

CALCULI

A calculus is a stone or a concretion occurring in the animal body and usually made of a mixture of mineral salts. The most common calculi are the gallstones, kidney stones, and bladder stones but of course calculi may occur in any tissue where calcium or other mineral material is deposited.

CALLUSES (See also discussion under *Feet*) A callus is a new tissue that is formed when a bone heals. Hardened tissue elsewhere in the body, such as a thickening of the skin due to friction, pressure, or other irritation, is called a callosity.

CALORIES Calories are units by which the energy intake of the body is measured. The usual calory is the amount of heat required to raise 1 cubic centimeter of water 1 degree centigrade.

CAMPHOR Camphor is a substance obtained from the camphor tree, applied to the mucous membranes and the skin as a mild irritant or antiseptic, occasionally used by injection to stimulate the circulation of the blood.

CANCER A baby keeps on growing within the body of its mother at an exceedingly rapid rate until it is born and then at a steadily diminishing rate until the child emerges into an adult. At all times the rate of growth is under control by factors within the body. Wornout cells of the human body disappear and are replaced by new ones which grow with sufficient rapidity to keep the body in repair. Sometimes, however, cells begin to grow wildly. They grow so fast that new cells appear faster than old ones disappear. This results in the accumulation of masses of cells in the form of a lump, which is called a tumor. If the lump grows so fast that it destroys other tissues near by and prevents their growth, it is a malignant tumor. Cancers do not stop growing in the vast majority of cases once they have begun. Most serious of all, however—portions of the cancer may get away from the original lump and spread through the body. These are called metastases and are secondary cancers,

frequently far removed from the original growth, which is called the primary lesion of primary cancer.

No one knows the exact cause of cancer. However, scientists have established certain factors that are important in stimulating the growth of cancer. Sometimes language is used to replace established fact. One can say that a cancer is a special condition in the body that causes tissues to grow with great rapidity and without regard to the health of the body. One can say that something disturbs the balance between the cells of different kinds so that some grow much more rapidly than others and without restraint. One investigator said that a cancer is a return of the cells of the body to their primitive state or to the type of cell that occurs in the body of the child before birth. Another has said that cancer appears because some factor in the body that regulates the growth of the cells ceases to function. These definitions, because certainly they are not established by evidence, may point toward the nature of the cause of cancer. Already, as will be explained later, substances are known that can stimulate the growth of cancer cells. These are called cancerigenic, which merely means they are substances that can cause the growth of cancer. In many instances, however, none of the substances that has been mentioned can be directly related to the growth of the cancer. Conceivably, although we know scores of cancerigenic substances, there may be many others of which we do not know. The possibility that there may be many different substances capable of stimulating rapid unrestrained growth of cells makes the problem of controlling cancer much more difficult.

MANY KINDS OF CANCER—Doctors classify cancers according to the nature of the tissue in the cancer, the speed of its growth, the portion of the body that may be affected, and sometimes even according to the chemical changes that take place in the cancerous tissue. One simple classification divides cancers into those that can be seen and felt, which are easily detected; those that are not seen or felt but which can be suspected because of unusual bleeding; those that cannot be seen or felt and which do not give any signs of their presence as by bleeding or an unusual discharge but which cause symptoms such as pain or failure of certain portions of the body to perform their functions, so that the victim becomes aware that something is wrong. Last and most difficult are the cancers that do not give any sign or symptom until they are so far along in their progress that nothing can be done about them. Fortunately the last group is the smallest.

A cancer of the skin, the mouth, or the breast can usually be seen or felt. Women are much less likely to die of cancer of the skin than men; women are careful about their appearance. Men have always suffered more from cancer of the mouth than women. Lately, however, the number of cases of cancer of the mouth found in women is increasing, and some investigators believe that this can be related to the more widespread practice of smoking by women.

Cancers of the breast are far more frequent in women than in men because of the nature of the tissue in the breast.

Most conspicuous of the cancers that cannot be seen or felt but which warn of their presence by unusual bleeding are cancers of the urinary bladder or kidney or of the organs of women that are associated with childbirth.

Most dangerous of all cancers are those of the stomach, brain, bowels, or lungs. These are likely to come on insidiously and therefore fail to be detected until any form of control is a major problem.

Ask any doctor today why modern medicine does not save more lives of people who have cancer; he will say that they came too late to the attention of competent surgeons, radiologists, or other physicians capable of giving modern treatment. Why do people reach the hopeless stages of cancer before seeking help? One reason is ignorance, even of the simple facts that are told here. Another is fear—fear that the condition may be cancer. Some people just do not like doctors or surgeons. Still others think that diagnosis and treatment may be expensive. In a recent study only 2 out of 150 people with far advanced cancer had delayed seeking attention for that reason. More than half the people who delayed too long did so because they just did not think the condition was serious.

In different parts of the body cancer indicates its presence in different ways:

THE MOUTH—Any sore in the mouth that lasts more than a few days without healing should be regarded with suspicion. When thick white patches form on the tongue and cheeks, the condition is called leukoplakia, which merely means thick white patches. These have been discovered, however, to have a relation to the formation of cancer and should be considered a warning sign.

THE LARYNX—Hoarseness that lasts more than a few days is a suspicion that there is something seriously wrong with the larynx or voice box and with the vocal cords. The doctor can look directly at the vocal cords, using suitable instruments that have been developed for the purpose. He can then determine the nature of the disturbance and give suitable advice about recovering the voice. If he finds that there is even a suspicion of a new growth, he has various technics for removing it.

THE BREAST—Any discomfort, pain, thickening, or lump in the breast of a woman or of a man, or any discharge from the nipple, either a bloody discharge or a thin serum, should demand an immediate expert examination.

THE STOMACH—Whenever a person finds it difficult to swallow, whenever there is loss of appetite, constant discomfort, nausea, diarrhea, or the appearance of black material in the bowel movements, careful study should be made as to the presence of cancer in the esophagus (the swallowing tube), the stomach, or the bowels.

THE FEMALE ORGANS—Irregular bleeding is always a sign that something is wrong; prolonged bleeding also means that something is wrong. Every woman after thirty-five years of age should be examined at least once each year to determine whether or not the tissues related to childbirth are normal. Such an examination is not too difficult, and it may mean the difference between life and death.

NEW AIDS TO DIAGNOSIS OF CANCER—The early diagnosis of cancer is aided nowadays by a variety of instruments and methods that were not available as recently as twenty years ago. All sorts of instruments, gadgets, and tests have been found which are applicable in such cases. Remember that every lump in the breast is not necessarily a cancer. The doctor will make this decision by asking the patient about her symptoms, by the use of the hands to determine whether or not there are lumps that can be felt, even though they cannot be seen, by looking at the surface of the breast to see if a lump is visible or if the nipple has been drawn back or if it is fixed in its position. He may use the X ray to find out whether the tissues of the breast are of a uniform density. He may look at the breast with a light that is cast through the tissues. If there are lumps or growths in the breast, the light will fail to pass through wherever a lump is present. When a suspicious growth is discovered a small section may be taken from the growth. This can be examined immediately under the microscope to determine whether or not it is cancer. The removal of pieces of tissue for examination is called biopsy; that merely means examination of living tissue. The cancer cell, when seen under the microscope, is quite different from ordinary cells. The difference is chiefly in the presence of changes that indicate rapid growth.

Among the most recent medical discoveries is a technic which has come to be known as the Papanicolaou test for cancer. In this test scrapings are taken from the surface of the cervix of the uterus or from the walls of the vagina. After treatment with proper substances, immediate examination under the microscope will reveal the presence of the abnormal cells of cancer. If there is a suspicion that there may be cancer of the lungs, material coughed up from the lungs is submitted to a similar examination. A tube may be passed into the stomach and material from the inside lining of the stomach can be examined. These tests have already aided the rapid detection of cancer beyond any technics previously known.

One of the areas in which the most important studies are now being made has to do with the attempt to develop a blood test for cancer that will be at least as positive in its decisions as the blood test that is made for the presence of syphilis. At present several such tests are undergoing study in different parts of the world. Not one of the tests thus far developed is considered sufficiently accurate to warrant its general application as a means of detecting the presence of cancer. Nevertheless, the methods used are well established and may yet yield positive information which will lead to an accurate test. Indeed one of the most recent technics under process of investigation is the attempt to use a device like the electric eye to separate cancer cells from normal cells. The idea is based on the fact that the cancer cell is different in appearance and that an electrical method of measuring variation in appearance may be more certain than is the eye of the physician who looks at the cancer cells under the microscope.

IS CANCER CAUSED BY A GERM?—Some investigators believe that cancer may be caused by a virus, a form of living growth too small to be seen under the microscope—small enough indeed to pass through the pores of a clay filter. Already there seems to be evidence that certain filtrable substances of this type may be able to produce cancers. A factor that passes through the milk, at least in mice of a cancer strain, has been indicted as being capable of producing cancer in other mice. This is known as the Bittner milk factor.

All sorts of studies are being made along these and similar lines by a vast organization known as the Committee on Growth of the Division of Medical

Sciences of the National Research Council. This committee is broken up into many subcommittees dealing with every phase of study of cancer. Their investigations point toward the development of far more knowledge of the chemistry, physiology, genetics, biology, and pathology than modern medicine has ever had previously.

Another technic that has aroused great interest is the attempt to grow tumors in the yolk sacs of developing chicks. This is the method by which viruses are grown and distinguished one from another. Already some success has been had with the growing of tumors from the breast and with another form of cancer called sarcoma. This inclines the investigators to the belief that cancer may be in some instances the result of a virus. However, there is also the possibility that whole living cells may have been taken from tumors and, since these are small enough to pass the filter, they might have duplicated themselves under proper conditions of growth.

Among the most interesting of recent observations, however, is the determination that hormones, or materials derived from the glands in the body that pass their secretions directly into the blood, may have the ability to stimulate the growth of cancers. These include particularly female and male sex hormones, called estrogen and testosterone respectively. Thus scientific evidence has already proved that an excess of the estrogenic hormone may stimulate the growth of cancer of the breast in animals and that conversely the female sex hormone may delay, if not stop, the growth of cancers of the prostate in men. A great study in which many clinics participated has proved that testosterone, the male sex hormone, can inhibit the growth of cancers in the breasts of women and indeed that it is of great importance in stopping secondary growths from cancers of the breast in women. Thus again, for emphasis, there may not be any single cause of cancer but that any factor which regulates growth of living cells may be a factor in stimulating the growth of cancers.

Is CANCER HEREDITARY?—Usually the question is asked, Is cancer hereditary? Studies made on innumerable strains of mice and on the family histories of great numbers of people have proved that cancer occurs more frequently in the families of cancer patients than in any other class of families. Thus tumors may develop only when the soil is suitable for their development, and such soil may be far more frequent in the bodies of families with a cancer history than in other families. For that reason women whose mothers or grandmothers have died of cancer of the breast are told to be careful about taking excessive quantities of female sex gland hormones. Certainly they should inform their physicians of the heredity so that the physician may be aware of the possibilities.

In addition to such cancer-stimulating substances as tars, X rays, and other unusual forms of radiation, sunburn, viruses, and hormones, other chemical substances may on occasion be related to cancer. Since cancer is a change in growth of an individual cell and since such changes are associated with changes in the chemistry of the body chemical substances may have a relation to cancer. Physical contributing causes are known, because continuous irritation of the skin by a rough collar at the back of the neck, by the stay of a foundation garment which constantly grinds at the breast or the tissues near by, by a rough tooth within the mouth, may stimulate excessive and unrestrained growth of the cells. Similarly a burn of the lip, constantly irritated by holding a pipestem or a cigarette or cigar at exactly the same place, may result in a sore that will not heal and which eventually may become a cancer.

Of special interest are various forms of overgrowth of the cells in the blood which are sometimes called cancers of the blood. If there is an excessive growth of red blood cells, the condition is called polycythemia. If the white blood cells grow rapidly, the condition is leukemia. If the glands that carry the lymph grow very rapidly, the condition may be Hodgkin's disease. All these are manifestations of rapid, unrestrained growth and may be cancer. In the examination for changes in the blood a recent step is the taking of a small amount of bone marrow by the use of a punch and the examination of the bone marrow under the microscope, since this will yield information as to the rate of growth of the blood cells which ordinarily are produced in the bone marrow.

TREATMENT OF CANCER—Not many years have passed since the only way of treating cancer was the use of surgery. Surgical removal of a cancer does not, of course, remove the cause except as that cause may be a part of the cancer. Nowadays the approach to cancer is varied, owing to great discoveries that have been made in many places. Surgery is still the recommended method of treatment for certain forms of cancer which cannot apparently be approached in any other way. There are, however, differences of opinion as to whether surgery alone, X rays alone, radium alone, or various combinations of two or three of these technics should be applied in different forms of cancer. Indeed there is now added the use of various chemical substances which have been proved to have positive effects on cancers. Thus a cancer of the prostate gland—of course the prostate is found only in men and not in women—may be attacked by surgical removal, by castration in order to remove the testicle completely and thus to get rid of the stimulating hormone which comes from the testis, or by the giving of the female sex hormone, estrogen, which is antagonistic to that of the male.

A cancer of the larynx may be attacked by the use of surgery or X ray or radium, or perhaps combinations. A cancer of the breast may involve the use of surgery and of X ray after the operation. In late cases the treatment may be X ray alone, and in severe cases the use of the male sex hormone may produce a palliation and lessening of pain.

Among the very latest of substances being applied in studies of cancer treatment is a product in various forms known as aminopterin and teropterin. A substance called folic acid has the power to stimulate the growth of blood cells. The substance called aminopterin opposes folic acid. Therefore it has been used in an attempt to control rapid growth of cells, and there seems to be evidence that in some instances it does delay growth because patients may say that they feel better and suffer less pain. In addition aminopterin has been applied with some success in attacking leukemia, which, as previously explained, means an excessive number of white blood cells.

Most exciting of all the recent approaches toward cancer are the uses of radioactive isotopes. Already medical literature shows instances in which radioactive phosphorus has been used with benefit in leukemia, in polycythemia, and in Hodgkin's disease. The isotopes have the special value of representing radioactivity combined with a chemical element. Since these chemical elements are likely to go, for the major part, directly to one tissue of the body, various radioactive isotopes are used for tumors in different places. By far most of the iodine in the human body is centralized in the thyroid gland. Already there are records of cancer of the thyroid treated successfully with radioactive iodine. Iron, sodium, potassium, chlorine, bromine, calcium, strontium, sulfur, carbon, and hydrogen have also been subjects of experiments in treating growths in various portions of the body. Radioactive phosphorus, incidentally, has also been applied externally to warts, moles, and other growths on the surface of the body and in some instances with apparent success.

During World War II it was discovered by the Chemical Warfare Service that chemicals known as the nitrogen mustards had the power to damage the formation of white blood cells. Now these nitrogen mustards have been tried on Hodgkin's disease, chronic leukemia, and various forms of tumors, and the results have been interesting, even though apparently the method is not curative. Quite recently also a substance called urethane, and scientifically known as stilbamidine, has been used in cancers particularly affecting the white blood cells. Thus the outlook for continued progress is better than ever before.

Much of the progress depends on intricate, complex chemical studies of the tissues that become cancerous. Out of such tissues chemical substances may be developed which will have the power of being antagonistic to the growth of cancer cells. In one series of investigations living organisms have been found which tend to localize in cancer cells but they have to be tamed so as not to destroy the patient.

Notwithstanding the fact that we are only at the very brink of knowledge related to the chemistry of cancers and of substances antagonistic to cancers, that knowledge may be the ultimate answer. It will provide a form of control over cancer that does not require the use of methods that destroy or remove tissues, such as surgery, radium, or X ray, which are now our chief reliance.

CANKER SORES This term usually applies to small ulcerations that appear on the inside of the mouth and lips and on the cheeks. They may be due to a variety of causes—sometimes wholly nervous, sometimes due to sensitivity to various substances that are taken into the body The exact cause of the canker sore is seldom determined since the condition tends to heal promptly with proper treatment, usually the application of some mild astringent substance. Whenever canker sores appear persistently, however, it is customary to make a scientific study of the patient, including a study of the blood, to determine whether or not there is present a sufficient amount of the substances involved in clotting of the blood. Tests are made of sensitivity to various foods. Occasionally also studies are made to determine the nature of the fillings in the teeth, since it has been shown that dissimilar metals used as fillings for teeth may create electrical currents which, in turn, are associated with the appearance of cankers in the mouth.

CANTHARIDES A substance derived from the dried bodies of Spanish or Russian flies and used as an irritant. Formerly cantharides were given internally to stimulate sex activity. Because of their poisonous character the internal use of cantharides is never justified.

CARBOHYDRATES Carbohydrates is the scientific name for sugars, starches, celluloses, and gums.

CARBON DISULFIDE One of the most widely used substances in modern industry is carbon disulfide. In the rayon industry it is used in the preparation of viscose; in the rubber industry it is used as a solvent for rubber and rubber cement; in fumigation it serves as an insecticide; in chemistry it is used to dissolve fats, oils, and phosphorus. It is also used in the manufacture of many other drugs. From time to time it has been used in the dry-cleaning industry and also on occasions for the care of the hair.

Carbon disulfide is so poisonous that it should never be used except under proper controls. If there is a high concentration of this substance in the air to the extent of 5000 parts per 1,000,000 by volume, death can occur from exposure over one half to one hour. With half that amount there is danger to life. With one fifth of that amount there may still be some symptoms.

When acute poisoning occurs, there is unconsciousness which may be preceded by delirium. Less severe exposure results in headache, dizziness, trouble with breathing, pain over the heart, and disturbances of digestion. More common, however, than acute poisoning with this substance is chronic poisoning. In the latter condition there are toxic effects on the nerve structures and the blood. Such symptoms as easy fatigue, loss of memory, heaviness of the limbs, and dizziness may occur. There may be insomnia during the night and sleepiness during the day, also loss of appetite, pain in the intestinal tract, and similar disturbances. Some people complain of foggy vision; others suffer from blinding flashes of colored lights.

Because of these dangers it is recommended that carbon disulfide always be handled in sealed rooms or vats so that the fumes cannot get in contact with the human body. Whenever it is used as a solvent, there should be forced ventilation, and all of the vapor should be removed as rapidly as it is formed by the use of exhaust ventilation. Because the gas is explosive, arrangements must be made so that it should not come in contact with hot pipes, hot plates, or hot electric bulbs. Workers in plants who may have to go into rooms where there is much carbon disulfide vapor should be provided with masks through which they breathe and with safety belts with which they can be drawn from the room.

There is the possibility of irritation through contact of the skin with carbon disulfide. Rubber gloves are not a protection because carbon disulfide dissolves and penetrates rubber gloves.

Any worker who has to be constantly in contact with this substance should have regular physical examinations, including studies back of the eye with the ophthalmoscope, and laboratory studies of the blood. Whenever a worker with carbon disulfide suddenly collapses as a result of acute poisoning, he should be transferred at once to fresh air, soiled garments should be removed, and the skin should be washed with large quantities of alcohol to remove the toxic material. A doctor should be called at once to take care of the breathing and of the heart.

CARBON MONOXIDE POISONING

Carbon monoxide gas is produced by imperfect oxidation of any carboniferous material. It therefore develops from the burning of charcoal, coal oil, illuminating gas, or other types of heating appliances which depend on combustion of coal or oil. The most frequent source of carbon monoxide gas in modern life is the exhaust of the automobile. The gas is especially dangerous because it is odorless and colorless, and insidious as a poison. When it gets into the blood, it unites with the red coloring matter so that it cannot carry oxygen. The blood of people who have been poisoned with carbon monoxide gas has a bright cherry color, due to the formation of the combination that is described. Sometimes the aftereffects of carbon monoxide gas poisoning are serious and result in permanent damage to the brain because of a lack of oxygen over a considerable period of time. Thus there may be serious disturbances of memory, vision, hearing, and speech or the appearance of unusual psychoses.

In an earlier day miners used to carry canary birds into mines because such birds are especially sensitive to carbon monoxide gas. Nowadays it is possible to buy carbon monoxide indicators which indicate by a direct reading of the meter how much carbon monoxide is present in the air.

When a person has been poisoned by carbon monoxide, he should not be permitted to make any physical exertion but should lie down and be kept warm. Inhalations of oxygen or of a carbon dioxide mixture are desirable since the inhaling of pure oxygen accelerates the release of the carbon monoxide, freeing it from the blood about four times as rapidly as would the inhalation of air.

From time to time various methods of injection have been suggested as a treatment for carbon monoxide, including the use of methylene blue. However, such substances are seldom immediately available.

The person with carbon monoxide poisoning, if the case is at all serious, should be taken at once to a hospital where proper medication and even blood transfusions may be tried.

CARBUNCLES A carbuncle is an infection of the deeper layers of the skin and of the tissues under the skin, usually caused by a germ of the streptococcus group.

When the resistance of the tissues to infection is weakened by such conditions as rubbing with a saw-edged collar on the back of the neck, the projecting edge of a broken corset steel, or some similar material, when the person has diabetes or Bright's disease, or a diet containing too much of some substances and not enough of others, the tissues fail to exert sufficient defense to prevent the streptococcus from setting up its infection.

When the infection starts, the tissues become inflamed and red; the white blood cells are brought to the part affected, where they attack the germs and pus is formed in large amounts. The tissues then begin to wall off the infected area; a pocket is formed with a center of degenerated and infected material. One of the great dangers of such a condition is the breaking down of the wall of resistance and the spread of the infection throughout the body.

When the physician is called to examine such a case, the first thing he does is to determine whether any of the contributing diseases that have been mentioned is present. If it is, he at once takes steps to control it, limiting the amount of carbohydrates and sugars that are taken into the body. He will relieve the pain by the application of hot moist dressings. These serve also to bring more blood to the part affected and aid the attack upon the infection.

When a considerable amount of pus or infectious material is present, the carbuncle or boil must be opened and the infection permitted to drain. The physician does this carefully so as not to break down the retaining wall and spread the infection. The pus should be withdrawn as rapidly and completely as possible.

Since a carbuncle represents an infection by a germ of the streptococcus group, treatment with sulfonamide drugs such as sulfanilamide powder or sulfathiazole or sulfadiazine, and treatment with penicillin will do much to control the infection. The nature of these drugs is such that the dosage to be used and the method of application should be prescribed by the physician.

If the infection seems to be spreading, it is customary to inject a local anesthetic around the infected area at a distance far enough to be in sound tissue and then to open the infected area widely so as to be sure that all of the infectious material is removed.

Nothing breaks down the health of human beings so quickly and certainly as long-continued infection. Hence it is advised that patients who have been suffering with multiple boils be provided with a good routine hygiene which will build their general resistance and prevent the continuous formation of new infected areas.

CARCINOMA See *Cancer*.

CARDIOVASCULAR DISEASES See discussion under *Heart*.

CARRIERS OF DISEASE Common terms used in discussing the spread of infectious diseases are not well understood by many people; for instance, "contagious" and "infectious." A contagious disease is catching; the term usually implies "spread by direct or personal contact," since the word "contagious" comes from a word meaning to touch. An infectious disease may be carried not directly but indirectly. The distinction is an artificial one. Many infectious diseases are contagious, and contagious diseases are infectious. A better term is "communicable disease," which means that the disease can be passed from one person to another.

The carrier is a frequent medium of communication. About one third of people who have typhoid fever continue to discharge the germs for three weeks after the beginning of the disease, and about 10 per cent continue to discharge the germs for from eight to ten weeks. From 2 to 4 per cent, however, may continue to discharge the germs permanently. These people are known as chronic typhoid carriers.

There are innumerable similar cases now available in medical literature which prove definitely that a person who is infected chronically with typhoid germs must exercise extreme care in the handling of food and water to be used by other people. Especially important are new attempts to control this type of typhoid carrier by operating on the gall bladder. In many such cases the chronic typhoid carrier may be cured by removal of the gall bladder, which today is done with a fair degree of safety.

The health department of Massachusetts, which has given special attention to this problem, reported 75 to 100 known carriers in that state and estimated that there are probably 1100 carriers in Massachusetts who could be detected by a careful investigation. This is an indication of how many thousands there must be in the whole United States.

The discovery of new drugs, like the sulfa drugs, and of tetraiodophthalein, which, for instance, can localize in the gall bladder, and the use of radioactivated drugs and dyes, has stimulated a great deal of additional research toward controlling carriers of disease.

Human beings suffer with diseases which are transmitted from animals, directly or indirectly by insects, and by other living species which carry the organisms responsible for setting up disturbances.

The human being also becomes infected from contact with germs that are transmitted to him from other human beings who have previously been infected. The organisms may come from the secretions of the nose, throat, and mouth; through coughing, sneezing, spitting, and kissing; through contamination with secretions from the eyes, such as may come when one uses a handkerchief or towel that has previously been used by an infected person; through contamination from the excretions of the intestines and of the urinary tract; and even from contact with organisms that are on the human skin.

These organisms are transferred from one person to another by direct contact, by contamination from sewage, food, water, air, dust, and dirt, and by contamination from towels and similar utensils. Finally, a human being may be bitten by an insect which takes his blood and later inoculates it into another human being. So far as the spread of disease is concerned, the human carrier is a constant menace.

Moreover, mass activities of mankind, such as attendance in tremendous numbers on motion pictures, baseball and football games, elevators, apartments, and office buildings tend to increase contact with diseased persons.

Among the diseases spread by secretions from the nose and throat are streptococcal infections, pneumonia, septic sore throat, meningitis, diphtheria, infantile paralysis, scarlet fever, measles, whooping cough, mumps, the common cold, influenza, tuberculosis, and Vincent's angina. Among the diseases of the eye transmitted are pink eye, trachoma, and gonorrheal ophthalmia. The intestinal disorders include typhoid, dysentery, cholera, amebic infection, hookworm, tapeworm, pinworm, and schistosomiasis.

Many of the organisms maintain special locations in the body; for example the typhoid organism in the gall bladder, and the various worms in the intestinal tract. The venereal diseases are spread by contact with carriers who have been previously infected.

Organisms that live in the blood and that are carried from one person to another by insects are the plasmodium of malaria, carried by the anopheles mosquito. Other diseases carried by mosquitoes are dengue, yellow fever, and filariasis.

The trypanosome of sleeping sickness is carried by the tsetse fly. Typhus fever and trench fever are transmitted by the louse. Bubonic plague is carried by the flea. Rocky Mountain spotted fever is carried by a tick. Other insects suspected of carrying disease, but not absolutely incriminated, include bedbugs, water bugs, cockroaches, and ants.

Among animal carriers of disease are the dog and various wild animals of the dog type which transmit hydrophobia; the cat, which has been incriminated with the transmission of diphtheria; the cow, which, by way of its meat, may transmit various worms, and by way of its milk, tuberculosis, septic sore throat, and undulant fever; the sheep is incriminated with the transmission of anthrax; the goat with Malta fever; various fish in connection with tapeworms; the oyster with typhoid; the hog with trichina and various worms; the rat with plague and ratbite fever; the rabbit with tularemia; and the parrot family with psittacosis.

Among human pets the cat and dog enjoy most intimate contact with man. They are likely to share not only his living quarters but in some families even his bed and board. Nobody knows how many dogs there are in the United States, but everyone knows that there are innumerable dogs and cats without any apparent owners, which move from one place to another, living on scraps of garbage, and which are a menace not only to man but to one another.

The chief danger from dog to man from the point of view of its severity is rabies, or hydrophobia. This is spread primarily by the bite of a dog, although other animals may be affected. In addition the dog is undoubtedly the source of certain tapeworms which spread to man, and occasionally certain forms of ringworm will be passed from dog to man.

Distemper and respiratory infections occur in dogs as well as in human beings but differ in their nature. It has been reported that the dog may act as a carrier of scarlet fever or diphtheria, but obviously the opportunity for such transmission is relatively rare.

The cat is fairly resistant to most human diseases, but apparently the cat can be infected with undulant fever and transfer it to man. It can develop hydrophobia. It carries around multiple parasites and tapeworms but is not likely to carry plague or tularemia.

The cat or dog may obviously be the carrier of various insects that transfer from them to man when opportunity offers. A pet animal in the household must therefore receive the same attentions from a hygienic point of view as are given to children.

Regular washing, prompt treatment of diseases, and similar hygienic procedures are necessary to avoid the transferring of contagions from animals to man.

CAR SICKNESS See discussion under *Seasickness*.

CASCARA Cascara is a laxative substance widely used for habitual constipation. It is made from the bark of a tree. Its action is mostly on the colon. Usually cascara is prescribed by doctors in the form of an aromatic extract of cascara.

CASTOR OIL Castor oil is one of the oldest household remedies for constipation. It is an effective and prompt cathartic but is likely to be followed by constipation and is, therefore, seldom used in chronic constipation.

CATARACT A cataract is a clouding of the lens of the eye which acts very much like the frosting on a glass. It prevents the suitable passage of distinct images. Thus the complete development of a cataract results in blindness. There are all sorts of classifications of cataracts, depending on their nature, their state of progress, and their possible causes. A person may have a cataract in one eye or in both, although it is rather common to have cataracts in both eyes, either developing at the same time or separately.

If you happen to be troubled with red eyelids, defective vision, inexplicable headaches which develop during the day, or drowsiness from reading or close work, consult a physician who specializes in diseases of the eye as soon as possible. A cataract is not a growth or a tumor.

Most cases of cataract occur in people between fifty and sixty years of age but occasionally the condition occurs in young people who may be born with cataract.

Because of the psychological factors associated with vision it has been possible for all sorts of quacks to offer special treatments for cataract that do not involve surgical operation. The desire to see better is so great that the person is willing to admit he sees better following any sort of medical treatment. Don't believe these charlatans. There are no drugs, no drops of any kind, no exercises or treatments which are successful in stopping the slow development of a cataract. There are, however, operations which are successful in the vast majority of cases and which are now capable of being performed by competent men all over the United States. In India trained operators remove cataracts from aged Hindus. When a cataract is removed, the effect is the same as the defrosting of a window or the letting up of a shade. Light gets in again, and the person is again able to see. The operation does not injure the front of the eye in any way, and the pupil of the eye is preserved.

After a cataract is removed the person wears what are known as cataract glasses, made so that they will help to fix the image properly on the retina. The person who has been unable to see for some time because of a cataract, who has been unable to play golf or to get about, and who then recovers his sight by the simple operation that any specialist in diseases of the eye can perform is usually most thankful for the benefits of medical science. Good vision follows 97 per cent of the operations for cataract. Ridley of London has developed an artificial lens of plastic that can replace the natural lens when it is removed.

CATARRH See *Colds, Rhinitis,* et cetera. The word "catarrh" is simply an obsolete popular term for an inflammation with secretion and therefore was most usually applied to a cold with a "running" nose.

CATHARTICS AND LAXATIVES

The chief danger from cathartics and laxatives is their use in the presence of severe pain in the bowel. Such pain may be the first sign of a beginning appendicitis or some similar inflammatory condition. Never take a cathartic of any kind for abdominal pain unless the cause of the pain is known. In its earliest stages appendicitis is just a little spot of inflammation or infection of a small tube which comes off the large bowel. If this infection becomes worse, it develops the way a boil develops from a pimple. Eventually an abscess forms with the danger of bursting and spreading the infection throughout the body. When infection is spread in the abdomen, the result is peritonitis. Peritonitis is an inflammation of the membrane which lines the interior of the abdominal cavity and covers practically all of the important organs. In many cases peritonitis is fatal.

Mildest among cathartics used nowadays are mineral oil and mineral oil modified with various substances. Mineral oil is a lubricant which relieves constipation by mixing with the material in the bowel, softening it, and permitting easier passage along the intestinal tract. It is not fattening, as are other oils, because it is not absorbed by the bowels. The usual dose is one or two tablespoons.

Sometimes mineral oil is modified by the addition of a substance called agar, a form of seaweed, or by the addition of psyllium seed or other mucilaginous materials which swell when water is added and thus increase the bulk of waste material. This helps to prevent possible leakage of the oil from the orifice of the body. Apparently too much mineral oil interferes with the absorption of vitamin A.

Mineral oil has also been modified by the addition of strong laxative materials like cascara and phenolphthalein. Cascara is a plant laxative made from the bark of a tree. It is available not only mixed with mineral oil and agar but also in the form of extracts and aromatic mixtures. Phenolphthalein is a laxative now widely popularized as the basis of most advertised laxative remedies. This substance, which is a coal-tar derivative, acts on the large intestines as a purgative. Some people are especially sensitive to phenolphthalein and respond to its use with eruptions on the skin.

It is not safe to develop the cathartic or laxative habit. Constipation is much better treated by determining its cause and eliminating that cause and also by the use of enough fluid and enough fruits, vegetables, and similar laxative material in the diet.

Severe and chronic cases of constipation should not be self-treated. Much quicker and safer results will be secured by consulting a competent physician.

CECUM A portion of the bowel on the lower right side of the abdomen. The appendix comes off the cecum.

CELIAC DISEASE Babies sometimes have a condition called celiac disease. These babies are unable to digest and utilize fats, starches, and some sugars. As a result they are undernourished, their growth is stunted, they become anemic, and sometimes they have little swollen bellies.

The exact cause of the condition is sensitivity to wheat and gluten. Usually the child has decrease in appetite and fails to gain weight. There is considerable nausea, swelling of the abdomen, and the appetite is bad. The child may cry for food and appear to be hungry and yet refuse it when it is given to him. Naturally the material that passes through the bowels is quite different from that which comes from a normal child.

Since these symptoms are relatively frequent in a wide variety of conditions, it is not safe for anyone to make a guess that a certain child has the condition. It is much better to have a specialist capable of recognizing what is wrong. This is also important because children vary in the extent to which they will respond to different forms of treatment.

Because the child does not get along well particularly with starches and also with fats, it is better to watch carefully the amount of such foods that may be given. Starches are improved by being heated so that the starch is broken up into sugars. However, milk sugar and other sugars will tend to increase the amount of gas and the diarrhea. Those sugars that are best tolerated are the ones that come from fruits. Orange juice and thoroughly ripe and baked bananas may be given in fairly large amounts.

The claim has been made that bananas exert a beneficial effect. This is apparently due to the fact that wheat is stopped when banana is fed. We know, however, that protein gives little disturbance to these children, so that milk protein, egg white, lean meat, fish, chicken, liver, or gelatin, and those vegetables that are high in protein may also constitute a part of the diet of children with celiac disease. Of special advantage for these children is a preparation of milk with protein milk, which has the advantage of a high protein content with a small amount of milk sugar and only a moderate amount of fat.

These babies have to avoid butter, cream, fats, ice cream, fried food, candy, and cake. Cooked cereals may cause them to have a return of their symptoms if wheat or rye gluten is in the cereal. The monotony of their diets can, however, be overcome to some extent by flavoring the foods with cocoa and fruit flavors.

In 1952 investigators found that feeding a diet free from wheat and rye increased absorption of fat. A high caloric diet can be given with biscuits made from corn flour or soybean flour instead of wheat. When vitamin B complex is given simultaneously recovery occurs promptly.

CELLULITIS Any inflammation of the cells of the body at any point can be called a cellulitis. However, the term is usually used to refer to a deep inflammation or infection of the tissues just under the skin. Frequently pus-forming germs like the streptococcus or the staphylococcus will get into this tissue and set up such inflammations.

CEREBELLUM The small portion of the brain (which see) at the back concerned with the co-ordination of movements.

CEREBROSPINAL FLUID The fluid which is in the ventricles of the brain and the spinal cord is known as cerebrospinal fluid. When there are various types of infection of the brain and spinal cord, it is customary to put a needle into the spinal column and to obtain some of this fluid for examination. This is known as a spinal or lumbar puncture. The doctor can tell by making a Wassermann test on the cerebrospinal fluid whether or not there is syphilis affecting the nervous system. By counting the number of cells in a certain amount of cerebrospinal fluid he can tell the extent of the infection; he can also find out the nature of the germs present. From the pressure under which the fluid escapes he can find out whether or not there is pressure on the brain. Blood in the cerebrospinal fluid is a sure sign of injury somewhere along the path that the fluid follows.

CEREBRUM A word used to mean brain (which see), but particularly the large front portion of the brain, as distinct from the cerebellum.

CHAFING The skin is frequently so delicate that it responds with chafing to the irritation that comes from the rubbing together of two skin surfaces. Scientifically this is called erythema intertrigo. The inflammation occurs most often between the thighs, under the breasts, between the buttocks, and in the skin folds of the abdomen of people who are very fat. The irritation is seen especially between the fingers, and very frequently it appears between the toes, particularly the third and fourth toes. Because ringworm of the feet, or so-called athlete's foot, is common, irritation of the skin between the toes is sometimes diagnosed wrongly as athlete's foot. The only way to determine with certainty that the condition is athlete's foot is to find the parasites on the skin.

When the skin once becomes seriously rubbed and chafed, infections of various kinds easily gain entrance; quite frequently there is secondary infection. The doctor will look at the material under the microscope and make cultures to determine the nature of such infections.

The usual appearance of the skin in the condition called erythema intertrigo, or chafing between two folds of skin, is the loss of the ordinary dull tone of the skin. Instead the appearance of the tissue is smooth, shiny, slightly reddened, and somewhat moist.

Obviously the first step in controlling this condition is prevention of further rubbing. The rubbing of the two surfaces must be prevented. Stop wearing shoes that are too tight. If the rubbing occurs because of overweight, reduction of the weight is exceedingly important.

Because the skin has been denuded of its upper layers by the rubbing, the use of caustic soaps of any kind is usually forbidden. The use of ordinary ointments, pastes, and lotions commonly advertised for skin cures is dangerous because most of these also contain irritating substances and are not applicable to a skin that is chafed.

The physician who looks at the skin under these circumstances will usually determine first of all that there is no infection present. If infection is not found, the use of dressings to keep the skin surfaces from rubbing together and the use of suitable powders and soothing lotions will bring about a cure.

CHANCRE The first sign that a person has been infected with syphilis is usually the appearance on the genital organs of a sore that is called a chancre.

There are several different forms of chancre—the name depending on the appearance. The name "soft chancre" is given to a sore which is not due to syphilis but to another type of organism. This type of chancre is more scientifically called chancroid. When syphilis is properly treated, the spirochetes which are the cause of syphilis disappear from the chancre and it heals.

CHAPPED SKIN When your skin gets chapped, it is merely reacting to physical irritation. In winter the air is dry and the glands of the skin situated just below the surface are relatively inactive. They produce less moisture than usual. This, together with the increased dryness of the skin, is responsible for chapping. The lack of moisture makes the skin unelastic and brittle. Under such conditions it is more easily attacked by irritating substances such as dishwater and certain irritating soaps. The scientific name is "asteatosis" but "chapping" will do for it.

When the fat secreted by the glands in the skin is present in sufficient amounts, irritants will not attack it. Chapping does not occur where there is much perspiration. Since, however, the fat of the skin is lessened, it is necessary to apply extra fat in such cases; this can be done by the use of suitable ointments. The ordinary ointments used to prevent chapping are cold cream and vaseline.

Soaps serve to dissolve the fats from the skin and to take them away from the surface. Therefore, when the skin is chapped, soap and water should be used in great moderation. When they are used, the skin should be dried immediately, preferably with a soft towel so as not to injure the damaged tissues still further by rubbing.

If chapping has already occurred, the cold cream or other ointment may be put on thickly at night and allowed to remain on the skin. During the day it may be put on lightly and rubbed in by the hands. If the skin of a woman's face tends to chap, it may be necessary for her to apply sufficient grease to the skin whenever she is exposed to the weather conditions which cause chapping.

Particularly when an area of the skin is chapped, the avoidance of irritating substances and the application of a sufficient amount of ointment will bring the condition under control. If, however, improvement does not occur promptly, there exists the possibility of some other condition being responsible for the symptoms, or perhaps the chapping may be complicated by a special sensitivity of the skin to cold or to the weather. This can of course be determined by a specialist in diseases of the skin after a suitable examination.

The humidity of the air indoors may be increased in winter; gloves should be worn and the use of caustic soaps and solutions stopped. If the skin breaks or becomes infected, treatment must be like that given to wounds of the skin generally.

CHICKEN POX Chicken pox, one of the most contagious of children's diseases, spreads as rapidly as measles. Almost invariably from fourteen to sixteen days after a child has been in contact with another child who has chicken pox, the blisters begin to appear.

All sorts of names have been applied to chicken pox. In some parts of the country it is called water pox, glass pox, sheep pox, and crystal pox. These names usually refer to a resemblance of the blisters to the substances mentioned or to a similar disease that occurs in animals. Doctors called the disease varicella. Once it was called "variola spuria" because it used to be mistaken for smallpox, which is called "variola."

The cause of chicken pox is an agent so small that it will pass through a porous clay filter—too small to be seen with an ordinary microscope. Such toxic agents are called viruses. Contact with the material in a blister during chicken pox will produce the disease in someone who has not had it. We do not know with certainty just how the disease is usually transmitted from one person to another. We know that it is probably transmitted directly, although it may be transmitted on soiled clothing or linens. A person who has once had chicken pox is not likely to have it again.

Most cases of chicken pox occur in children from five to six years old. Actually 52 per cent of people have had it by the time they are grown up. Girls have it more often than boys, and native white children more often than foreign-born or colored children.

The best way to protect a child from chicken pox is to keep him away from other children who have the disease. Children with chicken pox should not be permitted to go to school. Whenever there is smallpox in a community, the diagnosis of chicken pox to distinguish it from the more serious disease is of the utmost importance.

In chicken pox the blisters on the skin appear in groups, usually first on the back, chest, and face but most profusely on those parts of the skin that are covered by clothing. Nobody knows how long a person who has chicken pox remains infectious for other people, but it is best to keep the person who is recovering from the disease away from other people until the skin is free from the crusts.

Usually all the treatment that is necessary in most cases of chicken pox is to make certain that the child does not scratch the spots, as there is likelihood of secondary infection. The child who has the disease should have his fingernails cut quite short to prevent scratching. If scratching cannot be stopped in any other way, it is desirable to put mittens on the hands or to place metal tubes around the elbows so that the arms cannot be bent. When the itching is sufficiently severe, however, the child will scratch itself against the side of the bed or against any other object.

Ordinarily the blisters, if let alone, will last a few hours, break, dry up, and form crusts. The crusts will then disappear in from two to four days.

Many of the people you see with pock-marked faces nowadays had chicken pox when they were young. The marks result from scratching the blisters so that there is secondary infection. If the blisters are permitted to dry of their own accord and the crusts or scabs are allowed to fall off naturally, there is seldom any mark left from the disease.

When a child has chicken pox, the chief factors in treatment are its diet and the care of the skin. The diet is usually mild and soft. Mild warm baths are used. The doctor will prescribe for the skin various powders or ointments or antiseptic solutions which will prevent itching and secondary infection. One of the simplest common substances is a 5 per cent solution of bicarbonate of soda.

CHIGGERS See discussion under *Insect Pests.*

CHILBLAINS When the circulation in the skin is poor and the skin is exposed to cold, it may be damaged in such a way as to be exceedingly painful. Redness and swelling of the skin of the hands and feet occur in extremely cold weather, particularly among poorly nourished children who have been exposed to dampness. When the chilblain occurs, the spot appears bluish-red because of the stagnation of the circulation of the blood in that area. The color will disappear on pressure because the fluid material is forced out of the swollen area. Usually the spot feels cool but sometimes it has a clammy feeling because of the excessive perspiration.

Of the utmost importance in preventing chilblains is encouragement of the general health and the feeding of a proper diet to aid the improvement of the blood. The circulation of the blood in the tissues is benefited by regular exercise and massage. General health is of course benefited also by plenty of rest under conditions of warmth.

People with a tendency to chilblains should wear woolen socks and preferably thick shoes or boots in cold weather. The feet or hands may be kept warm by the use of the electric pad or by a heat lamp or by the use of the hot-water bottle if it is properly protected against the danger of burning the skin by covering with a towel or a portion of blanket.

Recently two new methods have been suggested for aiding people with chilblains. One involves the application of continuous heat by what is called a paraffin wax bath. The parts concerned are first cleaned thoroughly with hot water and then protected with a simple protective ointment. Thereafter the portion of the limb concerned is immersed in a bath of melted paraffin wax with a temperature of about 120 degrees. While the foot or hand is in the bath, the circulation is benefited by the retention of heat. Interesting is the fact that the foot or hand can remain in the melted paraffin wax bath at a temperature as high as 120 degrees for at least twenty minutes without complaint about the heat. If, however, the hand or foot is put in a bath of water at a temperature of 110 degrees, the person concerned frequently complains of burning.

CHILDBIRTH See *Prenatal Care.*

CHILD CARE GROWTH OF THE NORMAL INFANT—A normal baby will show the following characteristics as he grows:

1. Steady gain in weight.
2. A clear, soft, pink skin.
3. Peaceful sleep, with mouth and eyes closed.
4. A good appetite, without vomiting or spitting up.
5. Bright eyes when awake, and usually a contented expression.
6. Steady improvement in length, weight, and intelligence.
7. Springy muscle movements.
8. Regular bowel movements that are normal in color, frequency, and consistency.

The average baby weighs seven pounds at birth. However, a baby may weigh six, seven, eight, or nine pounds, and still be perfectly normal. A baby who weighs five pounds or less at birth is classed as irregular or premature and requires special care.

Length of the baby also is some indication of its growth but is not as significant a measurement as that of weight.

The baby's head grows rapidly during the first year, increasing two and a half inches in circumference. The bones of his skull are soft and easily molded in incorrect shape by permitting the baby to lie too long in one position. There are instances in which the shape of the baby's head was wrong because the mother did not take care to see that his position was changed frequently. The baby should lie on the left side after one feeding; on the right side after the next feeding.

SOFT SPOTS IN THE SKULL—There are two softs spots in the baby's skull at the time of birth. The small one in the back of the head is usually hardened by growth of bone at the end of the third month. The large one in the front of the head is usually closed at the end of eighteen months.

PROGRESS OF CHILD'S GROWTH—The following tables indicate the progress that a child should make from the time of his birth until he is six years of age:

At one year—
Weight—Boys, 21.5 pounds; girls, 20 pounds.
Height—Boys, 29.5 inches; girls, 29 inches.
Teeth—Should have six cut.
Muscles—Growing rapidly.
Speech—A few words.

At two years—
Weight—Boys, 28.4 pounds; girls, 27.8 pounds.
Height—Boys 33.1 inches; girls, 32.7 inches.
Teeth—Should have sixteen cut.
Muscles—Growing rapidly.
Speech—Vocabulary of 100 to 500 words; two-word sentences.

At three years—
Weight—Boys, 33.5 pounds; girls, 31.5 pounds.
Height—Boys, 36 inches; girls, 35.6

inches (gain of about three inches over previous year).

Teeth—Completion of the first set of twenty teeth.

Muscles—Growing rapidly; should like to skip and jump.

Speech—500 to 1500 new words; should begin to use pronouns.

At four years—

Weight—Boys, 36.4 pounds; girls, 35.1 pounds.

Height—Boys, 38.6 inches; girls, 38.4 inches.

Teeth—Full set of twenty milk teeth.

Muscles—Growing rapidly with increasing co-ordination.

Speech—500 new words and ability to make complete sentences.

At five years—

Weight—Boys, 41.4 pounds; girls, 40.2 pounds.

Height—Boys, 41.7 inches; girls, 41.3 inches.

Teeth—Twenty.

Muscles—Same as fourth year.

Speech—The articulation should now be nearly perfect, and an interest in rhyming developed.

At six years—

Weight—Boys, 45.1 pounds; girls, 43.6 pounds.

Height—Boys, 44 inches; girls, 43.4 inches.

Teeth—The child should have twenty-four teeth, four of which are permanent —especially important to preserve sixth-year molars.

Muscles—Growing rapidly; increasing correlation.

Speech—The articulation should now be perfect; the inflection of nouns and verbs nearly perfect.

Child should be interested in words and like to draw his ideas. Speech defects are recognized before six years; 80 per cent of stuttering occurs before six years.

All children are not normally the same size. Size and weight of parents should be taken into consideration in every case.

LEARNING TO WALK—A baby of nine to eighteen months of age begins to creep, to pull himself up by a chair, and then to walk. At fifteen months the child can climb upstairs by holding to the banister and creeping on all fours, and he can come downstairs by sitting down and sliding one step at a time. At eighteen months the baby can go upstairs in an upright position, by holding to the banister.

There are records of children who have walked at nine months, and occasionally there is one who can walk at seven months. Forty per cent of children walk at twelve months, and 67 per cent walk at eleven to fourteen months. Some children, who are otherwise normal, may not walk before they are eighteen to twenty months old, because of physical illness or lack of practice.

Babies have to learn to walk. They have to learn to co-ordinate and strengthen the muscles used for walking. When the baby does begin to walk, he has the thrill of accomplishing something.

If the child cries too much, or if he is afraid of falls and bumps, he will learn to walk slowly. Fears which he develops at this time may affect his entire existence.

Some children are delayed in walking because they weigh too much, because they have rickets, or because their nutrition is insufficient and they cannot trust the strength of their muscles. Or it may be because they are kept in a limited space, particularly in a pen that is too small. Sometimes the floors are too slippery or too dirty. If conditions are such that the child cannot practice walking easily, he will be slow in walking.

Other children fail to walk at the proper time because they are kept in dresses that are too long and shoes that are too soft. In a few instances the children's minds do not develop rapidly enough. A mother should not be disturbed if her baby fails to walk at fifteen months of age, merely because Aunt Susie walked when she was ten months old.

When a baby is born, his brain is a

well-developed structure, capable of learning, but the tissues have to develop sufficiently to carry the weight, and the muscle action must be co-ordinated before the child can walk.

SEEING AND HEARING—At birth the normal baby can cry, nurse, sleep, move the arms and legs, and sometimes lift his head very slightly. Babies at birth apparently are able to distinguish between light and dark, but they are not able to fix their attention on any single object. Inability to control the muscles of the eye may give the young baby a squint, or his eyes may even seem to be crossed. This, however, should not frighten the mother because it is only normal.

The sense of taste is not developed in little babies, but they seem to be able to distinguish between sweet, sour, and bitter. Our sense of taste includes not only these fundamental traits but also the odor of food and the feel of the food on the tongue. Such abilities develop later with education. A little baby can feel pain, but not so acutely as older babies.

An infant is startled by a loud noise but does not appreciate small variations in the sense of hearing. Babies recognize noises and voices very soon after birth, but they are unable to recognize particular sounds for two or three months.

THE FIRST FOUR MONTHS—The first three or four months produce the most remarkable progress in a child's existence. Almost every day marks some distinct growth or development in the baby.

The sense of cold and warmth is not well developed in little babies. For this reason mothers should protect them against cold and warmth with the right kind of clothing.

A baby one month old will look first at his mother. He will hold or grasp any object that is put into his hand. His eyes will follow moving light. Occasionally he will lift his head.

Mothers sometimes think they see a tiny baby smile. Cynics say that this is simply "gas on the stomach." Investigators find that one baby out of 375 can smile when one month old. When he is two months old, the baby will smile if he has anything to smile at.

By the age of two months most babies make cooing noises or gurgles. They can cry real tears. They will also yawn, stretch, and kick.

The eyes of the tiny baby must be protected from strong light. At the age of two months the baby will turn his eyes toward a bright light and learn to blink when the light is too strong. Babies of this age will also turn their heads in response to spoken voices, and sometimes be frightened by a voice that is too loud or too shrill.

At three months of age some babies laugh aloud. They also will learn to roll over, so that it is not safe to leave a baby unprotected in an open bed. At this age the baby should always be guarded against falls. A three-month-old baby will grunt or gurgle, and grasp objects in his vicinity.

As the infant grows, he begins to observe near-by objects. For this reason a four-month-old baby will study his hands and fingers, and want to play a great deal at feeding time. About this time the mother may begin to be exasperated with the difficulty of keeping the child's attention on his feeding.

The baby will be able to hold his head steady, so that he will turn away and begin to demonstrate will power, occasionally in opposition to the mother's idea of what he ought to do.

EARLY MENTAL DEVELOPMENT—The baby's mental development is especially significant. The type of mind indicates the activities which the child may undertake. A child with a slow mind will be interested in activities that require concentration but not speed. There are still other children who seem to care little about learning and whose minds are definitely superficial in character. Parents should study the traits of their child and make the most of the kind of mind that he has.

By the age of five months some babies will resent interference with their activities. This is an indication that training is necessary.

At the end of the sixth month the baby will sit for a moment without support for his back, reach for things that he wants, and pound on the furniture.

When the baby gets old enough and strong enough to be playful, he needs even more attention than he did previously. During the seventh, eighth, and ninth months the baby is able to express his satisfaction in various ways, and becomes more interested in sounds, so that he enjoys bells and pounding.

At the eighth month the mother will suddenly discover that the baby will play peekaboo and can be taught to clap his hands. This usually creates a great sensation in the home, but not nearly so great as that which occurs during the ninth month when the baby suddenly starts to crawl or to sit up alone, when he learns to wave "bye-bye" and to tell his family, by the tone of his voice, that he is pleased or satisfied.

A ten-month-old baby will recognize his own name, and, by the age of one year, other names as well.

MEASUREMENT OF INTELLIGENCE— Speech is an important means of testing development of the child. It is the chief distinction between man and the animals. At the age of one year a child can say a few single words, and at the end of two years he can begin to make sentences of about two or three words each. A two-year-old child may have a vocabulary of from 100 to 500 words. Dr. Arnold Gesell, child psychologist, says that a two-year-old child can fold paper, use simple sentences and phrases, name familiar objects, such as keys, pennies, and watches, listen to stories, look at pictures, and attempt to describe his own experiences. He will also ask for things by their own names.

There are various tests to show whether the baby is developing normally from the mental point of view. In the Binet-Simon tests, which are standard, the child of three is asked to show his mouth, nose, and eyes; he is asked to repeat two numbers which are not consecutive, and he is given three opportunities to repeat numbers in this way. If he succeeds once out of three times, he is considered as not below normal intelligence. A sample test is to show the child a picture in which there are four or five objects of importance, and have him name the important objects. A three-year-old child, if normal mentally, is able to pick out a boy, a dog, a tree, or a car.

By the time the child is four years old, he should know whether he is a boy or girl. A four-year-old child should be able to name successively three familiar objects shown to him, such as a spoon, a book, or a pencil, and to repeat three non-consecutive numbers.

A six-year-old child should be able to tell whether any particular time of the day is noon or evening. He should be able to define use of a fork, a chair, a knife, or a table.

Tests that have been developed will seem relatively simple to most grown-up people. Even so, these tests demand a certain amount of brain activity. The tests are based on the results of careful observation of thousands of children. Conspicuous failure in performance of any of these tests should demand special attention of the parents to the question of the child's education.

CRYING—Crying is as natural to a baby as complaining is to a good many adults. Even weak, premature babies will cry with a low, feeble whine that sounds like the mewing of a cat. Sometimes crying is the result of a display of anger, sometimes of fear. It is an emotional reaction. Few people realize that crying is one way in which the baby gets exercise, but by crying he also gets attention. Babies are just as eager for attention as are most grownups.

Physiologists recognize that crying helps to ventilate the baby's lungs, forcing out residual air and replacing it with fresh air, drawn in by the deep breathing that follows the crying attack. Moreover, crying is usually associated with active movements of arms and legs.

There are so many different reasons why babies may cry that it is impossible to try to diagnose each one separately. In many instances the baby cries because he is not comfortable. Certainly he is not comfortable if a sharp end of a safety pin is penetrating his skin at some concealed tender spot. The baby is not comfortable in winter if he becomes wet and cold. He isn't comfortable if his digestion is disturbed and he has cramps. And the youngster can't be comfortable if he has an infection in the ear.

A great deal of the control of crying in babies depends on the control of the mother. Mothers simply must learn to endure crying by the baby after it has been determined that there is no apparent cause for it.

Nobody loves to boss as much as a baby does. If he learns that he can boss by crying, he will do so as long as the trick works.

Remember, then, that when a baby cries it may be from hunger, from extremes of temperature, from colic or other pains, and, quite often, from fear. In a series of experiments it was found that fear is aroused in babies by loud noises, such as the banging of a dishpan or slamming of a door, by a loss of support, or by careless handling.

Anger, which babies express by stiffening the body and crying aloud, is caused by anything that hampers their movements and sets up resistance to their activities.

THUMB-SUCKING—Practically all babies indulge in the instinctive habit of thumb-sucking. Thumb-sucking in moderation probably does no harm. Dentists say that overindulgence in this habit causes a typical deformity of the jaws, in which the upper front teeth are pushed forward and the lower front teeth are tipped backward. They have found that, if the left thumb is sucked, the teeth are displaced toward the left; if the right thumb is sucked, the teeth are moved toward the right.

This serious possibility of malformation of the jaw should be a decided warning to parents to do something early about thumb-sucking. If the habit is broken before the child is five years old, the deformity may disappear within a year or two.

A dentist discovered that 70 of 170 children had developed such habits as sucking the thumbs, fingers, tongues, or lips. Thirty of the seventy sucked their thumbs. With the exception of two children who began the habit during their second year of life, all who sucked their thumbs had started it during their nursing periods. Twenty-one of the thirty children were easily broken of the habit, but nine persisted in it.

Although the practice in moderation may not be harmful, it is hard to draw the line between moderate and excessive indulgence. The safest plan is not to permit thumb-sucking to any degree which will indicate that it is apt to become an established habit.

All sorts of devices have been developed to cure a child of the habit. One of the simplest methods is to wrap some adhesive tape lightly around the thumb. This makes the sucking somewhat disagreeable and with a good many babies will prove to be sufficient to break the habit.

Another method is to place a stiff cardboard over the child's elbow, so that the arm cannot be bent. And still other ideas are the application of bitter medicine on the thumb, the use of wire rings, aluminum mitts, and similar devices. The elbow cuffs seem to be the most effective.

BED-WETTING—Bed-wetting is one of the habits of early childhood that is most difficult to control. Most babies learn control of the urine during the first two years of life; others within six months. If a baby fails to learn by the end of the third year, or if a baby once properly trained relapses into infantile habits, he should have special medical study, and perhaps also psychological examination, to find out just what is wrong.

While the baby is young, the act of releasing fluid from the body is not controlled by a center in the brain but is an automatic performance in which only the spinal cord takes part. Gradually the brain becomes involved, so that the child is able to learn control while he is awake. Later this control can be extended to cover the hours when the baby is asleep.

There are many causes for persistent bed-wetting. They include nervousness, infections, poor nutrition, inflammations, and other physical defects. When a child who persistently wets the bed is brought to a doctor, the latter first makes a complete physical examination to determine whether the child is physically sound in all respects.

Sometimes a child of three years may wet his clothes during the day because he is too interested in play and fails to go to the bathroom. Little is to be gained by punishing such a child. It is much better to instruct him intelligently and to praise him for keeping dry.

In training her child, a mother should consider the following points:

1. Do not give him any water, milk, or other fluid to drink after 5:00 P.M. See that the baby drinks water freely during the day.

2. If the child complains of thirst at bedtime, give him a piece of orange or apple.

3. Pick up the child at ten o'clock every night. Wake him thoroughly and have him care for himself just as he does during the day.

4. Protect the bed well but do not put on diapers at night after the baby has begun to go without them during the day.

5. Take the baby up just as soon as he wakes. Many children wet the bed a few minutes after waking in the morning.

6. In preparing dry suppers, omit milk for drinking or for use on cereals or puddings, and water or cocoa for drinking. Use milk when possible in cooking foods. Breads and cereals of whole grain are preferable.

Sometimes it is necessary to take the baby up a second time during the night. If so the mother should notice the time at which the baby wets the bed and awaken him just before. Then the period between the first awakening and the second may be gradually lengthened.

BOWEL CONTROL—Training the child to control his bowels is easier than training him to control his bladder. In teaching the baby bowel control these seven suggestions may be followed:

1. Begin during the first month to train your baby to use the chamber.

2. Hold him comfortably in your lap on the chamber. Do this at regular times: when he wakes up, when he is ready for his nap, and before each feeding.

3. Change diapers promptly when wet. This helps in his training. The baby soon learns to feel uncomfortable in a wet diaper.

4. As soon as the baby sits up easily of his own accord, have him use a chair in the bathroom instead of the chamber in your lap.

5. Leave him on the chair not longer than five minutes. Do not let him have toys to play with.

6. When the baby can walk successfully, take off the diapers and put him into jersey panties.

7. Do not use rubber panties—they injure the skin. When traveling, use the large, loose, rubberized diaper. Have an extra one to place in your lap or on the car or train seat.

It is important to teach the child not to delay after he gets on the toilet. If he is permitted to sit at the toilet playing with a toy or looking at a book, or otherwise amusing himself, without giving his main attention to the matter concerned, he will form a habit which may eventually result in constipation.

The baby must learn to attempt to have an action of the bowel just as soon as he feels contact with the toilet seat.

Many mothers, because of excess modesty, teach the child all sorts of tricks to indicate that he wishes to go to the toilet. Queer words are used for the purpose, and also strange gestures. The child should learn from the beginning the suitable words in relation to this activity.

EXERCISE FOR BABY—Babies need exercise exactly as do adults, but of a different kind. When a small baby lies on his back and kicks, he is really having strenuous exercise. Time should be allowed every day for this activity. Part of the time the baby should lie on his stomach and be permitted to lift his head or push himself up from the bed. Exactly as with grownups, a certain amount of exercise is a stimulus to hunger and appetite in the baby, and also creates enough fatigue to make him want to rest.

Children whose bodies are flabby in construction need more exercise than those who are solidly constructed. They should also have a physical examination, however, to indicate whether they are free from rickets or malnutrition.

Violent exercise should never be permitted immediately after eating. In warm or pleasant weather a half hour of exercise outdoors is exceedingly beneficial. Exercise, of course, is an excellent method of training. Children learn by practice. When a boy first gets on a bicycle, he promptly falls off. With a little practice he learns how to balance himself, co-ordinating his muscles in such manner that balance is maintained and he is able to go forward.

Especially important in getting suitable reaction to exercise is the feeling of satisfaction that comes from accomplishment. If the activity is successful and satisfying to the child, he is more likely to repeat the performance. Children are taught much more easily during early years of life than in later years. Mentally backward children, who suffer from lack of development of the tissues and organs, will not respond promptly to exercise.

Parents are often proud of the baby and like to show his accomplishments. This leads to forcing the child before he is really ready to carry on a certain activity. It also leads to repetition of such activity for long periods of time, which results in fatigue and exhaustion.

Babies are much more easily excited than grownups, and they respond more fully. Thus a baby will be greatly excited by a large variety of toys, by a long automobile ride, or by great excitement in the people around him. Any excitement which brings about fatigue or exhaustion is bad for him.

Remember also that the eyes of the baby are delicate and must be protected against accident and against direct sunlight, when the child is outdoors.

In exercising the baby, remember that he is not to sit up until the muscles of the spine and neck are strong enough. When the child is able to bring his head up with the rest of the body, the mother may help him gradually to sit up. A good exercise is to permit the child's legs to bend and straighten against slight counterpressure by the mother. As soon as the baby is able to sit up, he may begin new exercises, including bending and reaching for objects above his head. When the baby's muscles are able to bear the weight of his body, he will begin to crawl. In that stage he should be protected suitably by a pen, or in some other manner, against being burned accidentally and against falling downstairs.

BATHING THE BABY—A newborn baby should be cleaned, during the first few days of life, with oil and cotton, and should not be given a full bath until the cord has separated. During the first few months the bath should be given in a warm room at a temperature of 98 degrees Fahrenheit, which is about the temperature of the body. The bath should not last long, and the baby should be dried quickly by application of an absorbent towel, without vigorous rubbing. If the child's skin is exceptionally delicate, a handful of table salt to a gallon of water will make the water less irritating to the skin.

At six months of age the temperature of the bath is lowered to 95 degrees, and at the end of the first year it may be 90 degrees. Some doctors suggest that healthy children, after reaching the age of six months, may be sponged with water at a temperature of 65 or 70 degrees, for a second or two at the end of the bath, presumably with the idea of accustoming the child somewhat to cold.

As the child grows older, he should be given a warm bath, preferably at night, which will assure pleasant and restful sleep. The cooler bath is taken in the morning before breakfast. Ordinarily the bath should be a pleasant performance for both baby and mother. Everything for the bath should be prepared before the baby is taken up. The child should be handled as little as possible.

There are two ways of bathing very young babies: one, in the mother's lap; the other, on an especially prepared table or tray, covered with padding. It is important to remember that the baby must be kept warm and comfortable during the bathing period. The head and the neck should be supported as long as the baby's muscles are unable to do this.

It is not necessary to wash the baby's mouth or to use stiff instruments in cleaning the ears. The ears may be wiped with swabs of cotton dipped in mineral oil.

Any discharge from the ears or the eyes should be called immediately to the attention of the doctor.

If the scalp is not properly cleansed, the child may develop a slight irritation, due to oversecretion of the sweat and oil glands. The fat and the oil mix with dirt and form a crust. This crust may be removed with oil. If the head is kept clean, the trouble ends promptly.

Special pains should be taken in drying the skin thoroughly where there are folds or creases. Oil may be used on the parts of the body where there are likely to be irritations, and powder may be applied to keep the areas dry.

Following are some simple instructions:

1. In washing the baby, pay special attention to creases in the neck, under the arms, at the elbows, between the toes, and in the groin.

2. Put the baby in the tub, supporting his head with the left hand, spreading the fingers to support the shoulders.

3. With the baby sitting on the right hand, slide him into the tub gently, feet first. Plunging the baby suddenly into the water will frighten him.

4. Hold the baby so that his head and ears are out of the water.

5. Allow the baby to remain in the tub for two or three minutes after completely rinsing off the soap mixture.

6. Remove the baby from the tub, holding him as you did when immersing him.

7. Wrap in a bath towel and pat thoroughly dry

8. Oil irritations or creases, and remove excess oil with a soft towel.

9. Powder as desired.

BREAST FEEDING—The best possible food for a baby is his mother's milk, particularly during the early months of life. Increased responsibilities of modern woman, however, and the fact that so many women are helping to earn the family income, have undermined interest among mothers in this important duty.

Many experts claim it is possible to feed babies artificially and thereby produce just as healthful children as those fed from the breast. Few babies, however, can have the opportunity to secure their artificial feeding under the daily direction of competent experts.

In the vast majority of cases breast milk is the best food for an infant during his first three months of life, provided the supply is satisfactory and the baby gains weight as he should. In many cases the milk of the mother continues to be the ideal food for the baby up to six or even nine months. Most babies, however, will do well with complete weaning after the fourth to the sixth month.

When the baby cannot get at least half his food supply from the mother's breast, he may be weaned. In this way the mother will be spared the annoyance and dissatisfaction of combined breast feeding and artificial feeding. Under such circumstances it is necessary to be certain just how much food the baby is getting from the natural source. A healthy mother who is eating the proper diet will have in her milk all the food elements necessary for nutrition of a normal baby. There is little danger of overfeeding or underfeeding, provided the amount of milk is adequate.

The milk in the mother's breast rarely contains harmful germs. If she keeps herself reasonably clean, and if her breasts are not infected, the milk is safe as far as germs are concerned.

Breast feeding is not always adequate, because the total amount of milk may be insufficient for the baby's needs, the milk may not be of good quality due to illness of the mother or for similar reasons. The milk of the healthy mother usually agrees with the baby.

DIET FOR NURSING MOTHERS—There is a common belief that a nursing mother should stuff herself with milk, cocoa, or even beer, because it is felt that these substances will aid her in producing great quantities of good milk. The mother who follows this practice is likely to become unpleasantly fat, disgusted with the whole business of eating and nursing, and inclined to give up suckling the baby before she should. If her diet contains three or four glasses of good milk every day, and if she drinks her usual supply of water, she will get just about as much milk for the baby as she will by drinking great amounts of milk, cocoa, or beer.

At the same time the nursing mother should not encourage the loss of water from her body by taking substances which will stimulate the flow of fluid, such as doses of laxative salts, or substances which stimulate kidney action. These should not be taken in any event, unless the doctor directs.

Actually the opportunity of influencing the quality or quantity of the mother's milk by manipulating her diet is small.

There is the superstition that a nursing mother should avoid foods that are sour, and likewise salads, cabbage, and raw fruit. This also is without foundation. The substances mentioned are rich in vitamins and minerals, and there is no evidence to indicate that they can in any way harm the milk supply of the mother. If, however, the mother is sensitive to any particular food, and reacts to it with skin eruptions or digestive disturbances, she ought to avoid that food.

For ordinary work the average woman requires from 1500 to 2000 calories a day. In addition she must supply 600 calories to the baby. She should there-fore estimate the amount of calories she takes in and be sure to get a minimum of 2500 calories daily. On that type of diet she should be able to nurse her baby satisfactorily yet not gain weight unnecessarily.

The best flow of milk results from regular nursing of the baby. Milk flow will be regular and undisturbed if she remains calm and quiet.

The diet of the nursing mother should contain milk, butter, eggs, two green vegetables, and fresh fruit, including particularly tomatoes and oranges, which provide vitamin C. Butter helps to provide vitamins A and D; so at least one ounce of good butter should be taken daily. To provide a full supply of vitamins A and D, she may also take cod-liver oil, or halibut-liver oil, as her physician directs. The milk which she takes daily need not be in the form of liquid, if she does not like to drink milk, but may be used as cocoa, ice cream, or custard. A pound of evaporated milk equals a quart of bottled milk.

In general a mother may eat the food that she usually eats, including meat, potatoes, bread, cereals, or any other foods that she knows will not upset her digestion.

Mothers sometimes worry about taking medicine, for fear that it will appear in the breast milk. Few drugs taken by mouth appear in the milk in amounts sufficient to affect the baby. She will always do well, however, to ask her doctor before taking drugs of any kind.

The mother begins to secrete milk soon after her baby is born. Occasionally a few drops may come from the breast even before the child's birth. The milk is scanty during the first two or three days, but becomes profuse, in most cases, by the third or fourth day. Occasionally the milk flow may be delayed until the tenth or twelfth day.

If the supply of milk seems insufficient during the first ten or twelve days, it should be stimulated by encouraging the baby to nurse, by artificial pumping, or in some similar manner. The average mother will secrete from ten to sixteen ounces, or about a pint, of milk by the end of the first week. The amount gradually increases, so that by the sixth month she may be secreting a quart daily. The amount of milk usually parallels demands of the baby. Complete emptying of the breast helps to encourage the milk supply.

Milk from the mother's breast provides twenty calories for each ounce. During the early days immediately after the birth of the child the thin fluid which is secreted is called colostrum. This differs from the milk which comes later. It contains more protein than the later milk, and is also richer in minerals; but it provides less sugar and less fat. It has been established that the colostrum of the cow contains substances which protect calves from certain infections. It is not known whether these substances exist in human colostrum, but the latter does contain a high percentage of substances with which antibodies, affecting diseases that concern human beings, are usually associated. Doctors therefore insist nowadays that babies should have colostrum, if it is at all possible for their mothers to provide them with it.

Mature milk, which is secreted by the mother after the first month, is about 87.5 per cent water; 1.25 per cent protein; 7.5 per cent sugar; and 3.5 per cent fat. The amounts of these constituents vary in different specimens, most variable being the fat, which may be anywhere from 2 to 6 per cent. If the mother is getting an insufficient amount of food, the milk will be deficient in both fat and protein. If she gets too little fluid, the milk will diminish in quantity. The composition of the milk is influenced little by the mother's diet, except for the vitamins.

A question invariably asked is whether tea, coffee, tobacco, or alcohol affect mother's milk. Most doctors are convinced that these substances may be used in small amounts, but that excesses will be harmful. Alcohol taken in negligible quantities does not appear in the mother's milk. Mothers who are nursing babies, however, should not experiment with alcoholic drinks, because it is known that intoxication of the nursing mother may produce harmful symptoms in the baby.

HYGIENE OF NURSING MOTHER—The nursing mother must keep herself in good physical condition and eat proper food. Her diet has been described previously. To maintain good physical condition she must have plenty of sleep and some exercise in the open air. Worry and mental strain may affect the quantity and nature of the milk secretion. If the mother does not have enough milk, the baby remains hungry and gets fretful. In that case the mother gets less rest and becomes more worried. As a result she has less milk. It is a vicious circle.

The size of the breast and the size or weight of the mother do not seem to be of great importance in relation to the amount of milk that the mother may produce.

It is not possible for anyone to say, before the baby is born and the mother actually starts to secrete milk, whether any woman will be able to nurse her baby. However, any competent doctor can tell the mother after the baby is born whether she has enough milk to supply the baby with his necessary food.

A woman with active tuberculosis, or one who has had the disease in any form, should not nurse a baby. If she does, she will expose the baby to infection, and the added strain on her body will lower her resistance to disease.

Whenever a woman has severe complications after childbirth, such as hemorrhage, infection, or convulsions, she should not nurse her baby. After she has recovered, the doctor may determine whether she can resume nursing, but it is advisable to be cautious in permitting nursing of the baby after the mother has had any fever, signs of infection, or toxemia. If the breasts of the mother become infected, it is customary to discontinue nursing until the condition has definitely healed.

If the baby develops vomiting or colic, or fails to gain weight, the mother should not stop nursing. She should, instead, find out from the doctor whether she is feeding the baby often enough or too often. Her diet should be surveyed, and the doctor should determine whether the baby ought to have extra food in addition to what she can give him.

If the mother is suffering from any chronic disease, such as inflammation of the kidneys, heart disease, or cancer, she certainly should not nurse the baby. Indeed, if she is delicate, the doctor should determine whether nursing will do her harm, and whether it will be of any benefit to the child.

Physicians generally believe that mothers are more likely to nurse satisfactorily their first and second babies than later ones. In other words, the ability to nurse the baby tends to diminish with each successive child.

FREQUENCY OF FEEDING BABY—A baby is usually given his first feeding about twelve hours after he is born. During the next twenty-four hours, he may be fed every six hours. After the third day the baby may be fed from both breasts every four hours.

Doctors, however, differ widely regarding the technic of nursing. Some suggest that the baby nurse from each breast every three hours, others that the baby nurse from each breast every four hours, and still others suggest that the baby be fed alternately at each feeding from one breast or the other.

If a baby on a four-hour schedule cries because he is hungry at the end of two and a half or three hours, he may not be getting enough milk, or his stomach may be getting rid of the food too quickly. It may be necessary, in this case, to change from a four-hour to a three-hour schedule. Very rarely is it necessary to nurse a baby more frequently than every three hours.

Tests have been made by feeding the baby every time he seemed to be hungry. Most babies soon fall into the habit of three or four feedings in twenty-four hours.

Among the reasons which have been cited in favor of the four-hour nursing interval are the following:

1. The baby is hungry at the end of four hours.

2. The baby will nurse more vigorously and empty the breasts more completely at the end of four hours. This helps to stimulate milk production.

3. The stomach and the intestines have a chance for a suitable rest period.

4. The baby will take more food at each feeding and sleep longer after each feeding.

5. A baby fed every four hours is likely to vomit less than a baby fed at two- or three-hour intervals.

6. When the baby is fed at four-hour intervals, the mother has a chance to rest and does not have to spend all her time with the child.

In the course of two or three weeks a healthy baby will usually be trained to nurse and sleep with almost perfect regularity. If a baby cannot be placed on a four-hour schedule in three months, he requires some supplementary feeding.

Value of a long interval between nursing periods is relief for the mother from nursing the baby at night. It will also help her to maintain her health and permit her to nurse the baby to better advantage.

Whenever possible, the baby should not sleep with the mother. If the baby is in the same bed with the mother, and if he cries at night, the mother has a tendency to nurse the child to keep him quiet.

A mother with a tiny baby has no business taking the infant to a motion picture theater or to other places of public assemblage. Under these circumstances there is a tendency to permit the baby to nurse constantly, to keep him quiet.

DURATION OF NURSING—If a mother who is nursing her baby has plenty of milk, she will probably do well to feed the baby from one breast only at each nursing. Less frequent use of the breast lessens danger of infection and of sore or cracked nipples. If a mother does not have very much milk, she should use both breasts in nursing, because regular use of the breast for nursing stimulates the milk flow. If one breast only is used in nursing, the baby should not nurse much longer than ten minutes. If both breasts are used, six minutes' nursing should supply the baby with all the milk that will be useful to him. Scientific studies show that the food obtained by the baby after the first six to ten minutes is hardly sufficient to be of great importance in ordinary nursing.

Once a schedule of feeding has been adopted, it should be followed closely. Sometimes a baby fed every four hours gets unusually hungry at the end of three or three and a half hours, especially if he has been active or if the previous feeding has been small. In such case the baby should not be allowed to cry for a half hour, but may be fed a little ahead of time. The next feeding, however, should be given at the regular period.

SWALLOWING AIR—A baby who nurses too long at the breast will tend to swallow much air toward the end of the nursing period. After the feeding he will try to regurgitate this air. As a result he may vomit or have colic. To overcome this air swallowing the mother should sit up while the baby is nursing and hold the baby in a semierect posture. Just before nursing the baby she may hold him upright over her shoulder. If she will then pat him lightly on the back, he will be likely to belch up the air. After the nursing is completed, the same procedure should be followed for a short time.

Some babies swallow more air than others. If the baby tends to be an "air swallower," the nursing may be interrupted occasionally and the baby held over the shoulder. This will permit him to belch up some of the air he has swallowed, before he proceeds with nursing.

OVERFEEDING AND UNDERFEEDING— Underfeeding is the more difficult to correct. One method is to stimulate the breasts by means of a pump. Another is to improve the mother's physical condition. It may be advisable for the mother to be relieved of her child's care except for feeding. The child may be given some supplementary food. Nursing, however, should be attempted regularly so as to give the breasts the stimulation that comes from the suckling of the baby.

A baby getting too much milk will vomit, or regurgitate, some of the food. Sometimes he will have colic. Usually, however, the overabundance of milk lessens after the first few days. If the milk remains in overabundant amounts, the milk that the baby takes may be reduced by shortening the time of nursing.

In a few cases the baby may seem to be overfed due to the fact that there is too much fat in the milk. In this case the doctor may direct the addition of water to the diet before nursing. There are, however, few cases in which breast milk is unsuitable for digestion.

There are various ways of finding out how much milk a baby is getting. He may be weighed before and after feeding. This should be done at each nursing, until the mother knows how much milk the baby is getting regularly from the breasts. If the mother is unable to weigh the baby regularly, she may tell something from the way the child nurses. If a baby is hungry, he will nurse hungrily and with considerable "pulling power." If there is plenty of milk, the baby will seldom nurse more than five or six minutes. If, however, the milk supply is insufficient, he will nurse for a half hour or more; when he stops he does so because he is exhausted rather than because he has had enough milk. If a baby is getting no milk at all or exceedingly small amounts, he will try to nurse vigorously for a few minutes and then stop.

USE OF COW'S MILK—Cow's milk is used most generally in the United States as a substitute for mother's milk. It is essential that the milk come from healthy cows, that it be handled only by healthy people, and that it be clean and fresh. Milk from different types of cows varies in its composition. The rich milk that comes from Jerseys and Alderneys is usually not so satisfactory as that from average grade cows. Ordinarily the best milk is that taken from a herd and mixed.

Nowadays milk production and distribution are largely under state control. The milk taken from the cows is mixed and put into sterilized pails. The cows have been tuberculin tested. The milk is pasteurized, or perhaps first certified as to its freedom from harmful germs and then pasteurized.

In country homes and in districts where milk is obtained fresh from the cows, the fluid should be boiled at once. Then it may be strained through several thicknesses of cheesecloth into jars or milk bottles which have been boiled. After being filled with the milk, these bottles should be covered and cooled immediately. Milk for older children should also be boiled, unless it has been pasteurized. Pasteurization or boiling destroys the germs by heat. Most of the germs in good milk are not dangerous to human health. Occasionally, however, the streptococcus which produces septic sore throat may get into milk, and more rarely such dangerous germs as those of typhoid, diphtheria, or scarlet fever. In general it is believed that heating milk does not injure it seriously so far as its nutritional value is concerned. Moreover, some specialists believe that heating makes the milk more digestible by altering the curd.

Because the vitamin C necessary for the child may be destroyed by the heat process, it is customary to begin giving orange juice early in life.

Directions for artificial feeding of any baby should be given by a doctor who understands this work. Cow's milk alone will not provide the baby with the food elements that he requires and in the proper proportions. It is necessary to change the composition to meet the needs of the individual baby. Only a thorough understanding of these requirements can bring about proper modification for the individual child.

When cow's milk is fed, the gastric juice of the baby will increase in acidity to take care of the difference in the reaction between the cow's milk and human milk. To bring cow's milk

to the optimum acidity for digestion, three times as much acid must be added to obtain the amount that is had with ordinary human milk. One part of cow's milk diluted with two parts of water makes the milk more like the human variety. For this reason it is customary to add water to the cow's milk in preparing the baby's formula.

PREPARING THE BABY'S FORMULA—If the formula for the baby is made up at home, all materials used, as well as the bottles and the nipples, should be washed thoroughly and boiled daily. The top of the bottle in which the milk is delivered should be washed with boiled water and wiped off with cotton. The ingredients should be mixed and measured in sterilized vessels. The bottles into which the formula is poured should be washed thoroughly and boiled, and they should be closed with non-absorbent cotton or sterilized rubber, or cork stoppers. It is much better to pour the mixture for the baby's food into individual bottles than to keep it all in one big bottle and measure it out into smaller bottles as needed. The wise mother will always make one extra bottle for the twenty-four-hour period, to provide for accidents, such as dropping the bottle or contaminating it in some way.

After the individual bottles have been filled and stoppered, they may be kept in the icebox.

Nipples should be made of thin rubber and be washed thoroughly and boiled before using. All nipples may be washed and boiled at one time and kept in a covered dish ready to put on bottles as they are used.

As soon as the feeding is ended, bottle and nipple should be washed in cold water. The bottles may be filled with water and left standing until ready for preparation the next day.

The person who is to give the feeding should wash her hands thoroughly before handling the bottles. In picking up the nipple, it should be touched only at the edge and if possible not at the part that goes into the baby's mouth. Just before feeding, the bottle should be placed in water heated to about 100 degrees Fahrenheit, which is just a little more than the temperature of the body. Never put a bottle which has been in the refrigerator into a vessel containing boiling water or very hot water, as the bottle will probably break.

When the milk seems to be warm enough, a drop or two should be tested on the inside of the mother's wrist. This part of the skin is very sensitive, and the mother may tell in this manner whether the milk is warm enough or too warm. The milk should drop from the hole in the nipple in fair-sized drops and rather regularly. It should not run out. If the drops come too small or too slowly, the hole in the nipple may have to be enlarged.

Nowadays there are all sorts of inventions, in the way of specially constructed nipples, which are said to make nursing easier and to prevent the baby from swallowing air. The baby should take just about as long for an artificial nursing as he would for nursing from the breast. The same rules may be followed, relative to preventing the baby from swallowing air, as were suggested in relation to breast feeding.

USE OF WATER AND SUGAR IN BABY'S FORMULA—Babies who live on cow's milk are more likely to have digestive disorders than those who live on mother's milk. Until recently a good part of the trouble, no doubt, was due to invasion of the milk by germs. Modern methods of cleanliness have eliminated this possibility.

Most modifications of cow's milk involve a reduction of the amount of protein and fat, and an increase in the amount of sugar. A diet which contains too much protein, as compared with sugar, will lead to an increased amount of bacterial action in the bowels and in that way cause trouble with nutrition. Too much protein also will increase the amount of water needed by the body. Most babies can take a fair proportion of the fat in cow's milk. However, it is customary nowadays to cut down on the fat also. A baby getting cow's milk with a high degree of fat

sometimes develops an intolerance for fat. The fat of cow's milk is not so easily absorbed by the human body as that of mother's milk.

All sorts of mixtures and variations of cow's milk have been devised to overcome difficulties such as have been mentioned. Sugar is added to the milk in many forms. Milk sugar is one of the most frequent forms, as are also malt and cane sugar. The latter is inexpensive and is widely recommended by most doctors who specialize in infant feeding. Many doctors recommend a mixture of dextrin and maltose, such as is found in many proprietary infant foods.

The common method of preparing artificial feeding for the baby involves the adding of water and, later, of carbohydrate or sugar. Another method is merely to add sugar to the whole milk and to reduce the total quantity of food that is taken. In such cases a good deal of additional water is given between feedings. This adds to the amount of nursing necessary for the baby.

An average mixture is one which contains about seven ounces of whole milk, three ounces of water, and half an ounce of sugar. Such mixture may be made with boiled, fermented, or acidified milk. In certain climates it may be preferable to use dried or evaporated milk. This mixture will give about 20 calories to the ounce and contain about 15 per cent of protein, 35 per cent of fat, and 50 per cent of carbohydrate. The feeding may be prepared with boiled, pasteurized, skimmed, dried, evaporated, sweetened, condensed, or fermented milk. There are also special preparations called protein milks, acidified milks, and all the different proprietary foods.

The mother should ask her doctor what to use and how to use it. Babies vary in their reactions to these different mixtures.

BABY'S WEIGHT AS GUIDE TO FOOD— When a mother is feeding a baby with artificial milk mixtures, she will have difficulty in determining whether to increase the food or to diminish it, whether to change the food because of various reasons, and when to begin adding other foods.

If the baby seems healthy and continues to gain in weight regularly, there would seem to be no reason for increasing his diet. The main reasons for increasing the supply of food are that the baby is not gaining weight satisfactorily and that he seems to be hungry. It is not well to estimate the necessity for increasing the food by the weight curve alone. If the mother does this, she will be increasing the amount of food all the time, because mothers like to see the baby gain weight.

A baby's gain in weight is not always continuous. Many healthy babies will remain stationary in weight for a week or two without any visible cause. On the other hand, it is fairly easy for any intelligent mother to know when the baby is hungry. If he drinks greedily and rapidly, if he cries for more, if he gets fretful long before feeding time, the baby needs more food. Remember, however, that babies sometimes cry merely because they are spoiled. Furthermore, a baby who is hungry and does not get enough food will keep on sucking and swallowing air, and this will be associated with regurgitation and vomiting.

Overfeeding of the baby may occur with artificial milk mixtures as well as in breast feeding. The baby who eats too long or too much will tend to regurgitate, or vomit. The doctor can tell whether the baby is getting too much to eat by finding out how many calories the child is receiving per day in relation to his weight.

The growing baby is a little machine. He can handle just so much fuel daily with a certain output of energy. A baby who gets too much to eat may become nauseated and refuse food. The baby who lacks certain essential substances in the diet, such as vitamins or cod-liver oil and orange juice, will not grow satisfactorily. A baby who is eating too much concentrated food and not enough water may take more food to satisfy thirst. If, however, he gets too much water, his stomach becomes distended and his appetite satisfied before he gets enough food.

For this reason the doctor is likely to recommend a formula which will have just about the same ingredients as are possessed by mother's milk.

WATER ESSENTIAL FOR BABY'S GROWTH—Among the most important considerations in feeding a baby is its requirement for water. The child being fed by the breast usually gets enough water in the milk. The infant being fed artificially should receive water between feedings. This is of special significance in warm weather because of the increased evaporation from the surface of the body. In winter, with our overheated and dry apartments, it is also well to be certain that the baby is getting the water he needs.

The water requirement of a baby is about three times that of a grownup. The reason is that there is much activity in the baby's tissues because of its rapid rate of growth. Its output of heat is greater, in proportion to its weight, than that of a grownup.

Large amounts of water taken into the body require a constant circulation of water from the blood to the intestines and back again, to take care of digestion and absorption of the food constituents. Since the amount of food taken is large, the amount of waste material also is large. This waste material is not all excreted in solid form but is largely dissolved.

Of the water taken into the body, about 50 to 65 per cent goes out through the kidneys; 30 to 35 per cent in evaporation by the skin and the lungs; and 5 to 10 per cent by way of the bowels. Two per cent is retained by the body to carry on the necessary chemical processes.

If a baby cries a great deal and exercises his limbs, the amount of water lost from the skin and the lungs will be increased. If the baby has diarrhea, the amount of water lost from the bowels may equal or even exceed the amount of water taken into the body. If the baby vomits, water taken by the mouth may be returned directly and so be of no benefit to the body. Hence one must be certain that the baby not only gets sufficient water but that the water is retained and in that way is useful to the child's system.

It is also possible for large amounts of water to be lost by way of the lungs, when there is an increased rate of breathing, such as occurs in pneumonia or in severe conditions of acidosis.

The average normal baby receiving breast milk should obtain daily, for the first year of its life, about two and a half ounces of water for each pound of its body weight. This helps to take care of its needs during hot weather or when some of the water is lost by diarrhea or vomiting. A small excess of water will not produce any serious disturbance, but too much water given with food will interfere with absorption.

Incidentally, if the amount of milk given is too great, or if the dilution is too great, the baby is likely to vomit. When babies are fed artificially, the proteins and salts in the diet are usually higher, and there is increased elimination, so more water is required to take care of the output from the kidneys.

USE OF PREPARED BABY FOODS—Modern proprietary foods are results of attempts to take advantage of new facts discovered in relation to essentials of the human diet. The proprietary foods of a previous era frequently lacked vitamins and mineral salts. They were also over-rich in carbohydrates. As a result the producers were able to show pictures of very fat babies, which, however, may not have been healthy babies. When properly diluted with water or when made up with milk, some of the prepared foods now available approximate the composition of breast milk. In some the fat is a mixture of vegetable and animal fats, in an attempt to imitate the physical and chemical qualities of the fat found in breast milk. These proprietary foods, in most instances, are somewhat more expensive than the milk mixtures which may be made up at home, their chief advantage being their ease of preparation.

Specialists in infant feeding do not quite agree as to whether the synthetic mixtures of fat are more easily absorbed or digested by the baby than the fat of cow's milk.

Other baby foods consist largely of dried milk in addition to sugars. Some contain milk, cane sugar, starch, dextrin, maltose, vitamins A and B, and a variety of mineral salts. Malted milk also is used in infant feeding. This consists of one third dried skimmed milk and two thirds extra sugars, such as dextrin and maltose. There also are malted foods which are chiefly mixtures of dextrin and maltose. Physicians frequently recommend these as supplementary foods because of their value in furnishing calories and in aiding the baby to gain weight.

Other special preparations, such as lactic-acid milk, milk powder, protein milks, and various cereal and gruel feedings, should be used only when prescribed by the doctor.

Sometimes you may hear that your neighbor's child is doing remarkably well with a special type of proprietary or patent food. That should not be taken as evidence that your baby will do equally well. Every baby is a special problem. It is not wise to experiment with strange foods without knowing that they are especially fitted for your baby.

FEEDING FROM A SPOON—Even tiny babies can learn to take orange or tomato juice from a spoon. Merely put a drop or two of the juice on the tip of the spoon and hold it to the baby's mouth. It is natural for the baby to make a sucking motion, which will draw in the juice. If the baby learns to like the food, it will soon be eating satisfactorily from a spoon.

By the time most babies are six months old, they can learn to drink from a cup. The cup, however, must be broad enough so that the baby's nose will not bump the opposite rim. As the baby gets older, he will soon put his hand out to help in holding the cup. By the time a baby is ten or eleven months old, he will be used to holding a cup, and feeding will be much easier.

If the baby refuses to drink from a cup, you should adopt about the same procedure that you use when the baby declines to accept feedings except from the breast. It is necessary to be firm and to keep taking away the food until the child is hungry enough to want it. This means a great deal of patience. It will require holding the cup to the baby's lips over and over, time after time, without any strain or emotion, until the baby begins to eat. If the child finds out that he can create considerable disturbance simply by refusing to have anything to do with cup or spoon, he is likely to use that fact to get his own will enforced in opposition to that of the parent. Sometimes a change in size of the cup, or in shape or color, will encourage the baby to eat when other methods fail.

After the baby has become used to orange juice and cod-liver oil taken by the spoon, he goes on to cereals and sieved vegetables. A bland cereal such as farina is used most frequently as the first solid food. It should not be given in large amounts, and should be thin until the baby is accustomed to it.

After the cereals have been established, the vegetables are tried, one by one, using carrots, peas, and string beans, one at a time, to determine which foods meet with the child's preference. There is no use forcing spinach or any other vegetable on the baby, since the variety available today is exceedingly great and various combinations will provide all essential factors.

FIRST USE OF SOLID FOODS—Whenever a new solid food is added to baby's diet, always begin with a small amount —not more than a teaspoonful. As new foods are added, the baby of course will take less of the foods that he has been getting.

The refined or white cereals are given first, because they are more easily digestible and less likely to be laxative than the whole-grain cereals. Cereals should be cooked with salt and water or with milk, according to the instructions accompanying the specific product,

if it is packaged. If not, the proportion for farina is about one part of the farina to six or eight parts of water or milk. Such mixtures are brought to a boil and cooked in a double boiler for one or two hours. When made with milk, farina will provide about 30 calories for each tablespoonful; with water, about 20.

Potato may be substituted for some of the cereals. Potatoes also should be well cooked and mashed. In this form the vegetable usually is as digestible as other forms of starch. Later spaghetti or macaroni may be used.

Crackers, zwieback, dried bread, or toast may be given when the teeth have started to appear and it is possible for the baby to chew these substances satisfactorily.

Use of new puréed green vegetables frequently is begun as early as the fifth or sixth month, and by the ninth month may occupy an important place in the diet. They are prepared preferably by boiling or baking. The water in which the vegetables are cooked should not be discarded, because it contains some of the valuable salts.

Remember that the substances eaten by the baby may appear in the bowel movements. The mother should not be worried if the red pigment of the beets or the fibers of some of the other vegetables are visible in the excretions.

Broths are frequently given to the baby in the sixth month. They include beef, veal, mutton, or chicken broth, and to these broths barley, rice, and vegetables may be added occasionally. Broths have the special virtue of providing minerals and extractives of meat useful in stimulating appetite and digestion.

About the ninth or tenth month the child may receive beef juice, and, finally, chopped liver and chicken.

Young babies also will be able to use cooked fruit in the diet if it is properly mashed. Fruits have laxative qualities and are useful for food value. Bananas may be given baked, or raw if they are ripe.

Remember that a healthy baby can digest a variety of food substances but that he cannot chew until he has molar teeth. The mother, therefore, must make certain that the food is properly divided or broken up if the baby is to be spared indigestion.

The appetite is a good guide not only to the kind of food but also to the quantity. Experiments made with many babies show that infants will grow well if guided to a great extent by their appetites, provided they eat enough food during the growing period. Experiments of this kind, however, should not control mothers in training their babies. Make certain that the baby gets a good variety and do not indulge too greatly his fanciful notions and appetites.

SCHEDULE FOR THE ONE-YEAR-OLD BABY—When the baby is a year old, he will be taking a diet approximately as follows:

At six o'clock in the morning he should have from seven to eight ounces of milk.

At ten o'clock he may have some cereal, about four tablespoonfuls; seven to eight ounces of milk, some of which may be placed on the cereal; and a cracker or piece of toast.

At two o'clock the baby may have from four to six ounces of vegetable or meat broth, or he may take one egg, or, as a third alternative, some scraped or chopped meat.

To this may be added some white vegetables, such as two tablespoonfuls of potato or rice, and from two to four tablespoonfuls of a green vegetable, such as string beans, peas, or spinach. The baby should also receive from five to eight ounces of milk, the smaller amount if he has some broth.

Then at six o'clock in the evening he may have four tablespoonfuls of cereal with seven to eight ounces of milk, some of which is placed on the cereal. He may also have, at this time, a cracker or a small piece of toast, and one or two tablespoonfuls of cooked fruit, which has a slight laxative quality.

Babies thrive best on a strict daily schedule. If you compare the life and character of a baby who has been suitably trained with those of a child who has been allowed to develop in a haphazard manner, you will realize at once the importance of a definite routine. Babies become accustomed to a fixed schedule. They will act almost like an alarm clock in notifying those who take care of them that the time has arrived for some definite procedure. A baby who is fed irregularly will be yelling most of the time for food.

The baby on a regular schedule is fed at six o'clock in the morning; gets some orange juice at eight-thirty, and at nine o'clock is put on his chair for action of the bowels. At nine-fifteen he has a bath, and at ten o'clock another feeding and some cod-liver oil. From ten-thirty until one-forty-five the baby may be outdoors in his carriage, presumably asleep. If he is a normal baby and comfortable, he will not cry during this period.

At two o'clock the baby is fed again, and from two-thirty until about five-thirty the baby again may remain outdoors in his carriage. At five-thirty he will be undressed, sponged, and made ready for bed.

At six o'clock, he will be given another feeding, with some cod-liver oil. At six-fifteen he may be put to bed.

When the baby is a year old, the feeding at six o'clock in the morning is substituted by one given at seven or eight o'clock.

ESSENTIAL HEALTH HABITS FOR THE ONE-YEAR-OLD—The essential habits include those which affect eating, cleanliness, sleeping, and exercise.

One of the important habits concerned in eating is feeding oneself. Most children can be taught to feed themselves by the end of the second year. For a child to be fed by another after this time is abnormal and unfortunate.

The child should be taught to eat a variety of foods and not to make an entire meal of one or two substances. While children may be sensitive to one or two articles of diet, there still remains a vast variety of foods from which to choose. Children should be taught to eat foods that are proper for them and not to want coffee, candy, or other foods of their own choosing, in amounts not suitable to their years.

Children should eat slowly and chew thoroughly. They can be taught to chew by giving them solid food and such substances as hard, dry crackers, zwieback, crisp toast, and similar substances.

Finally, the baby, according to his needs, should drink water several times a day between meals, as well as the water which regularly accompanies the meals.

Especially important is emphasis on the baby's feeding himself and eating without too much trouble. The baby who lacks appetite learns to play with the food. Parents encourage this by feeding the baby and amusing him during the eating. The child develops less and less desire for food and will probably learn to vomit, just to avoid eating.

Most experts now advise that the food should be given at regular hours and be taken away in fifteen or twenty minutes, even though none has been eaten. The child should not be offered more food until the next regular meal. It is hardly worth while to spend much time talking to him, because coaxing only makes matters worse.

TRAINING IN CLEANLINESS—Habits of cleanliness include a full bath at least twice a week, and preferably once a day, regular washing of the hands and face as needed, and invariably washing of the hands before eating and after going to the toilet. Habits of cleanliness also include brushing of the teeth, preferably every morning and every night before going to bed.

Finally, there is the habit of internal cleanliness, which involves regular bowel movements, established preferably as a habit each morning immediately after breakfast.

Mothers should establish a routine of cleanliness for their children. This does not mean that a child should remain immaculate all day long. If he plays as he should, he is likely to get dirty at frequent intervals. But he must learn that cleanliness invariably precedes eating.

Cleanliness will include not only the daily bath but also brushing of the hair, cleaning of the fingernails, and a suitable shampoo. A child who plays outdoors at the beach may need to have his head washed every three or four days. After such head washing, the soap is rinsed out. If the scalp is too dry, some olive oil may be rubbed in.

Cleanliness is much more likely to become habitual if it is made easy. The washstand should not be too high, the soap should be easy to reach, the mirror should not be so high that the child cannot see himself washing, and the towel should be readily available. This does not mean a midget-size bathroom for every home. It does mean, however, suitable boxes or steps on which to stand and a towel rack exclusively for the child. It is remarkable how much can be accomplished in establishing good habits if they are made easy rather than hard to acquire.

DIET FOR THE TWO-YEAR-OLD—In the second year the child's diet still should consist chiefly of milk, cereals, vegetables, fruit juices, or cooked fruit, some meat and some eggs. A suitable diet for the two-year-old will be about as follows:

7 to 8 a.m.—Cooked cereal, three to six tablespoonfuls, with milk and a little sugar; milk, six to eight ounces; dry bread, toast, zwieback, or cracker, plain or lightly buttered.

10 a.m.—Juice of an orange. (This may be given with one of the meals instead.)

12 to 1 p.m.—Meat broth, vegetable soup, ground meat, or egg; white vegetable: potato, macaroni, spaghetti, rice, or hominy; green vegetable: peas, beans, beets, spinach, asparagus, onions, carrots, squash, et cetera (mashed or strained); cooked fruit or banana; dried bread, zwieback, or toast, lightly buttered. A drink of milk or a cracker may be given in the middle of the afternoon, provided this does not disturb the appetite at mealtimes.

6 p.m.—Same as breakfast. In addition, soft-cooked egg, junket, custard, or some simple dessert may be given. A white vegetable (see above) may be

substituted for the cereal, and soup for the milk.

Up to the age of nine or ten years the child may have a midafternoon lunch, but after that he should have three regular meals with the family.

Thick cream should not be given to small children, because it is commonly associated with disturbances of digestion and with coated tongue, foul breath, and similar difficulties.

Fresh cottage or cream cheese may be given to children of three or four years of age, but other forms of cheese are not especially suited to children before the youngsters are ten years of age or older.

Eggs may be given at all ages, but the nature of preparation varies. Fried eggs should not be given to very young children. Before the age of seven they should get only plain omelet. Most children from five to ten years old may have a fresh egg for breakfast and another for supper, unless they happen to be sensitive to eggs.

COD-LIVER OIL—Cod-liver oil is used primarily for its content of vitamins A and D, and for treatment of the disease called rickets. In rickets there is softening of the bones due to failure of the body to use properly the mineral substances, calcium and phosphorus. Vitamin D apparently is the substance which controls this utilization. Vitamin D is created by the human body when it is exposed to the ultraviolet rays of the sun. Strangely, rickets did not appear prominently among human beings until the development of window glass. Ordinary window glass does not permit the ultraviolet rays to pass.

There was a time when rickets affected as many as 50 to 80 per cent of all children. Their long bones did not grow properly. Their muscles were flabby and they developed characteristic potbelly. Along the sides of the chest where the bones of the ribs meet the cartilages, little knobs appeared. This gave the appearance of what is called "rickety rosary." The head bones did not develop properly and the rickety

children had a square-headed appearance. The bones of the arms and legs bent and such children became knock-kneed or bowlegged, while some even developed twisted spines.

Now cod-liver oil is the substance in nature which is richest in vitamin D, and physicians soon found that use of cod-liver oil prevented rickets. Most doctors prescribe five drops of fluid cod-liver oil three times a day for babies two weeks old, and increase the dose, after three weeks, to ten drops three times a day. Later the baby should get two teaspoonfuls daily, this dose beginning at three months. From four months onward, it is common to prescribe three teaspoonfuls daily.

Modern cod-liver oil, however, is more potent in its content of vitamin D than that available even four or five years ago, so that now only two teaspoonfuls daily are required for the prevention of rickets in most children.

USE OF IRRADIATED FOODS—So important has cod-liver oil been found for growth and development that it is commonly given to chickens, cattle, dogs, and other animals as well as to man. It is especially important for the prospective mother, since she must supply vitamin D, calcium, and phosphorus not only for herself but for the growing baby.

In addition to taking cod-liver oil, however, there are other ways in which the baby may get the vitamin D that he requires. Most specialists in diseases of children still feel, nevertheless, that babies are better off with cod-liver oil than with some other method of getting vitamin D into their bodies. Babies in general do not object to the taste of cod-liver oil, which is usually best given just before feeding. In rare instances babies object seriously to the oil and sometimes have indigestion. Moreover, premature babies need much more vitamin D than normal babies, and in such cases it may be desirable to use some of the other preparations.

Among preparations which may be prescribed are irradiated ergosterol or viosterol. This form of vitamin D is much more potent than cod-liver oil. Because of its potency it is best that it be prescribed by a doctor according to the baby's individual needs. It is understood, of course, that the baby also gets some vitamin D by exposure to sun rays. Sun baths should always be given to babies when the climate permits. They should be exposed gradually, however, permitting only a portion of the body to have the sun for a few minutes at first, and gradually increasing the area exposed until the whole body is tanned. Not more than ten or fifteen minutes' exposure should be given at first. This may be increased later until the whole body is exposed to mild sunlight for as long as an hour.

In winter, when the rays coming from the sun have little vitamin D value, the doctor may recommend instead the use of artificial ultraviolet rays.

Most recently vitamin D has been prescribed in the form of irradiated milk products. Those examined and passed by the Council on Foods and Nutrition of the American Medical Association will bear labels indicating the amount of vitamin D units that they contain, and it is possible to compare these units with those of cod-liver oil. But even though a quart of milk will provide the same number of units of vitamin D as are provided by two or three teaspoonfuls of cod-liver oil, you should see that the baby actually gets all the milk, to be certain that he gets all the vitamin D he needs. For children who cannot take this amount of milk, it may be better to rely on cod-liver oil or viosterol.

Halibut-liver oil, when reinforced with viosterol, has a high content of both vitamins A and D. Certain food substances, such as egg yolk and butter, also contain considerable amounts of vitamin D, but it is not well to depend on these substances alone to provide the child with sufficient insurance against rickets.

SLEEP FOR THE BABY—Newborn babies, with good digestion and good appetite, and with the proper food, will usually sleep about nine tenths of the time. Gradually they require less and less sleep, so that by the age of six months they sleep about two thirds of the time. From four to six years of age a child will sleep twelve hours a day; from seven to ten years of age, eleven hours a day; from eleven to fourteen years, ten hours a day; and from fourteen to sixteen years of age, nine hours a day. Up to six years of age, a baby should also have a nap during the day, lasting from three quarters of an hour to an hour and a half.

Children seldom sleep too much. They are usually, if well, too full of vim and vigor to sleep too long or too often. In fact, excess sleep may be a sign of a disturbance about which parents should consult the doctor. Children between two and ten years of age are likely to be intensively active during every wakeful moment.

Some children require more sleep than others, and consequently like to sleep late in the morning. If growing children stay up late, they should not be accused of being lazy when they oversleep in the morning.

If a child lies in bed, awake, for a few minutes after being aroused in the morning, he may be lazy; but if he immediately falls asleep again and sleeps soundly, he may be trying to get the sleep he actually needs.

Sleep is distinctly a habit. If good sleeping habits are established early in life, they tend to persist.

Hunger, pain, sudden noises, flashes of light, and sudden changes in temperature will awaken a small baby. Obviously, if the baby is kept warm, if he is put into his crib in such manner as to permit muscular activity, if his digestive tract is kept free from discomfort by proper feeding, if his clothing is not too thick, and if the room is not too warm, the baby probably will sleep well.

Children can be taught to disregard slight noises, slight changes in lighting, and similar external factors. Training in sleep must begin early. The child who once has formed the habit of wakefulness, or the child awakened by the slightest noise, is difficult to control in matters of sleep. Mothers must learn to disregard slight wakefulness and not rush into the child's room every time he turns over. For this reason it is inadvisable for the mother or the nurse to sleep in the same room with the child, and certainly not in the same bed. If the infant sleeps with his mother, there is a tendency to nurse the baby frequently.

It is argued that children will sleep better if they are allowed to stay up at night until they almost "fall asleep on their feet." The child who is unusually tired before he goes to bed will be irritable and excited.

AIDS TO SLEEP—For babies, as for grownups, the conditions of sleep make a great deal of difference. Everybody knows that two factors most necessary for sound sleep—darkness and quiet— are exceedingly hard to achieve in our modern times.

Use of artificial light has become so universal that it is exceedingly difficult to find places to sleep in which there is complete darkness. Even tiny rays of light may be sufficient to serve as a stimulus to awaken a sleeper.

It is even more difficult to secure quiet. We have one motorcar for every four or five people, and at least one radio for every family. This means plenty of noise. In the large cities the rattle of streetcars and the roar of railroad and elevated trains all serve to make sleep difficult, even for those who can easily adapt themselves to disturbances. One specialist has even recommended the use of nightcaps, to serve the double purpose of keeping the head warm and shutting out noise.

The mattress on which the baby sleeps should be firm, but soft enough to be comfortable. The baby should be covered lightly, but well enough to be warm. The clothing should be sufficiently loose to permit the baby to move freely, but tight enough to keep him from falling out of bed or getting into trouble. Pillows usually are unnecessary for small babies.

If the baby's feet become cold, if he is not warm enough, if there is too much clothing, or if there is lack of fresh air in the bedroom, the baby's sleep will be disturbed. Most mothers now know that babies ought to have fresh air, but few of them know just how much fresh air the baby should have and, for that matter, may have no idea of what constitutes fresh air.

Babies ought to be put outdoors to sleep at as early as two weeks of age, if born in the summer months; if born in the winter months, they should be taken outside at six weeks of age.

Since it is difficult for people living in modern city apartments to put the baby outside, the best substitute is to put him, dressed as if he were going out, in his carriage in front of an open window. Then the door of the room should be closed to prevent a direct breeze or draft from blowing over the baby's head. If the weather is very cold, some cold cream may be rubbed on the baby's face before he is taken outside, to prevent chapping. There is little to be gained if the baby is put outdoors, swaddled in heavy clothing and his face covered with a veil. A veil keeps out the beneficial rays of light and keeps in the moisture from breathing. Under such conditions the child soon becomes damp and uncomfortable.

Among other causes of disordered sleep is obstruction of the nose by adenoids, infection, or a cold. Obviously these conditions will prevent a child from sleeping, and certainly should be called to the prompt attention of a doctor.

CLOTHING FOR THE BABY—Most mothers make the mistake of dressing their babies too warmly. As a result of being overdressed, a child perspires freely. If he then kicks off his covers or some of his clothing, he will become chilled.

There is increasing evidence that sudden changes in temperature are harmful to health. Of course a child must be protected against cold and should be suitably covered when he is taken out in cold weather. On the other hand, during very hot days or nights many babies sleep better while wearing only a diaper and flannelette or cotton gown. There has been much discussion as to whether babies should wear cotton, wool, silk, or rayon, or mixtures of these fabrics. In general cotton is not a warm material, as it readily conducts, or carries off, heat. It can be boiled or sterilized, however, without damage.

Wool is a warm material because it is a poor conductor of heat. It is sometimes more irritating to the skin than cotton, and is usually more difficult to wash. Wool must be cleaned with lukewarm water, because boiling water and strong soaps harden and otherwise harm its fibers.

Silk is not a warm material, and some babies are sensitive to it. Rayon is not warm, either, and must be washed with the same care that is given wool or silk.

To overcome the irritation of woolen fabrics, and yet retain their heat value, clothing now is made with cotton on one face and wool on the other.

Tests made by investigators showed that ribbed knit cottons stretch from one third to one half in washing. Cotton flannels and fleece-lined garments lose much of their fuzz in washing. Woolen fabrics, rayon, and bird's-eye are not changed much by washing if carefully done. In hospitals knitted diapers have been found to outwear other varieties.

Most people nowadays must consider the costs of various fabrics. Cotton is the cheapest. Cotton and rayon mixtures cost slightly more. Wool and cotton, or wool and rayon, are next most expensive. Pure wool is still more costly, and silk and wool is the most expensive mixture.

SLEEPING BAGS AND ACCESSORIES— Among the most important articles of clothing for babies is the sleeping bag. All sorts of sleeping bags have been developed and many have been given extensive trials under various conditions.

A few instances are on record in which babies have suffered harm from sleeping-bag necks that are too tight and loose tapes which wind around the baby's limbs. Mothers, therefore, should be extremely careful in using these articles. A good sleeping bag should be wide enough to cover the crib and somewhat longer than the baby. Materials may be sheeting, canton flannel, French flannel, or light blanketing, depending on the season. There usually are tapes which fasten to the sides of the crib. These serve to hold the bag in place and also to keep it from winding around the baby. Such a sleeping bag should permit freedom of movement for hands and legs. Some of these bags are made with special materials around the neck, to keep the bag from becoming too tight and restricting the breathing in any way.

Rubber pants sometimes are convenient when a child is taken on a trip, or under other special circumstances. They should not be used continuously, however, because they result in less frequent changing of the diapers and subsequent chafing of the skin. Sometimes they restrict the legs so tightly that circulation of the blood is disturbed.

Tests have been made on babies who wore diapers with a waterproof covering as contrasted with babies who wore diapers without such protection. Six babies of each type were compared. At the end of a week the babies without the coverings had used approximately four hundred more pieces of laundry than those with the coverings. Moreover, extra time was required by nurses in changing the entire bed. The children with the waterproof coverings seemed to have no more irritation than those without the coverings. It was the opinion of those who made the test that the irritation came from the excretions and not from the fact that they were held rather longer in contact with the skin.

Modern manufacturers of infants' garments now prepare sun suits which consist simply of a covering for the lower portion of the body, with two straps to go over the shoulders. On some suits there is mesh material which permits ready passage of the sun's rays.

EXERCISES FOR BABIES—A muscle which is used has a feeling of life and elasticity that scientists call "tone." A muscle that is not used becomes flabby. Exercise is needed to give muscles good tone. For this reason exercise of the baby is desirable. Merely playing with the child for a few hours each day will be beneficial. When the baby waves his arms, kicks his legs, and attempts to use his body in various ways, he is taking exercise. When the baby cries, he is exercising his lungs. Every baby should be permitted to lie and kick for a half hour after his bath in the morning, without any restriction except a shirt, diaper, and stockings.

Following are some exercises recommended by a specialist:

TRAINING IN POSTURE—As soon as the baby is able to sit alone, he begins exercises that are useful in developing good posture. These involve bending, reaching for objects held in front of him and over his head, and, associated with this, a certain amount of relaxation.

When the child enters school, he will get regular exercise there, but it may be advisable to continue the exercises at home to insure good development and good posture. In good posture the abdomen is well in and flat, and the buttock muscles do not protrude in the back. In other words, the back should have a normal curve and not be hollowed. The weight of the body is carried on the front of the feet.

Here are a few simple exercises that help the baby develop good posture:

1. In a warm room, with plenty of fresh air, have the child take several long, deep breaths through the nose, inhale and exhale slowly.

2. Stretch the baby's arms overhead with hands apart. Bend his body forward from the waistline, touching the floor with the tips of his fingers. This exercise may be repeated ten times each morning.

3. Lay the baby face downward, raise his body with the hands flat on the floor, then lower. This may be repeated five to ten times.

4. Lay the baby flat on his back, bring hands to shoulders and arms as near to the body as possible, then stretch legs to their utmost, at the same time

extending the arms and bringing them down to the sides. This may be repeated four or five times each day.

Simple exercises of this type demand no special apparatus and are exceedingly useful in maintaining good physical conformation and posture. It is understood, of course, that the modern child indulges in outdoor sports, as well as swimming, badminton, volleyball, and similar indoor activities during the winter.

Clothing worn by growing children should be adapted to such exercises.

CARE OF BABY IN HOT WEATHER— Problems involved in the care of infants and children in summer are related primarily to the change in temperature. Heat makes changes not only in our bodies but in the foods that we eat and in the conditions which surround us.

Probably most significant of the factors to be controlled in summer are those concerned with the food supply. Milk should always be put in the refrigerator as soon as possible after it is delivered. In the summer it is safer, for the health of babies, to boil all milk, whether it has been pasteurized or not. Boiling will destroy harmful germs which may be present.

Ability of the baby to digest food is diminished during hot weather. It is, therefore, customary to cut down somewhat on the amount of food given the child. This may be done safely, because there is less demand on the body for production of heat. The amount of the feeding is reduced anywhere from one sixth to one fifth of the usual quantity. With very small babies it is usually better to cut down the strength of the feeding rather than its total amount.

You should realize, of course, that in summer the baby will require more fluids than are needed during colder weather. If a baby is receiving eight ounces of whole milk at each feeding, the strength of the mixture may be changed by adding two ounces of water to six ounces of whole milk.

He may not gain weight so rapidly under the reduced diet, but this is in the direction of safety. It is understood,

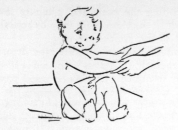

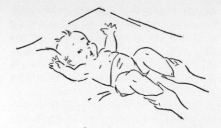

Exercise 1—The baby is laid on his back with his feet toward the mother. The mother then grasps the baby's hands and pulls him toward her. The exercise should be repeated two or three times. The baby tries to help himself up, which strengthens the arm, shoulder, neck, and abdominal muscles

Exercise 2—The baby is laid on his back with his feet toward the mother. The mother then grasps both feet and gently resists any movements that the baby may make. This resistance usually stimulates the baby to kick all the more. The exercise should be continued one or two minutes. It serves to strengthen the leg muscles

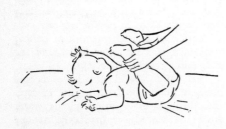

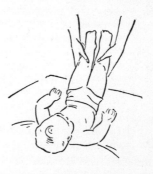

Exercise 3—The baby is laid on his back with his feet toward the mother. The baby's legs are raised and the calves grasped near the ankle. The feet are brought toward the child's nose with knees straight and thighs in contact with the abdomen. This exercise should be repeated three or four times. It tends to strengthen both leg and abdominal muscles

Exercise 4—The baby is laid on his back with his feet toward the mother. The legs are grasped by the mother midway between the knees and the ankles. The legs then are raised until body and legs are almost vertical, with only the baby's head and upper part of the shoulders on the table. The baby then is returned to his original position. The exercise should be repeated two or three times. It tends to strengthen the trunk and spinal muscles

Simple exercises for the baby

of course, that the doctor who is in charge of the baby's feeding should be consulted before any significant changes are made.

The child's food in summer should contain less fat than during the winter because fats are heat-producing.

Mothers frequently ask whether the baby may be given ice cream in hot weather. Sometimes babies are sensitive to frozen milk or cream when they do not have trouble with ordinary milk or cream. Certainly ice cream for children under five years of age should be given in small amounts, and mothers should be certain of its source and character. For older children, ice cream is a useful summer dessert but should not be given in unlimited amounts.

First manifestations of difficulty with food are in the form of diarrhea and vomiting. In hot weather, if the baby begins vomiting or if he shows signs of unusual looseness of the bowel, all food should be omitted immediately and plenty of plain boiled water given instead. After the symptoms stop, milk weakened one half to two thirds with plain boiled water may be used, and if no other symptoms occur, this formula may gradually be increased in strength until it equals the one the baby has been taking regularly.

In older children who suddenly develop vomiting or diarrhea without apparent cause except that related to food, it is advisable to stop food at once and to give nothing but orange juice and water or similar mild drinks.

Remember that babies require a great deal of water at any time but particularly in hot weather. It has been estimated that, if a grown person were to drink the same amount of water as the baby drinks in proportion to his weight, he would consume as much as twelve and a half quarts every day. Remember also that all water given to the baby in summer should be boiled.

CLOTHING FOR SUMMER—Again let me point out that babies should never be overclothed, particularly in summer. In very hot weather they may be clad in only the thinnest type of cotton undervest and a diaper. Remember that the hottest time is at midday and that it may be much cooler in the morning and in the evening, so that the baby will require extra coverings at these times. With too much clothing, the baby's skin will become moist; a sudden drop in temperature would result in chilling of the body and possible frequent colds. On very hot days a sun suit may be worn as the simplest type of easily washable clothing.

A good test of the temperature condition of the child and of the suitability of his clothing is the moistness of the skin. If the skin is moist and particularly if it is moist and clammy, the baby is probably wearing too much clothing. If, on the other hand, the feet and hands are cold and the lips are blue, the baby is cold and requires more clothing. If his clothes are not comfortable, the baby will show his resentment in the usual way—by irritability and crying.

BATHS IN HOT WEATHER—On exceedingly hot days frequent baths do much to keep babies comfortable. These may include not only the full tub bath, which is given for cleansing purposes, but also the sponge bath. For sponging purposes a solution of one teaspoonful of baking soda to a pint of water helps cool the skin and prevent irritations.

The baby should not have a cold bath. A lukewarm bath is just as cooling, through evaporation of the water from the surface of the body, as one which is considerably colder.

After the skin of the baby is dried, it may be powdered liberally with any of the good baby powders. Then, as has been mentioned, the child may be dressed in a light cotton undervest and diaper and allowed to kick or to fall asleep.

There has been a question as to whether babies should be permitted to swim in the sea or in fresh water. Children under five years of age should not be allowed in the water. Children under ten should not go into the water more than once daily, and the water should be warm.

It is important to protect the nose, throat, and ears of children because of the possibility of infection. A child finds it exceedingly pleasant to play on the beach and to paddle in the shallow water near the shore. On the other hand, this may be dangerous for small children if there are waves and undertow.

Some children react more seriously to cold water than others. Some may remain longer in the water than others. The mother who is familiar with her child's constitution and general condition will realize these variations.

EXPOSURE TO THE SUN—Summer sunshine is exceedingly desirable for all babies. There is no danger to the eyes or to the skin of the baby if exposure to the sun is begun moderately and increased gradually. Fresh air and sunshine help to improve the diet and the digestion and actually produce visible signs of improved health.

On hot summer days the best hours for airing the baby outdoors are in the morning and late in the afternoon, rather than in the extreme heat of the sun in the middle of the day. Small babies may be put outdoors in summer when they are one week old. In winter or fall small babies should not be put outdoors unless they are at least three to six weeks old.

It should be remembered that the child is helped not only by the direct rays of the sun but also by the reflected rays or by what sometimes is called "sky shine."

One may begin exposing an infant from three to four weeks of age to five minutes of reflected sunshine and fresh air and gradually increase this by two minutes daily until the baby is receiving from one half to one hour of exposure each day. With older children it is satisfactory to dress the child in a sun suit and permit him to play in the sun for fairly long periods.

While sunstroke is a fairly frequent condition in adults, it is not so common among children. They are not compelled to stay in the sun when they are not comfortable, and they are likely to avoid blisters and too much sun. Children may become acutely ill from an overdose of exposure to the sun. This illness is manifested not only by redness and blistering of the skin, which is painful, but by fever and even delirium and prostration.

The only thing to remember in preventing such disturbances is the necessity of safeguarding the child by having him acquire the sunburn gradually. There are various lotions and creams which serve the purpose of protecting the child from sunburn.

Heat prostration, of course, is more common than sunstroke. When the condition of the child indicates that he has been overexposed to heat, he should be put to bed and a physician called. Before the doctor comes, the child's feet should be kept warm. He may be given plenty of fluids—not too cold—and may be kept cool by forced ventilation with a fan.

SUMMER CAMPS FOR CHILDREN—A large hotel devoted primarily to the recreations and dissipations of adults is not the best place for a child in the summer. Under these conditions the child's food cannot be supervised properly because the menus are planned primarily for adults. For the child's welfare a summer cottage or a small hotel is preferable to the great summer resorts. Many mothers and fathers arrange to give themselves a two-month vacation in summer by sending the children to camps. These are now under state supervision in many places. The best camps also have doctors and nurses in constant attendance as well as suitable educational and recreational instruction.

In selecting a summer camp, parents should make certain whether the camp provides sanitary conditions, food, and medical attention, and social conditions at least as good as those the child has at home. Parents should make certain that health hazards are under suitable control. A good camp provides for proper disposal of sewage, elimination of dust and crowding, and prevention of fire hazards. In areas where there are many insects, particularly mosquitoes, good camps will be provided with mosquito netting and other methods of controlling insect life. Particularly important in the summer camp is the water and food supply.

There is a great tendency in summer camps for children to overexercise and overwork to obtain high ratings in camp activities. Parents should be certain that fatigue is under control and that the children are given enough rest to enable them to recuperate from both physical and mental excesses.

Hundreds of camps do not have even an infirmary for children who become ill. In such camps there are records of children who have broken arms or legs, or who have suddenly developed infectious diseases, appendicitis, or similar ailments, and have not had immediate medical attention because of inability to obtain a physician promptly. While the parent delegates the responsibility for the care of his child to the camp authorities, he must at the same time make certain that these officials have available the necessary professional and medical advice to protect against such hazards.

TRAVELING WITH BABY—The best advice regarding travel for a small baby is —"Don't." For such infants travel should be avoided as much as possible.

The chief risks of travel, like those of vacations, involve the difficulty of control over temperature, food, and water; the hazards of meeting people who may be subject to infections easily transmittable to children; and the dangers of dust and accident, if one is traveling by motorcar. In general, a motorcar is as good as a train for a short trip. For longer trips the motorcar introduces the extra danger of accident and the difficulty of regulating satisfactorily the temperature inside the car.

If it is necessary to travel with a baby and if the trip is to be made by train, the mother should provide a pillow on which the child may rest; also, if the infant is small enough, a large basket in which the pillow may be placed. If the train trip is short and the baby is being fed by the bottle, a sufficient number of bottles should be filled with the formula in advance and taken along. Porters on trains now are quite accustomed to putting such bottles in the refrigerator and bringing them out as they are required by the baby. If there is any chance that refrigeration will not be available, a small bucket may be filled with ice and the bottles put in this bucket before the mother boards the train. Large amounts of the formula should not be made up and put into a thermos bottle with the idea of pouring small amounts from the thermos bottle into the small one as required. It is impossible to keep the milk cold enough by this method, and it is hard to prevent contamination of the material as it is used.

If a trip is to be over a long distance, so that it is necessary to prepare food for the baby while traveling, mothers usually find it better to depend on evaporated or powdered milk or on some of the special milk formulas now available. In most hotels and even in dining cars on the trains arrangements may be made to heat the formula and to prepare it suitably for the baby as needed. Be sure, however, that on the trip children are not permitted to eat all sorts of extra food substances to which they are not accustomed, since this may lead to disorders of digestion.

THE CHILD'S TEETH—Children differ considerably in the ways they develop their teeth. They differ even in the difficulties they have during teething. But even the healthiest children may be fretful and sleep poorly for two or three nights when the first teeth come through. They have a disposition to put fingers in their mouths and to indicate discomfort in other ways. Sometimes there is considerable drooling, or flow of saliva, with loss of appetite. There may also be slight fever and looseness of the bowels and the appearance of undigested foods in the excretions. In most instances these symptoms will last only three or four days, and there may be no gain in weight for three or four weeks. If symptoms of teething are severe, the mother should consult her doctor promptly for aid in prevention of pain and in encouraging development of the teeth.

It is useful also to know the sequence in which the teeth usually appear. First come the two central lower teeth during the period from the fifth to the ninth month; next the four upper central teeth, which come in from the eighth to the twelfth month. The other two lower central teeth and the four front double teeth follow in the twelfth to the eighteenth month. Altogether there are twenty teeth in the first set. The remainder appear between the eighteenth and the twenty-fourth month, except the four back double teeth, which usually appear between the twenty-fourth and thirtieth month but may be even later.

The importance of teeth for health and long life cannot be overestimated. Few mothers realize that first attention to the teeth of the child must begin before the baby is born. The mother should visit her own dentist early. She must keep her own teeth clean and take care of any cavities or decay which develop. She must always eat the right foods, so that the child's teeth will develop properly. Proper foods for the expectant mother include plenty of milk, fresh vegetables, eggs, cooked fruits, cereals, and a sufficient amount of calories to provide energy. The foods to be avoided are sweets and meat in excess, pastries, and highly seasoned substances.

DIET FOR GOOD TEETH—Research workers have emphasized the importance of an adequate supply of minerals, such as calcium and phosphorus, and particularly of vitamins A, C, and D, for the proper development of sound teeth. Such essentials are included in a diet which provides plenty of milk daily or its equivalent in butter or cheese, eggs, leafy green vegetables, and fresh fruit. For growing babies this is supplemented by cod-liver oil.

Many doctors and dentists feel that coarse foods strengthen the jaws and help to harden the gums. When a new tooth is coming in, the coarse foods serve as a resistance against which the gums may work, to permit the teeth to cut their way through.

Among the substances in the diet likely to be deficient, calcium is most prominent. Phosphorus is fairly abundant in the tissue of meat and in eggs. Milk is the best source of calcium, as are also milk products, such as cheese. It is necessary, however, to have both vitamins A and D in sufficient amounts to make certain that the body will suitably utilize the calcium and phosphorus for purposes of growth. The appearance and the development of the teeth are an indication of whether the child is being fed properly.

Of the vitamins that are necessary, vitamin A, as has already been mentioned, is found most plentifully in halibut-liver oil and cod-liver oil, also in butter and eggs. Vitamin D is found particularly in cod-liver oil and in the halibut-liver oil preparations which are reinforced with vitamin D. Vitamin C is found plentifully in orange and tomato juice as well as in other fruit juices.

Until the first teeth of the baby appear, the mouth does well if it is let alone. After the first teeth appear, the gums and teeth may be wiped each day with a soft clean cloth dipped in water to which a little salt has been added. This should be done very gently because of the tender character of the tissues of the child. At about eighteen months a soft brush may be substituted for the soft cloth. As the child becomes older, he should be taught to take pride in the appearance of his teeth and to learn to brush them for himself each morning and evening. If the child likes the taste of toothpaste, he may have toothpaste. If he prefers water with a little salt, he should be given that solution. Most dentists feel that toothpastes, tooth powders, and similar preparations are equally efficient so far as concerns any possibility of preventing infection. Their chief purpose is to cleanse and polish the teeth. Claims for prevention of acidity, or other similar medical claims, are not warranted.

THE SICK CHILD—When a baby is

sick, the first thing to do is to make certain of the nature of the ailment. For this a doctor must be called. Do not take illnesses lightly, as most of the common infectious diseases begin in just about the same way. The child who is listless, drowsy, flushed, and breathing with difficulty is obviously a sick child. The one who is alert, smiling, and playful is more likely to be healthy. A child who looks well probably feels well. It is not absolutely safe, however, to trust merely to the appearance of the child as a sign of his physical condition. It is much better to know with certainty than to take a chance.

An adult is able to say something about the state of his health; not so the child. The examination of a sick baby, therefore, is much more difficult than the examination of an adult. Specialists in diseases of children are compelled to make their diagnoses on the basis of their own observations, helped somewhat by the advice of an intelligent mother or nurse. Some people are inclined to "pooh-pooh" the help of a mother or nurse, but because of their familiarity with the condition of the child they know better than the doctor, who is called for the first time, whether changes are taking place.

If the baby's face is swollen, if his eyes are almost closed, and if he has all the appearances of acute illness, anyone can tell that something is wrong. The real art of scientific observation is applied when conditions are merely beginning to be wrong. If a baby is ill, he has a fretful and moaning cry which differs from that of the healthy baby.

The moment a child shows signs of illness, he should be put to bed. If the child is an infant, the food should be cut down to half strength; if he is older, only fluid food should be given. If the skin seems to be hotter than usual, the temperature should be taken. In the presence of a fever it is well to call the doctor immediately. Do not give any medicine—even a cathartic or a laxative —until the doctor orders it. Until the doctor comes, all other children should be excluded from the room.

PREVENTION OF INFECTIONS (See also *Diphtheria, Scarlet Fever, Typhoid Fever, Smallpox, Whooping Cough, et cetera*)—Certain diseases can be prevented in most instances by inoculations. These are smallpox, diphtheria, scarlet fever, measles, typhoid fever, and chicken pox.

Even though smallpox is rare, every child should be vaccinated against it by the family doctor. The best time for this is usually from the third to the sixth month. For delicate children vaccination against smallpox may be postponed until the child is better developed. If a child happens to be suffering from a skin disease of any sort, vaccination may be temporarily postponed also.

The best place for vaccination is that portion of the body which is most easily protected and which may be kept at rest. For small babies, who have not begun to crawl on the floor, the leg is preferred, particularly in girls. Modern physicians must be far sighted in regard to matters of dress and must look forward to the time when the young lady will be wearing an evening gown. For boys, the arm is just as satisfactory as the leg. When vaccination is done on the legs of older children, they should not be allowed to walk while the vaccination is sore or painful.

If a vaccination does not succeed, this does not necessarily indicate that the child is immune to smallpox. It is rather to be taken as an indication that vaccination will again be necessary in two or three weeks.

Vaccination against smallpox may be repeated at intervals of seven to ten years. It should also be repeated at any time that smallpox is prevalent in the community. We know now that vaccination eradicates smallpox. It is, however, impossible to secure universal vaccination, and because of danger of occasional outbreaks children must be vaccinated regularly.

Against diphtheria we now have available a highly useful inoculation with toxoid. It is so mild in its reactions and so certain in its effects that physicians in general have discontinued preliminary tests of the skin to see whether the child is immune to diphtheria and, instead, recommend universal application of the toxoid inoculation. It is best given to children before the time of their entrance to school. In children who live in cities toxoid inoculation is best given between the sixth and twelfth month. In children housed in institutions, such as orphan asylums or protective homes, inoculation against diphtheria may be practiced in the third month. Millions of children have been inoculated with toxoid without harmful results.

Inoculations against scarlet fever, typhoid fever, and other infectious diseases that have been mentioned are not generally recommended as a routine. Whether such inoculations are to be applied should be left to the family doctor, who will make his decision on the basis of the prevalence of the disease in the community and the likelihood of infection of the individual child.

HYGIENE FOR THE SICK CHILD—When a child is sick, he should be placed in a room with plenty of fresh air and, if possible, sunshine. In cold weather the room should be kept warm; in country districts a room with a fireplace is helpful. Provisions must also be made to prevent drafts by use of suitable window boards or screens. The bed or crib should be freely movable and should be placed in such relationship to the windows that the child will not have to lie and stare at the direct sunlight.

If there is an infectious disease, all unnecessary drapes, carpets, pictures, or other materials should be taken out of the room, as it might afterward be necessary to destroy the materials with which the sick child has been in contact. This applies also to toys and books. Such materials should be inexpensive and easily washed or destroyed. Sick children should not be allowed to play with toy animals made of fur or cloth, since these accumulate discharges and will in any event have to be burned when the child recovers. For the same reason it is not advisable to have upholstered furniture in the sickroom, but preferably hardwood or metal pieces.

When possible the child's sickroom, as well as the adult's, should be adjacent to a bathroom, as this will lessen greatly the amount of work necessary in taking care of the child.

The mother or the nurse who is responsible for the care of the child should keep available a smock or a wash dress to be worn whenever the person is in attendance on the invalid. If there is an infectious disease, it is also advisable to have a cap which covers the hair. The hands of the attendant should always be washed on entering and leaving the sickroom.

Those who are taking care of invalids will find it exceedingly convenient to keep a large paper bag by the side of the bed. In this bag may be placed paper towels, gauze, cotton, and other materials used around the sickroom, and the entire sack and contents burned each day.

No one except the physician who has made the diagnosis and who is familiar with the condition of the invalid should attempt to prescribe food or treatment for a sick child.

All medicines should be kept in stoppered or closed bottles or jars. They should be kept in one place and should be destroyed after the patient recovers, since it is not possible to use the same medicine six or eight months later for other people.

BATHING THE SICK CHILD—The sick baby or child must be suitably clothed to provide for his temperature and to permit the necessary attention. In summer the materials next to the skin should be thin, and the warmth of the body may be regulated by covers. In colder weather a nightdress or simple pajamas may be worn. In the hospital it is customary to have a typical hospital jacket, which makes fairly easy frequent examinations of the chest. In the case of a sick child the doctor will want to listen repeatedly to sounds of heart and lungs. Arrangements must be made so the child will not be too greatly exposed to changes of temperature during this process.

Many mothers fear bathing the child during illness. However, a bath is of greatest importance not only for cleanliness but for control of temperature. When a baby is sick, he must be bathed frequently. Sometimes, unfortunately, the baby will be so ill that he has to be bathed in bed instead of in a tub. When this is necessary, the first step is to see that the room is properly heated, that there are no drafts, and that an hour has passed since the child has had a meal. Fresh bed clothing, towels, and washcloth should be placed at the foot of the bed. The utensils used in washing should be on a table beside crib or bed. When everything is ready, the bath proceeds as follows. The sick child is covered with a blanket and undressed under it. The soiled clothing is placed either in a laundry bag or on sheets of paper ready for wrapping. A bath towel is spread under the child's head and neck, which are then washed with the washcloth wrung out of water and with soap if desirable. After the face, neck, ears, and upper arms are washed, they are dried with the face towel, and the bath towel is removed from under the head. It is then placed lengthwise under the patient, and chest and abdomen are washed carefully.

If turning does not cause pain, the child is turned to the side, and his back is washed while the bath towel is placed lengthwise, close to the back. Then the bath towel is spread lengthwise under each leg separately, and the legs are washed and dried. The child must be well protected by being covered with the blanket during the changing procedure.

After the bath the child may be rubbed with alcohol, or, if too young for this, powder may be applied generously. Then the patient is dressed under the blanket in clean sleeping garments. If the child has been having much fever, cold cream or vaseline may be applied to the lips to overcome dryness and crusting.

FEVERS IN CHILDREN—Fever usually is a sign that a child is ill. A slight increase in temperature, however, is not of itself alarming.

Many babies and children with temperatures just above 99 degrees may be more dangerously ill than babies with 103 degrees. The temperature of the child is not so steady as that of the grownup and varies frequently within large limits.

Baby's temperature usually should be taken with a large bulb thermometer made especially for taking rectal temperatures. The range in babies is between 98 and 99.5 degrees Fahrenheit but not infrequently will vary between 97.5 and 100.5 degrees.

To be certain of a correct reading, the thermometer is shaken well and left in place at least two minutes. Usually it is best to leave in the instrument for one minute longer than the time printed on it.

There are many different causes of fevers in young children. A sore throat, a cold, or a disturbance of digestion may bring about a fever or may indicate the onset of any of the common infectious diseases, such as scarlet fever, measles, diphtheria, whooping cough, or chicken pox.

As has been mentioned already, the physician should be called immediately when there is a fever. No attempt should be made to give strong cathartics or to clean out the bowels with castor oil until one is certain of the nature of the disturbance.

Many feverish babies feel better after a sponge bath with lukewarm water. An icecap or an ice bag around the neck is helpful in cases of sore throat or severe headache. The diet should be restricted. In the presence of severe bowel disturbance all food should be stopped until the physician is in charge of the case. In complaints without bowel disturbance light materials, such as cereals, broths, and finely ground or sieved foods, may be served. Water may be given in large quantities, as well as drinks such as orangeade and lemonade.

The fever is likely to be particularly high in cases of earache or in other conditions in which infectious material is accumulated under pressure at some point in the body. In such cases a release of the infectious material usually brings about a prompt fall in the temperature. It is not well to temporize even slightly with a severe earache.

COLDS IN BABIES (See also *Bronchitis, Colds, Coughing, et cetera*)—The most frequent illness of babies is the common cold. Usually this is not serious, but everything possible should be done to prevent secondary bronchitis, pneumonia, or an infected ear.

Children who are well fed and well taken care of, with proper attention to hygiene, are much less likely to catch cold than those who are undernourished and constantly exposed to changes in temperature and crowded conditions. The child who has plenty of sleep, exercise, fresh air, and sunshine is more likely to resist colds than the one who is subjected to improper hygiene.

Air in the child's room should be suitably moistened by evaporation of water from the radiator or by use of a humidifying device. It is now possible to purchase at small cost an instrument which tells the humidity of the room. The average house is about 20, when it should be 45 or 50 in winter.

People with colds should not be permitted to come near babies, particularly those who are delicate, for they catch cold much more easily than adults who are accustomed to colds.

Large tonsils and adenoids also seem to make children more susceptible than adults to sore throats. If a child is found to have large or infected tonsils and adenoids, these should be removed. It is the universal opinion that children who have had infected tonsils and adenoids removed suffer less frequently with sore throats than they did before.

In preventing colds in children the diet should contain adequate amounts of cod-liver oil, and the amounts of carbohydrates should be lessened. The clothing should be of medium weight, and care should be taken to avoid chilling after perspiration. The sleeping room should be cool.

The child should have a lukewarm or slightly cool sponge bath in the morning, given in a warm room and with the feet in warm water. This bath should be quite short—less than a minute—and should be followed by a brisk rub with a towel. The warm bath should be taken at night.

Use of shots or injections to prevent colds is not yet established as really useful, although many physicians are inclined to believe that these injections help. When adults in homes in which there are small babies develop colds, they may wear gauze masks to cover nose and mouth and in that way prevent transmission of colds to the babies.

At the first sign of a cold the child should be put to bed, his food lessened, and his bowels regulated. If there is fever, the doctor should be called. The child should not be permitted to get up until one day after he has recovered from the cold. Then he should be permitted to play in the house but not to go outdoors until he has certainly recovered. He may then go outside for brief periods until he is free from secondary symptoms, including discharges from the nose.

When babies are sick with colds, they should not be overdosed with widely advertised cold remedies, since many of these remedies contain drugs which may be dangerous.

RUPTURES IN BABIES (See also *Hernia*)—Not infrequently a child is born with a weak place in the wall of the abdomen which results sometimes, even at birth, in the appearance of what scientists call hernia and what the public commonly calls a rupture.

The rupture usually is seen as a swelling, because the intestines or other materials within the abdomen have pushed their way through the weak place in the muscle wall. The most common place for ruptures to appear in babies at birth is somewhere in the middle line around the navel. In older children ruptures usually are seen in the groin, and not infrequently in boys they may push down into the genitals.

When the child coughs or cries or strains, the rupture is seen more easily because of the pressure which develops in the abdominal cavity. If the child lies down and stops straining, the material in the rupture will disappear or can be pushed back easily.

One way to prevent ruptures at the navel is to make certain that the abdomen is given extra support during the first few months. For this reason an abdominal band is worn. Babies may wear this band for five or six months, if the doctor indicates necessity for it.

Ruptures in the groin are much more serious than those in the middle line of the abdomen. A child with such a rupture should be under the immediate care of a doctor, who will advise the proper procedure to be followed.

Various devices have been developed for controlling ruptures, including usually a simple pad over which a piece of tightly drawn adhesive tape is placed. This should always be arranged by the doctor, since it is possible with the wrong kind of a pad to enlarge the opening rather than to aid its closure.

In cases of whooping cough in young babies it is desirable occasionally to put on an abdominal binder quite soon because of the danger of rupture due to the increased strain brought about by constant coughing.

Rupture is a fairly frequent condition among adult Americans. Ruptures in the groin were found in 5.1 per cent of 17,000 men who were given periodic physical examinations.

A rupture is an injury which may be corrected without much trouble if it is seen, diagnosed, and treated early. If it lasts for a long time, however, suitable care becomes more and more difficult.

TONSILS IN BABIES (See also *Tonsils*) —Tonsils are removed simply because they are so greatly enlarged as to interfere with swallowing and breathing. In many instances, however, they are found to be filled with infectious material, and for that reason constitute a menace to health and life.

No one has ever determined just why we have tonsils. Apparently they serve some purpose in taking care of infectious germs that get into the throat. When the tonsils become infected, they swell and there is pain, soreness, difficulty in swallowing, swelling of the glands in

the throat, high fever, rapid pulse, general weakness, and an appearance of illness.

The germ most frequently responsible for tonsillitis is the streptococcus. A germ of the same general nature also is responsible for various forms of heart disease, rheumatism, erysipelas, and scarlet fever. Once the tonsils have been seriously infected, they are likely to become infected again and again.

A child with tonsillitis should be put to bed immediately. When a physician is called, he will usually apply suitable antiseptics directly to the throat to destroy the germs on the surface. He will do what he can to control the fever, and he will prescribe helpful remedies. Application of an ice bag or of hot packs will give relief from the pain and soreness. A gargle with a small amount of baking soda will help to clear the throat of mucus and will make it feel more comfortable. Doctors do not, however, place much confidence in gargles for eliminating infection.

Bear in mind that tonsillitis is especially dangerous because of its secondary effects. The condition itself is seldom fatal, but the possibility of an infected ear, infected joints, or heart disease is so serious that a sore throat and chronically inflamed tonsils should never be neglected.

Removal of the tonsils is not dangerous. It has been well established that such an operation will lessen the incidence of sore throat and make less likely the occurrence of scarlet fever and diphtheria. Wholesale removal of tonsils, however, is not warranted. At present most doctors are convinced that the correct method for removing the tonsils usually is the surgical method rather than their slow destruction by electric coagulation.

ADENOIDS IN BABIES (See also *Adenoids*)—The adenoids lie in the cavity behind the nose. Like the tonsils, they may be seriously infected and transmit infection to other parts of the body.

When the adenoids become infected and swollen, they block nasal breathing, the mouth is kept open, and the person afflicted often appears to have a stupid expression. After breathing continuously through the mouth, the child with infected adenoids is likely to develop an unusual appearance. The upper lip is shortened and turned out, the lips are thickened, and a line is formed between the cheeks and the lips. This is a result of the narrowing of the dental arch of the upper jaw.

When there is infection in the adenoids, the germs pass through the tubes that connect the throat to the ear and may infect cavities of the internal and middle ear.

Since the nose is blocked, the speech of a child with adenoids has a nasal sound. Children with obstructed breathing are restless at night; they snore, gasp, and toss about. Furthermore, difficulty in breathing may interfere with development of the chest, which becomes narrow and flat.

There is no fancy way for prevention and treatment of adenoids that are infected and swollen. They can be removed by a minor operation. Whenever they are enlarged or seem to be infected, they should be removed. The time of the operation is determined by the symptoms. Thus it may be necessary to remove the adenoids in babies under one year of age. In general, however, the operation should be postponed until the child has passed the age of two or three years. The chance of new growth of adenoid material is less after the age of two or three years than it is before. Somewhere between 10 to 15 per cent of the cases in which the adenoids have been removed require a second operation.

The improvement which follows removal of the adenoids usually is almost miraculous. The child begins at once to gain weight, his breathing is easier, his voice improves, and he is no longer irritable or restless.

CARE OF BABY'S EARS (See also *Mastoiditis, et cetera*)—When your child gets an infected ear, call the doctor. That is the safest thing to do when so tender a part of the head as the human ear is concerned.

Even in the simple matter of cleaning the baby's ears, you must be extremely careful, and you should know the proper technic to use so as not to harm the baby. It is safe enough to go further and wash out accumulated and hardened wax or other material that may have gotten into the ear by accident. For this purpose use a solution of boric acid —two teaspoonfuls to a pint of water. Old hot-water bags which have been lying about in closets and which have filled all sorts of purposes should not be used until they have had a thorough cleaning by repeated rinsings with boiling water. The tube attached to the bag also should be cleaned before any attempt is made to wash the ear. The hard rubber tip should be cleaned thoroughly in alcohol.

The bag filled with the solution may now be hung at a height of about six feet from the floor. If the child to be treated is sitting on a bed or a chair, this will give a fall of about three feet, which is sufficient pressure for the purpose. If more pressure is used, there may be pain from the force of the solution against the eardrum or the inflamed tissue.

If a large syringe filled with water or with the boric acid solution is used, the tip should be held at an angle so that the water will not strike directly against the eardrum but against the side wall of the tube leading to the eardrum.

Temperature of the solution should be tested by dipping the elbow into the water or by dropping some of the solution on the inside of the wrist. If it is too warm for the elbow or wrist, it is too warm for the ear and is likely to be painful.

The head may be bent so that the water will run in and out. However, if there is much hardened wax in the ear, more force may be used to loosen it than is ordinarily necessary for washing the ear canal. Repeated washing with warm water will take care of such conditions. When the canal is inflamed, washing three or four times a day with a lukewarm solution will help.

PAIN IN THE EAR OF BABY—When a

small child has a pain in the ear, he will usually indicate the condition by putting his hand to the ear or crying whenever the ear ; touched. The pain of earache is generally severe, prolonged, and continuous. Immediate relief may be given in such cases by application of heat. This may be done in various ways. You may cover the ear with a piece of cotton and then put a small hot-water bag or a hot application over the cotton. The child may lie with his head on the hot-water bag or on an electric pad. It is not advisable to drop any medicine into the ear unless the doctor has prescribed it.

Infections of the ear frequently follow infectious conditions in the nose or throat and acute infectious diseases.

When a doctor is called to see a child suspected of having an infected ear, he will take the child's temperature, which is usually high in these cases. He will also look directly at the eardrum with a magnifying device and a light. This apparatus is called an otoscope, which merely means a device for seeing the ear. If the doctor finds that the ear is infected severely, he will arrange to open the eardrum promptly, particularly if it is bulging as a sign of pressure within. Opening the eardrum will relieve the pain immediately and will also help prevent the likelihood of infection spreading from the ear to the mastoid.

Sometimes the pain of an earache may be relieved in an early stage by dropping into the ear some warm ear drops, composed usually of glycerin with a small percentage of boric acid or phenol. Such a solution should not be used without advice of the doctor, who will determine also the strength of the mixture to be used in each case.

When the condition spreads from the ear to the mastoid, a much more serious infection, called mastoiditis, develops. In this condition great pain and tenderness are noted behind the ear over the region of the mastoid. From the very first, the mastoid bone may be sensitive to pressure because of the swelling inside.

Puncture of the eardrum is not dangerous. If it is done sufficiently early, there will be no interference with hearing because the eardrum will heal promptly and hearing will be just as good as it was before. It is far less dangerous to puncture the eardrum than it is to postpone the operation too long.

CAUSES OF EARACHE—Sometimes an earache is caused by a boil or an infection in the canal which leads from the exterior down to the eardrum. When a boil begins in the canal that leads down to the eardrum, the tissues around the boil promptly swell. Swelling means pressure, and pressure means pain. A boil in the ear canal will come to a head, just as it does elsewhere. When it comes to a head, it bursts, and the swelling is relieved. With relief of the swelling, there will be relief from the pain. Whenever there is a boil or even a large pimple in the ear canal, the pain will be accentuated if one pulls on the ear or presses on the skin in front of or behind the ear. Even moving of the jaws, as in chewing, may exaggerate the pain.

In some cases nothing may be visible from the outside of the ear. If, however, the doctor looks into the canal, he will find a swelling which partially blocks the view to the eardrum. Under such circumstances the doctor will apply antiseptic substances to stem the growth of the germs and hot applications to eliminate tenderness. When the boil comes to a head, he can puncture it to expedite the removal of its contents and to bring about a more rapid cure.

Remember that boils inside the ear, like boils elsewhere, begin where the skin has been broken or irritated. This is particularly true of boils on the back of the neck which follow irritation by the rough edge of a stiff collar.

Any manipulation of the ear canal for the removal of wax, or of the inside of the ear with hard instruments by those who do not understand the delicate nature of these tissues, may be the first step toward breaking the skin and starting formation of a boil.

FOREIGN BODY IN EAR OF BABY—Two serious dangers affecting the ears require particular care and attention of parents. One concerns the introduction of foreign bodies into the ears. The other results from immersion of the head in water.

A foreign substance in the ear canal will seldom cause much discomfort unless it is a live insect. Cases are on record in which bugs of various kinds have gotten into ears and remained for many years. They die and are surrounded by hardened wax. There are cases in which people have been deaf in one ear for many years as a result of such blocking of the eardrum. Then, when the wax and the foreign body are washed out, the hearing returns.

Persons without experience should not try to remove foreign bodies from the outer ear if the substances cannot be washed out by use of a syringe. Several interesting technics have been developed for this purpose. One includes use of a probe with some adhesive material at the end, to which the foreign body sticks. When the probe is removed, the foreign substance comes with it.

CUTS AND BRUISES OF CHILDREN— Little children frequently suffer cuts, bruises, burns, and similar injuries of the skin which carry with them the possibility of infection. In such cases the first aid given at home is of the greatest importance in preventing secondary infection or dangerous complications.

Whenever germs get into the body and begin to release their poisonous products, the human being may react with fever and chills and usually with an increased number of white blood cells. In a severe infection there is swelling and redness of the part as well as pain and tenderness. However, if suitable first-aid treatment is given promptly, there is no reason for the occurrence of a general reaction affecting the body.

A great many different antiseptic substances are available for use in first aid for children. The child may object seriously to use of any antiseptic substance which burns on application. For this reason many infants refuse to have cuts or infections painted with tincture of iodine. Among other first-aid antiseptics which have been found of value are mercurochrome and metaphen as well

as a solution of hexylresorcinol. From the point of view of antiseptic efficiency, iodine usually is believed to be safer than any of the others, but all have been found to have virtue, particularly as they are applied to human tissue. Effects on the human body are not quite the same as the results shown by comparative tests of various antiseptics made with germs in a test tube.

Danger to fingernails from being mashed or caught in a door also is worthy of attention. Infection underneath the fingernail or destruction of the matrix from which the fingernail grows may result in sufficient damage to the nail plate to produce a crooked fingernail for the rest of the person's life. If a doctor is called to see a patient having a fingernail under which there is infection, he will likely bore a hole through the nail to permit the infection to escape or else cut away that portion of the nail which is over the infection. After the infected material is removed, hot fomentations and hot antiseptics may be applied until the infection clears up completely. Then the fingernail will grow again, and recovery will be complete.

Ordinary small bruises hardly demand more than a casual amount of attention and care, since the blood and the natural mechanism of the body are able to bring about healing. Pain is relieved in most such conditions by application of heat or cold.

CONVULSIONS IN BABIES—Infants have convulsions much more frequently than adults. The nervous system of the child is so sensitive that frequently an acute infectious disease will begin with convulsions. If there is an associated rapid rise in the body temperature, convulsions are more common than otherwise.

In ordinary convulsions the child loses consciousness and becomes rigid. Then there may be a spasmodic jerking of the face and of the arms and legs. It is, of course, necessary to distinguish between ordinary mild convulsions and those which are the result of epilepsy. It is important also to know as soon as possible the cause of the convulsions. This can be determined only by a competent doctor. Even he, however, may not be able to make a diagnosis immediately, since it may require several days for the disease involved to develop. Nevertheless, convulsions should be checked as soon as possible because of the damage they may do to the body.

It is known that warmth is quite sedative, so a hot bath is often used to control mild convulsions. Wrapping the baby in blankets and applying hot-water bottles or electric pads will also lessen the convulsions. You should be certain, however, that the heating equipment used is tested before being applied to the baby's sensitive skin because of the danger of burning.

In a study of convulsions in children made some years ago it was found that boys and girls were affected almost equally. In only one fifth of the cases were the convulsions apparently due to epilepsy.

It is particularly interesting to know that many parents have found the convulsive disorders to be frequently associated with constipation, and that the number of fits were increased by meals which were unusually large or rich. Parents are prone to blame all the disorders of infancy on constipation or on teething. These, however, are rarely actual causes. For this reason a diagnosis is of great importance.

It is well established that deficiencies in calcium in the body will produce a type of convulsive disorder called tetany, which is in a way related to rickets; occasionally, in fact, a complication of rickets. Victims of tetany are promptly benefited if the doctor prescribes suitable amounts of the necessary drugs, including calcium and vitamin D.

CHILLS Anyone who has ever come home from work feeling tired and apprehensive, got into bed, and then suddenly succumbed to the shaking, throbbing, tremulous feeling called a chill knows that it is a nasty symptom. This symptom was known to medical writers thousands of years ago. When the chill

was associated with malaria, it became common to call it "ague."

Now, after these many years, scientific experts have begun to study the chill to find out why it happens and what it means. Nowadays many physicians feel that a chill has a real importance in overcoming a disease and that it ought to be considered from that point of view.

When a chill occurs, there is an increase in the chemical activity going on within the body and, therefore, a rapid rise in the production of heat by the body. The net result of a chill is to raise the body temperature. A person with a chill is usually quiet, lies doubled up, has a pale, cool skin, and sometimes "goose flesh." This is due to the fact that the superficial blood vessels under the skin are constricted—sometimes so greatly that the skin appears blue.

Some degree of voluntary control can be applied, particularly if the chills are mild. When, however, there is a severe chill, it comes on regardless of the will power of the person concerned.

One of the examples of the manner in which a chill functions to maintain the heat of the body is the constant trembling of a hairless dog.

The application of heat, with blankets, warm bed clothing, hot drinks, hot-water bottles, and electric pads, is one of the ways to make a person with chills feel better.

Chills can be induced in patients by injecting non-specific protein substances. They can also be prevented by the giving of drugs which act as sedatives and as controls of the body temperature. It is believed that the action of these drugs, which are known as anti-pyretic or anti-fever drugs, is to depress the shivering center in the brain.

CHIROPRACTIC Chiropractic is a technic for treating disease described about 1894 by D. D. Palmer, of Davenport, Iowa. This system of treatment is based on the belief that the nerves which emerge from the spinal column are pressed on by the bones of the spinal column and that interference with the function of the nerves results, so that eventually the tissues are damaged. Innumerable investigations made by dissections of the spine, the use of the X ray and all of the other technics known to medicine have not been able to show any really scientific basis for the method of treatment called chiropractic. Nevertheless such practitioners are licensed to practice chiropractic in many states and, having once embarked in the field of healing, they undertake to advise concerning diet, massage, physical treatments, colonic irrigations, and similar procedures.

CHLOASMA This is a term applied to discolorations of the skin which appear as yellowish-brown patches and spots. They appear sometimes following exposure of the skin to sun or heat, occasionally in pregnant women, occasionally when oil of bergamot (used in perfumes) is put on the skin, which is then exposed to the sun. Chloasma is also a scientific name for so-called liver spots. A new drug called Benoquin has been used successfully in many cases to relieve pigmentation. It is applied as an ointment. However, specialists in diseases of the skin sometimes remove them by surgical or skin-peeling procedures.

CHOLECYSTITIS See discussion under *Gall Bladder;* cholecystitis is the scientific name for inflammation of the gall bladder.

CHOLELITHIASIS See discussion under *Gall Bladder;* this is the scientific term for gallstones.

CHOLERA From time immemorial a disease has existed in India which has now spread widely throughout the world, probably traveling by way of the caravan routes into Europe and by water along the trade routes of Arabia and Egypt. Some fifty years ago the germ that causes cholera was described by Robert Koch. The organism gets into the bowel and causes an acute infection chiefly involving the small intestine. The main symptoms are a severe, constantly flowing diarrhea, vomiting, collapse, cramps in the muscles, and suppression of the flow of urine from the kidneys. Cholera spreads most in moist, warm climates.

Being an intestinal disease, it spreads in much the same way as does typhoid fever. The germs that cause cholera get out of the body with the material that is vomited or passed from the bowel. The disease can be controlled in various ways, most important being complete control of the supplies of food and water. The material that is passed from the patient must be destroyed by heat. People can protect themselves by making sure that they use only cooked food and boiled water. Sometimes people make the mistake of cooking food or boiling water and then allowing it to stand for long periods of time. During the cooling-off period it may become contaminated again and be just as dangerous as if it had not been heated in the first place. There is also available to those who are going to travel or live in cholera-ridden areas a vaccine against cholera made from the killed bodies of the specific germs that cause the disease. All American troops going into such areas have been inoculated against cholera, and the incidence among our troops has been exceedingly low.

About five or six days after a person has been infected with cholera he develops a severe diarrhea with violent purging and eventually begins passing practically pure mucus and water. Then vomiting begins and then comes collapse. The skin loses its elasticity, the muscles cramp, the eyes are sunken, the voice is feeble. As more and more water is lost, the thirst becomes intense, the pulse becomes rapid and weak, and the blood pressure falls. As the blood loses its oxygen, the skin develops a blue, cyanotic tinge. Then as the patient's condition improves, the reverse of the process occurs.

Whenever large amounts of fluid are lost from the body without replacement, there is danger of death from acidosis. Therefore the chief step in the treatment is restoration of the fluid, which is accomplished by giving large quantities of normal or physiologic salt solution by injection into the veins. Frequently it is necessary to give one or two quarts of this solution every six or eight hours for two or three days. The acidosis is overcome by giving large doses of sodium bicarbonate. Usually the patient with this condition is glad to remain in bed. Warmth is sustained by the usual application of blankets and hot-water bottles. The doctor can help to control the vomiting by prescription of proper remedies.

CHOREA An extraordinary disease of the nervous system is known as St. Vitus' dance, or Sydenham's chorea, after the man who first described it. Nowadays it is believed to be due, in some perhaps indirect way, to infection by a germ of the streptococcus type. Perhaps some of the poisons developed by this germ in the body get into the brain and nervous system and by their action produce their characteristic symptoms.

Sometimes the first appearance of the symptoms is associated with a fright, an accident, or an emotional shock. Children who frequently mimic the actions of other people may seem to have this disease, but a habit spasm is not to be confused with the twitching that is associated with the true chorea.

Girls suffer with this condition about two and one half times as often as do boys, and more than 80 per cent of all of the cases occur during early childhood. The cases appear more often in certain families, probably because of the special construction of the nervous system in those families.

Frequently St. Vitus' dance is associated with rheumatism or rheumatic infections, probably because both conditions are related to an infection by the streptococcus type of germ. Occasionally there may be a period of illness with headache, vomiting, and even a slight fever before the symptoms first appear. Then come the spontaneous movements, the dizziness, and the weakness, which are the chief mark of the disease. The person who has St. Vitus'

dance makes involuntary but conscious muscular jerks and twitches, and because of this has difficulty in co-ordinating his actions. When the twitching movements affect face muscles, they are, of course, much more noticeable than when they concern the arms or legs.

The typical twitching movements are quick, beginning suddenly and passing rapidly. No two movements are exactly alike, as is usually the case with a habit spasm. The movements usually stop but in severe cases may appear during sleep, and in some cases the trouble may be so severe that the patient cannot sleep.

In about one fourth of the children with chorea the speech is disturbed because of the difficulty of articulating during the movements. Simply because of the presence of the disease the child becomes irritable and restless and later may have carelessness, dullness, loss of memory, or inability to pay attention. There are also mild emotional disturbances.

In many instances the condition comes and disappears in six months. In the United States cases seldom last much beyond twelve weeks. There are cases, however, in which the twitching becomes chronic, and sometimes a habit spasm follows the twitching.

Since chorea is a condition affecting the body generally instead of just the nerves and muscles, it is customary to put these children to bed for three to six weeks and to insure plenty of rest. Occasionally they improve greatly with suitable baths and with drugs which help to lessen the severity of the symptoms. Physicians prescribe other drugs which seem to attack the organisms within the body. From time to time various new remedies are tested, but as yet none seems to be specific. In some cases the application of heat appears to help, but here again experience is inadequate to speak with certainty.

Certainly a child with any streptococcic infection within the body demands most careful study and attention. If there are infections at the roots of the teeth or in the tonsils and the adenoids, these must be eliminated. The heart must be watched carefully because such streptococcus infections may reach that organ, where they are much more serious than elsewhere in the body. For this reason the child with symptoms of St. Vitus' dance should be put to bed and should rest for a long time.

During convalescence it is important to build up the nutrition of the child and his reserve. This may be done by giving plenty of food, well balanced with suitable amounts of vitamins and mineral salts, so that the child will not necessarily become too fat, but rather will have the substances necessary for the best possible growth.

In the aftercare of this condition the exercise must be regulated as well as the rest, and the child must have plenty of relaxation, including supervised play. With this type of attention there is little danger of permanent residues from the disease.

CHROMOBLASTOMYCOSIS Blastomycosis is a form of fungous infection of the human body which has long been recognized in the United States. Chromoblastomycosis, however, is a fungous growth in which similar granular tumors occur but in which they are of extraordinary colors. The condition is not wholly rare in tropical areas but cases in the United States itself are so unusual as to command special attention whenever one is found. So far only six cases have been reported in medical writings in the entire United States.

In a case recently found in Atlanta, Georgia, a farmer became suspicious of a growth on the back of his left wrist. It was a vivid bluish-red in color. When doctors took a specimen from this growth and raised it by the methods used for growing living organisms, a dark-colored fungus developed which was known to be the one that causes chromoblastomycosis. These fungous growths are like molds which grow on spoiled food, resembling yeasts in their manner of development. Naturally if such a fungus gets into a vital portion of the body, like the lungs, it may be the cause of death. In the case of the farmer it was possible, by use of the X ray externally and by giving suitable drugs internally, to cause the fungus and the growth to disappear from the body.

As the airplane makes interchange of population between our country and various tropical islands much more frequent, unusual cases of tropical diseases will begin to appear more and more frequently in the United States. A specialist in diseases of the skin in Havana has seen twenty cases of this type in the last two and one half years. Many more cases are seen in Brazil.

In one instance reported in this country the condition had occurred in a man who was a log handler. The physicians who studied this case believed that the fungus occurs most frequently as a saprophyte on plants and wood.

CIRCUMCISION This procedure, originally established as a religious rite among Jews, Mohammedans, and South Sea Islanders, is an operation which involves cutting off of the foreskin of the penis. Nowadays the operation is performed as a routine by many people as a preventive method which permits cleanliness and diminishes the possibility of contracting venereal disease. Inflammation and irritation under the foreskin are also associated with various nervous manifestations like bed-wetting. The operation is most frequently done with a local anesthetic except in exceedingly nervous and high-strung boys or men. When the operation is done in early infancy, it represents a minor procedure. However, it should always be done under the strictest surgical or aseptic precautions. The proper repair of the tissues after the extra skin has been removed is important in securing a good result.

CIRRHOSIS (See discussion under *Liver*) This term is used to describe a hardening of any tissue but most frequently for a hardening of the liver, called cirrhosis of the liver.

CITRIC ACID Citric acid and the citrates are employed as an acid flavor and in effervescent drinks. They are not an effective substitute for orange juice or lemon juice. Citric acid has an alkalizing effect but does not have any vitamin effect.

CLEFT PALATE (See also *Lips*) Sometimes a child is born in whom the tissues of the head have not come properly together, so that there is an opening in the palate and the roof of the mouth. This condition is called cleft palate. Occasionally the lip will have failed to come together, producing what is called harelip. In such cases modern medicine provides surgical procedures which, in the majority of instances, produce complete recovery. These procedures are in the field of oral and plastic surgery. Obviously the operation is only to be done by someone who specializes in this field. In the operation it is customary to bring the separated parts together and to fix them firmly so that they will heal together.

CLIMACTERIC See *Menopause*.

CLIMATE The most ancient of peoples were convinced that there was some relationship between climate and health. The ancient Egyptians and Greeks, Romans and Babylonians wrote down their ideas on the subject. Some of those ideas are well established today, but others have been modified since that time. Modern medicine approaches the subject of climate scientifically, collecting evidence and analyzing its observations, so that some definite facts can be recorded.

For years it has been known that rickets is more frequent in poverty-stricken slums. Recently doctors have learned that rickets is due to failure of the sun to act on the naked skin of the body. Out of this observation came the use of sunlight to produce vitamin D and the prevention of rickets by the administration of vitamin D.

Physicians knew for many years that goiter occurred much more frequently in some areas of the world than in others. Now it is known that goiter occurs most frequently in areas in which the water and soil lack sufficient iodine. Nowadays we give iodine in small doses regularly to people living in such areas and thus prevent goiter.

The ancient Greeks and Romans recognized that malaria affected people who lived in low marshy areas. They blamed the malaria on sleeping in the night air. Nowadays science recognizes that the mosquitoes that carry malaria grow in the swamps and marshy areas. The drying up of the swamps and the prevention of the entrance of the mosquitoes through unscreened windows will control the malaria.

Hippocrates, more than three hundred years before the beginning of the Christian Era, wrote a book called *Airs, Water and Places,* in which he insisted that "the inhabitants of a region which is mountainous, rugged, high and watered, where the changes of the seasons exhibit sharp contrasts, are likely to be of big physique, with a nature well adapted for endurance and courage." This was the first recognition of the temperate zone as the best area in which to live. Hippocrates also said, "If there be no rivers, and the water that the people drink be marshy and stagnant, the physique of the people must show protruding bellies and enlarged spleens." He, of course, did not know that the protruding belly and the enlarged spleen were the result of the malaria which was prevalent in marshy areas.

Climate in its relation to disease includes temperature, humidity, winds, sunshine, the amount of dust in the air, the altitude, the water supply, and many similar factors. Some of the conditions for which changes of climate are frequently recommended are the rheumatic conditions, tuberculosis, and infections of the sinuses and the lungs.

It used to be thought that people with tuberculosis had to go to a high and dry climate in order to be relieved of their condition. We now know that tuberculosis can be successfully treated in any climate and that the attention of a competent doctor, the services of a good sanatorium, and a sufficient amount of rest and good food, the use of artificial pneumothorax and proper drug remedies are much more important than the climatic factor alone.

People with rheumatic conditions frequently do better when they are free from exposure to cold and dampness. Some basic research done on rheumatism has shown that changes occur in the composition of the body tissues, including the blood, when there are changes in the barometric pressure. Similar changes have been discovered with regard to rickets and other ailments. Changes in the blood supply to the joints are associated with sudden changes in temperature. In general, chronic rheumatic conditions attack people in the latter half of life, which is particularly the time when the physical activities of the body tend to become more sluggish and inactive. Quite likely changes in temperature, humidity, and sunlight cannot be regarded as the cause of rheumatic disease. However, it is possible that undesirable combinations of these factors may lower the resistance of the person so that variations may result in more involvement of the tissues by rheumatic fibrosis.

Persons with heart disease do not do well at high altitudes because of increased difficulty in getting enough oxygen for the circulation. People with disturbances of the nervous system and with undue fatigue do badly at busy summer resorts or at the seashore because they receive neither rest nor relaxation but instead indulge in unnecessary activity.

Climate itself is just a part of the whole environment, which includes not only the weather but also the living conditions, the people, and similar factors.

For years the belief has been prevalent that dampness and drafts are associated with catching cold and with the incidence of pneumonia. Careful statistical studies seem to prove a definite relationship between these factors and the incidence of colds and respiratory infections. The explanation may be found in the fact that the changes in temperature and the dampness bring about changes in the circulation in the mucous membranes and that under these circumstances the invading viruses and germs are able to produce infection when otherwise this would not occur.

The question is repeatedly asked as to what climate is best suited to persons with infections of the nose and throat or with chronic infections of the sinuses. In general it is advised that a warm dry climate is preferable to one that is damp and cold. However, the belief that is so tenaciously held by people generally that the Southwest and Southern portions of the United States possess more health-giving and health-restoring virtues than the more rigorous regions of the North has been controverted by the fact that the men and women at Stanford University, where the climate is mild and soft, have just about as many coughs and colds as students at Harvard, where the climate is cold and rigorous. Women students at Stanford and women at Wellesley also had about the same number of infections of the nose and throat when the statistics were accumulated.

The class of patients most benefited by a change to a warm, dry climate is the one whose resistance is low, who takes cold easily, and who suffers more or less constantly from some inflammation of the nose, throat, and sinuses from the first frost in autumn to the last frost in spring.

A warning is justified: never make a permanent change from the climate in which you are established to a new climate until you have made certain by a fairly long residence and an actual trial in the new climate that you are going to feel better and be healthier than in the place where you are living. A change of climate is in most instances a rich man's experiment.

CLOTHING (See also discussion under *Hygiene, Personal*) The fundamental needs of the human being include food, fuel, clothing, shelter, medical and dental care. Much is written about the hygiene of the body from the point of view of housing, nutrition, and warmth. Seldom is serious consideration given to the hygiene of our clothing.

Some scientists insist that human beings first adopted clothing for decorative purposes in order to call attention to themselves or to certain portions of their bodies. Others insist that clothing came because of the development of a sense of modesty. A final view says that we wear clothing to protect us against exposure to cold and the elements.

Probably clothing came first as a decoration; exactly as various animals have highly colored plumage to attract the opposite sex, primitive man probably began fastening things to his body as a means of attraction.

In earlier days most men lived in warm climates, so that clothing was not needed for protection against the elements. It is reasonable to believe that human beings could not have spread from these warm areas to the cold areas without the development of clothing. Man is a warm-blooded animal. He must sustain the warmth of his body if he is to live. Clothing is one means by which the warmth is held within his body. The coverings do not create heat; they do diminish the rate at which heat is lost from the body.

We lose water from the body through the skin. By the evaporaton of this water we also lose heat. When there is too much heat lost from the surface of the body, chilling occurs; hence clothing must be changed from one season of the year to another to meet the conditions necessary for health and comfort.

Various fabrics vary in their ability to retain heat and moisture and to permit ventilation. Cotton and linen garments permit heat to pass off rapidly and thus help to keep the body cool. Silk and wool do not conduct heat rapidly and are, therefore, better suited to winter than summer wear.

Of special importance is the choice of underclothing. In summer all cotton or lightweight silk or mixed silk and cotton garments are more suitable than woolen garments. Some types of clothing permit ultraviolet rays to pass through them more easily than others. A fabric with open mesh not only permits the circulation of air and irradiation of heat but also permits more sunlight to pass through than a fabric with closed mesh.

From the health point of view garments should in general never be so tight as to constrict the tissues. Any garment that is so tight as to prevent circulation of the blood and a free expansion of the organs of the body is not a healthful garment. Garters, belts, and bands which are so tight that they leave red marks on the skin and dents in the flesh interfere with the circulation of the blood and should not be considered suitable.

One of the chief difficulties in modern clothing is the necessity of adapting its use to both indoor and outdoor conditions. In winter women wear fur coats for outdoor use but customarily wear thin clothing both summer and winter for indoor use. The average man wears heavy clothing both indoors and outdoors.

Most hygienists are inclined to recommend to both men and women that all clothing not necessary for warmth or modesty should be eliminated for indoor wear. Nevertheless fashions have much more to do with the choice of clothing by both men and women than hygienic considerations. When it is the custom for men to wear overcoats indoors, they will do so; when it is the custom for women to do without protection to the feet, legs, and chest, they will go without the clothing necessary for warmth.

Change of clothing according to the season of the year is much less necessary in the modern city than was the case in a previous generation. The use of the closed motorcar for transportation, the heated street-car and bus, the heated and air-conditioned schoolroom, assembly hall, and theater make it possible for most people to wear clothing that is reasonably light and to plan only for a single heavy garment for protection against the elements.

From the health point of view this is about all the consideration that can now be given to the subject of clothing. However, the growing boy and girl may well be cautioned again following every foolish fad in clothing that comes along. Zoot suits, bell-bottom pants, tight sweaters, and similar garments have had their day.

Students are often responsible for beginning unusual fads such as autographed jackets, saddle shoes, and similar styles which have come and gone. The intelligent student will consider carefully whether or not the wearing of clothing of a disreputable appearance for the attraction of momentary attention is worth while. Over the centuries it has been proved that cleanliness, orderliness, neatness, and the most nearly perfect fitting that is possible are most important in producing attractiveness.

CLUBFOOT Clubfoot was first described by the father of scientific medicine, the great Greek physician Hippocrates. He recommended that a child born with twisted feet be subjected to repeated manipulations and that bandages then be applied to hold the foot in place until it healed properly.

As time went on various surgeons studied the question more scientifically with a view to producing not only a foot that looked well but also a foot that would be as useful as possible. The methods of treatment of clubfeet have varied and changed from early operative methods, which involved removal of portions of bone and cutting of tendons, to manipulative methods which involved forcing the foot into proper position, and finally to a gradual change in the position of the foot brought about by a series of plaster casts and wedgings.

Today hundreds of children born with clubfeet have been treated by the modern methods with exceedingly successful results.

The exact cause of clubfeet is not known. Apparently heredity has some influence in the matter, because it is found in some 4 to 5 per cent of cases in the family that has had trouble with this deformity previously.

Each year after a child has begun to walk, a longer and longer time is required to correct this type of deformity. Children treated during the first year of life could have their treatment completed within 23 weeks; during the second year of life, 24.5 weeks; the fourth year, 32.3 weeks, and the sixth year, 41.7 weeks.

It is one of the marvels of modern science that children who would formerly have hobbled through life, the subjects of pity, are now enabled to walk about with feet that resemble those of the normal child and are thereby given opportunities for success and happiness.

COCAINE Cocaine is the oldest known drug used for local anesthesia. It is habit-forming and poisonous and should never be used in any way except when prescribed or administered by the doctor.

COCCIDIOSIS In several areas of the country, including particularly California, parasitic organisms of fungal type infect the human being. When they get into the body they cause swellings like tumors and damage to the tissues so that secondary infections may also occur. The organism is called the coccidium and the condition that it causes is known as coccidiosis. The portions of the body infected may include the bones, joints, lymph glands, lungs, or skin. About one in a thousand cases is fatal.

COCCYX The small bones at the lowermost end of the spine are called the coccyx. They are interesting to medicine chiefly when they become bruised by a fall.

COD-LIVER OIL Cod-liver oil is used for the prevention and cure of rickets, to provide vitamins A and D where they are needed in the body whenever there is a deficiency of such vitamins in the diet. Nowadays it is recognized that every growing baby must have cod-liver oil or the equivalent in vitamins A and D. The amount of cod-liver oil usually recommended is a teaspoonful daily of the best preparations or two teaspoonfuls of those that are not so highly concentrated.

COFFEE A cup of coffee made with a tablespoonful of coffee contains from one and a half to three grains of caffeine. The caffeine is the substance in coffee which is stimulating. Some people find their nervous systems overstimulated by the amount of caffeine they get in a cup of coffee. The majority of people, however, do not get such overstimulation, so that for them it is comparatively harmless. Every person can determine for himself the extent to which he is stimulated by coffee so that it interferes with sleep. If it does interfere with sleep, it should be eliminated from the diet. There are now available coffees which have the caffeine greatly reduced.

COITUS The scientific term used for sexual intercourse.

COLDS The common cold is a highly contagious condition which comes on somewhere between twenty-four and thirty-six hours after one has been in close contact with someone else who has a cold. Recent research on the common cold shows that the person who has one can transmit it to other people only during the early stages of the disease—that is, during the first day or two after the cold appears. The most infectious period is the first day. One of the reasons colds spread so rapidly is that a person can infect another with a cold from four to six hours before he himself begins coughing and sneezing.

In the United States there are three seasons of the year when colds are most prevalent. The first is January and February, the second April and May, and the third September and October. The epidemic in the spring is the mildest; that in January and February the most serious.

The common cold and other infections of the tissues concerned in breathing are responsible for more loss of time from industry than any other single group of disorders. Colds are no respecters of persons. Studies made in various portions of the United States and in all sorts of schools, colleges, and industries show that people average between two and three colds each year.

Most experts now agree that the common cold is caused by a virus—one of those toxic organisms so small that it can pass through the pores of a clay filter. When this virus sets up a cold, other germs attack the areas in the nose and throat that have been damaged. These germs include particularly the one that causes pneumonia, the streptococci which produce sore throats, the staphylococci related to pus infections, and the influenza germ.

When one has scarlet fever or diphtheria or measles, a single attack seems to protect against a second attack, at least for many years. However, the immunity of resistance to another infection following a cold is short. Studies made on animals show that it lasts about a month. An extensive investigation made in human beings indicated that it was probably not less than twenty-three days but averaged about seven weeks.

Recently Professor Chester S. Keefer reviewed the entire subject in an effort to find out why common colds occur in cycles. He says that it is completely mysterious why sudden outbreaks of this condition occur and spread rapidly, and then are followed by long periods with a much lessened incidence.

Experience certainly shows that sudden changes in temperature and excessive chilling or wetting of the skin promote conditions of the mucous membranes in the nose and throat that permit the virus of the cold to invade some individuals and from them to spread throughout the community. Chilling alone will not produce a cold, since the organism necessary for the infection must also be present. There have been innumerable means suggested for preventing colds but none of them is now accepted by the medical profession as really effective. If it were possible to prevent the spread of the virus from one person to another, the incidence of colds could be greatly decreased. However, we do not know of any way to prevent such spread. Artificial vaccines do not seem to be of any special virtue in resisting ordinary colds but are effective against influenza. People who are deficient in some vitamins apparently catch colds more easily than those who are on a diet containing the essential substances. There does not seem to be any reason, however, to believe that the taking of extra vitamins will prevent colds or that they will cure a cold once it has begun. The suggestion has been made that one could be hardened against colds by taking cold shower baths every morning and exercising outdoors. However, a careful study made by experts in the United States Public Health Service did not show any lower incidence of colds in people who followed these procedures than occurred among those who did not.

Apparently the virus that causes the cold may be present on the membranes of the nose and throat for a long time and not produce the symptoms until a sudden chilling or cold breaks down the resistance of the tissues.

Although everybody has a cure for a cold, most doctors simply try to make the patient comfortable. Some well-established treatments consist of the so-called "grippe capsules" which usually contain aspirin, phenacetin, and caffeine and which are known as APC tablets. These may be modified by adding antihistamines or even codeine, but such additions require a physician's prescription. The standbys in the treatment of a cold are rest (preferably in bed) and keeping warm but sitting up to aid nasal drainage when necessary. Elimination is usually encouraged by taking plenty of water or the citrus fruit juices because they have an alkalizing action and keep up the sugar of the body. If the bowels tend to clog, mild laxatives (preferably the one the patient is used to) are taken. Many people with colds lose appetite but if hungry can take food.

One of the most disturbing symptoms of a cold is the clogging of the nose. This is helped by hot packs over the frontal sinuses at the base of the nose. Such packs are kept in place about twenty minutes several times a day. The nose can be washed out with simple salt solutions or alkaline antiseptics. Nasal inhalers have been developed which tend to shrink the membrane, and there are solutions for shrinking the membranes if prescribed by the doctor. Oily nose drops have fallen into disuse because of the danger that the oil may be inhaled and cause symptoms.

The medical profession seems to disagree on whether or not to prescribe antihistamine drugs early in the cold. Many believe that the antihistamines can have an effect, if given sufficiently early, in stopping the congestion and reaction of the nasal tissues.

The antibiotic drugs will not affect the viruses that cause colds but are effective in overcoming what the doctors call "secondary invaders" such as staphylococci, streptococci, and other pus-forming germs. Penicillin, aureomycin, or terramycin are most frequently given. They are helpful in preventing the secondary complications affecting the nose, throat, ears, sinuses, and lungs which in the past have been the worst features of the common cold.

Some people who suffer frequently from colds are convinced that something may be wrong with the construction of the nose and incline toward operating on the nasal septums. Operations should not ordinarily be undertaken primarily with a view to decreasing the frequency of colds. A sufficiently long residence in a hot dry climate with adequate nutrition and rest will do more to build the resistance than any operative procedure now recognized.

Much research is now being done on the common cold. Likely specific viruses are responsible and these will be found in the near future. When they are found, specific methods of treatment are likely to come also.

Indeed, carrying the evidence a little further, we come to the conclusion that the vaccines will not even shorten the course of a cold or prevent secondary infections. Professor Chester Keefer says, "We are forced to the unhappy conclusion that at present there are no effective methods available for the prevention of the common cold."

The avoidance of exposure to colds is important although not always practical. Every person should practice hygienic measures such as washing the hands before eating and avoiding direct contact with people who have colds. Once the colds have developed, relief may be secured more promptly by rest and by taking care of the ordinary symptoms as they develop. Good personal hygiene and the avoidance of excessive chilling, and particularly of sudden changes of temperature (especially at the time of year when colds are prevalent), may aid in reducing the total number of colds in some people.

COLD SORES See *Herpes Simplex*.

COLIC The word "colic" refers to an acute pain in the abdomen which may be due to a variety of causes. The word "cramp" refers to a sudden constricting pain which may be in the abdomen or in muscles anywhere in the body. In most cases of colic in babies the trouble is gas or air in the bowels. Usually the air has been swallowed but occasionally gas is due to fermentation in the bowels. Accumulation of air can be prevented by holding the baby up against the shoulder after feeding, patting him gently on the back, and giving him an opportunity to eruct the gas or air. A little warmth to the abdomen helps to relieve ordinary colic. If colic is severe, the doctor has to determine the cause, the kind of pain reliever to be prescribed, and, most important, make certain that obstruction or some serious surgical condition is not present.

Colic occurs in grownups due to any one of a variety of causes. One of the most frequent is a stone caught in the tubes that carry bile from the gall bladder to the bowel or in the ureters that carry the urine from the kidney to the bladder. Gallstone colic may also occur in cases of chronic gall-bladder inflammation even when gallstones are not present. Gallstone colic is usually due to spasm of the muscle in the wall of the gall bladder, to the distention of the gall bladder by an overaccumulation of bile, and, as has already been mentioned, to the lodging of a gallstone in any of the tubes or ducts that carry the bile.

In the colic due to the attempted passage of a stone from the kidney the pain strikes suddenly in the kidney region, then radiates down into the abdomen, the thigh and the leg, and the genital organs. The symptoms include nausea, vomiting, and gaseous distention while the attack is on. The attack may last from a few minutes to several days. Usually the duration is from four to twelve hours. Heat is helpful in relieving this type of colic, but the doctor must make certain of the diagnosis; he has available powerful drugs of the narcotic variety that can be used to control the pain once the diagnosis is certain.

A special form of colic related to the bowel is mucous colic, associated with a spasm of the muscles of the large bowel or colon. In this condition there is intermittent pain or spasm on the right side of the lower abdomen, usually worse after meals. This kind of colic has to be differentiated from inflammations or tumors of the bowels and its dependence on functional or nervous conditions definitely determined. Such cases require the most careful and detailed study by an expert physician involving usually the use of the X ray, examination of the material excreted from the bowel with laboratory and microscopic tests, experiments in feeding different diets, and in many cases also a complete study of the patient's life and record to get at the possible environmental, social, and mental causes.

COLITIS The human bowel is a long tube beginning with the duodenum, immediately following the stomach. The bowels are comprised of the small intestines and the large intestines. As food passes through the human body it is digested. Thus materials important in body nutrition are taken up by the blood and carried to the individual cells and to the storehouses for various ingredients of the muscles, the nervous system, the blood, and the other tissues.

The waste matter or indigestible residue is passed along until it is eliminated from the body. Early in life children are taught that such elimination should take place at regular intervals. Most of us develop some regular time of the day which is devoted to this purpose. Obviously the time of elimination comes to be a habit.

Amazingly, the human being may go along for several days without exercising this function and with little disturbance. However, many a human being becomes overaware of the habit early in life, so that he achieves a mental state described as being colon-conscious.

The colon is a portion of the large bowel in which material accumulates and in which water is absorbed from the waste matter to be eliminated so that it assumes in the colon its final form. Many a doctor has recognized excessive attention given to this function of the human body and is inclined to dismiss it with scant courtesy.

However, people who fix their attention too seriously on the matter of elimination begin, sooner or later, to

urge undue activity by all sorts of procedures. They may take irritating substances in the form of drugs, use large amounts of salts, water injected above or below, massive vibrations, oils, and innumerable other materials and technics. Frequently the result of such urging is the induction of irritation and of overactivity; indeed, even the breaking down of resistance and invasion by bacteria. The result may be an attack of irritation called colitis or inflammation of the colon.

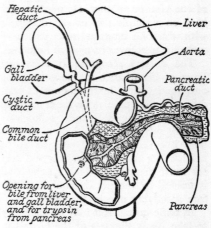

Here are shown the relationships between the liver and the gall bladder and the tubes known as the hepatic duct, the cystic duct, and the common bile duct, which carry the bile to the intestines. From the pancreas comes another duct which carries a digestive fluid called trypsin into the intestine

In other instances the urging is so persistent that eventually the person concerned loses the ability to function without artificial aid. This may be called habitual constipation.

The psychoanalysts who have given most serious and detailed study to the relation of the human mind to the physical functions of the human body are inclined to believe that many a disorder of the bowel and its action is related to some mental disturbance in the life of the person concerned. For that reason Dr. Walter Alvarez has suggested to doctors that they look most carefully into the mental aspects of the lives of people who come to them with such conditions as nervous indigestion, dyspepsia, or colitis.

Sometimes these people are benefited simply by learning that it is better to settle as best they can with the amount of disturbance they have than look for some sort of "quick cure." In many instances the person with nervous indigestion or colitis has developed the habit of taking more and more roughage of one kind or another. He needs to get back on a simple diet of soft materials with which his intestinal tract will have a chance to recover its normal functions.

The doctors recognize at least two types of disturbance in the colon. For one, food with a large amount of residue or indigestible material is needed. For the other, a bland, sufficiently cooked, soft material is better, since it does not distend the bowel so as to heighten its activity. Obviously the doctor must determine which special diet is needed by the person concerned before specifying one or the other.

In some instances it may be necessary to take X-ray pictures of the bowels in action after the patient has been given barium or other materials which are opaque to the X ray. In many instances lack of certain vitamins definitely associated with activity of the bowel may be the important factor in their failure to act suitably.

It is unwise for anyone with these conditions to resort to the habit of bowel washing. The ancient Egyptians used to try that technic and the reports indicate that they were no more successful with it on a routine basis than are people today.

Certainly it is unwise to get into the cathartic habit. If you have become colon-conscious, with constipation, the most important step in recovery is to realize the nature of the condition, then practice good mental hygiene. Treatment of this condition demands less attention to the colon and more attention to the body as a whole. Stop hurrying; stop overworking; stop being anxious about the future; stop excessive stimulation, including tea, coffee, tobacco, and alcohol; stop also excess stimulation of the bowel by large amounts of bran, psyllium seed, or other roughage. These may serve merely to irritate the lining of the bowel still further.

Diets in colitis vary according to the nature of the disturbance. The form of constipation in which the bowel simply lacks stimulus to move demands a diet containing large amounts of food that yield undigested residue. These are the leafy vegetables, the whole-grain cereals, and fruits, both fresh and cooked. Here, for instance, is a menu for the day, developed by Dr. B. D. Kenamore, indicating the foods that are useful:

Breakfast—
Orange, grapefruit, applesauce, baked apple, prunes, figs, or stewed peaches.
Cereals: Whole-wheat cereal, rolled oats, oatmeal, with cream.
Eggs: Soft-boiled, poached, or seven-minute cooked.
Whole-wheat or rye bread, plain or toasted.
Coffee with half cream or milk.

Luncheon—
Vegetable soups.
Vegetables: Tomatoes, corn, spinach, cauliflower, eggplant, string beans, asparagus, turnips, rutabagas, squash, parsnips, beets.
Salads with mayonnaise or French dressing.
Whole-wheat, rye, or corn bread, or corn muffins, with butter.
Tea, weak, or milk.

Dinner—
Celery, olives, or pickles.
Meat: All roasted, stewed, or broiled meats.
Vegetables as at noon.
Desserts: Raw or canned apples, pears, peaches, grapes, cherries, or pineapple. Dates, figs, or melons in season.
Coffee with half milk or cream; or milk.

Combined with this should be the attempt to establish the regular habit, to increase the amount of fluid taken during the day by mouth, and to avoid cathartics.

If the physician considers it necessary, extra roughage may be added as he prescribes. Mineral oil is sometimes used in such cases, though it is not a cure for the condition, but merely an aid to securing the proper consistency of the material to be eliminated.

In the majority of cases of irritation of the colon and of associated constipation the most important dietetic consideration is that the diets be free from unnecessary roughage or stimulation. Here are the suggestions of Dr. Walter Alvarez on the smooth diet and the hygiene:

If you are to give this diet a fair trial, eat no coarse foods with fiber, skins, seeds, or gristle. Avoid particularly salads with celery, tomatoes, cucumbers, and pineapple, many of the green vegetables, raisins, berries, jams full of seeds, nuts, and many of the raw fruits. Beans, cabbage, onions, green or red peppers, melons, cucumbers, and peanuts are notoriously gassy. If you are living in a boardinghouse, you can stick to this diet by simply avoiding the forbidden foods and eating more of the digestible ones which are put before you.

Avoid sugar in concentrated form and take no candy or other food between meals. Hot cakes and waffles might not be bad if they were not eaten with so much syrup. Fried foods are not bad if they are properly fried, that is, totally immersed in fat at the right temperature. Avoid eating when in a rush and when mentally upset. Family rows should be banned from the table. Chewing gum may cause distress, as much air is swallowed with the saliva. Digestion is greatly helped by a good chewing surface. If there are any gaps in your teeth, have your dentist fill them with bridges. Purgatives often cause flatulence and distress in the abdomen.

The following are suggestions for breakfast: Orange juice, grapefruit (avoid the fiber in the compartments). Cantaloupe and melons are inadvisable. Coffee, if desired, is allowed in moderation, but it sometimes causes flatulence. If you are sensitive to caffeine, try a caffeine-free coffee, or Instant Postum. Chocolate, cocoa, or tea; one or two eggs with ham or bacon (avoid the tougher part of the bacon); white bread, toast, or zwieback, with butter; any smooth, soft mush such as farina, cream of wheat, corn meal, or rolled oats; puffed cereals and cornflakes are also allowed. Shredded-wheat biscuits and other coarse breakfast foods are not allowed. Bran is particularly harmful. Graham bread is permitted, but not the coarser whole-wheat bread.

Suggestions for lunch and dinner: In fruit cocktails, avoid the pieces of orange and pineapple. Broths, bouillon, cream soups, and chowder are allowed; also meat, fish, chicken, squab, or game, except duck (avoid the fibrous parts and gristle). Veal may be tried; it is not digested well by many persons. Eat no smoked fish or pork. Crab and lobster had better be left alone. Oysters and sausage may be tried later.

Bread and butter are allowed, and hot biscuits if they are made small so as to consist mainly of crust. Rice, potatoes— mashed, hashed brown, or French fried —are allowed; and later, sweet potatoes, hominy, stewed tomatoes (strained and thickened with cracker or bread crumbs), well-cooked cauliflower tops with cream sauce, asparagus tips, Brussels sprouts, squash, beets, turnips, creamed spinach, Italian pastes, noodles, macaroni, and spaghetti cooked soft, purées of peas, beans, lentils, lima beans, or artichoke hearts. All skins or fiber should be removed by passing the food through a ricer. Sweet corn may be used if passed through a colander. There are almost no other vegetables that can be puréed to advantage. String beans are allowed if they are young and tender. Large tender string beans which can be used as a vegetable or salad can now be obtained in cans.

No salad should be taken at first. Later you may try a little tender lettuce with apples or bananas, tomato jelly, or boiled eggs. Mayonnaise and French dressing are allowed. Potato salad without much onion may be tried.

Suggested desserts are: Simple puddings, custards, ice cream, jello, plain cake, and canned or stewed fruits, particularly pears and peaches. Cottage cheese is permissible; other cheeses often cause trouble. Apple, peach, apricot, custard, and lemon-cream pie may be tried if only the filling is eaten.

In case of constipation stewed fruit may be taken once or twice a day. In winter the dried pared fruit may be used for stewing. Prunes are probably the most laxative of fruits and if eaten every other morning they will relieve the average case of constipation. They should be cooked slowly until they almost go to pieces. If the skins are still tough they should be discarded. Applesauce is much more palatable if made from unpared and uncored apples. The sauce is strained later. It may be mixed with a little tapioca or sago. The apples may be baked. Apples, even when cooked, often cause distress. Blackberries and loganberries can be stewed and strained and the sweetened juice thickened with cornstarch. This makes a delicious dish with the full flavor of the berries. Later you may try fully ripe pears and peaches.

Make no effort to drink water. Be guided by your thirst. Avoid excessive use of salt or other seasoning. If you wish to gain in weight, eat as much cream, butter, fat, and starch as you can. If you wish to lose or to stay thin, live largely on vegetables, fruits, and salads, with a moderate amount of lean meat.

The regular elimination of waste material from the body, as I have said previously, is a habit. Simply because the habit factor is so important, I cannot emphasize too much the necessity for regularity whenever that is possible. Far too often the man is busy in the office with a conference, the housewife is attending to her daily work or possibly occupied with her early morning telephone interchange of gossip.

However, it is not well to put too much emphasis on this matter, because grim determination may overcome the purpose by defeating relaxation. As Dr. Harry Beckman has said, the necessary elimination is accomplished only with maintenance of a nice balance between contractions and relaxation.

Physically the body may be helped by placing the feet on the rounds of a chair so that the thighs are flexed on the abdomen. Savages who attend to their wants under the conditions of nature assume a posture of squatting on their heels, in which this scientifically sound position must be assumed. Many a person is helped in his elimination by reading, smoking, or other attention to relaxation. Exercise to improve the muscles of the abdomen may be helpful, but certainly massage of the muscles or rolling a heavy ball over the abdomen is dangerous.

After one has tested the smooth diet and brought the walls of the intestines back to their normal tone, a gradual change to the material with more roughage may be desirable. There is, however, no justification for excessive roughage. The amount has to be carefully balanced. The determination of the correct amount may be calculated by adding bran in the form of muffins, cookies, or in a similar manner to the morning cereal. Most important is the warning against the statement "If a little bran is good, a lot is better." There are actually records in which overindulgence in this roughage brought about complete obstruction of the bowel.

The situation is complicated further by the fact that a person may have an excessive amount of intestinal fermentation and react to cellulose material with the formation of gas. The roughages that are advisable include bran, agar, psyllium seed, and such materials as lettuce, celery, spinach, carrots, figs, dates, raisins, and prunes. Some of the remedies now promoted over the radio for constipation include materials of the type of a substance called karaya gum, which has effect due to bulk.

The enema and suppository are

widely known as a means of inducing action of the bowel, and have been urged by many a promoter because they are said to be harmless. The enema habit is just as vicious as any of the other devices that have been described and some enemas containing soap or other irritants may produce inflammations of the bowel.

When the bowel has been irritated with the development of large amounts of mucus—mucous colitis—repeated washing may result in more than the presence of mucus. The mucus may be considered ordinarily as the secretion of the lining of the bowel, tending to facilitate the passage of hard, dried material.

There is a condition of the bowel that is exceedingly severe and presumably something quite removed from the ordinary type of irritation that has been described. In ulcerative colitis there is inflammation of the wall of the large bowel and the formation of ulcers. This usually comes on after long periods of disturbance.

With the appearance of ulcers there may be all the symptoms of serious disease, including fever, loss of weight, anemia, persistent diarrhea, and prostration. Such a disease demands the most prompt medical attention and often may require considerable time in the hospital under the care of a competent doctor before a cure can be brought about. Authorities are unanimous in their opinion that people with ulcerative colitis should stay in bed as long as there is fever and as long as there are two or three movements of the bowel daily.

In this form of colitis the diet is of the utmost importance because recovery may depend on the feeding of the best possible foods. Protein is necessary to maintain the cells of the body for growth and health. Red meats, liver, kidneys, sweetbreads, and lean pork are often prescribed, properly cooked, for such patients.

One must be exceedingly careful about extra amounts of fruits and vegetables because of the fact that they may stimulate the number of bowel move-ments by irritating the walls of the bowel. Since, however, these foods ordinarily would provide large amounts of vitamin B complex and vitamin C, extra amounts of these vitamins may be necessary to make up the deficiency. These patients may also require extra amounts of liver and iron to control the anemia.

In case an infection is found, it must, of course, be treated by the appropriate remedies. The sulfa drugs and those that are used particularly for the parasitic dysentcries are prescribed by the doctor as specifically needed.

In some instances the loss of material from the body may be so great that transfusion of blood or of blood plasma is necessary. This has been reported as life-saving in many instances. If the patient has lost much blood along with the material from the ulcerated and irritated bowel, these transfusions of blood are especially important.

Many attempts have been made to reach the ulcers with medicine of one type or another, by the use of enemas and material injected high into the bowel. In other instances surgery may be necessary to reach areas of the bowel which have been well-nigh destroyed by the disease. All of these procedures are serious medical processes which are undertaken only after the most careful study of the individual patient to determine exactly what is needed in his case.

COLLODION Collodion is a mixture of substances which, when painted on the skin, acts as a protective membrane. Sometimes it has been sold as a proprietary medicine under the name of "New Skin."

COLOR BLINDNESS See discussion under *Eye*.

COMA The word "coma" describes a state of complete loss of consciousness from which the person cannot be aroused even by the most powerful stimulation. The forms of coma most frequently seen are those following alcoholic intoxication and that which occurs in diabetes. The treatment of such forms of coma is so serious that it should never be undertaken except by a physician.

COMEDOS (See discussion under *Acne*) This is the scientific term for blackheads.

CONJUNCTIVITIS The tissue which lines the eyelids and runs out over the eyeball is called the conjunctiva. An inflammation of this tissue is known as conjunctivitis. When the conjunctiva becomes inflamed, there is burning and smarting of the eyelids, formation of pus, and reddened eyelids. Usually the eye, when inflamed, becomes exceedingly sensitive to light, and tears flood it constantly. In the morning the eyelids will be found crusted together. Doctors treat this condition according to the character of the germ that causes the inflammation and according to the severity of the infection.

Pinkeye is a common type of conjunctivitis. Shortly after this special type of germ gets into the eyes, they become reddened and the lids are swollen and puffy, and usually glued together in the morning. Pinkeye is usually spread by the use of a common towel, and sometimes by soiled hands.

In some instances the eyes become inflamed by germs which get in from contaminated swimming pools. Physicians are able to prescribe much more powerful germicides than boric acid, and antibiotic lotions and ointments bring dangerous infections under control.

It is easy to transfer germs of this character from one person to another. The safe step is for people with infected eyes to use individual towels and to make certain that the hands are always thoroughly washed with soap and water whenever any contact is made with the eye.

CONSTIPATION When for any reason the residue of food taken during any one day fails to be excreted within the next forty-eight hours, the person is said to be constipated. The failure of the residue to pass from the body may be due to some delay in the passage of the material through the large bowel or failure of the terminal portion of the bowel—that is, the sigmoid and rectum —to empty itself. The technical name "dyschesia" has been given to the second type of constipation.

Some people have thought that constipation existed when a person had only one bowel movement in twenty-four hours and urged as many as three as a regular habit. However, the vast majority of experts are convinced that regularity and the nature of the action are more important than multiple actions.

The normal baby has three or four actions of the bowel in twenty-four hours. However, the child who has fewer than three is not necessarily constipated, provided the eliminated material is normal in character and consistency. If the child remains well and gains weight, the physiology of his digestion and elimination is likely to be normal. Much depends on whether the child is fed at the breast or artificially. Much depends on the nature of the training given to the child. Children whose bodies are flabby in construction and those who have rickets and bulging abdomens find it difficult to expel waste material.

If there is an excess of fat in the diet of the baby, the bowel may react either by exceeding slowness of action and hardness of the excreted material or in other cases by exceeding looseness of the bowel and by greasy-looking material. One of the main causes of difficulties among children is the taking of insufficient amounts of water. Another cause is underfeeding.

In older children training is much more important than in infants. Sometimes children go to schools in which attention to the bowel action is made so difficult because of bad discipline that a child develops constipation rather than submit himself to criticism by the teacher or school attendants. Psychologists believe that children sometimes develop defensive reactions against adult control or criticism by symptoms related to the activity of their bowels.

This type of constipation frequently is controlled by a complete change of environment.

In general, addition to the diet of stewed fruits, especially apples and prunes, the taking of plenty of water, and suitable control of food will relieve constipation in children.

Sir Arthur F. Hurst, one of the leading British authorites on gastrointestinal diseases, divides most cases of constipation into two varieties. In the first the colon or large bowel is at fault, and in the second the condition is related to the lower portion of the bowel, including the sigmoid and rectum.

Delay in passage of material through the colon may be due to deficient motor activity or to the fact that the nature of the material to be moved requires excessive force. When the food contains too little indigestible residue and when an insufficient quantity of material is formed on an adequate diet, it is difficult for the muscles and nervous system of the bowel to act efficiently. In very old people and in those who are undernourished, the muscle of the intestinal wall fails to develop or to keep its normal physical condition. Investigations show also that a lack of some of the vitamins of the B complex may be related to undernourishment and to failure of the bowel to act properly. When the material passing through the bowel is abnormally dry, due either to insufficient consumption of water or to overproduction of sweat because of hot weather, there may be constipation because of the failure of the muscles of the bowel to have proper material on which to exercise their activity.

In the second type of constipation the proper nerve-muscle relationships fail to occur in the lower portion of the bowel. The baby can be trained so that the simple act of exposure and placing it on the pot will cause it to evacuate. Older people develop a series of habits that are much more complicated. There is the matter of getting up, taking a bath, dressing, having breakfast and, finally, the question of access to the toilet, the provision of suitable reading matter and a pipe or a cigarette. Already it is known that interference with any one of this involved series may disturb the whole mechanism.

The complication of nerve and muscle reaction is called a conditioned reflex. In most cases this kind of constipation or dyschesia results from neglect in responding to the call because of laziness, false modesty, bad discipline, or any one of a number of similar factors. Eventually failure to respond to the call to empty the bowel will result in loss of sensation. Unfortunately, however, by this time the person concerned has begun to fix his mind on his difficulties and is likely to begin indulging in laxatives, enemas, colon washings, or similar procedures which create new habits and result ultimately in a complete loss of the possibility of normal emptying of the bowel. There are rare instances in which dyschesia may result from weakness of muscles, the fear of pain because of some disease in the area concerned, or even difficulties involving the nervous system, but these are rare compared with the vast majority of cases which result from bad habits.

In many instances people who are constipated have developed a fixation on the time, the amount, the shape, the color, or other factors associated with evacuation of the bowel. One of the first steps in overcoming constipation due to such a fixation is to convince people that there is no standard size, shape, consistency, or color. Sir Arthur Hurst indeed suggests that these people should be educated to the example of the dog rather than that of the cat, and never look behind them.

The people of the United States probably spend more than $50,000,000 a year to avoid constipation. Most of this is probably wasted, since it should be possible for practically everyone to have a normal action of the bowel with proper habits of diet and bowel training. Doctors know that the excessive use of cathartics tends to establish a habit which in the end damages the digestive tract. When the bowels get used to artificial stimulation, they are like a horse that will not run and requires more and more whipping as time goes on.

A good mixed diet with proper proteins, carbohydrates, fats, mineral salts, and vitamins, and enough indigestible residue is probably the most important single factor. People inclined toward delay in action of the bowel should take fruits, fresh or preserved, raw or cooked, with each meal and green vegetables or salad with both lunch and dinner. Stewed prunes for breakfast are considered particularly useful.

The various foods which contain excessive amounts of bran are to be avoided, as they may irritate the bowel and they do not seem to have much advantage over fruits and vegetables. Indeed, foods with large quantities of bran should be considered medicinal foods and should be used only when prescribed by the doctor.

Among the drugs most commonly used to stir the bowels to action are saline and vegetable cathartics, organic and mineral preparations, mechanically acting substances and water in various forms. The continued use of strong salts may so irritate the lower portions of the bowel as to produce colitis. The vegetable cathartics like cascara, senna, aloes, rhubarb, and jalap act by irritating the bowel. Since irritation is abnormal, it is not well to make a habit of using any such cathartics. The mechanically acting substances include mineral oil or liquid petrolatum, agar-agar (which is a seaweed), psyllium seeds, flax seeds, and bran. One of the chief arguments against the continued use of mineral oil is the fact that it absorbs vitamin A and may produce a vitamin A deficiency if used too constantly in connection with a deficient diet. Sometimes the use of mineral oil is unfortunate because of leakage of the material from the bowel. Mixtures of mineral oil with agar-agar or other substances, psyllium seeds, and flax seeds develop a mucilaginous, bulky material useful in cases when failure of the bowel to act is the result of insufficient residue. In any event it is necessary to know the nature of the constipation before deter-

mining which preparations are desirable in any specific case.

The majority of cases of dyschesia require re-education to get a good result, but in many such cases the first step is to develop a habit through the use of a mild enema, a mild laxative, or suppository. Just what is to be used in any case should be determined by the doctor. Regular exercise helps to keep the bowels active and is important particularly for people who are confined to a desk most of the day. For such people a five-minute walk before or after breakfast may be a good habit to establish. Exercise of the abdominal muscles may be ordered when the failure of the bowel to act seems to be due to weakness of the muscles involved in the act of emptying the bowel.

CONTACT LENSES See discussion under *Eye*.

CONTRACEPTION (See also *Pregnancy*) Increasing interest has attached in recent years to various technics for the preventing of conception with a view to spacing childbirth and to its prevention where there are good medical reasons for it. The technics most commonly used involve the wearing by the male of a sheath or condom or the use by the female of a protective rubber pessary and the injection into the female of any one of a variety of ointments or suppositories. Frequently used also are douches of various kinds which are employed following intercourse. Thus far, none of the methods suggested for prevention of conception has had complete success or perfection. Nevertheless the wearing of a sheath by the male or the combination of pessary and ointment used by the female insures success in well over 90 per cent of cases.

Much attention has been given recently to the so-called rhythm technic, which is based on the fact that the ovum, or egg cell, passes from the female ovary once each month. There is for each woman a fertile period during which the likelihood of conception is much greater than at other times in the month. In contrast to the fertile period, there is a "safe" period. Should a woman expect to menstruate, for instance, on the ninth of the month, the fertile period would be between the twentieth and twenty-seventh of the previous month. The fertile period is estimated at a maximum of eight days. When a woman menstruates regularly every twenty-eight days, the "safe" period begins with the first day of menstruation and lasts nine days. Then come eight days of fertility, after which there are eleven more days of the "safe" period until the next menstruation. Thus the safe period is most easily calculated as the week before and the week after menstruation. When menstruation is irregular, it is much more difficult to calculate and the woman will do well to consult her physician in order that he may advise her in relation to conception and contraception.

By the temperature method the woman takes her temperature each morning on arising before any food or fluid is swallowed. Concomitant with ovulation, there is a drop in temperature followed by a rise. Intercourse is omitted for three days before and three days after ovulation.

CONVALESCENCE After a long illness, a surgical operation, or a childbirth, the body requires some time to repair damaged tissue and to return to the habits of health. Certainly it is not desirable for anyone to get up and try to go about the daily work at once. The mere disappearance of the fever and the depression asssociated with an illness is not an indication that the patient is well. At such times, in fact, the human body is particularly susceptible to secondary infections. Following a long period of illness or disability, the digestive system, the nervous system, and the various organs of the body are in such a weakened state that any slight extra stress may result in breakdown. Convalescence after any serious illness should be slow. For this reason the guidance of the doctor as to just how

soon the ordinary activities of life may be undertaken is necessary.

Formerly it was the custom to keep people in bed for long periods of time. More recently physicians are tending toward the idea that fairly early return to activity is valuable in hastening the process of convalescence. There is, indeed, coming to be the impression that rest may be abused. Nevertheless damage to the heart, the kidneys, or other vital organs may result from too much stress after infectious disease.

As soon as possible after recovery has begun, it may be desirable to change the patient from the room in which he has been living and to give him opportunity to see other portions of the house if he is at home, or perhaps to spend some time on a sun porch or in a recreation room if he is in a hospital.

Although visitors may have been forbidden during the illness, an occasional visitor may now see the patient. The choice of visitors is of the utmost importance because the maintenance of the patient's morale is vital. Only visitors who are cheerful and entertaining should be permitted, and none of them should be permitted to stay long. Unfortunately there are some people who come to enjoy invalidism. This attitude is enhanced by visitors who are overly sympathetic and whose whole tone tends to induce the patient to make much of suffering. Such visitors encourage patient complaints and may lead to a permanently harmful mental attitude.

It is well for a person who has a protracted illness and a long convalescence to develop a fixed routine of life. In the morning, after attending to the usual needs of the body, the patient should have opportunity for cleaning the teeth. It is perhaps well to take the temperature regularly each morning until it is certain that there is not going to be a relapse. Until the patient is able to wash himself, he should be washed in the morning by someone familiar with the manner of washing a patient in bed. Only a small part of the body should be exposed at any one time. The windows should be closed during the washing period.

If the patient complains of cold, a warm drink will be helpful to sustain the temperature of the body. When the patient has been in bed for a long time, it is important to look after the hair and scalp. An occasional shampoo will improve the patient's feeling of health.

As soon as the patient has been bathed, it may be desirable to turn the mattress.

A patient who has been long in bed should not try to get up all at once. The first day he may merely be able to sit up on the edge of the bed for five or ten minutes. If he gets dizzy, he should be put back immediately in a reclining position. If the patient is able to sit up on the bed without support, he may try sitting in a chair for a while. A sudden resumption of activities may throw strain on the heart so that permanent recovery would be impossible.

CONVULSIONS See discussion under *Child Care;* also *Epilepsy.*

COPPER SULFATE Copper sulfate is used in swimming pools to destroy fungi or bacteria. It has little use in medicine.

CORNEA (See also *Eye* and *Conjunctivitis*) The membrane over the front of the eye.

CORNS See discussion under *Feet.*

CORONARY THROMBOSIS See discussion under *Heart.*

CORYZA A term sometimes used for colds and rhinitis.

COSMETICS A manuscript written in Egypt in 1200 B.C. provides numerous recipes for beauty which were in vogue thousands of years ago. There are remedies for moles, treatments for gray hair, and suggestions for overcoming baldness. More than three thousand years have passed and still hope springs

eternal in the brain of the bald-headed man.

The Egyptian woman of four thousand years ago had a dressing table with just about as many fancy mirrors and jars filled with all sorts of colored pastes as does the lady of today. Cleopatra used to shape her eyebrows and tip her eyelashes. The ancient Egyptians used to dress their hair every ten or twelve days. Recently an American businessman bought a beauty shop because he said his wife put in most of her time there.

Galen, one of the fathers of modern medicine, who lived about eighteen hundred years ago, developed the first formula for cold cream, consisting of four ounces of white wax and a pound of oil of roses mixed with some water and perfumed. Today cosmeticians offer not only the cold cream that Galen described but thickening creams, thinning creams, protective creams, foundation creams, vanishing creams, and dozens of others in little white jars with brass lids. In this uniform it is quite possible for a quarter's worth of cold cream to be sold for two dollars.

Face powders available today include materials of various origins. Vegetable powders come from rice, wheat, corn flour, acacia, and tragacanth. Mineral powders come from chalk, talc, kaolin, magnesium carbonate, bismuth nitrate or carbonate, and zinc oxide. Orris root has been used frequently to "fix" face powders.

The vast majority of substances used in face powders are harmless.

No doubt the chief reason for powder on the skin is protection against wind and weather and the removal of the shiny appearance which women consider unfavorable from the point of view of beauty. Powders have an added usefulness in relief of irritation of the skin, in the absorption of moisture and in their cooling effect. Moderate use of powder will not clog the pores sufficiently to interfere with perspiration.

Some people are especially sensitive to orris root. Others are sensitive to aniline dyes. Such people may suffer from eruptions, asthma, hay fever, inflamed eyes, or sneezing following the use of powders containing materials to which they are sensitive. Otherwise there is little if any danger in the common face powders now sold.

Most cold creams are made with formulas somewhat like the one that Galen developed. Once upon a time creams contained dangerous salts of lead or mercury. Today such substances are seldom, if ever, found in the creams sold in drugstores and beauty shops.

Occasionally there may be sensitivity to the dyes in rouges, lipsticks, eyebrow preparations, or creams. Creams that are supposed to bleach or peel the skin may contain dangerous substances. Vanishing creams are made, for the most part, without much fat. They are chiefly potassium or sodium stearate and glycerin together with rose water or perfume. Sometimes the fat is replaced by almond oil, wax, or gelatin. The chief value of creams of this type is that they are rubbed in, which aids the circulation of blood in the skin and acts as a mild massage.

Particularly dangerous are wrinkle removers and skin-peeling solutions. No wrinkle remover thus far available is effective. Most of these are astringent lotions which give a sense of contraction of the skin on drying but really do not contract the skin at all. Preparations have been made with egg white which stiffens on the skin and gives the woman the impression that her skin is being straightened out.

Recently preparations have been developed which contain estrogen, the female sex hormone. If there is enough of the estrogen to have an effect on the body, its use may be dangerous. If there is not enough to have such an effect, the preparation obviously is fraudulent. Furthermore, there is no evidence that the use of such a preparation will really restore elasticity in the tissue of the aged.

Most skin specialists are convinced that creams are valuable for exceedingly dry skins. The skin is a living tissue and has certain automatic powers of regulation. The circulating blood keeps the skin in health. The most valuable step in care of the skin is encouragement of circulation and nutrition. This is accomplished by proper diet and hygiene.

COUGHING A cough is not a disease. It is a symptom of changes that have taken place in the tissues of the nose, throat, or lungs, interfering with the free passing of the air in and out of the lungs. The purpose of a cough, therefore, is to get the irritating or obstructing materials out of the breathing passages. You cough if your breathing is being obstructed by a feather, a fishbone, a piece of bread, or anything else that you may have swallowed or inhaled and which obstructs the passage of air.

In the vast majority of cases coughing is due to a collection of dust or broken-down tissue or mucus or other secretions that may come from the cells that line the breathing passages. Germs which infect the membranes can cause swelling and irritation and the pouring out of secretions. One of the reasons for the pouring out of such secretions is the removal of the germs that are causing the inflammation.

Thus a cough serves a double purpose. It removes the secretion or obstructing materials and removes infectious germs at the same time. Coughing, therefore, is a means of spreading germs and for that reason one of the most famous rhymes in the field of public health is the following:

Cover up that cough and sneeze.
If you don't, you will spread disease.

Another form of coughing is due to constriction of the breathing tubes in the chest and lungs by an asthmatic attack. Such constriction does not permit a sufficient amount of air to pass through with each breath and gives the feeling of obstruction. By the use of a stethoscope a physician can tell that there is interference with the passage of air through the tubes and the points at which the difficulty occurs. By use of the X ray he can obtain a picture of the breathing mechanism. Substances like lipiodol can be blown into the bronchial tubes; then the X ray gives an accurate picture of the smoothness of the lining of the breathing apparatus.

Some diseases like tuberculosis or silicosis cause fibrous changes in the lungs which may be associated with a feeling of obstruction. Occasionally there are inflammations of the membranes that line the cavity of the chest, known as the pleura. Such an inflammation is called pleurisy. An irritation of this lining may be associated with a cough.

Certain diseases are especially likely to produce coughing—most particularly whooping cough, or pertussis. Following a cure of the whooping cough, a child may have developed the habit of coughing; even though he is well he continues to whoop and cough for months. Sometimes the child feels that the whoop or cough makes him the center of interest and uses the cough as a means of holding attention. In such cases the doctor will, of course, by a careful examination determine the nature of the condition.

Any cough must be considered a symptom that demands attention. Any material that is coughed from the body will be examined by the doctor to determine the nature of the infection and the kind of secretion that is being poured out. Examination will indicate whether there is infection in the nose, the adenoids, or the sinuses, with infectious material dropping back into the throat which, in turn, must be coughed or hawked out of the throat. Like the pain in an ulcer of the stomach, a cough is to be considered not as a disease but as a warning signal to indicate danger.

If a cough is caused by an obstruction that can be detected and removed, the treatment of the cough involves such removal. This happens when a foreign substance has been caught in the throat or in the breathing tubes. If there is an abscess in the lung, emptying of

the abscess and its healing will stop the cough. The presence of a cancer in any part of the breathing apparatus may cause a continuous cough as will the presence of tuberculosis with the production of material that has to be coughed out of the lungs.

The vast majority of coughs are not, however, to be credited to such serious conditions as tuberculosis, cancer, or foreign bodies in the lungs. Most coughs are less serious and are likely to be associated with conditions like inflammation of the linings of the bronchial tubes or windpipe associated with infections with the virus of the common cold, measles, scarlet fever, or any of the common infectious diseases.

Almost every mother knows ways to relieve a cough. One of the most common home procedures is to inhale steam from water to which a few drops of the compound tincture of benzoin have been added. This merely relieves the tension in the tissues and soothes them. Such procedures will not cure the basic cause of the cough. The taking of hot drinks may produce relaxation of the tissues but is certainly not a cure for the cough.

Relief of a tight cough will lessen the discomfort in the chest. The story is told of a doctor who always treated patients with a moist cough by giving them remedies which would dry up the secretions. Those who had a dry cough were given remedies which would increase the secretions and moisten the cough. Here again, however, the relief comes by the pouring out of secretions which get the infectious and irritating materials out of the body.

When the bronchial tubes become chronically inflamed so as to produce chronic bronchitis or bronchiectasis, the treatment must be directed toward the cure of that condition. Frequently there is associated with a cough a continued irritation of the vocal cords, since both air and the infectious material are propelled with an explosive force through the larynx and vocal cords. The result may be an inflammation of the larynx with the production of hoarseness. In such instances it may be necessary for the doctor to prescribe sedative drugs which will tend to quiet the coughing through lessening the attention that the person will give to the irritation.

The final emphasis must be placed, however, on the point that a cough is, after all, a symptom and not a disease. Because of the danger of coughing as one of the means of spreading disease, health officers have recommended that people wear gauze face masks in times of epidemics so as to stop the spread of infectious materials by coughing. Pictures have been taken to show that a sneeze will project billions of germs into the atmosphere near the body, and a series of coughs can propel infectious material for many feet.

Another jingle frequent in the annals of medicine accurately describes the significance of the cough:

*It isn't the cough that carries you off.
It's the coffin they carry you off in.*

CRAMPS See discussion of pain in the stomach and abdomen under *Child Care, Dysmenorrhea* and *Menstruation.*

CRESOL Cresol is a poisonous substance that has antiseptic qualities. Its chief use in medicine is as a disinfectant.

CROSS-EYES See discussion under *Eye.*

CROUP The disease that used to be called croup is nowadays likely to be called acute laryngitis, diphtheria, or occasionally streptococcus sore throat. The word "croup" really refers to a single symptom of throat infection, since the word is used to describe any condition in which the breathing is difficult or in which there is a spasm of the larynx with a wheezing sound.

The laryngeal cords or the vocal cords are inflamed and swollen, so that the breath comes through with a wheezing sound and the patient coughs constantly to try to rid himself of the obstruction. In some instances there is spasm of the cords, which makes them red and pulls them toward each other without the presence of any obvious infection. This is called spasmodic croup.

The most important measure in croup is to determine exactly what is wrong. The most serious form of the infection in the throat is that due to the germ of diphtheria. In diphtheria a thick, adherent membrane forms in the throat. In very severe forms of streptococcus throat a membrane forms also, but it is usually not so thick and white as that of diphtheria. In the worst forms the fever is high, the breathing labored, and the patient exceedingly ill.

In the simplest cases of croup the doctor usually advises that the child be put promptly to bed; then he is given plenty of fluids. A good deal of relief can be had by inhaling steam, which may or may not be medicated with benzoin or other soothing oils, according to the doctor's orders. If coughing is exceedingly severe, the doctor will prescribe sedatives which will relieve the cough. If the throat is sore and painful, an ice bag is sometimes used to relieve the pain.

The dangerous cases of croup are those in which there may actually be complete obstruction to breathing, so that the immediate attention of the doctor is of the utmost importance. In such cases the doctor may arrange to supply oxygen for breathing so that the supply of oxygen will be increased in passing through the small opening that is available because of the croup. A tube, known as an intubation tube, may be put into the throat. This makes certain that the air will pass suitably through the larynx or voice box. In the most severe cases a tracheotomy is done. This means that an opening is made directly into the windpipe from the outside, so that the breathing will go on until the patient has a chance to overcome the inflammation. Any case in which there is great swelling in the throat and difficulty in breathing should be considered serious. Breathing **is** necessary to life, and even sudden blocking for a few minutes may result fatally.

CRYING See discussion under *Child Care*.

CURES The human being is a credulous animal. Before the time of modern medicine he was always seeking a panacea or specific sudden cure for anything that troubled him. In the Bible there are stories of healing by the laying on of hands or even of raising from the dead by such technics. During the Middle Ages it was believed that a king or any similar personage had the special virtue to heal disease by touching sick people. This was known as the "king's touch." Many a monarch owed his popularity to his willingness to spend at least a part of each day in touching the royal finger tips to the diseased, the poverty-stricken, and the malformed who applied to him for such purposes. When there were great epidemics, like the plague that devastated Europe from 1400 to 1600, the kings were kept busy with this performance.

The use of the "king's touch" for healing disease in France began with Philip I around 1100. Both Henry I and Henry II in England are credited with starting the practice in that country. Indeed it was thought that the condition called scrofula, which might have been any form of skin disorder, was supposed to be especially susceptible to relief by this method. It is now believed that scrofula was associated with malnutrition and poverty.

Modern evangelistic healers of all types still continue to urge their power to accomplish cures by this method. There seems to be no doubt that any disease which is entirely in the mind of the patient may sometimes be relieved by technics which convince the person that something is going to happen. Some of the most widely publicized healers of modern times accomplish their so-called miracle cures in the same way.

The American people are not the only ones who crave miracles. The French some years ago sent us a healer named Coué, who healed disease by so-called autosuggestion, in which people were supposed to say, over and over, "Every day in every way I'm getting better and better." Who remembers Emile Coué now? Nowhere in the world, apparently, is there anyone who now uses the Coué method.

In Spain there was a miracle healer named Asuero at San Sebastian. Outside the gates of his home thousands of crippled swarmed for him to apply his magical method. He used to pass a hot wire up the nose and touch the nerve endings as a means of curing pains and all sorts of paralysis. Who remembers Asuero now? And where in the world is there anyone who practices the Asuero system?

These cures—which depend for such success as they may have on making people think they are better—are on a par with carrying a buckeye in the pocket to relieve rheumatism and burying a cucumber in a graveyard at night to relieve warts.

CYANOSIS Cyanosis is a term used to describe blueness of the skin. It is derived from a Greek word meaning blue. The chief cause of cyanosis is a change in the blood resulting from a lack of oxygen. When a person has blueness of the skin, he is said to be cyanotic.

There are many different causes for blueness of the skin, which may be temporary or permanent. If for any reason the blood is temporarily deprived of oxygen, as in strangulation, asphyxia, or shock, the skin will appear to be blue. If the heart is so weak that it cannot force enough blood through the lungs to permit a sufficient amount of oxygen to come in contact with the blood, the blue appearance will be permanent. There are various diseases of the blood in which an exceedingly large number of red blood cells, associated with a need for large amounts of red coloring matter, make it impossible to supply all of the red blood cells with a sufficient amount of hemoglobin or red coloring matter.

Sometimes the inhalation of illuminating gas or carbon monoxide will produce a combination of the carbon monoxide with the hemoglobin of the blood, since this substance has a greater affinity for the blood than does oxygen. Hence suffocation with illuminating gas or carbon monoxide is invariably associated with a blue or purple color of the body.

In some cases of congenital heart disease the blood passes directly from the veins to the arteries without circulating through the lungs and thus fails to get oxygen by proper passage through the lungs. This produces blueness in babies who have this heart difficulty.

Anything that will relieve the cyanosis and reduce the demand for oxygen in the tissues or anything that will stimulate the circulation of the blood will be helpful in controlling cyanosis. Rest is of the greatest importance, since it lowers the amount of oxygen demanded by the tissues and gives them opportunity to recover from the deprivation of oxygen that is associated with cyanosis.

CYCLOPROPANE Cyclopropane is a new gas anesthetic said to be somewhat less irritating than ether. It is inflammable. Apparently the stage of excitement which follows the induction of ether anesthesia is less with cyclopropane.

CYSTS (See also discussion under *Ovary*) Any sac or small cavity in the body surrounded by tissue which contains a liquid or semisolid substance is called a cyst. Most frequent location of cysts which demand surgical care are those in the skin and in various glands. Whenever the opening of the glandular cell or organ is blocked, the accumulation of fluid produces a cyst. Since the urinary bladder is of the nature of a sac of fluid, inflammation of this bladder is called cystitis. Inflammation of the gall bladder is called cholecystitis.

CYSTOSCOPY (See *Bladder Conditions*) Term meaning examination of the interior of the urinary bladder.

DANDRUFF (See also discussion under *Hair*) Dandruff is usually the result of a condition called seborrheic dermatitis. It is the most common of all skin diseases. Sometimes dandruff is said to be dry and scaly; in other cases it is moist and greasy. Innumerable remedies have been suggested for dandruff from time immemorial. The recent introduction of drugs based on selenium has brought about the first effective treatment of dandruff. These ointments are beneficial in controlling seborrheic dermatitis and oily skin. It has been thought from time to time that the taking of too much fat or too much sugar in the diet was associated with excess oil in the skin. Now, however, there does not seem to be any proof that such a relationship actually exists. Many of the remedies for the control of seborrheic dermatitis include drugs like mercury, salicylic acid, sulfur, and resorcin. Thorough washing of the scalp will remove dandruff, which, however, usually returns. The antiseptic substances, if used in sufficient strength, can also be harmful and should not be used unless prescribed by a physician. Many of the common treatments used in barber and beauty shops depend for their effect on the presence of alcohol and salicylic acid.

DEAFNESS (See also *Otosclerosis*) Deafness, commonly referred to as hardness of hearing, involves the functions of the ear. The ear itself includes the external ear, the middle ear, and the internal ear. The external ear is all of it down to the eardrum. Then comes the cavity behind the eardrum and the small bones of the ear commonly described as the hammer, anvil, and stirrup because of the shape and manner in which they function. Last of all, there is the internal ear. This is a highly complicated structure and close to the brain, connected with the nervous system and containing several smaller structures which are concerned not only with hearing but also with the sense of balance.

The external ear serves as a trumpet to collect and gather the sound waves, which are then passed on to the ear-drum. The eardrum vibrates and transmits the vibrations to the small bones that have been mentioned. These take up the vibrations, amplify them, and pass them on to the tissues which connect with the nerves of hearing. Damage to any part of this mechanism may interfere with hearing. It is so delicate that, like a fine watch or a very sensitive radio, it is easily deranged.

Infections which destroy the tissues or inflame them will damage the hearing. Because of its position, the mechanism of hearing is more likely than any other part of the body to suffer serious effects when there is a disease like an infection of the whole body. The ear can suffer also in relationship to disturbances of the brain. Most dangerous of all, however, are the infectious diseases like measles, meningitis, scarlet fever, and the like, but also minor infections like inflammations of the adenoids and tonsils, colds in the head, infections of the sinuses, and similar disturbances.

Deafness or impaired hearing may also result from accidents like a blow on the head, from rupture of the ear-drum, or from the entrance of some foreign substance into the ear. In some instances people are born without hearing due to infections which have damaged the nerve of hearing or to conditions which have brought about degeneration of the structures involved in hearing before birth.

A recent study of pupils in schools for the deaf in the United States showed that almost 15 per cent were found to be suffering from loss of hearing because of meningitis, more than 7 per cent because of scarlet fever, and more than 5 per cent each from measles and from falls and blows. Then came whooping cough, abscesses in the ear, and pneumonia—all around 4 per cent.

Just how many people in the United States have defective hearing is not now known. Estimates vary, depending on the definition of the condition. Hearing loss or impairment of hearing in persons of advanced years are becoming more frequent because there are more people living longer. Among the aged the conditions related to the ear and associated with loss of hearing may include also dizziness and ringing in the ears. Most serious, however, is progressive deafness, or otosclerosis. In this condition the tissues of the ear become hardened and, as the condition proceeds, hearing disappears completely.

A child who does not hear well uses his eyes much more than the child who does hear well. The child who does not hear well will fail to get enjoyment from the use of a rattle. He will not respond to a spoken word unless there is movement associated with the speaking. These are simple tests that any parent can make. When it is determined that there is trouble, the attention of a specialist should be had as soon as possible.

A certain percentage of inability to hear is apparently due to inheritance of structure which makes hearing impossible. The available evidence indicates that hereditary deaf-mutism and the tendency to otosclerosis are inherited. Such inheritance is, however, recessive and tends to be bred out rather than in. If deaf persons are able to marry those who hear well, the tendency toward hardness of hearing will gradually disappear. When people who are hereditarily deaf marry people who are also hereditarily deaf, one third of the children are also likely to be deaf.

Hearing is one of the most suggestible of all of the human senses. Even children try the playful experiment of holding a watch that is not going near the ear and asking the subject of the experiment to say when he first hears the watch. Great numbers of people will "hear" the watch tick even though it is not going.

One of the greatest problems of medical diagnosis is to determine the exact amount of deafness that is present. This requires a number of highly technical scientific tests which specialists in diseases of the ear can make but which are difficult for anyone who is not thoroughly conversant with the factors involved.

During war there are many instances of hysterical deafness which develop in association with air raids and bombings. A British physician found that eardrums perforated after an explosion usually healed. If mental symptoms failed to develop, there was no impairment of hearing. If deafness after the explosion lasted longer than a few days, it was frequently mental rather than actual. The person affected did not hear because the shock associated with the explosion convinced him in his own mind that he could not hear. The initial hardness of hearing which follows an explosion usually makes such an impression on the minds of both soldiers and civilians that the first thought after an explosion is always for the hearing.

When a person is temporarily deafened by a loud noise, he finds he is unable to hear no matter how hard he tries. Then he may give up trying. Because he knows he cannot hear, he stops listening. A British soldier in a German prison developed hysterical deafness because he could not understand what was said to him. Finally he stopped listening and paying attention to what was said. When he was returned home, he was rapidly cured of his hardness of hearing by psychological treatment.

For the person who is actually hard of hearing due to progressive loss of this sense, devices like the audiometer are used to determine the extent of the loss. People who work in industries in which there is a great deal of noise may develop some impairment of hearing associated with the character and intensity of the sound. Occupational deafness in the trades of boilermaking and drop forging is a constant hazard. One investigator found that 52 per cent of train dispatchers suffered from diminished hearing in the telephone ear.

Most important, therefore, in relationship to loss of hearing is the prevention of deafness. This means, of course, the prevention of the infectious conditions which result in damage to the ear. When pus or infectious material forms in the internal ear, the pressure should be released at the earliest possible moment by having the doctor puncture the eardrum so that permanent damage will not occur. Minor infections in the throat which spread to the Eustachian tubes and by that route to the internal ear are a special hazard. Therefore prompt attention should be given to every infection in the back of the nose and in the throat if for no other reason than to protect the hearing. Any slight loss of hearing, even though temporary, should have the prompt attention of a specialist in conditions affecting the ear so as to stop the progress of the condition before it becomes permanent.

If anyone needs glasses for defective vision, his first step is to find out the extent of the damage and then to purchase glasses that will fit his case. Eyeglasses have been used for many hundreds of years. The development of the hearing aid is within the memory of living man. Now the manufacturers have been able to achieve success in the control of pitch and to devise hearing aids at reasonable prices which will fit the various types of hearing loss. A hearing device cannot be fitted with the precision that an eye specialist uses in fitting the eyes but the thousands of people who now use such hearing devices are an indication of their helpfulness. Indeed the time will come when it will be quite as common to see people wearing hearing aids as it is to see them wearing eyeglasses for defective eyes, braces for weak backs, and supports to correct defective parts of the body.

Hearing aids are in general of two types: those which act by air conduction and those which act by bone conduction. Tests made by the specialists can determine the nature of the loss of hearing and to that extent determine which type of device is most favorable. Because of the subjective element involved, the real test, however, is the patient's own determination, by the actual use of the device, of the extent to which it is helpful to him.

Life for those who suffer partial deafness or even complete deafness can be made quite happy and complete. In some occupations impairment of hearing may be an asset rather than a liability. The deafened bookkeeper or machine operator minds his job and does not spend time gossiping with those about him. Deafness decreases distraction, fosters constructive thought, and aids reason.

The cultivation of lip reading is also helpful in enabling the person who is hard of hearing to carry on most of the work of daily life. There is no reason to feel discouraged or defeated if you happen to be hard of hearing. Among those who have become famous despite this handicap are Beethoven, Sir Joshua Reynolds, Oliver Goldsmith, George Meredith, and Lord Chesterfield. Martin Luther was troubled by hardness of hearing, ringing in the ears, and dizziness. Nevertheless his name lives forever because of his contribution to philosophy.

Quite recently there has been developed for the benefit of victims of otosclerosis, or progressive deafness, an operative procedure which seems to constitute a considerable advance in the control of this condition. A window is made into the labyrinth and this seems to supply the function lost in the fixation of the small bones of the ear by the otosclerosis.

DEATH, SUDDEN Most dramatic of all of the occurrences in life is sudden death. Anyone who has witnessed such a case is likely to remember it ever after.

Nowadays one of the most frequent causes of sudden death is coronary thrombosis, which produces a sudden stopping of the heart. Death due primarily to sudden stopping of the heart occurs when the heart has had a prolonged struggle against overwhelming difficulties or when there has been a sudden obstruction in the flow of blood to the coronary arteries which supply the muscles of the heart with oxygen. At least one half of all of the sudden deaths that occur in this country are due to changes in the small blood vessels or coronary arteries which supply the heart with nutrition.

For years there has been a superstition that human beings are more likely to die at the coming of dawn than at any other time of the twenty-four hours. After he had examined 13,000 records of death, Dr. Emil Bogen found that there were 1632 deaths in the period between two and five in the morning against an average of 1645 deaths for the eight three-hour periods into which twenty-four hours can be divided. More people die in the daytime hours from six in the morning to six at night than in the corresponding nighttime period. More people die of drunkenness in the afternoon and night than in the morning, as might be expected. Deaths in childbirth occur more frequently in the hours from four to six in the morning, the period associated with the exhaustion that may follow a night of severe effort during childbirth.

There is a common impression that most suicides occur during the lonely hours of night and early in the morning. This is related to the passing of a sleepless night. However, a scientific study of the records does not support this opinion. The actual records indicate that the time of death in the vast majority of suicides and murders is unknown.

The majority of deaths from automobile accidents occur on Sundays with a record 20 per cent greater than that of any other day and nearly double that for Wednesday.

In addition to sudden deaths which follow blocking of the blood vessels to the heart, other causes of sudden death include hemorrhages into the brain or abdominal cavity following the breaking of a blood vessel or the perforation of an ulcer, also injuries to the skull and brain from blows or falls.

DECIBEL A decibel is a measure of hearing. One decibel is the lowest intensity of sound at which any given note can be heard. Therefore it has become possible to determine the number of decibels developed by a motor horn, a train on a track, or any other sound.

DEFICIENCY DISEASES With our knowledge that the human body requires many substances in the daily diet in order to be healthy, and indeed to live, there developed a term for describing the conditions of ill health associated with a lack of certain essential substances, namely deficiency diseases. The most important of such diseases are: rickets, due to an absence of vitamin D from the diet; scurvy, due to a lack of vitamin C; and pellagra, associated largely with a lack of nicotinic acid. There are, however, many other deficiency diseases, such as xerophthalmia and night blindness, associated with a deficiency of vitamin A. Certain forms of neuritis are related to a lack of thiamine, as is the disease known as beriberi.

Since the gradual development of our knowledge of deficiency diseases related to a shortage of various vitamins in the diet, knowledge has accumulated regarding the effects of deficiencies of other substances, including proteins and the individual amino acids, sugars, fats, and many mineral salts. We now know that some of the individual amino acids are absolutely necessary to health and growth. Quite certainly eight and perhaps ten of the known twenty-two amino acids are essential to human health and growth. They are particularly important in relation to our resistance to infection.

A lack of iodine in the diet is associated with the production of simple goiter. A deficiency of sugar results in a condition known as hypoglycemia, which means less than the normal amount of sugar in the blood. This results in weakness and fatigue.

Indeed all of these discoveries point to the importance of adequate nutrition. The people of the United States have a high standard of living and therefore suffer less from malnutrition than people in most of the other countries of the world.

If malnutrition is understood to mean a lack of a sufficient amount of food to sustain life, there is probably very little malnutrition in the United States. If, however, malnutrition means inability to utilize food properly or a wrong selection of food, so that the body lacks certain definite ingredients, then there may be much malnutrition in this country. By this understanding of deficiency disease the term may be applied to any stage or sequence of events leading to changes in the body and ultimate failure of portions of the body to act properly. The changes that occur in rickets, such as the bowlegs and the beading of the ribs, the irritated skin and the red tongue found in pellagra, and the bleeding from the gums that is a sign of scurvy are easily detected. Much more certain in the detection of a deficiency disease is an examination of the blood and of the urine to determine the amount of the essential substance that is present and the amount that is being excreted from the body. Whereas rickets is gradually being brought under control, at least 20 per cent of children of preschool age still show some of the signs of this disease. It would perhaps be better to speak of these conditions not as deficiency diseases but as dietary deficiencies.

DEGENERATIVE DISEASES Conditions resulting from breakdown or wearing out of organs like the heart, liver, and kidneys.

DELIRIUM TREMENS When a person has been for a long time addicted to alcohol and then abstains, or even sometimes when he does not abstain, he develops an acute disorder of the mind and body to which the name "delirium tremens" has been given. This condition does not develop in a normal person following an acute spell of drunkenness nor is it seen frequently in chronic beer or wine drinkers. It usually appears after a long or prolonged debauch associated with lack of food and sleeplessness. The situation is carefully depicted in a book called *The Lost Weekend*—in which the psychosis proceeds, however, only to the initial stages.

An ordinary case of delirium tremens lasts from two to ten days, during which time the victim displays disorientation as to time and place, great fear, disturbances of vision and hearing, sensations of pain, and sensations of the skin that are called paresthesias. These reactions are summarized in the word "horrors." The disturbance of vision produces monkeys, cats, mice, snakes, and lice. The symptoms referable to the skin include itching, burning, and prickling. Not infrequently there are muttering and tremor of the muscles. Delirium tremens is worse at night and is likely to clear up after a long sleep.

At present no specific method of treatment is known that will control every case of delirium tremens. The multiplicity of symptoms involved makes impossible the simultaneous treatment of all of them.

The mental aspects of the condition are of the utmost importance, since the alcoholic approaching delirium tremens may make accusations related to sex or crimes which are exceedingly serious. The lack of food in the person who has been on a long debauch is of the utmost importance, particularly the vitamin deficiencies which result. Since thiamine is used up rapidly in the human body, thiamine deficiency is a serious condition in chronic alcoholism. Therefore the two most helpful measures for delirium tremens are rest, which may be brought about by the use of proper drugs, and concentrated feeding, particularly of vitamins.

Because of the danger of depression to the whole body, large doses of sedative drugs or sleep producers are given only under the most careful supervision by the doctor. In most instances such drugs are best given by injection directly into the blood or under the skin. The doctor will, of course, determine the types and amounts of drugs that are to be used. It has been found that another portion of the vitamin B complex—nicotinic acid—is of great importance in clearing up some of the nervous and muscular manifestations that appear during delirium tremens.

Of exceedingly great importance is attention to the circulation of the blood. Formerly anywhere from 5 to 15 per cent of people with delirium tremens died in the attack, due, in most instances, to collapse of the heart and the circulation. Improved treatment has now greatly reduced this death rate. It has been learned that many patients were formerly fatally exhausted by struggling against restraints when they were in the course of an attack. Nowadays the administration of proper drugs, rest, vitamins, nourishment, and other methods of management have tended to yield more rapid recovery.

DELUSIONS False beliefs which cannot be corrected by reasoning. Frequently these are symptoms of mental disturbances.

DEMENTIA (See discussion under *Mental Disease*). A name for various forms of mental disurbance.

DENGUE From the tropical areas where our soldiers have fought come reports of occasional outbreaks of dengue, which is not, however, peculiarly a tropical disease. Dengue is also known as "breakbone fever." Epidemics of this disease occurred in the latter part of the eighteenth century, and there was a great outbreak in Philadelphia around the time of the American Revolution.

This disease is caused by a virus, a toxic agent so small that it can pass through a clay filter, so small that it cannot be seen with an ordinary microscope. This virus is transmitted from person to person by mosquitoes, of which there are plenty in the South Pacific. The particular mosquito concerned in most instances is known as the *Aëdes aegypti*. Dengue occurs wherever there are lots of these mosquitoes and where the climatic conditions are such that the virus can survive in the mosquito. Occasionally there have been epidemics in the Southeastern and Gulf states of the United States, but most frequently they occur in Australia, Egypt, and Greece. Incidentally, it has been determined that epidemics occur at intervals of about five years, affecting anywhere from 50 to 60 per cent of the people in the area, so that apparently some resistance to the disease is developed for this period of time. Already it is known that airplanes may carry contaminated mosquitoes, so that our public health authorities are now on the watch for them and carefully decontaminate airplanes on arrival in this country.

About four to ten days after a mosquito has inoculated the virus into a susceptible human being, there begins severe headache with pain behind the eyes and pain on moving the eyeballs. There is also a good deal of backache and prostration. The temperature rises rapidly to anywhere from 102 to 106 degrees. The heart rate becomes slowed and the blood pressure low. All the large joints, particularly those of the knees, hips, and back, become painful, and motion is difficult, if not impossible. Sometimes a rash appears, and because of the fever and inflammation the face is flushed and the eyeballs congested. Frequently the glands of the body are enlarged.

After three or four days the fever drops rapidly, there is profuse sweating, and all the symptoms become greatly improved. There may then be a second rapid rise in temperature, recurrence of the symptoms, and the appearance of another brilliant rash like that of scarlet fever. Peeling may occur also, such as follows scarlet fever.

The doctors may by their examination of the blood determine changes that take place in the blood. Because of the inflammation that may involve the kidneys, the flow of urine must be carefully watched and the nature of the urine studied.

Dengue is, fortunately, not a fatal disease in most instances. Less than one person in 10,000 people affected dies of this condition.

Of course the way to avoid dengue is to avoid the mosquito. Therefore our

soldiers are now provided with mosquito nets, and a mosquito repellent is used in the rooms and on the mosquito netting, so as to prevent as far as possible being bitten by the contaminated mosquito.

It is customary to treat the disease by relieving the symptoms of pain, giving rest and good nursing. Liquids are forced, solid foods decreased, and sedatives prescribed.

DENTIFRICES (See also *Teeth*) At least fifty different mouth washes are sold to the public with a variety of claims. In most instances the antiseptic powers of these mouth washes or dentifrices are due to small amounts of alcohol that they contain. Sometimes there may also be added some boric acid or other antiseptic. Occasionally dentifrices contain astringent substances which are compounds of zinc and which are designed to stop bleeding of the gums. Sometimes hydrogen peroxide is used to cleanse infectious conditions in the mouth. Many of the mouth washes contain baking soda flavored with peppermint water.

Actual studies show that no mouth wash can do much more than wash. The antiseptics are in contact with the infectious material for so short a time that they have little, if any, effect in destroying germs. Furthermore, the mouth wash is likely to be in the mouth for so short a time that it certainly cannot change the reaction of the mouth from acid to alkali or back again.

Dentists cure serious infections in the mouth by applying germicidal solutions directly to the infected areas. The normal gums and teeth do not need any antiseptics. Merely rinsing the mouth with water will serve just about as much purpose as an ordinary mouth wash. However, many people like a flavored mouth wash. They can select according to their taste—either peppermint, lemon, or orange flavors.

In certain instances the mouth may be infected with fungi. Occasionally there are recurrent canker sores.

Most of the common mouth washes

and gargles follow a fixed formula, such as the liquor antisepticus or the liquor aromaticus alkalinus of the National Formulary.

When ulcers appear in the mouth due to infection of canker sores or blisters, it may be necessary to use stronger materials such as hydrogen peroxide or sodium perborate, which the physician or dentist can apply. When the mouth has been infected by the parasite of trench mouth or Vincent's angina, the use of the ordinary mouth wash is entirely without effect. The physician or dentist will apply to the infected areas the specific remedies in sufficient strength to kill the parasites.

According to the *Journal of the American Dental Association,* scientific studies have shown that decay of the teeth called dental caries can be controlled in about 90 per cent of people by definitely reducing the intake of sugars. The editorial in the dental journal points out that this method of control of dental decay requires a high degree of co-operation by the dentist and the patient and lots of self-control by the child and adult suffering with dental decay. Since the body requires a certain amount of carbohydrates in order to carry out its work, it is impossible to eliminate them entirely.

New methods which have been developed for controlling dental decay include careful and repeated brushing of the teeth, the use of sodium fluoride and other dentifrices which include ammonia, penicillin, and chlorophyll. Many investigators believe that the addition of certain amounts of sodium fluoride to drinking water will control dental decay and still others assert that the application of a properly diluted solution of sodium fluoride to the teeth of children will reduce the incidence of new decay by at least 40 per cent.

Announcements of the new ammoniated dentifrices has created hope but some years will have to pass before it can be proved that these methods actually can reduce dental decay. This criticism applies also to the use of penicillin and chlorophyll in toothpastes.

Obviously the control of dental decay is a matter of the greatest importance to both dentists and the public health but the kind of scientific evidence necessary to establish that any of the methods here discussed actually will do it is not yet available. While the scientists are continuing their studies, people will do well nevertheless to make sure that concentrated sugars are not kept long in contact with the teeth. Thorough brushing of the teeth after eating sugars and regular brushing of the teeth morning and evening with the use of a suitable dentifrice is undoubtedly helpful in controlling dental decay. Moreover, evidence seems to be accumulating that the eating of a diet that is adequate in proteins, carbohydrates, mineral salts, and vitamins, and especially adequate in vitamins A, C, and D and calcium, is helpful in securing the growth of good teeth.

DEPILATORY A depilatory is a substance used to remove hair. Most modern depilatories include mechanical technics like the use of the razor, waxes that are put on and allowed to harden and then pulled off so that the hair comes off with the wax, and the X ray. The depilatory of the past included caustic substances and poisons which were dangerous because of the possibility of damage to the skin and even more dangerous because the material could be absorbed and poison the entire body. Some of our modern depilatory creams have been found safe when properly used.

DERMATITIS (See discussion under *Skin*) Inflammation of the skin.

"DEVIL'S GRIP" This is the name given to an infectious condition in which the patient is seized suddenly with excruciating pain in the side, the back, or anywhere in the chest wall.

The scientific name is epidemic pleurodynia, which merely means an epidemic condition of pain in the pleura and in the nerves to the intercostal muscles. The pleura is the membrane that lines the chest wall. The condition is now recognized to be caused by a virus like the Coxahackie virus which resembles mild poliomyelitis.

DEXTROSE Dextrose is one of the sugars developed by digestion of starches. Dextrose is readily absorbable in the body and is frequently used by injection into the blood vessels or in the form of enemas to supply food to the body both before and after operations and in the presence of diseases. It is also used in some instances to prevent circulatory failure.

DIABETES The word "diabetes" is derived from a Greek word meaning "fountain." The essential feature of the disease is the pouring out from the body of considerable amounts of urine containing sugar. To the physician, the essential feature is the failure of the gland called the pancreas to do its work in providing a substance called insulin that takes care of sugar in the body.

Before the discovery of insulin, diabetes was treated usually by lowering the amount of food eaten, particularly the amount of sugar. It is still customary to take some of the burden from the incapacitated pancreas by control of the diet. However, the use of insulin permits the person with diabetes to take some carbohydrates and to substitute the insulin for the material that the pancreas fails to supply.

The number of cases of diabetes and the number of deaths from the disease have risen steadily. All diabetics in previous years used to die young. Now even children with diabetes may live to a reasonable age, get married, and have children of their own. Since most diabetes comes on late in life and since more people live longer, more people die from diabetes rather than from infections. Since diabetes is definitely hereditary, those with diabetes may give birth to others who will develop diabetes. Before the discovery of insulin, children with diabetes invariably died young. This explains why there are more cases of diabetes, and more deaths than formerly even though we know much more

about the disease and the use of insulin in its treatment.

With the discovery of insulin we have not discovered a cure for diabetes. Insulin merely substitutes for the material that the incapacitated pancreas fails to supply. This material from the pancreas is the important substance necessary for the suitable utilization of sugar by the human body. Sugar is absolutely necessary as fuel used by the body in its activities. When the heart beats, sugar is used up. When the muscles act, they use up sugar.

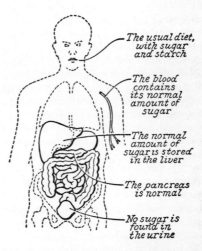

The normal sugar metabolism

The blood of every living person contains from 80 to 120 milligrams of sugar for each 100 cubic centimeters. The blood of a person with diabetes contains much more sugar, simply because his body is not using sugar as it should. Because of the increase in the amount of sugar in the blood, the diabetic is usually thirsty and hungry. With this thirst and hunger, however, he is usually underweight, because he fails to benefit from the food that he eats. In the normal person the sugar taken into the body is stored in the liver, muscles, and skin, or burned by the body in order to keep us warm and to furnish energy. In diabetes this sugar is eliminated from the body in the urine.

In 1674 an English physician named Willis found that the urine in diabetes is sweeter than normally. One hundred years later another doctor found that the sweetness was due to sugar. The diabetic is weak because he is unable to use sugar for energy.

Diabetes is not so menacing a disease as any of the infections. It is not contagious. It is not associated with chronic fever, unless there is a secondary infection. The patient who learns the rules of treatment and follows them can keep his diabetes under control and live almost as long as any normal person. Some diabetics who are exceedingly careful will live longer than normal persons who are not so careful. Two thirds of the cases of diabetes begin after the age of forty. It is not usually a disease of the young. If one happens to come from a family in which there is a tendency to diabetes he must, of course, be a little more careful than those whose family records are without any trace of this disease.

One of the most important factors in diabetes is overweight. The people of previous generations worked hard outdoors and ate to supply the energy needed for the kind of work they did. There were no automobiles to cause a discontinuance of walking and no elevators to carry them upstairs. Today improvement in cooking and the sophistication of foods, as well as modern advertising, encourage us to eat even when we are not hungry. The new machine age prevents the use of muscles for the burning up of food. Hence overweight is increasing.

A famous Viennese physician classified diabetics into two types—those who are blamable and those who are blameless. Most people who develop diabetes are fat before they get it. Dr. E. P. Joslin says that any ten diabetics put together weigh a ton before they develop the disease. He calls these fat people blamable diabetics because they would not have had diabetes if they had kept their weights down to normal. The blameless diabetics are the children who develop the disease, and most of those are under ten years of age.

INHERITANCE OF DIABETES—Fortunately the inheritance of diabetes is recessive; that is to say, it tends to breed out of the family rather than to multiply. Because of the hereditary character of diabetes, the question is constantly asked as to whether or not people with this disease ought to marry. In making the decision, it is well to recognize the nature of the heredity. If two people who are diabetic get married and if their histories show any considerable number of cases among their ancestors, it is quite likely that all of their children will have the disease. If two people marry who do not have diabetes but their records indicate that the disease is prominent in the ancestries, the chances are that one in four of their children will develop diabetes. If, however, a person with diabetes marries someone who does not have the disease and whose family shows no record of the disease, there is no reason to expect that any of their children will have diabetes.

If a person has diabetes which is severe and difficult to control, he will realize that his life expectancy is not so great as that of a normal person, and he will take this fact into account before getting married. It must be remembered also that the woman with diabetes who becomes pregnant has a special risk in relation to childbearing that does not concern the woman without diabetes.

HYGIENE OF THE DIABETIC—Certain general rules of hygiene should be practiced by every diabetic. They will, in fact, be useful also to other people. By the aid of modern scientific medicine the person with diabetes may look forward to a long and useful life. Eight to ten hours of sleep each night and, if possible, a rest each day after luncheon are advisable. Fresh air and sunshine will help to invigorate the body and improve nutrition. The diabetic must, however, avoid the danger of sunburn because his skin lacks resistance. Any damage to the skin may result in a severe infection. In order to avoid excessive dryness of the skin, it may be rubbed occasionally with cold cream or lanolin cream. The person with diabetes should avoid strong soaps because these will increase dryness of the skin and also the danger of infection.

Difficulties with the feet are exceedingly serious for the person with diabetes. Watch the feet carefully; wear proper shoes; consult the chiropodist about the care of corns and calluses; have medical attention for every cut or bruise. Never wear tight garters because of the danger of gangrene due to disturbances of circulation. Do not try to treat any slight wound of the skin with iodine or a caustic of any kind.

Exercise in moderation. The amount of exercise should depend on the age of the patient, the duration of the diabetes, and the amount of food that he is able to take together with his insulin. Exercise must be scientifically regulated in relationship to the total number of calories used each day.

Bathing should be in water of moderate warmth. Scalding must be avoided because of the danger of damage with subsequent breakdown of tissues.

The diabetic frequently asks whether or not he may indulge in alcoholic beverages. Here again he must know definitely the amount of calories that are provided. One gram of alcohol yields approximately 7 calories. The diabetic should, however, avoid the use of sweet, soft drinks, such as pop or ginger ale, because of the sugar content.

Smoking in moderation is not harmful for the diabetic, but excessive smoking may increase the blood sugar. Moreover, there seems to be some evidence that excessive smoking of cigarettes may interfere with circulation of the blood, particularly in the legs, and the diabetic must not take chances.

The following seven rules for the avoidance of the dangerous acidosis or unconsciousness which occurs in diabetics when they are getting too much sugar have been suggested by Dr. A. M. Sindoni:

1. Do not be careless about your diabetes.

2. Do not overeat or break dietary rules.

3. Do not miss insulin injection when scheduled.

4. Avoid infections because any trivial infection may prove serious.

5. Tell the dentist, the chiropodist, the barber, and the surgeon that you are a diabetic so that the necessary precautions may be taken.

6. Test your urine for sugar frequently if you have broken a diabetic rule; otherwise at least twice a week.

7. Keep the urine sugar-free and you will help to prevent acidosis or coma.

If you feel sick, take no chances. Go to bed, call the doctor, get someone to care for you, and keep warm.

DIET IN DIABETES—When we come to diet for diabetics, the problem is to provide the necessary substances for health and growth, and yet not to overtax the weakened ability of the body to take care of sugars. In diabetes care must be taken of the weakened pancreas. The sugar in the diet must be controlled. Of course the patient can be given insulin, which helps to take the place of the materials that the pancreas does not supply; but even with insulin it is necessary to watch the diet.

The person who has diabetes should keep the body weight a little under the general average for age, sex, and height. Overweight must be avoided. At the same time he should always feel satisfied, because it is known that the use of a low-sugar diet for long periods frequently causes such people to become dissatisfied and discouraged. Therefore the diet must be sufficiently liberal to eliminate hunger.

It is hardly possible for any person with diabetes to calculate his diet for himself. When the doctor calculates the diet, he determines first the number of calories that the patient must have for his age, weight, and the amount of work that he does. Then he determines the ability of the person to take care of sugar. Following that, the physician may decide how much he wants to supplement this weakness by insulin, and how much of it is to be controlled through diet.

A person with diabetes should have a scale for weighing food. In order to determine his tolerance for sugar, he begins with a diet composed almost exclusively of green vegetables containing 5 per cent of carbohydrates. Among these vegetables are lettuce, spinach, cauliflower, sauerkraut, canned string beans, celery, asparagus, Brussels sprouts, tomatoes, rhubarb, eggplant, cabbage, radishes, and artichokes. Although these vegetables contain but little nutriment, they have a large bulk and will fill the stomach and thus allay the pangs of hunger. The person is given from 150 to 200 grams of these vegetables, about 5 grams of which will be available carbohydrate or sugar.

If there is no sugar in the excreted fluids on this diet, he is given a diet on the second day which contains 5 more grams of carbohydrates, and this is increased until 20 grams of carbohydrates are being taken. Then the diet is increased by 5 grams of carbohydrates every other day until the sugar appears, or until the patient is receiving an amount of sugar equivalent to 3 grams for every 1000 grams of his body weight in twenty-four hours.

After the first two or three days vegetables containing 10 per cent of carbohydrates, such as onions, squash, turnips, carrots, beets, or canned peas, may be added to the diet in order to make up the increased amount of sugar. Subsequent to that, foods containing 15 per cent of carbohydrates, such as canned lima beans or parsnips, or 20 per cent, such as beans, corn, potatoes, and succotash, are used.

The vegetables should be cooked preferably by steaming in a double boiler, as in this way all the juices are retained.

Bread is seldom included in the diet of a diabetic, because it contains large amounts of starch. There are on the market special breads made of gluten or diabetic flours, with the amount of carbohydrates and proteins usually mentioned on the label.

When sugar appears in the patient's urine, the physician realizes that the patient's ability to assimilate has been exceeded. It then becomes necessary to cause him to fast briefly until the sugar disappears, or he may be given insulin, which aids in causing it to disappear.

In the past many patients did not do well on the diabetic diets because the amount of food taken was not sufficient to provide proper nutrition. As a result there was a marked loss of weight and strength and the patient could not resist disease. The discovery of insulin has made it possible to feed the patient a more varied diet, to avoid fasting, to combat complications, and thereby to prolong life.

DIABETIC COMA—According to Dr. E. P. Joslin, patients with diabetes need never go into coma or unconsciousness if they will live on their diets, watch the output of sugar, and be careful about their insulin. They must remember, however, that an infection will make a person with diabetes much worse and make necessary an increase in the amount of insulin required.

The first symptoms of unconsciousness associated with diabetes, called coma, include such sensations as nausea and vomiting. Sometimes an infection or seasickness will precipitate the attack; occasionally extreme exercise or lack of food. Usually the period of sickness is preceded by a sense of weakness, irritability, and fatigue. All this comes on slowly. Therefore anyone who has diabetes should go to bed immediately if he feels sick, get a doctor, and take precautions against the onset of coma until the doctor makes certain that the condition is not actually that.

Diabetic coma comes on slowly but acts fast once it has occurred. Death or recovery will take place in twenty-four hours. Once the patient becomes unconscious, the doctor and nurse must stay on the job constantly to bring the patient out of the unconsciousness. He may then have to spend another week or two recovering completely. As Dr. Joslin said, "An hour of prevention or early treatment saves a week of stay in the hospital."

DIABETES INSIPIDUS—A peculiar disease characterized by the frequency and profuseness of action of the kidneys in pouring fluid material out of the body, associated sometimes with weakness and emaciation, is called diabetes insipidus. The actual cause of this condition may be some damage to the pituitary gland, as a result of hemorrhage, injury, infection, or the growth of a tumor. Modern medicine is convinced, however, that in the vast majority of cases a disorder of this portion of the brain is responsible.

In diabetes insipidus excessive amounts of water are poured out through the kidneys. Since the body must have water in order to carry on its functions and permit comfort, such people drink large quantities of water. Obviously the amount of fluid taken in and given out will vary according to the seriousness of the condition. Since so much fluid passes through, the urine is seldom of high concentration but far more often is exceedingly pale yellow in color.

In some instances people with diabetes insipidus give out many quarts of fluid. Instances have been known of as much as twenty pints or more passing from the body in twenty-four hours. People with this disease frequently lose weight and become broken down because of loss of sleep due to frequent emptying of the bladder and inability to take sufficient food.

Sometimes there is difficulty in distinguishing between this type of diabetes and diabetes mellitus, which is more commonly known as "sugar" diabetes. The latter condition is, of course, associated with inability to handle sugar properly, so that large amounts of sugar are in the blood and also get into the urine.

If the diabetes insipidus is not due to a tumor or serious abscess in the region of the pituitary gland, the patient may get along well throughout life. When, however, there is such a destructive condition present, the patient is likely to die of that rather than of the diabetes insipidus, which is the result of the condition.

It has been discovered that injection into the body of material from the posterior portion of the pituitary gland will control the excessive flow of fluid for hours; sometimes for six hours at a time. In some cases this substance has been used in the nose as snuff in the form of dry powder, which also seems to control the excessive flow of fluid. The material from the pituitary gland, taken by mouth, does not seem to be equally effective.

In severe cases, when there is a tumor or other growth found on the pituitary gland, surgical operations have been performed for the removal of the tumor which have resulted in control not only of the growth but also of the serious symptoms.

DIAPER RASH See *Intertrigo.*

DIAPHRAGM (See also *Hiccups*) The large muscle which lies between the abdominal and chest cavities is known as the diaphragm. It is important in breathing and in the circulation of the blood. Any disturbance of the action of the diaphragm resulting from an injury to the nerves will produce serious symptoms. Occasionally the muscles of the diaphragm become inflamed and the infection can extend from the diaphragm to the organs which lie near it.

Any inflammation or infection of the diaphragm will be accompanied by a shortness of breath, a feeling of soreness, and a sense of pressure over the lower part of the chest. Hiccups especially are a sign of disturbance of the diaphragm. The most common form of spasm of the diaphragm is the hiccup.

Occasionally the diaphragm will be paralyzed because of injury to the nerve. A paralysis of the diaphragm is an exceedingly serious condition because breathing may be so greatly disturbed as to cause asphyxia.

A condition which became exceedingly important in medicine following the discovery of the X ray is diaphragmatic hernia, or rupture of the diaphragm. When any portion of the diaphragm is weak, so that an abdominal organ or part of the abdominal tissue

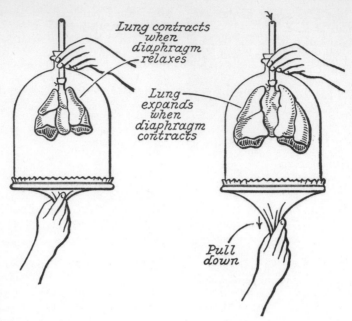

Demonstration of method by which motion of the diaphragm expands the lungs

protrudes from the diaphragm and into the chest cavity, symptoms related to that condition promptly occur. While the condition is not frequent, it is also not unusual. Out of more than 13,000 people whose chests and abdomens were examined by X ray, hernias through the diaphragm were found in 290 cases. The most prominent symptoms are shortness of breath and a blue color. This is due to the fact that the heart may be displaced and beat with great difficulty. It is also due to the interference with the movement of the lungs that occurs.

If a rupture of the diaphragm occurs suddenly, there may be all of the symptoms of shock with severe pain in the lower part of the chest, hiccups, shortness of breath, and vomiting.

Obviously from the description of these conditions it is clear that a disturbance of the diaphragm demands the most careful study that the physician can give to it. Among the most important steps in making such a study is the introduction into the stomach and esophagus of material which is opaque in appearance under the X ray. Then when the X-ray picture is taken, the line of the diaphragm will be observed and also the point where an organ that has been displaced protrudes through the diaphragm. Modern developments in surgery have made possible operations on the diaphragm for control of the hernia, or rupture, exactly as a rupture anywhere else in the body would be treated.

DIARRHEA Diarrhea is a symptom and not a disease. It was once defined by a doctor as "the too rapid evacuation of too fluid material." Usually the acute diarrheas are due to some poisonous material of either dietary or infectious origin that has gotten into the bowel. Since the action of the bowel washes this material out, the diarrhea disappears promptly. Occasionally, however, the actions of the bowel and the amount of fluid material poured out are so prolonged that the condition becomes chronic; that is to say, it persists over long periods of time.

One classification of chronic diarrhea included eight main headings with forty subheadings. There were, for instance, those due to conditions in the stomach involving a lack of acid in the stomach; operative procedures on the stomach which caused it to empty too rapidly; conditions related to the intestines, such as infections with germs and parasites, also ulcers and cancers. Then there were the cases associated with the taking of all sorts of toxic drugs like mercury, arsenic, and alcohol; next, diseases of the gall bladder and the pancreas. Then came the diarrheas which were related wholly to emotional or nervous causes and, finally, those which were constitutional, as in the case of diarrhea associated with excessive action of the thyroid or with diabetes.

In the order of frequency, the excessive action of the bowel associated with nervous and emotional causes is most important. Then come chronic ulcerative colitis and cancer of the large bowel. Obviously it becomes necessary, therefore, whenever a diarrhea occurs, to consult a physician who will make a careful study of the patient and of the material that is eliminated from the body and of the circumstances under which the diarrhea appeared, so as to be able to treat the condition according to its cause. In such a study it is necessary to get a thorough report on the emotional reactions and the family situation of the patient. A state of tension, anxiety, or mental conflict often occurs in so-called emotional diarrhea. The record of the relationship of the movements of the bowel to the taking of food may be important. The length of time during which the diarrhea has occurred is significant. The pain that may be present and the portion of the abdomen involved may indicate whether or not the diarrhea is due to some disturbance in the colon, like mucous colitis, ulcerative colitis, or diverticulitis, or whether the disturbance is chiefly associated with some other part of the large intestines. The occurrence of diarrhea repeatedly after eating certain foods always suggests the possibility that it may be due to sensitivity to some special food substance. Often the eating of roughage like bran or cabbage or celery, the eating of highly seasoned foods or the drinking of alcoholic beverages will precipitate the onset of diarrhea. With some people the eating or drinking of food that is very hot or very cold may bring on an attack. Such cases may be associated with a sensitivity to heat or to cold. In every such case the treatment will be directly related to the cause that is found.

DIET *See Weight, Over- and Under-.* See also diets used under various diseases.

DIGITALIS A drug used principally to stimulate the heart because of its effects in slowing and strengthening the heartbeat. Digitalis is a poison and should never be taken except when prescribed by a physician and in the dosage prescribed.

DIPHTHERIA Diphtheria, once most serious of all the infectious diseases that threaten children, is now known to be a wholly controllable disease.

Anyone who has seen a child suffering in the advanced stages of diphtheria and who has then seen the marvelous effects of the antitoxin can appreciate what a tremendous blessing the discovery of diphtheria antitoxin has been for mankind. So dramatic was this strangling disease before the discovery of modern methods that many a great writer of the past pictured its development and the attempts of the doctors of that day to control it. Often the doctor would be called in the middle of the night to the bedside of the gasping child. He might try to suck the membrane from the throat, using a tube, or in severe cases even by direct mouth-to-mouth suction. It the most severe cases he would open the windpipe with a knife to permit the child to breathe through that opening so that he would not strangle to death. Then in the 1880s came a series of great discoveries, including the announcement of the germ that causes the disease and the antitoxin that can be used to control it.

The modern physician has accurate methods for determining with certainty that the disease is really diphtheria. This is known as the culturing of the germs. Practically all health departments provide the doctor with assistance for this purpose. The doctor merely inserts into the throat of the child a rod on which there is some cotton. This is rubbed thoroughly over the infected area; the material is then transferred to a tube which contains some material on which the diphtheria germs grow readily. This is called the culture medium. The culture is put into an incubator, and after eight to eighteen hours the material is examined. By that time the diphtheria germs have grown on the culture medium, and the expert in bacteriology can determine not only whether they are the germs of diphtheria but also whether they represent any special type of that germ.

Quite recently it has been found that diphtheria germs vary in their virulence in different epidemics. People may carry the germs of diphtheria in their throats without themselves being ill. There are germs which resemble the germ of diphtheria and which are nonvirulent. The diphtheria germ gets its effects in the body by producing a poison known as the toxin of diphtheria. When this poison or toxin is injected into animals, it kills them, provided the dose of the poison is sufficient. The virulence of the germ can be measured by the amount of poison necessary to destroy an animal of standard weight.

In the United States more than two thirds of all the cases of diphtheria occur in children below five years of age and over 80 per cent in children below ten years of age. Now that great numbers of children are inoculated against diphtheria by the use of diphtheria toxoid, there is a tendency for the disease to occur more frequently in older rather than in younger children.

Diphtheria is spread by direct contact of a child who does not have the disease with one who does have it or with a carrier. Possibly there are indirect contacts, such as occur from coughing and spitting or from contact with infected materials such as handkerchiefs, towels, cups, pencils, and toys. If the germs are coughed out with the sputum or with pieces of membrane, they may remain alive for many weeks under suitable conditions of moisture. Before pasteurization of milk was adopted, infected milk sometimes spread diphtheria, but nowadays that source is no longer a menace.

Usually from two to five days after he has been exposed to the germs a child who is infected will develop a slight fever, going up to 102 degrees Fahrenheit, a sore throat, general illness, and weakness such as is frequent with the beginning of almost any infectious disease. The congestion and the growth of the membrane begin usually in the upper part of the throat or pharynx and then spread downward into the larynx, or voice box, and perhaps also to the nose. The membrane is a thin, grayish film which then thickens. Associated with the swelling and redness there may be enlargement of the glands in the neck and increasing fever. Therefore, whenever a child appears to be ill with fever, complains of pains in the throat, seems dull and apathetic, a physician should be called at once to examine the throat. The more the throat is involved, the greater the spread of the membrane in which the germs are found. The longer the time the poisons developed by the germs are permitted to get into the body generally, the more danger there is of death or of serious complications. An early diagnosis is of the utmost importance in diphtheria. If the diagnosis is not made promptly and antitoxin in sufficient amount given promptly, the swelling in the throat becomes larger, hemorrhages begin, the voice becomes high-pitched and strangled, and there is a fetid odor from the throat. If the continuous absorption of the poisons goes on, drowsiness is followed by delirium, and the danger of death is great.

When the membrane in the larynx becomes large enough, breathing becomes impossible. The child will be blue, will have a croupy cough, and may pass into collapse. Many years ago a physician named O'Dwyer developed a method for helping people with diphtheria in the larynx to breathe. A series of gold tubes were developed called intubation tubes. The physician can pass such a tube through the throat into the larynx and thus permit the child to breathe. The use of such a tube requires expert knowledge, and they have been lifesaving in many cases.

Before the discovery of antitoxin, 35 per cent of children with diphtheria died of the disease. In cases where the larynx, or voice box, was involved, 90 per cent died. Today that rate has been reduced to 5 per cent for diphtheria in general and 15 per cent for cases in which the membrane has clogged the larynx. Whereas the death rate from diphtheria in Massachusetts was 155 for every 100,000 of the population in 1880, it is now less than 1 for every 100,000 population in that state.

These results have been brought about by several factors. First, diphtheria is now controlled by the use of inoculation against the disease with the diphtheria toxoid. Formerly it was customary to test children for susceptibility to diphtheria with the Schick test. This is simply a method of injecting a small amount of the poison of the diphtheria germ into the skin. Those people who have antitoxin in their blood against the poison will have a negative test. Those who do not have antitoxin or who cannot develop it will have a positive Schick test. In a positive test the skin becomes red and slightly raised within twenty-four to forty-eight hours. The use of the Schick test showed that about 8 per cent of newly born babies and young infants are susceptible to diphtheria, which means that they are likely to become infected if they are exposed to the disease. The remainder are not likely to have the disease at this early

age because they have from their mothers a certain amount of resistance to the disease, which means that they have in their blood substances which prevent the effects of the germs and the toxin. Such natural immunity is gradually lost, however, so that from 30 to 40 per cent of children are susceptible at one year of age and about 65 per cent at five years of age. In order to increase the resistance of the child, he should be inoculated in most instances with the diphtheria toxoid before he is one year old.

Millions of children have been inoculated without the slightest harmful reactions, and it is customary in most of our large cities to recommend inoculation of all children against diphtheria. The toxoid is sometimes given in three divided doses, sometimes in two doses, and sometimes in one dose. The optimal results are apparently produced by successive doses, but in inoculations of great numbers of children it is customary to use either the single-dose or the two-dose method.

If all of the knowledge we now have relative to the prevention of diphtheria could be generally applied, this disease coud be eliminated entirely. Utica, New York, has not had a death from diphtheria in six years; Rochester, New York, none in five years. There are many other large communities in the United States which have not had a death from diphtheria in several years. In 1920 Michigan had 25 deaths from diphtheria for each 100,000 population; today this state has less than 1 death from diphtheria for each 100,000 population.

In preventing the spread of diphtheria, it is necessary that all who have the disease and all who carry the germs in their throats be isolated. This means that they must not have direct or indirect contact with other people and that dishes, linens, and other utensils which they use must be sterilized. The people who take care of the patient should be protected by the wearing of gowns and masks. The person who has had diphtheria is not released from control until he has been shown to be free of the germs by cultures of the throat taken two days in succession and proven negative.

When a child has diphtheria, he should be put to bed at once and kept as free from exertion as possible. There is always danger to the heart in infectious diseases and particularly in diphtheria. The diet in diphtheria is usually liquid but must contain enough sugars to overcome loss of material from the body because of the fever. There must also be enough of vitamins B and C.

Most important in the control of diphtheria is the use of the antitoxin. The value of the antitoxin depends furthermore on giving an adequate amount early in the disease. The figures show that patients treated on the first day of infection practically always recover. The longer the time that elapses before the antitoxin is given, the less chance there is of recovery. In any area where it is not possible to get a culture of the throat made promptly, the physician is likely to want to give the antitoxin immediately on the basis of his knowledge of the way the throat looks when diphtheria is present. The antitoxin cannot overcome destruction of tissue that has occurred before it is administered.

In very serious cases the antitoxin may be given directly into the veins. In milder cases it is customary to inject the antitoxin into the muscles of the buttocks. The amount of the antitoxin administered is determined by the doctor on the basis of the severity of the infection, but in general it is the tendency nowadays to give much larger doses than used to be given.

The only possible danger from the antitoxin relates to those cases in which there is a sensitivity to serum. It is quite possible to determine whether or not a person is sensitive to serum by injecting a tiny amount into the skin. If there is sensitivity, a positive reaction will appear within a few minutes. Another test is to drop a little of the diluted serum into the eye, which will react promptly

in case the person is sensitive. If the person is found to be sensitive to the serum, the antitoxin is nevertheless of the greatest importance, so that desensitization is done by giving increasing doses under the skin, beginning with a very small amount and continuing at thirty-minute intervals. Obviously the control of diphtheria in this way demands the most experienced care that can be secured.

When a child becomes a diphtheria carrier, so that he continues to give off germs after he has recovered, he remains a threat to the population. It has been rather well established that removal of the tonsils of diphtheria carriers is one of the most important steps to be used in freeing them from the presence of the germs. Outdoor living and exposure to the sun are of great value. There is much less tendency for a child to become a carrier in the summer than in the winter. If there is an infection of the sinuses, that must also be controlled because the germs can be in the material coming from the sinuses. A great variety of antiseptics have been used to treat the throats of carriers. When they are inefficient, it is perhaps associated with the fact that it is difficult to get the antiseptics directly on the area from which the germs come.

DISC The cartilage between the bones of the spine. Soft material in this cushion, called nucleus pulposus, may be pinched and result in severe pain in the back.

DISINFECTION After there has been an infectious disease in the home, it is necessary to make certain that all infectious material is removed from possible contact with those who are well. One hundred years ago it was customary to put pieces of camphor about the clothing of those who were not sick, and occasionally to throw camphor on a hot stove with a view to killing infections that might be present. Still later sulfur used to be burned in the rooms of those who had been infected. Occasionally sheets used to be hung in such rooms and moistened with solutions of formaldehyde so that the formaldehyde vapor would clear the air of germs.

Nowadays we have learned to rely on fresh air, sunshine, and dryness as a means of destroying germs in places where infectious disease has been present. During the course of infectious disease disinfection must be carried on constantly to prevent transmission of the disease from the infected person to others. Materials discharged from the eyes, ears, nose, throat, skin, or other parts of the body can be disinfected by burning after being collected in a paper, cloth, or cotton container. Those who attend sick people should avoid touching materials from the body of the infected person. Towels, bed clothing, and linens should always be gathered up with the infected side inward and should be handled by the noninfected corners or edges.

The infectious materials vary in different diseases. In chicken pox the source of the infected discharges is the mouth, nose, throat, and skin lesions. In measles, meningitis, pneumonia, septic sore throat, and whooping cough it is usually the mouth, nose, and throat that give rise to infectious material. In dysenteries, typhoid fever, and paratyphoid fever and in infantile paralysis it is the material from the bowels that probably carries the virus, although it is quite likely that in infantile paralysis the virus may come also from the mouth, nose, and throat. In scarlet fever and in diphtheria, infectious material may come from the eyes, mouth, nose, throat, and wound surfaces.

Following recovery of a sick patient, it is usually desirable to disinfect the sickroom and its contents. Cleanliness of the sickroom must be maintained at all times. A sickroom should be limited preferably to just what it necessary for the patient's care and comfort. When there is an infectious disease, upholstered furniture, carpets, curtains, draperies, and ornaments, whenever practicable, should be removed from the room before putting the patient in it.

At the end of the illness bedsteads, chairs, tables, and woodwork should be thoroughly scrubbed with soap and hot water. All linens and other washable articles should be thoroughly boiled for at least fifteen minutes. Clothing and other material that cannot be boiled should be put out of doors and exposed to direct sunlight for at least twenty-four hours. Rubber goods, such as sheets, hot-water bottles, and icecaps, should be thoroughly washed with soap and water and aired outdoors for at least two hours. Toys should be thoroughly washed and cleaned. Material like magazines and toys that cannot be washed and cleaned should be burned.

After the contents of the room have been thoroughly cleaned, all the windows of the room should be thrown wide open to admit fresh air and sunshine and—weather permitting—should remain open for at least twenty-four hours.

A disinfectant is any substance that is used to destroy germs in or on material that has been contaminated. Such disinfectants include heat, solutions of creosol, chlorite of lime, or milk of lime.

DISLOCATION The displacement of any part of the body from its usual place, particularly pulling bones out of proper place in a joint, as in the elbow, shoulder, or hip.

DIURESIS Excessive action of the kidneys is called diuresis. Drugs to produce diuresis are given in instances in which accumulations of fluids in the blood vessels need to be lessened or removed.

DIVERTICULITIS The intestinal tract of the human being is a long tube which begins at the end of the stomach and continues for a good many feet. The small intestine is 23 feet long and about 1.3 inches wide; it holds about 3 quarts of material. The large intestine is 4 feet 8 inches long and is about 2 inches wide at its commencement and 1½ inches wide at its termination.

Usually the intestine is a smooth-walled tube with slight indentations. However, there are cases in which a small pouch or tube will come off from the smooth walls of the intestine. The most frequent, as far as the small intestine is concerned, is a diverticulum, or pouch, that develops around the middle of the small intestine near the navel. This was described by a man named Meckel and is known as Meckel's diverticulum. If this pouch is present and becomes infected or inflamed, it may cause symptoms like those of appendicitis.

About 5 per cent of all adults develop pouches along the walls of the large intestine. Ordinarily these are without any symptoms. When they are found present, the condition is called diverticulosis. If, however, the linings of such little pouches become infected or inflamed, symptoms occur which demand medical attention. Such inflammation is called diverticulitis. Occasionally an ulcer may form in a diverticulum, so that the wall of the bowel will be perforated.

Doctors are able to determine the severity of diverticulitis by taking an X-ray picture of the bowel after the person has swallowed a mixture which contains barium, a substance that is opaque when viewed with the X ray. With this kind of X-ray picture the contractions and pouches of the bowel can be seen clearly. The X-ray picture will show also whether or not there has been a narrowing of the bowel by destruction of tissue or twisting of the intestine, so that food does not easily pass along the bowel.

One of the dangers of diverticuli, particularly in old people, is the danger of chronic irritation with the possible beginning of cancer.

Usually the doctor who believes, following his examination, that the diverticuli have become inflamed will prescribe a rather soft diet, the use of rest and enemas as necessary to help empty the bowel, and sometimes the use of mineral oil to aid the passage of hardened material. Occasionally the application of heat in the form of hot packs, an electric pad, or hot-water bottle is recommended to relieve the pain. If, however, there is persistent obstruction as a result of diverticuli, or constant inflammation and pain, surgical treatment may be necessary. At the time when the operation is done, the surgeon makes his decision as to the extent of the operation and the kind of operation that is needed.

DIZZINESS Dizziness is one of the most common symptoms of which patients complain when they come to see a doctor. Like a cough, dizziness is a symptom and not a disease. Like a cough, dizziness is a symptom that demands careful attention because it may be one of the first signs of an exceedingly serious disease.

Dizziness occurs after all kinds of illnesses. It may be associated with poisoning by drugs. It follows any condition in which there is an insufficient supply of blood to the brain. It may be associated with disturbances of vision. Dizziness accompanies sensitivity to foods. One of the most common forms of dizziness is related to changes that take place in the mechanism in the inside of the ear that is associated with the sense of equilibrium, or balance. In the internal ear there are the semicircular canals, which are small rings of bone containing fluid. In this fluid there are solid substances. These rings are in different planes or levels. For instance, when we stand erect, one is perpendicular; another horizontal. From these rings sensations pass to the brain, indicating to us whether we are standing erect, lying flat, moving forward or backward, or falling down.

When we ride rapidly forward and stop suddenly, we have for a while the sensation that we are still moving. This is due to the fact that a brief time is required for the fluid in the semicircular canals to readjust itself to the new situation.

Anything that interferes with the

mechanism of the semicircular canals will produce attacks of dizziness. Sometimes people will feel that everything else is moving, while they are standing still.

If the sensation of dizziness is transitory and yields promptly to hygiene, such as suitable attention to the diet and digestion, the action of the kidneys, and correction of disorders of vision, one need not be particularly disturbed. However, repeated dizziness, which may be the result of an insufficient supply of blood to the brain or an insufficient action of the heart or any disturbance involving the semicircular canals or some portion of the brain, demands the most careful scientific study. A spell of dizziness, like a cough, is then a danger sign. Unless the warning is heeded, disaster may follow.

New drugs such as Dramamine, Bonamine and Marezine have been found especially useful in seasickness, air sickness, and other instances of dizziness.

DROPSY See *Edema.*

DUODENAL ULCER See discussion under *Stomach Ulcers.*

DUODENUM (See also *Stomach Ulcers* and *Intestines*) The first portion of the small intestine directly after the stomach.

DUST Dust is disastrous to human beings. No doubt man would live much more healthfully in an atmosphere free from floating dusts of all kinds.

Dust is not a single substance. Dusts arise from industrial processes involving grinding, crushing, cutting, or drilling. Such dusts are similar to the substances from which they are derived. Fumes and gases that occur in industry are the results of chemical action.

Most dusts contain some carbon and other materials of animal and plant origin. Such dusts are developed in the textile industry, in manufacture involving flour, sugar, wood, leather, and feathers. Many people are sensitive to dusts and have skin reactions when the dusts come in contact with the skin. When such dusts are inhaled they cause irritation of the windpipe and the bronchial tubes. Some wood dusts are important in relation to irritations of the skin. This includes particularly Brazil wood, satinwood, teak, some mahoganies, and the California redwood. The organic dusts like carbon differ from the inorganic dusts in that they do not cause the changes in the lungs that are associated with silica. Organic dusts do not cause the blackening and fibrous changes in the lungs that are associated with the condition called pneumoconiosis. Their particles do not penetrate lung tissue. Much of such dust is absorbed by the body. Coal dust, when it gets into the lungs, causes pigmentation and may stimulate the production of fibrous tissue but will not cause the kind of changes that occur in silicosis.

The inorganic dusts are mostly metallic and mineral. Those that contain free silica produce a special form of change in the lung which is known as silicosis. The action of silica is to produce nodules which are distributed through the lungs and which produce a characteristic appearance when seen by the use of the X ray. A lung thus damaged becomes easily infected secondarily with various germs, including those of tuberculosis.

Asbestos also has a dust, known as magnesium silicate, which produces fibrous changes in the lungs somewhat different from those produced by pure silica. These changes are called asbestosis.

In the prevention of harm from such dusts, engineers recommend the use of exhaust systems or suction devices which trap the dust, the use of water or oil to keep the dust out of the air, the use of enclosed systems for any operation which produces much dust, increased ventilation which will dilute the dust in the air, and finally the wearing of helmets or breathing devices such as have been developed by the United States Bureau of Mines to protect the breathing apparatus of the worker from taking in the dust.

The immediate hazard to human health from the inhaling of dust during dust storms such as occur in the United States is not particularly great. Most of the dust that gets into the nose and throat under such circumstances may be washed out, blown out, or coughed out. Ordinarily such dust storms are more dangerous to property, furnishings, and clothing than they are to health. The worst effects of such dust are the mental effects and the occasional association of the dust storm with secondary pneumonia.

DWARFISM See *Achondroplasia.*

DYSCHESIA See *Constipation.*

DYSENTERY Dysentery is a term used to describe any one of a number of disorders in which there is inflammation of the bowels with diarrhea. No doubt the most common form of dysentery is that caused by definite germs of a number of varieties.

Although dysentery is chiefly a problem of the tropics, the condition also occurs in the United States and is apparently increasing. With American travelers scattered all over the globe and likely to bring back with them various infections of the bowel, the problem of controlling dysentery is increasingly important. In the Far East dysentery is caused chiefly by the use of contaminated water. In the Middle East the water supply, in general, is safe, but dysentery is spread by flies which contaminate both food and water. Uncooked vegetables are also likely to be contaminated by the use of fertilizers and by careless habits in regard to the preparation of foods, particularly salads.

Dysentery may be so serious in some areas of the world that it will kill 26 per cent of those infected in a single epidemic. The names of the Japanese investigator Shiga and of the American investigator Simon Flexner have been attached to some of the germs most frequently found in various forms of dysentery.

In ordinary dysentery the lining of the large bowel is swollen and red, and the infection may be so severe that bleeding occurs directly from the wall of the bowels. If secondary infections occur, large ulcers are formed. This form of dysentery usually begins with a mild fever and with diarrhea. There is a griping pain in the abdomen, the symptoms increase in severity, and soon the bowel movements are full of mucus, which is poured out by the bowel in an attempt to alleviate the condition. After twenty-four hours the typical bowel movement contains mucus, pus, and blood, and actions may occur from five to ten times a day or even more frequently. Associated with the infection and the loss of water from the body are headache, vomiting, drowsiness, and a general feeling of serious illness. Because of the great loss of fluid, thirst is excessive.

The prevention of the disease depends on the sanitary disposal of material from the bowels, on the prevention of contamination of food and water by flies, and particularly on the proper handling of raw fruits and vegetables. The bacteriologic experts have been trying to develop vaccines which will be helpful in these conditions, but thus far they are still used experimentally.

The moment anyone gets severe abdominal pain with numerous actions of the bowel, such as occur not only in dysentery but also in food poisoning, the person affected should go to bed and have as quickly as possible the attention of a physician.

Repeated actions of the bowel, particularly with the passing of blood and mucus, are a sign of serious sickness. Enough water must always be given to relieve thirst and to take care of the fluid that has been lost from the body. If the person is too sick to take fluids in the usual way, they may be injected into the body either by way of the blood or under the skin. An intestinal tract that is seriously infected and perhaps ulcerated should not be given the extra task of handling hard or fibrous foods. Only liquid foods, such as hot tea, are to be taken, and in addition anything taken into the body must be prescribed by the doctor. The doctor will also prescribe remedies which will control the infection and lessen the irritation to the bowel.

Fortunately the treatment of the dysenteries has been revolutionized by the discovery of the sulfonamide drugs. One of the newer derivatives, called sulfaguanidine, is particularly valuable in the dysenteries. Also important is succinylsulfathiazole, which is useful because it is not absorbed rapidly and therefore can act for a longer time in the bowel. Sulfa drugs should never be taken except when prescribed by a doctor.

Because of the frequency of the dysenteries in many tropical areas the suggestion has recently been made that people going into such areas be given a small dose of sulfa drugs each day with a view to preventing dysentery.

AMEBIC DYSENTERY—One of the most serious forms of dysentery, second in importance in its distribution to dysenteries caused by germs, is that form which is caused by a parasite called an ameba. The amebas are larger than the bacteria. The one that causes dysentery is known as *Endamoeba histolytica*. The symptoms are likely to resemble those of bacillary dysentery and ulcerative colitis.

Since an epidemic of this condition occurred in Chicago at the time of the exposition in 1933, many people have become aware of this disorder, which was formerly considered wholly a tropical disease. Although this condition at one time was unheard of in the northern portions of the United States, examinations of great numbers of people show anywhere from 5 to 10 per cent of all the people infected with this germ, although in many instances they simply carry the germ and do not seem to have any symptoms themselves from it.

The ameba which causes this disease gets into the bowel and multiplies and gives off daughter cysts. These cysts are passed out of the body with the excretions, and if they happen to reach food or drink, they are then taken into the body of some other person, passed through the stomach and small intestine, and get into the upper portion of the large intestine, where they divide and multiply, producing organisms which invade the wall of the bowel.

The symptoms begin with frequent scanty evacuations of the bowel, often containing mucus and blood, associated with severe abdominal pain and depression. There is an incubation period of from nine to ninety-four days after the organisms get into the body before the severe symptoms appear. As the infection goes on, there may be toxemia with high fever. The abdomen becomes exceedingly sensitive. In some cases the symptoms become progressively worse, so that the patient may die in less than a week. In the majority of instances, however, there is a tendency toward recovery.

Sometimes the symptoms affecting the bowel are so severe that the condition is diagnosed as appendicitis or inflammation inside the abdomen, and surgical operations are performed. Most cases begin to improve toward the fourth or fifth day after the illness begins, but even in these cases it may be many months before the organisms disappear from the bowel.

The control of amebic dysentery is relatively simple, if care is taken to prevent contamination of food and water and if the sewage system is sufficient to provide for sanitary disposal of all excretions from the body. There must also be adequate measures for protection and purification of water supplies. Food handlers in public places must be properly supervised; thorough washing of the hands of food handlers with soap and water should be demanded. All foods ordinarily eaten raw, particularly the leafy vegetables, must be given proper supervision, which means inspection before purchase and thorough washing and cleansing before serving.

In the outbreak that occurred in Chicago it was demonstrated that there had been severe contamination of the water supply from mixture with sewage. Fortunately modern chemotherapy has developed drugs which can control amebic dysentery. These include particularly the drug called emetine, which is derived from ipecac; the oxyquinolines, which are known as chiniofon and vioform and other names; also a drug called carbarsone. All of these drugs are exceedingly poisonous and are never to be taken except when prescribed by the doctor. Carbarsone is a derivative of arsenic.

One of the greatest dangers in dysentery is the possibility of spread of the organisms to the liver and the formation of a secondary abscess in the liver.

DYSMENORRHEA (See also *Menstruation*) The average age at which girls mature in the United States varies between twelve and sixteen years. Normal girls may mature before twelve or after sixteen in exceptional instances. Menstruation, which is the characteristic reaction of maturity, begins at adolescence. The average interval between such periods is twenty-eight days, although it may be as short as twenty-one or as long as thirty-five. Slight variations should not cause any mental distress. If, however, the periods have occurred with great regularity and there is a sudden change, a physician should be consulted.

Pain at the time of menstruation is called dysmenorrhea. Discomfort in the lower part of the abdomen, pains in the thighs, and a general sense of pressure are not infrequent during such periods. Whenever pain is severe enough to interfere with normal routine, a physician should be consulted. Frequently mental factors are responsible, especially among young girls who have received inadequate preparation for the role of womanhood. When the pain is not severe, the use of mild doses of ordinary sedatives is frequently helpful.

Young women often inquire whether they may exercise immediately before, during, or right after their regular functions. Most physicians believe that strenuous exercise is to be avoided at such times, but normal activities need not be curtailed. In some instances it has been observed that strenuous exercise at such times is followed later by painful periods.

Physicians are sometimes asked whether it is safe for a girl to take a tub bath or even to go swimming at such times. Many women have tried the experiment without harmful results, but in general it is not considered advisable to take a tub bath for at least the first two days of the cycle.

All sorts of medicines are sold to women to relieve difficulties in connection with the periods. Most doctors believe that the use of simple pain-relieving drugs is not harmful. But all doctors naturally condemn the use of habit-forming drugs. Physicians also warn of the dangers that may lie in taking remedies containing amidopyrine or pyramidon without adequate control. Too many cases have been reported in which women who used such drugs without medical direction had difficulty with the formation of the white blood cells.

The practice of hygiene, including plenty of rest, hot drinks, the use of hot-water bottle, and a correct mental attitude, is sufficient to make the cycle uneventful in the vast majority of cases.

In many instances new information that has been developed regarding the action of various glands in relationship to the sex functions permits the physician to prescribe endocrine or glandular products which are helpful in controlling these conditions.

DYSPEPSIA See *Indigestion*.

DYSPNEA (See *Breathing*) Breathing such as occurs in shortness of breath.

EAR There is much more to the ear than just the portion that is outside the skull. This the doctors call the external ear. It is the internal ear that takes care of our hearing and helps us keep our sense of balance. The external ear is most noticeable when it is absent but it can extend or protrude on occasion so as to be exceedingly unsightly. Modern plastic surgery takes care of this condition by a number of operative procedures which aid in holding the ear back toward the skull.

The external ear because of its construction and position is subject to a good many bruises, abrasions, and infections. The doctors include, incidentally, in the external ear that portion of the canal which extends up to the eardrum. An infection in this canal or a boil occurring in that area can be one of the most painful conditions that affect the human body. Such infections arise frequently from the hair follicles, occasionally also from the use of metallic instruments, toothpicks, or other hard objects in scratching or removing foreign bodies from the canal. Occasionally infection follows swimming when the tissues are softened by the water.

One of the first signs of infection is continuous pain which is aggravated by movement of the jaw. When the doctor looks at the ear, he sees swelling and redness, which are signs that infection has occurred. A boil or pimple in the external ear acts just the same as a boil or pimple elsewhere in the body. Seldom does the swelling become so great as to block the channel entirely and interfere with hearing.

The most that can be done by the doctor to hasten relief of the condition is the application of heat as with the infrared lamp. The application of the X ray may help break up the infection. Sometimes a strip of gauze soaked with an astringent solution will help to soften the area and hasten breakdown of the infection. The application of gauze soaked with sulfathiazole has been tried. For the pain the doctor can give aspirin or a stronger sedative if that seems necessary.

When the swelling comes to the point at which evacuation of the pus is possible—"when it comes to a head"—the doctor can incise it with the kind of knife especially used for this purpose, after which healing should occur promptly. Since, however, the infection may spread when the pus is released, it is well to continue application of the sulfathiazole solution until it is certain that no secondary infections are going

to occur. There may be further itching after the abscess has been opened. Anyone should realize that an attempt to scratch the area with a hairpin or a fingernail can only bring about the possibility of another serious disturbance.

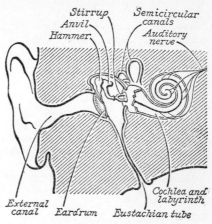

Mechanism of the ear

All sorts of organisms, insects, or fungi can invade the external ear and occasionally the results are serious in the form of infection and swelling. A doctor can look into the external ear with a suitable instrument and discover the nature of the disturbance promptly. He may wish to take some of the material and look at it under the microscope in order to determine its nature. Once this is done, he can clean the area by syringing and afterward apply remedies directed specifically to the nature of the infection.

ECCHYMOSIS This term is used for any extravasation of blood outside the blood vessels. It is also used to apply to discoloration of the skin when there is hemorrhage under the skin. The black and blue spot after a bruise is called an ecchymosis.

ECLAMPSIA The woman who is going to have a baby sometimes develops symptoms of an acute disturbance with convulsions leading to unconsciousness, which is the chief symptom of the condition called eclampsia. There has been a tendency to give the name "eclampsia" to all of the symptoms of toxemia that occur during pregnancy or to characterize some of them as pre-eclampsia, meaning that they come before an attack of eclampsia.

The first danger signal may be a headache or failing vision. The doctor finds on examination that the blood pressure has risen suddenly very high and that albumin has appeared in the urine. It is because of the importance of early detection of such symptoms that prenatal care is now carefully practiced by every physician who takes care of a woman in the period before childbirth.

Whenever these symptoms appear, steps must be taken to prevent the occurrence of eclampsia itself. It is customary to put such a patient immediately in the hospital, to restrict the intake of salt, and to prescribe only a soft diet, thus doing everything possible to prevent any extra burden on the kidneys. The physician prescribes methods of treatment using various drugs to control the tendency to convulsions. When there is a failure to respond to the methods of treatment, it may become necessary to end the pregnancy. Occasionally similar symptoms may occur immediately following childbirth.

Eclampsia occurs to women of any age. Fortunately in most cases the premonitory symptoms develop slowly. In some cases, however, the outbreak of a convulsion follows closely on the first symptoms.

The cause of eclampsia is not known. There are many different views as to its nature, most of them inclining toward the belief that certain substances are developed during the course of the pregnancy which have a toxic reaction on the patient. This reaction may affect certain organs of the body much more than others.

In recent years prenatal care has been the most important factor in pre-venting the occurrence of eclampsia and in reducing the mortality from that cause. Frequent routine checking of the blood pressure, of the urine, of the increase in weight, and of the general condition of the prospective mother leads to early recognition of the pre-eclamptic state. The treatment of the condition involves the most careful attention of the doctor, who watches the progress of the condition, controlling the tendency toward convulsions with proper sedative drugs, seeing to it that the patient has adequate nursing care, and watching indeed every aspect of the functioning of the patient's body.

Once the treatment of eclampsia was exceedingly radical, involving immediate removal of the child. Nowadays the conservative approach is followed in most instances, particularly when it is possible to get the patient immediately into a hospital, where all of the facilities of modern medical care can be provided.

ECTOPIC PREGNANCY Any pregnancy outside the uterus as for instance in the fallopian tube.

ECZEMA Once upon a time the term "eczema" was used for every eruption of the skin. Now it is limited by specialists in such diseases to any non-infectious inflammation in which a definite cause cannot be established and in which the chief disturbance is redness, swelling, blistering, oozing, and scaling of the skin. Similar appearances occur when the skin is inflamed after exposure to poison ivy or when there is inflammation following the washing of dishes with caustic substances. However, that kind of inflammation is commonly called dermatitis, which merely means inflammation of the skin.

Eczema may be due to a variety of causes, many of them concerned with changes in the body internally rather than externally. Since the distinction between eczema and dermatitis is so difficult, it is likely to be made properly only by someone who has specialized in a study of diseases of the skin.

The nature of the inflammation in eczema may be to some extent conditioned by factors like the weather and the extent to which the tissues are exposed to the weather. If there is a secondary infection in the inflammation, pus may form, in which case the eczema is known as pustular eczema. Also the eczema may be modified by changes in the skin, like the growth of warts or hardening of the skin due to repeated irritations, or by secondary infections with ringworm; in each instance the eczema appears somewhat different from other types.

Again eczema varies according to the portion of the body affected, whether it is the scalp, face, the lips, the eyelids, the genital regions, or the groin. Since the skin of babies differs from that of adults, eczema in babies may appear different from that which occurs in an adult. Eczemas are said to form from 20 to 40 per cent of all cases of diseases of the skin that come to a specialist's office.

One variety of eczema is quite certainly due to a hypersensitivity to substances either taken into the body or to which the skin may be exposed. There may be sensitivities to foods. In babies quite often a sensitivity to milk is responsible. When the eczema is due to a sensitivity to foods such as eggs, milk, pork, tomatoes, strawberries, or seafoods, elimination of such substances from the diet results in improvement. The external causes of eczema include chemical substances, mechanical irritants, heat, or even light.

Regardless of the cause of the eczema, cases are benefited by treatment of the body as a whole as well as treatment of the skin. The diets are regulated to meet individual requirements in sensitivities. Usually such foods as shellfish (except oysters), cheese, pastry, sweets, hot breads, pork, pickles, and pickled meats are avoided. Occasionally the treatment of such cases is begun with the use of laxative substances or cathartics, but no special remedies to be taken internally are known to be especially valuable as specific remedies against eczema.

A specialist in diseases of the skin treats the eczema according to the condition of the skin as it is first seen by him. He may use powders, lotions, ointments, or pastes, depending on the nature of the inflammation. Some remedies are used to control itching, others to control infection, others to dry lesions that are overmoist. Some are used to overcome thickening in the skin. Cortisone and hydrocortisone ointments have been found especially efficient in controlling eczema.

Frequently eczema appearing in babies will disappear after two or three years as the constitution of the child changes with age.

EDEMA Swelling of the tissues of the human body due to accumulation of water may occur in a variety of conditions. The general scientific word for such swelling is edema. The popular term is "dropsy."

Edema is likely to be noted first in the legs and ankles or dependent portions of the body. It occurs sometimes associated with allergic changes and often when the heart is not strong enough to force the blood through the blood vessels and back again. Sometimes edema appears when there is an insufficient amount of thiamine in the diet. Often it is associated with inflammations of the kidneys.

Actually there may be water in the tissues inside the body as well as in the skin and muscles near the surface. Occasionally deficiencies of certain glands are associated also with an accumulation of water in the tissues. Probably among the most common causes of swelling are disturbances of the heart and of the kidneys.

If the underlying condition is a deficiency of the heart, this must be controlled by rest and by treatment to strengthen the heart's action. The kidney condition has given great concern to medical science, and much more has been learned in recent years than was formerly known. Evidently the collection of fluid in the tissue spaces is associated with a low amount of protein in the blood. There are changes in the osmotic pressure or interchange of fluid between the blood vessels and the tissue spaces around them. The interchange of fluid is affected also by the state of the walls of the capillary blood vessels. Thus swelling of the tissues due to the accumulation of water may be due occasionally to difficulties with the diet. Such cases respond very promptly to a change in the diet. In the conditions in which the kidney is primarily responsible scientific laboratory tests may be performed which will determine definitely whether the condition is due to the kidney rather than to the diet or the heart. The kidney condition is commonly called nephrosis.

When the accumulation of fluid, particularly swelling of the feet, is related to a disturbance of the heart or the kidney, it is folly to attempt to overcome the condition by more walking or exercise, by massage or by bandaging or by anything that can be put on from the outside. The symptom is a serious one, and the making of a proper diagnosis as to the cause of the swelling is the most important single measure that can be recommended. The fluid in the legs will disappear when the person rests with elevation of the legs. The use of elastic bandages helps to control the swelling, but this is only a temporary remedy and is not in any sense of the word a cure for edema.

EGGS Eggs are among the products of high nutritive value and they are therefore included in every list of recommended foods for health and growth. The basic-foods lists suggest one egg a day for everyone. Eggs are rich in protein and fat, in phosphorus, iron, and riboflavin. In fact they are relatively rich in all known requirements for growth except calcium and vitamin C. Research has shown that one egg yoke per day is especially effective in balancing the intake and output of iron in the child. Eggs come nearer to milk than any other food as a source of good nutrition.

Another reason for the popularity of eggs is the fact that they can be included in the diet in so many different manners. For people who are anemic or undernourished, and especially for the tuberculous, the egg is a useful article of diet although nutritionists recommend that the eggs be balanced by correspondingly liberal amounts of fruits and vegetables. The digestibility of eggs is such that they are absorbed about as well as the proteins of milk or meat, which means about 98 per cent. The fat content of egg is digested about as well as the fat of milk. Actual tests show that eggs cooked soft at a temperature below that of boiling water are digested most rapidly and easily. However, the completeness of the digestion is not greatly influenced by the method of cooking. Hard-boiled eggs would naturally be chewed. Even raw egg whites are well utilized by the human being. Eggs contain a considerable amount of cholesterol and are therefore somewhat limited in diets for people over forty years of age. That is to say, they are not recommended in large amounts and in general people over forty may limit themselves to one egg a day.

ELBOW (See also under *Joint Disturbances*) This is the joint in the middle of the arm where three bones come together—the humerus, which is the large bone of the upper arm, and the radius and ulna, which are the smaller bones of the lower arm.

The elbow joint may suffer any of the serious conditions that affect other joints, including dislocation, in which case there should be an X-ray examination and the joint properly attended to by a competent surgeon. Sometimes it is necessary to put on a splint or a plaster cast to hold the tissues in place until healing occurs.

As a result of serious infections or inflammations in the joint, it may become ankylosed, or locked in place. This again requires the attention of an orthopedic surgeon and subsequent manipulation, massage, application of heat, and similar methods to bring about free movement.

Any condition affecting a joint of the body is important because of the danger of permanent crippling. Conditions around the joint are important, as in the case of so-called "tennis elbow," resulting from overactivity in playing tennis.

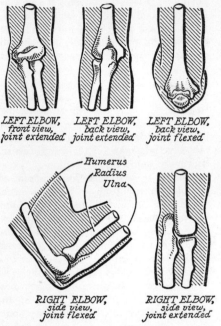

LEFT ELBOW, front view, joint extended   LEFT ELBOW, back view, joint extended   LEFT ELBOW, back view, joint flexed

Humerus
Radius
Ulna

RIGHT ELBOW, side view, joint flexed   RIGHT ELBOW, side view, joint extended

Relationship of the bones in the elbow

At the end of the elbow joint is a structure commonly called the "funny bone." In this area the pressure of the bone against the nerve will cause considerable pain. The small portion of the bone at the very tip of the elbow sometimes becomes detached. Again the treatment involves replacement and holding in place until healing occurs.

ELECTRICAL INJURIES Electricity is a powerful force. It can do great damage to the human body either by electrical discharge which enters the system or by burning the skin. It attacks the human body in two ways—naturally, by way of lightning, and artificially, by accidental contact with electrical current used in industrial or household devices. The majority of fatal electrical accidents are due to industrial accidents affecting workmen who are associated with electrical machines, switchboards, and cables. In the household such accidents are associated with faulty insulation or careless handling of lighting, heating, or refrigerating equipment.

When a person has been electrocuted either by lightning or by accidental contact with high-voltage electricity, the first step is to determine the path of the current through the body, if that is possible, and the quantity and form of the electrical energy. Obviously little can be known about a lightning stroke.

Dry skin offers a high resistance to the passage of an electric current. Therefore when the skin is dry, the local heating effects are greater and the general effects on the body are less. Moistened skin lessens the resistance to about one twentieth of the resistance of dry skin. Therefore moistness of the skin means that the shock is more likely to affect the body generally and to cause death. When the current passes through the head, the whole nervous system is likely to suffer from the shock effects. Nowadays electric shock is used in the treatment of certain disturbances of the brain, including dementia praecox and various melancholic states.

The immediate effects of a stroke of lightning are rather generally known. When a man is struck, he falls to the ground and is likely to say that he felt as though he had received a stunning blow on the head. The skin will be burned and there will be areas in which the clothing will be completely broken, particularly where any metallic object has been carried. If a group of men are struck by lightning when they are standing close together—as sometimes occurs on a golf course—they will be found thrown apart in different directions. If a person is struck when standing close to some rigidly fixed object, such as a tree or a pole, he will be flung directly away from this rigid object.

After the shock there may be pains

in various portions of the body, visual hallucinations like seeing flashes of light, and hallucinations related to hearing, with either blindness or deafness in some cases. After an electric shock the most dangerous symptoms are those affecting the nervous system with paralysis of various portions of the body, pains in the limbs, and sometimes hemorrhages.

The first step when a person has been shocked by electricity is to remove him from contact with the source of the electricity. If the source of the electricity cannot be readily cut off before removing the person who has been shocked, handling should be done only through some insulating material; otherwise the shock may pass into those who are trying to give first aid. If the person who has been shocked is unconscious, he should be given artificial respiration immediately, using some of those methods which do not require extra apparatus because delay is dangerous. The doctor should be summoned immediately in order to do what can be done to aid the work of the heart and the lungs so that life can be sustained. The body temperature should be properly maintained. The treatment of the injuries to the skin can wait until one is certain that life has been properly maintained by treatment of the shock.

ELECTROCARDIOGRAPH A machine which makes tracings of the electric current produced by contraction of the heart muscle. The upward and downward deflections permit the doctor to determine which portion of the heart tissue may be damaged.

ELEPHANTIASIS (See discussion under *Filariasis*) A chronic disease which is characterized by inflammation and obstruction of the lymphatic glands. Following this inflammation the skin becomes thickened and the tissues under the skin become swollen. The disease occurs most often as a secondary effect of filariasis. The filaria, which is a parasite, gets into the lymph ducts and blocks them. However, any blocking of

the lymphatics due to another cause could produce elephantiasis.

EMBOLISM An embolus is a piece of material which floats loose in the blood, usually detached from a clot of blood somewhere in the body. The great danger of an embolus arises from the possibility that it may get into an important blood vessel and block the supply of blood to a tissue on which life depends. An embolus in the brain, heart, kidney, or lungs is an immediate threat to life.

Most of the body is supplied with blood not only by one blood vessel but by several. In such cases the stopping of one blood vessel will cause only a temporary disturbance until the other blood vessels take up their function of supplying blood.

There are several different kinds of emboli. In addition to portions of a blood clot, an air bubble may circulate through the blood and, if sufficiently strong, may block a blood vessel. Following a fracture of a large bone, a small piece of fat may get loose in the blood vessels. Occasionally a collection of germs from an abscess may get into a blood vessel and be carried to other portions of the body, where they may block the blood vessel and set up a secondary abscess.

Fortunately modern medicine has developed several methods of attacking this condition when it occurs. In an ordinary case the early symptoms of an embolus blocking a blood vessel may be only a slight rise in fever and a rapid rise in the pulse rate. Usually within twenty-four hours, however, the temperature and pulse rate rise abruptly, breathing becomes rapid, and the patient has great mental anxiety and the symptoms of shock. After a surgical operation the release of an embolus into the blood stream with blocking of a blood vessel may be indicated by sudden pallor, perspiration, dilation of the pupils, rapid pulse, and collapse.

Usually embolism appears in people past middle life. The condition is more likely to appear in those who have had disturbances of the heart than in those whose blood circulation operates normally. In the condition called endocarditis, which is an inflammation of the lining of the heart, there may be encrustations and growths on the valves of the heart which break off and get into the blood stream.

Among the new methods of attack on embolism developed in recent years is the immediate surgical operation to release the blocked area when the embolus happens to be in the arms or the legs or in some spot where it can be reached. In the laboratories of medical investigation three substances have been developed in recent years which are now used in embolism. They are called heparin, tromexan, and dicumarol. These substances have the power to prevent clotting of the blood. They are remedies which can only be used for special purposes under controlled conditions. The operation for removal of an embolus must be done within eight hours after the embolus has lodged.

EMOTIONS Few people realize the fundamental effects of emotional reaction on the functioning of the various internal organs of the human being. The human being in a state of severe pain, fear, or anger gets pale because the blood vessels on the surface of the body contract; the skin feels cold and clammy; the mouth gets dry because the saliva stops flowing, and the tongue sticks to the roof of the mouth. The heart beats rapidly and sometimes so strongly that the pulsation can be seen in the blood vessels of the neck. The eyes widen, and the pupils dilate, while the tiny hairs all over the body may actually rise or stand on end. The breathing becomes fast. Moreover, there may be little twitchings of the muscles around the mouth and the other parts of the body, indicating the loss of the inhibitions that exist when the body is under control. All this is the effect of emotional reaction.

Some time ago a man saw his cousin fall out of a third-story window. He rushed her to the hospital. When he got there, he was nervous and upset, his knees were shaking, and his eyes watered for two hours. When his doctors examined the blood, they found that the amount of blood sugar had risen considerably. That is another serious effect of the mental reaction that is called emotion.

In the examination of young men by draft boards a far higher percentage are found with sugar in the urine than would be found under ordinary circumstances. The natural fears associated with such an examination cause an increase of sugar in the blood in many cases and an overflow of this sugar through the kidneys.

In the case of high blood pressure the pressure rises when the person becomes angry. People with high blood pressure are warned not to get angry or excited because a further rise in the blood pressure might result in hemorrhage into the brain and death.

A rise in the amount of sugar in the blood was found in the case of a man who had just had a motor accident during which his wife gave birth to a baby. In another instance a very high rise in sugar occurred when a woman was told that she had cancer. Sometimes a sudden noise, a peculiar odor, or the touch of the skin will produce a fainting attack. In these cases some memory of an incident of the greatest importance in the life of the person concerned is associated with the sensation of hearing, of touch, or of sight, and the combined effect on the nervous system is carried over to tissues and organs of the body with the result that a reaction like that of shock occurs.

Among all of the emotions, worry is probably most important as a cause of physical symptoms. When a person reaches the state in which he gets pleasure out of worry, he is called a hypochondriac; that is to say, he enjoys ill health.

Emotions are of many types—those which are pleasurable and those which are unpleasant, those which arouse fright, disgust, courage, calmness, or anger. There are the fundamental emotions of love and hate. All of these have their effects on the body by way of their effects on the mind.

EMPHYSEMA In the condition called emphysema the little cells in the lung are dilated and the walls are over-distended. There are many different types of emphysema, most of them re-lated to different causes. When there is obstruction to breathing due to any persistent cause, such as asthma or chronic bronchitis or the persistent coughing that is associated with various diseases of the lungs, there is a tendency for the walls of the small cells in the lung to be stretched and for air to ac-cumulate. In asthma, for instance, when the bronchial tubes are narrowed, the obstruction may be sufficient to cause greatly increased pressure inside the lung. Then when the person coughs, the walls in the lung are subjected to a great strain.

The stretching occurs most along the margins of the lung and along the upper edge, where the lung is less ade-quately supported by muscular and bony frameworks. The overstretching tends to destroy the elasticity of the breathing cells. As the elasticity is lost, the lung becomes distended.

Among the chief symptoms of em-physema are breathlessness on exertion and cough. The cough is usually due to the associated chronic inflammation of the bronchial tubes. These are irritable, so that exposure to cold air, dust, or exercise may start a spell of coughing. The usual appearance in a case of em-physema is a large barrel-shaped chest with prominent bones. When the doctor thumps the chest, the sound is much higher-pitched, as when thumping an empty barrel in contrast to thumping a full one. When the doctor takes an X-ray picture of the chest, the whole shape of the chest is found to be changed.

It is necessary in such cases to remove the cause in order to bring about a cure. The treatment of asthma, bronchitis, or any other chronic condition will relieve the emphysema. Since the cough tends

to stretch the tissues much more than they would be otherwise, medicines are prescribed to relieve the cough. Some-times a binder, properly fitted to cause a minimum of interference with the movement of the ribs and yet to sustain the walls of the chest, helps to control the condition.

Old people suffer with emphysema because of the gradual weakness of the tissues associated with advancing age. There is not much that can be done for emphysema that comes with exceeding old age. The cough is seldom as severe as it is in younger people.

EMPYEMA Associated with infec-tions of the lung of many different varieties is empyema, also known as suppurative pleurisy. This condition has been known since the earliest times, not only because of its frequency but be-cause it can be fatal if not promptly recognized and properly treated. The name refers to a collection of pus in the lung cavity. The condition affects chil-dren more often than it does adults. It occurs frequently in epidemics of in-fluenza, particularly when the infection with the virus of influenza is accom-panied by a secondary infection with streptococci. Occasionally, however, the staphylococcus or other pus-forming germs will be found. In about 10 per cent of all cases of empyema the germ of tuberculosis is present, but that germ may be concealed by a multiplicity of other pus-forming germs. Occasionally fungi of various kinds are found, such as the fungus of actinomycosis or blas-tomycosis. Occasionally also empyema may follow an injury to the lung like a wound of the chest. Thus empyema is not infrequently a war injury.

The doctor diagnoses empyema by a number of symptoms, but largely by taking into account the whole picture of the attack of illness. If there has been influenza or pneumonia during or after which there suddenly comes interference with movements of the chest, pain, fever, and similar signs of the presence of infection, and if the X ray shows an accumulation in the chest, the doctor is quite certain of his diagnosis. Added to this, of course, he uses the stethoscope to determine the extent to which the sounds of breathing are interfered with or changed. He can also thump the walls of the chest to find areas of dullness due to the presence of fluid.

Obviously the presence of the empyema is determined with certainty when a needle is put through the wall of the chest and thick, creamy pus escapes. Occasionally it is possible to withdraw most of this infectious material and to bring about a cure of the empyema by reinjection into the cavity of antiseptic or other substances that will control the germs. Rarely, however, is surgical operation necessary to get out the fluid. Prompt removal of the fluid is absolutely necessary whenever the amount is so large that it pushes the organs of the chest out of place and produces pressure on the heart and lungs. Repeated removal of the fluid with a needle or cannula at frequent intervals will often permit the patient to overcome the condition. In the most severe cases, however, a surgical operation may be necessary.

Fortunately modern methods of treating infections in the body by way of the blood, using the sulfa drugs and penicillin, have made unnecessary operations to the extent that they were formerly used for serious empyema.

ENCEPHALITIS   Encephalitis means, literally, an inflammation of the contents of the skull—that is, the brain. No one knows when the first epidemic of encephalitis occurred. Hippocrates, who wrote hundreds of years before the Christian Era, described an epidemic of this character that began in the spring and continued on into the autumn, at which time it was more fatal. Near the end of 1890 an epidemic occurred in southern Europe and was called "nona."

The condition recognized as epidemic encephalitis was described in Vienna in 1917 during World War I and given the name of lethargic encephalitis, or sleeping sickness, because drowsiness and somnolence were associated with the inflammation of the brain.

Until recently the cause of this condition was not known. However, studies that have been made on the disease since 1917 permitted the isolation from the brain of a virus; various forms of virus are now recognized as the specific cause of epidemic encephalitis. Incidentally some forms of epidemic encephalitis in human beings are associated with a similar outbreak among horses, so that the name "equine encephalomyelitis" is given to that type.

Another form of the infection appeared in a large outbreak in St. Louis in 1933. That form is now called St. Louis encephalitis.

There has been much confusion between African sleeping sickness, which is caused by a large organism called the *Trypanosoma* and is carried by the tsetse fly, and the epidemic encephalitis that is caused by a virus.

During World War II there have been several outbreaks of epidemic encephalitis in the Far East, particularly in Egypt, and several viruses have already been isolated in connection with those outbreaks.

Scientifically the viruses that cause encephalitis are known as neurotropic viruses because they seem to have a special affinity for the nervous system. Apparently the virus gets into the nervous system by way of the nose and sometimes by way of the gastrointestinal tract. This seems, incidentally, to be the same path that is followed by the virus of infantile paralysis.

Encephalitis begins like other infectious diseases with fever, headache, dizziness, and pains in the trunk and limbs. Sometimes there are vomiting and hiccups as secondary symptoms. The typical character of the disease is made manifest, however, by the signs and symptoms that are related to the nervous system. Among these are double vision and particularly the lethargy or sleepiness. Sometimes the whole rhythm of sleep is disturbed, so that these people are awake at night and sleepy during the day. Convulsions occasionally occur.

The doctor makes his diagnosis by the examination of the patient and the record of the disease. He makes laboratory studies including study of the spinal fluid.

The most serious aspect of encephalitis is, however, the permanent changes that may occur in the nervous system, resulting in symptoms like those of shaking palsy or Parkinson's disease, involuntary movements and paralyses, and sometimes deterioration in intelligence and behavior which is permanent. Depending on the extent and severity of the infection with the virus, there may be disturbances of breathing and of the action of the heart. In some epidemics death rates may be as high as one third or even one half of all of those affected within a few weeks of the onset.

Unfortunately scientific medicine has not yet developed a specific form of treatment for the attack on this disease. There are no serums or vaccines that are helpful. Certainly thus far the sulfa drugs and penicillin have not been proved to be specifically valuable. The doctor can, however, sustain life in many instances by taking care of dangerous effects as they develop. Most important is continuous care by specialists after the acute disease has run its course, in order to give the person who may have had a deterioration of the brain and nervous system every possibility to make the most out of the normal tissue that remains.

ENDOCARDITIS (See discussion under *Heart*) An inflammation of the lining of the heart.

ENDOCRINE GLANDS (See also *Glands*) These are the glands of internal secretion, such as the thyroid, the adrenals, the pituitary, the sex glands, and others.

ENDOMETRITIS (See discussion under *Uterus*) An inflammation of the wall of the uterus.

ENEMAS In connection with cathartics and laxatives, we must also con-

sider the enema. This has been greatly popularized in recent years, although it is one of the oldest methods of treatment known to man. An enema is a means of introducing fluid or drugs into the bowels from below, either to secure the action of the drugs or to secure the action of the bowel.

For very small babies, enemas or injections are given with a pear-shaped, soft, rubber-tipped ear syringe. These are also made with hard rubber tips, but for little babies the soft rubber tip is better than the hard rubber tip. These syringes hold about a wineglass of fluid, which is about as much as should be injected at any one time into the bowels of an infant. In these injections the bulb is squeezed as slowly and gently as possible.

For grownups the ordinary fountain syringe is used. The best types are those of glass or tin, graduated so that the amount of the material and the rate of the flow can be estimated. Enemas are given with material which is retained, for the treatment of the bowel, or with drugs which will be absorbed for the effects on the body generally.

There are nutrient enemas which contain food, given to people who cannot take food in other ways. There are also enemas which are planned to fill the body with fluids.

In place of laxatives or cathartics one uses enemas of plain water, of soap and water, of glycerine and salts, of soapsuds and salts, or of other irritants. Strongly medicated enemas should never be used except under the specific directions of a doctor.

Enemas are especially useful when the obstruction is in the lower part of the bowel. If the enema is planned merely to empty the lower part of the bowel, a pint of fluid injected rapidly with the patient sitting down will do the work. If a complete cleaning of the bowel is the aim, one or two quarts of water, preferably warm, introduced with the patient either lying on his side or in the knee-chest position (that is to say, kneeling with the chest touching the bed) will do the work.

Soapsuds are irritating to many people. For such cases a teaspoon of baking soda to a pint of water may be useful.

ENTERITIS (See *Dysentery, Diarrhea, Food Poisoning*, et cetera) A term referring to inflammations of the intestine which may be due to a variety of causes.

ENURESIS (See discussion under *Child Care*) A scientific term for bedwetting.

EPHEDRINE This substance is derived from a Chinese alkaloid called *ma huang*. It has the effect of constricting the smooth muscle tissues of the body. It is therefore used to constrict blood vessels in the nose when there is a cold. It is also used for low blood pressure, shock, and hemorrhage.

EPIDIDYMITIS Over the testicle at the upper end there lies like a hood a structure known as the epididymis. When this is infected, as occurs frequently when there is infection with gonorrhea, the condition is known as gonorrheal epididymitis. Inflammation of the epididymis may also be associated with other infections. The treatment of this condition is obviously the treatment of the original infection, for which nowadays the sulfa drugs and penicillin are most frequently used.

EPILEPSY In the time of Julius Caesar many spoke of the falling sickness; today we call the disease epilepsy. Ever since that time we have searched for the mechanism by which the convulsions come and for some means of preventing them.

The word "epilepsy" means a seizure. Epilepsy is a convulsive disorder. There is nothing disgraceful about epilepsy any more than about any other disease. The scientists call it "Cerebral dysrhythmia," which means that the normal rhythm of the cells in the brain is disturbed.

In the United States about 500,000 people have epilepsy, nearly half as many as have diabetes. The number is about the same as that for tuberculosis.

In the ordinary epileptic attack about half the patients have a premonition a few seconds before the convulsion that they are going to lose consciousness. This enables them, after one or two experiences, to get immediately to a place where they can lie down without being disturbed. It is fortunate to have such a symptom rather than to have the attack come on without a premonitory sensation. People frequently refer to this sensation as a "queer feeling" or a sense of dizziness or sickness.

The doctor inquires carefully about the nature of this sensation. Information as to the feeling during the attack may indicate to him the portion of the brain in which the attack begins. Doctors have recognized in the brain certain areas for certain symptoms. If an abnormal sensation starts in the hand or in the foot or in some portion of the face, that will indicate to the doctor the area in the brain most concerned.

Attacks of epilepsy are divided into two types which indicate the severity of the condition. We talk about petit mal (pronounced petty-moll), which merely means small illness. There are cases of epilepsy in which the symptoms are so slight that they are not noticed by people in the vicinity. They may include merely a rhythmical jerking of the shoulder or arm or eyelid. This type of condition is more frequent among young people than it is among older ones. Moreover, these attacks occur much more frequently than attacks of severe epilepsy and are seldom associated with any change in the mental powers of the person concerned.

Severe convulsions are called grand mal. Once a person has seen such an attack, it is not thereafter easily mistaken. There are other conditions in which consciousness is lost and in which there may be convulsions, but they do not represent true epilepsy. For the doctor, it is important to distinguish between the various types of cases because the diagnosis indicates the methods to be followed in treatment.

Many people who have epilepsy live a normal span of existence, although in others the condition may be so severe as to interfere with life itself. Sometimes the condition is responsible for death when it causes a serious fall or an accident.

Epilepsy, as other diseases, may be associated with heart disease, brain hemorrhage, tuberculosis, or any other disease. When patients with epilepsy are greatly overcrowded in public institutions under conditions that are not of the best, they become more subject to infection with tuberculosis or other conditions associated with overcrowding than does the public generally.

For a long time there has been the belief that epilepsy was necessarily associated with impairment of the mind. Experts have listed many people who had epilepsy and who achieved importance in the world, beginning with Julius Caesar, and including Peter the Great, Czar of Russia; Charles V of Spain; a number of relatives of Queen Victoria; Lord Byron; the great Russian novelist Dostoevski; the French writer Flaubert; the English poet Swinburne; the great writer of limericks and poetry, Edward Lear; the violinist Paganini, and the French composer Berlioz.

Only about 7 per cent of people with epilepsy are definitely deteriorated mentally, almost 70 per cent are completely normal, and about 23 per cent may be somewhat less than normal.

There may be a definite relationship between the mentality and the seizures, since both conditions concern the brain. Thus injury to the brain may be the principal cause of both the mental difficulty and the convulsive seizures. In such cases medical or physical treatment does much to alleviate the effects of the injury and thus to control both the mental impairment and the convulsive attacks.

Recently medical science has learned a great deal about epilepsy through the development of the apparatus called the electroencephalograph. The doctor does not, however, depend on any one device in making his study. He finds out all about the patient's record and about his heredity—that is to say, whether or not other people in the family or his ancestors have had attacks. He examines the whole body for the presence of other diseases. He takes an X-ray picture of the skull and also injects air into the open spaces in the brain to make other X-ray pictures which outline the interior of the brain.

The new device is a means whereby electric pulsations which occur in the brain are transferred to a record on a moving roll of paper. These are records of brain waves. The form of the brain waves is individual with individual patients. It has been found that about half the near relatives of the patient with epilepsy may also have brain waves which differ from normal brain waves. These people may not themselves have epilepsy but a study of these brain waves helps the doctor to determine the nature of the attacks.

The treatment of epilepsy demands continuous care by the doctor. Nowadays there are many remedies that can be used to control and lessen the attacks. These include not only the bromides and the derivatives of barbituric acid but also dilantin sodium, tridione, and milontin.

In many cases the convulsions are diminished by using a special diet called the ketogenic diet, which produces an acid tendency in the blood. The diet must be worked out by the doctor individually for each patient.

EPINEPHRINE This is a scientific term for the active principle of a portion of the adrenal gland, also called adrenalin. It has the power to constrict blood vessels and is employed in medicine as an astringent to stop the flow of blood and to increase the blood pressure in anesthesia.

EPISTAXIS (See discussion under *Nose*) The scientific term for bleeding of the nose.

EPITHELIOMA (See also *Cancer*) This term describes cancers of the skin or other epithelial tissues.

ERGOT This is a fungus that grows on grains and cereals. From it are made extracts which have the ability to contract powerfully the unstriped muscle fiber of the body, such as occurs in the wall of the uterus and the intestine. It is therefore used to check hemorrhage after childbirth by causing the uterus to contract. It is also used to arrest internal hemorrhages. Because of the poisonous character of the drug, the proper dosage must always be determined by the physician.

ERYSIPELAS Even in ancient times men suffered with erysipelas, a condition of inflammation of the skin due to a streptococcus. In the Middle Ages this condition was called St. Anthony's fire because the inflammation of the skin was brilliantly red and rapidly spreading.

Erysipelas may appear on any part of the skin. It occurs most often during the months from October to March rather than in the summer. The infection usually takes place where there has been a wound, a fissure, or an abrasion of the skin too small to be visible to the naked eye. The germs get into these little breaks in the skin and begin to multiply.

Men have erysipelas more often than do women because of the nature of their work and because they are more frequently exposed to physical injuries and bad weather conditions in the winter months. The cracking of the skin associated with exposure to the air and weather is predisposing to erysipelas.

There used to be great epidemics of erysipelas in hospitals, where the infection would be carried from one person to another by careless attendants. Nowadays the great danger of erysipelas has been recognized, and that type of spread is controlled. Nevertheless, everyone can learn from this experience. Since erysipelas is spread by contamination of the hands of the person who is taking care of the patient with the disease, there should be thorough washing of the hands with soap and water and perhaps also with an antiseptic solution like alcohol each time one leaves a patient who has the disease.

Erysipelas begins as an irregularly round or oval patch on some portion of the skin where there has been a small cut or fissure that has become infected. The patches of erysipelas are livid red, slightly swollen, hot, and tender. Erysipelas frequently stops when it reaches the line of the hair or any natural boundary like the nape of the neck or places where the skin is tight over the bones.

Ordinarily erysipelas is not fatal. In babies and in old and sickly people it may be sufficiently serious to cause death. In general there are about 3 deaths every year for every 100,000 in the population.

Fortunately most of the remedies that have been developed in recent years are specific against infections with the germs that cause erysipelas. The introduction of the sulfonamide compounds has rendered all other forms of treatment obsolete. Sulfanilamide, sulfathiazole, and sulfadiazine are used. When these drugs are given to a patient, the temperature drops, the spread of the inflammation is checked, and the condition is under control. It is customary to give some sodium bicarbonate at the same time to prevent any harmful effects from the sulfa drugs on the kidneys.

Formerly it was customary to put on the skin of a person with erysipelas a large number of different antiseptic substances. Nowadays that has been discontinued because they hide the lesions, so that it is impossible for the doctor to tell the extent of the spread. Moreover, the control from inside with sulfa drugs is better than any control that can be put on from the outside. Formerly antistreptococcus serum was used in serious cases, but that too has been discontinued because of the wonderful results secured with the sulfa drugs.

Because erysipelas, like other infectious diseases, will break down the blood and weaken the patient, people who are sick with erysipelas are given plenty of fluids and good nourishing food. They are asked to drink at least ten glasses of water daily.

A person who has once had erysipelas may have it again and again. Such people should be particularly careful about scratching the skin or irritating it.

ERYTHEMA A severe redness of the skin associated with some inflammation. Many forms of skin disease are classified as erythemas.

ERYTHROCYTES The red blood cells are called scientifically erythrocytes. Conditions affecting them are described under the heading of *Anemia,* et cetera.

ESOPHAGUS The tube which passes from the bottom of the throat or pharynx to the stomach is known as the esophagus. Like other portions of the intestinal tract, it may be the subject of a variety of complaints. Anything which interferes with the passage of food into the stomach means that the person concerned will be undernourished and even starved.

There is very little of the esophagus that a doctor can see by looking down the throat. Therefore he is compelled in cases of difficulty in the esophagus to use other methods, such as the X ray, and direct inspection of the esophagus by a device called the esophagoscope. This is a tube which is lighted at the end and provided with a system of reflecting mirrors. Passage of this tube into the esophagus permits the doctor to look directly at the walls of the organ. In some instances there may be little diverticuli or side tubes which grow off the esophagus or which are an accident of birth. If these become filled with food or other material that is swallowed, symptoms result from pressure. There is also the possibility of decomposition and infection in the area concerned.

The esophagus may become inflamed because of infections of its wall by a wide variety of germs. Such infection produces inflammation, and this in turn results in burning pains, pain on swallowing, extra amounts of mucus, vomiting, and occasionally in coughing of blood.

The swallowing of caustic substances or irritating substances may cause inflammations in the esophagus which will result in having the walls grow together. Under such circumstances it may be necessary for the doctor to open the swallowing tube by the use of devices which gradually stretch the constricted area.

The esophagus is also subject to reactions related to the nervous system. There are instances in which people find it difficult to swallow because of some emotional reaction. Instances are known in which people have actually starved to death wholly because of mental reactions against swallowing. Nowadays such starving is less frequent because methods are known of keeping the body nourished by other routes.

The valve at the bottom of the esophagus, where it enters the stomach, is known as the cardia. Spasm of this valve is called cardiospasm.

There is a condition called hysterical dysphagia, in which again because of some mental condition there is inability to swallow. Failure to obtain proper food results in a secondary anemia and the other symptoms that are likely to appear when essential substances like the vitamins, calcium, and iron are not taken into the body.

The advancement of medical science by the development of apparatus which permits the doctor to look directly into the esophagus, to withdraw foreign bodies through a tube, or to treat the esophagus directly through a tube have all resulted in tremendous improvement in relation to this organ. Moreover, modern surgery now permits physicians to operate on the esophagus, utilizing methods of anesthesia and safety devices for controlling breathing which did not exist in a previous century.

ESTROGENS (See also *Ovary*) The secretion of the female sex glands is a hormone or glandular substance called estrogen. This subject will be discussed under the heading of Ovary. The estrogenic hormones have control over such functions as menstruation and other activities related to childbirth. They are important in the treatment of the menopause.

EUCALYPTUS A tree or shrub which gives rise to leaves which, in turn, develop an oil that has astringent and antiseptic properties.

EUNUCH This term is used to describe a man or boy deprived of the external genitals or sometimes merely deprived of the testicles.

EXANTHEM A scientific term used to describe an eruption or any diseases in which there is an eruption on the skin.

EXERCISE Many people believe that the road to health lies in exercise. This strange notion has led to the development of innumerable systems of exercise, as well as to the sale of all sorts of extraordinary springs, bicycles, walking machines, dumbbells, and similar apparatus alleged to lead the user directly into vim, vigor, and vitality.

Actually, of course, exercise itself is merely a means of stimulating the action of the muscles, improving the coordination of nerve and muscle, and improving the circulation of the blood. The chief value of exercise is to stimulate the general chemistry and physiology of the body through its effect on the circulation and on elimination.

Various authorities have suggested the proper amounts of muscular activity for persons at various ages. One suggestion is that there be four hours of muscular activity at the age of five years, five hours daily from the age of seven to nine, six hours from nine to eleven, five hours from eleven to thirteen, four hours from thirteen to sixteen, three hours from sixteen to eighteen and two hours from eighteen to twenty. An-

other authority has said that one hour should be given daily to activities involving the use of the large muscles of the body after twenty years of age and that anything less will result in physical deterioration.

However, man does not live for his muscles alone. Certainly there is not the slightest evidence that big muscles are necessarily associated with good health. Such cynics as Henry L. Mencken and Robert Hutchins have said that whenever they get the urge to exercise they lie down on a couch with a good book and that pretty soon the urge leaves them.

Actually everyone should have sufficient strength of muscle to carry on the ordinary activities of life and to permit some exceptional use in time of emergency. For young people exercise has the value of stimulating body growth. Competitive sports of a vigorous kind, such as running, tennis, handball, football, and baseball, are available and useful up to the age of thirty. Serious overactivity after that age may do more damage than good.

The use of calisthenics, setting-up exercises, so-called "daily dozens," and similar performances is valuable within limitations. Such systems are not, however, to be considered as the single road to good general health.

Incidentally, it is the regular use of exercise in moderate amounts that maintains health, rather than the occasional overindulgence to the point of muscle strain and exhaustion. Among muscular activities suitable to people of all ages are swimming, walking, golf, horseback riding, fishing, and gardening.

EXHAUSTION (See also *Fatigue*) The speed and intensity of modern life tend to make people tire as they have never tired before. Almost everyone works as hard as possible without the periods of relaxation that were so frequent in a previous era. Once the world was tending toward a five-day week and a six-hour day. Perhaps that trend will return. Today, however, the forty-hour week seems to be about the minimum and the majority of people are putting in much more. When people work too long and too hard, they get tired. They are tired not in the sense of the fatigue or exhaustion that comes after a strenuous race, a game of tennis, or a workout. They get tired in the sense that they feel less inclined to work. People who are tired or exhausted are irritable; they awaken in the morning with the feeling that they would rather not go to work; they have no eagerness for their job.

Medical science now recognizes a condition of exhaustion called asthenia or weakness. This is sometimes modified as neurocirculatory asthenia because the condition is sometimes characterized by disturbances of the nervous system and manifests itself by fatigue, shortness of breath, palpitations of the heart, and occasionally pains over the heart. The precise mechanism by which this form of weakness develops is not known but it is believed to be associated with actions of the glandular mechanism of the body and of the nervous system.

People do not die of neurocirculatory asthenia but they can become so exhausted as to be unable to contribute much to the life of the family or the community.

Associated with this condition there is often anxiety and fear. When the causes are primarily mental, the condition has to be approached from the mental point of view. In many instances, however, there appear to be physical changes in the body associated with the mental difficulties. These are manifested by lowering of the sugar in the blood, sometimes by changes in the functioning of the liver and difficulties with the digestion and absorption of food. Not infrequently an insufficient intake of certain vitamins may be a part of the development of this exhaustion. The symptom of tiredness or exhaustion should not, therefore, be lightly dismissed. It demands instead, if persistent, a prolonged and careful investigation of the functions of various organs of the body and treatment applied not only to the physical changes that are found but also to the mental aspects. In this form of exhaustion rest alone will not always bring about relief. However, control of the diet and rest and change of work and the elimination of various causes of anxieties will usually yield recovery.

EXHIBITIONISM A form of sexual disturbance in which the person affected publicly exhibits the sex organs.

EXOPHTHALMOS This is a term applied to any bulging or forward displacement of the eyes. It is usually caused by an increase in the pressure within the eye or by changes in the muscle of the eye. It is seen most often in connection with the form of overaction of the thyroid gland resulting in exophthalmic goiter.

EYE DISTURBANCES OF THE EYE— The eye of man is one of the most remarkable organs of the body; it is like a camera but more intricate and efficient than any camera ever devised. Marvelous as the human eye is, the eyes of many another species surpass it in certain qualities. Many insects have eyes with far more facets, so that they may see instantly all around them. One form of lobster has an eye mounted on a movable stem, which may be pointed in any direction. Some reptiles have eyes which can look at two different objects at the same time. Other animals have eyes protected by a bony casing because of the nature of hazards to which these animals may be submitted.

The eye in man is relatively small in relation to the total size of his body. If his eye were comparatively of the same size that the eye assumes in certain birds, an average-size man would have an eye weighing five pounds.

A newborn baby is farsighted and for that reason pays little attention to objects that are close to him. By the age of two months he is able to use his eye muscles so as to bring his eyes into range for things he wishes to see. The baby does not, however, see small objects well until he is at least six months old. Because the eye of a baby is so delicate, it should be protected against strong light, against injuries from various objects, against the sun and irritants.

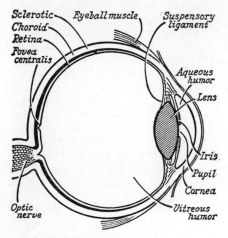

Sclerotic
Choroid
Retina
Fovea
centralis
Eyeball muscle
Suspensory
ligament
Aqueous
humor
Lens
Iris
Pupil
Cornea
Optic
nerve
Vitreous
humor

The anatomy of the eye

As we grow older, our eyes change —the most significant changes being those in which the lens becomes clouded, resulting in cataract. The muscles associated with changing the shape of the lens to accommodate various distances do not respond so well as formerly. Therefore people as they grow older—past forty—may require glasses when previously they had been able to do without them. Moreover, all of the tissues concerned with the nutrition of the eye, especially the blood vessels, will also change with increasing age, and the eye becomes functionally a less competent organ.

Our eyes are used almost constantly from the moment of birth to the time of death except for the hours spent in sleeping. Like any other organ, overwork results in earlier exhaustion. Hence it is important for the conservation of eyesight to facilitate vision in every way possible. The eye may be rested exactly as any other organ or tissue of the body may be rested, and it is desirable to give it regular rest periods. Moreover, it is possible to place less strain upon the eye by giving it suitable working conditions.

The eye has been called the window of the soul. It may be used also for measuring the general state of health. Conversely, the body sometimes reflects to a considerable extent trouble with the eyes. If your doctor finds the eyes clear and bright, he will feel less concern about any immediate danger to general health. When you have a severe cold, a fever, or general weakness due to any cause, the eye seems to lose its luster. The eyelids become heavy. Eye movements are sluggish. Jaundice gives the white of the eye a yellowish color.

SYMPTOMS OF POOR VISION—Nearsighted people are inclined to be stoop-shouldered because of a tendency to bend too closely to their work. People with astigmatism sometimes twist their whole bodies to see properly.

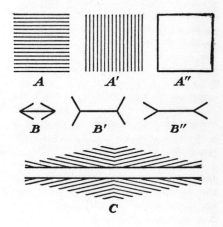

A   A'   A"

B   B'   B"

C

While the eye is one of the most perfect instruments known, it is subject to optical illusions. Figures A, A', and A" are of exactly the same size but appear to be of different sizes because the horizontal and vertical lines give a wrong impression. The lines shown in B, B', and B" are of exactly the same length, but again the rulings produce an optical illusion. The lines shown in C are exactly parallel, but the lines make them seem to diverge at the center

Children with difficult vision frequently try to intensify vision by closing the eyelids. People also attempt to bar excessive light in an irritated eye by keeping the eyelids partly closed. Such habits mean you need a special eye examination.

COLOR OF THE EYES—The color of the eye is apparently governed largely by our heredity. Eye color is a characteristic that descends from our ancestors. If a pure blue-eyed person should marry a brown-eyed person and there were four children, one probably would be blue-eyed, one brown-eyed, and two might be blue-eyed with traces of brown. Brown-eyed parents may produce not only children with brown eyes but also blue-eyed children. The color of the eyes is helpful in determining paternity but is not at all conclusive.

EYE REFLECTS UNSUSPECTED DISTURBANCES—The eye may also reflect general disturbances of the body such as hardening of the arteries, anemia, and diseases of the kidney, as well as diseases of the nervous system. A tumor in the brain is sometimes discovered first because of difficulty with eyesight. Sometimes double vision is the first symptom of inflammation in the brain. The pupils of the eye may be constantly contracted or constantly dilated or sometimes unequal in size because of the effects of drugs on the body.

In certain forms of anemia there are frequently hemorrhages in the back of the eye which the doctor sees by the use of an instrument called an ophthalmoscope. The little blood vessels in the back of the eye are thus seen at close range. When there is hardening of the arteries generally, those in the eye will be found twisted, narrowed, and sometimes broken, when studied with the ophthalmoscope.

MECHANISM OF VISION—The mechanism of vision is complicated. It is difficult to understand without an exact knowledge of the construction of the eye. Actually we do not see with the eye but with the brain and the nervous system. The chief factors involved in seeing are the optic nerve and the center in the brain for vision. Next comes the retina, a tissue in back of the eye which is a part of the nervous system and which conveys things seen to the optic nerve. The lens is actually a lens and serves to focus objects on the retina. The muscles control the size and shape of the lens in its focusing. There are also accessory muscles which move the eyeball. The iris makes up the pupil. By dilating and contracting, the iris controls the amount of light which enters the eye.

The eye, when functioning normally, has the ability to adapt itself to various conditions of light; even this mechanism of adaptation may be exhausted by overuse. It is better to provide suitable lighting than to strain the eye by insufficient light. The eye may also be strained by too much badly distributed light or glare. The effects of glare and of eyestrain result in fatigue of the eye with increased danger of accident.

Devices for measuring the amount of light in use at any point in the office, shop, or home are now available. Shades are made to distribute light suitably and thus prevent glare. Walls are painted and ceilings enameled to reflect a maximum amount of good light where it is most needed. Attention to these factors may mean many more years of good vision for those who otherwise would soon be incapacitated.

FATIGUE PREDISPOSES TO OTHER TROUBLES—An eye which is fatigued and unable to work satisfactorily becomes easily irritated. Moreover, it is more likely to be invaded by foreign bodies like cinders and dust, simply because the tissues do not react to get rid of such foreign material. People with bad eyesight frequently have red rims on the eyes, swollen eyelids, and constant watering. The eyelids will be crusted together in the morning. The appearance of any of these signs should be an indication that the eye needs attention by a doctor.

GUARDING EYESIGHT—These few simple rules are helpful in guarding your eyesight:

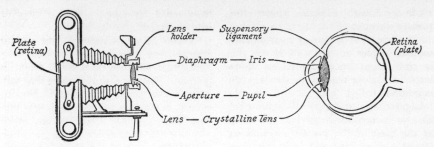

The eye is like a camera. Here are shown a camera with its main portions and the portions of the eye that correspond

Do not face bright windows or bright light when at work.

Never clean the eyes with a towel used by others.

Do not place hooks, doorstops, or other projections in the wall at the level of children's eyes. If these are placed near the floor or above the level of children's eyes, the eyes are less likely to be punctured by a hook or a nail.

FUNCTIONAL DISTURBANCES—Because of the construction of the eyes, there are several disturbances of vision which do not represent actual defects but are merely tricks of eye function. If you look up at the sky or look suddenly at a white ceiling after the eyes have been closed, you will probably notice a number of minute specks that move in front of the eye. These specks are the blood corpuscles moving in the smallest blood vessels at the back of the eyes. If the heart beats faster because of exercise, the blood corpuscles will move faster and the specks which represent the corpuscles will also be seen to move faster.

COLORED RINGS—When we look at bright lights at night, as for example street lamps, they may seem to be surrounded by areas of color or colored rings—blue on the inside and red on the outside. This is not a disturbance of the eye. These colors are due to the tissues and the cornea of the eye, the cornea being the membrane over the eye. These tissues are not seen in ordinary light.

When the eye is irritated or threatened, we blink. The blinking sensation is a protective mechanism. For every human being there is apparently a regular blinking rate, the blinking being associated with the protection of the eye. If you try to hold your eyes still without blinking, you will find that within 10 to 20 seconds the desire to blink is almost uncontrollable. You may then avoid blinking for a moment or two, but eventually you will have to blink.

How OFTEN Do You BLINK?—The average man blinks every 2.5 seconds. If he gets angry, he may blink every second. Some people form a habit of blinking more rapidly when they speak. If the attention is fixed, blinking will occur less frequently than at other times. In a reading room it was found that women would blink every 5 seconds and men every 11.2 seconds. Apparently women are not able to fix their attention as definitely as are men. Irritation of the eye from smoke during smoking may also increase blinking.

EYEGLASSES—With a few exceptions, eyeglasses are worn in order to correct errors in the anatomical construction of the eye which prevent it from seeing well, to correct errors in the pull of the various muscles of the eye which may unbalance the vision, or to take the place of decreasing ability of the eye to accommodate itself to distance. Sometimes eyeglasses are worn to protect the eye against glare from too much light. Such use of glasses has probably become more of a habit than reason and circumstances warrant.

The eye that is wrong anatomically so that it does not see well is one that is nearsighted or farsighted or shortened in such a way as to develop the condition called astigmatism. In the farsighted eye the rays of light come to a focus behind the retina, the tissue at the back of the eye with which we see. A convex lens will bring the rays to a focus on the retina and correct this condition. The nearsighted eye focuses the rays in front of the retina so that a concave lens is used to bring the focus on the retina itself.

ASTIGMATISM (See also *Astigmatism*) —Practically everybody has some astigmatism. This is a change in the curvature of the outer surface of the eye, and the use of a proper lens will correct this curvature in most cases. In some cases, however, the curvature may be so irregular that lenses cannot be adapted to the curve.

When the muscles of the eye are unbalanced to such a degree that the action of the two eyes is dissociated and one eye tends to deviate away from the point at which vision will be correct, a number of possibilities exist for correction. One method is, of course, training to improve the strength of one muscle or another. Another method is operation on the muscles, shortening them or lengthening them to make conditions more balanced. A third possibility is the use of correct lenses to overcome the imbalance of the muscles.

EYES LESS ADAPTABLE WITH AGE— As we grow older, the lens becomes less elastic, so that the muscles which adjust the lens have more and more trouble focusing properly. Therefore people past forty years of age who have never worn glasses previously may be required to wear lenses to focus on ordinary print. Some people who can still read print although far advanced in years may brag about that ability. A nearsighted person who boasts of his power to read without glasses at seventy and of never having worn glasses for any purpose

may never have had a decent view of the countryside in all his life.

VISION OF THE CHILD—When a child reaches one year of age, parents may determine whether or not his vision is perfect. There are simple tests that any parent may make for himself. For instance, a bandage may be tied over one eye. Then a block, a ball, or any other toy that the child uses may be put close by. If the vision of the child is normal, he will pick up the toy when either eye is bandaged, showing that each eye is for itself sufficient. If, however, there is slowness to detect the toy or inability to recognize the presence of the object, a physician who specializes in conditions affecting the eyes should be consulted.

The next important occasion for testing vision will come when the child begins to read. At such a time difficulties with vision may be determined by the fact that the child holds the book too close to the eyes or too far away. Again, the book may be held at some peculiar angle. An intelligent parent will observe this matter and at once make arrangements to have the child's vision tested.

There are certain elementary symptoms which are quickly apparent. If the child has a pronounced degree of astigmatism, he may frown when he reads. There may be an aversion to reading because it is associated by the child with headache and other difficulties. One eye alone may be farsighted, and the child will be able to get along by using just the other eye.

Unfortunately the child who is nearsighted will have few symptoms that are easily apparent. In the first place the child can see things that are close and will not be disturbed about objects that are far away. This difficulty may become apparent for the first time when he attempts to play baseball, basketball, or some other game, or goes for the first time to the motion picture show.

Parents must realize that the simple prescribing of glasses or the kind of automatic fitting of eyeglasses that goes on at some bargain counter or at the hands of some itinerant eyeglass fitter does not represent scientific study.

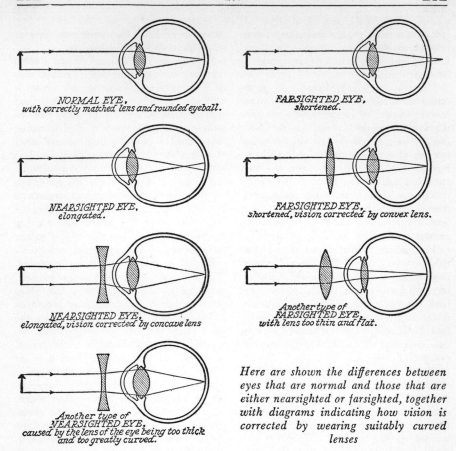

NORMAL EYE,
with correctly matched lens and rounded eyeball.

FARSIGHTED EYE,
shortened.

NEARSIGHTED EYE,
elongated.

FARSIGHTED EYE,
shortened, vision corrected by convex lens.

NEARSIGHTED EYE,
elongated, vision corrected by concave lens

Another type of
FARSIGHTED EYE,
with lens too thin and flat.

Another type of
NEARSIGHTED EYE,
caused by the lens of the eye being too thick
and too greatly curved.

Here are shown the differences between eyes that are normal and those that are either nearsighted or farsighted, together with diagrams indicating how vision is corrected by wearing suitably curved lenses

There are many other difficulties with the eyes besides those that can be controlled simply by glasses. A complete examination by a specialist in diseases of the eye is basic to proper management.

THE DOMINANT EYE—The eye is one of the most important organs in the human body, since it functions in relation to practically every activity having to do with learning or pleasure. The eye is only one of the instruments dealing with perception, but it is perhaps the most important of the instruments.

At first it was thought that each eye was just like the other eye, but now we know that eyes may differ, one from the other, and that the function of the brain in relation to the eye may be as important as the eye itself. There is an image

in each eye, and these images are fused by a higher center in the brain.

When a person sees everything with one eye and depends on the image from one eye only he is called a monocular person. If he sees with both eyes and the images are properly fused, he has binocular vision.

The psychologists have determined that a person may be right-eyed or left-eyed exactly as he may be right-handed or left-handed, and the one on which the person depends is called the dominant eye.

If anything happens to the dominant eye, the one that has not been dominant is forced to function. If the person is able to work satisfactorily with the new type of vision, there may be little difficulty. If, however, the other eye cannot assume the dominance, a variety of symptoms may result, including some related to vision but others related to fatigue, stuttering, or various types of hysterical attacks.

Many animals are organized on a one-sided basis, so that the eye, the hand, and the foot on the same side work together in order to achieve the best possible results. Obviously throwing the eye out of function on that side will interfere with the activities involving the foot and hand as well.

Various tests have been devised to determine which eye is dominant. One test is merely to ask the person concerned to look through a cylinder-like roll of paper. The eye that he uses for this purpose is the sighting eye. He uses the sighting eye when shooting. Another test is to ask the person concerned to look through a hole in the middle of an 8×10 inch piece of cardboard. He will look through the hole with one or the other eye and that will be the dominant eye.

If the person is found to be using the left eye for most such purposes and the right hand for other functions, the question of harmony between these activities needs investigation. Thus a right-handed person with a dominant left eye may represent a problem. If a person's natural left-handedness has been changed so that the hands no longer work in harmony with the dominant eye, many difficulties will be understandable.

COLOR BLINDNESS—A Quaker bought himself some scarlet stockings when he thought he was purchasing dark brown. His name was John Dalton, and his is the first scientifically recorded instance of color blindness. Dalton was an eminent English physicist. It is said that he was walking down the street wearing his cap and gown and the red stockings at Oxford when the degree had just been conferred upon him and that one of his brother Quakers promptly took him to task for wearing such colors in public.

Color blindness is more common in boys than in girls. It is exceedingly

important today because the signals on the railroads and on street corners are most frequently red, green, and yellow, but occasionally also blue, and these are the colors most frequently concerned in color blindness. Certainly no one who happens to be handicapped with this condition should attempt to drive a motorcar in modern traffic. The difficulty of distinguishing between red and green is the most common form of color blindness. The blue-yellow difficulty is much rarer. People who have color blindness see objects as lighter or darker but are unable to distinguish the shades. Sometimes they distinguish between the red and the green lights on roadways by their difference in brightness.

There is no specific cure for color blindness, since the defect is one of structure of the eye. However, as has already been mentioned, there are various ways in which the color vision may be developed or substitutions found. In testing for color blindness, the most common test involves the sorting of a number of colored worsteds. The person who is being tested is given certain pieces and asked to match them with others. There are other tests in which colored strips of paper are employed.

One woman who was an excellent seamstress was able to do sewing provided her family would tell her the colors of the thread. She was able to remember them by having each color in a different place in the workbox.

So significant is color blindness today in relationship to accident that every person who attempts to drive a motorcar or to indulge in any other occupation in which color detection is significant should have a test as soon as possible. The Navy and the Air Force do not admit men who are color-blind. A few have gained admission by learning the tests. There is no cure for color blindness. If a boy is smart enough to learn the tests so that he can pass them, the Army can probably find a place for him.

EYESTRAIN—Eyestrain is one of the conditions that everyone talks about. Unsuspected eyestrain may be associated with twitching of the eyelids and face. It may be responsible for nausea and vomiting, for headache, bad nutrition, loss of appetite, and many other similar conditions. Yet the only way to determine whether or not eyestrain actually exists is to make a suitable examination of the ability of the eyes to see and then to overcome the condition by rest and the provision of eyeglasses.

There is also the stress placed on the eye by glare or bright light, and the kind of strain that is associated with overwork. The printing trade particularly places great stress on the use of the eye. Modern printing plants look carefully into the provision of proper light, suitable type, and other conditions which will relieve stress on the eye.

Motion pictures have been incriminated as a cause of eyestrain and tiredness. Under normal conditions moving pictures do not cause serious fatigue of the eye. However, the wrong type of lighting in a motion picture house, films that are jerky or spotted or badly lighted, and long periods of projection without change in the light will produce serious fatigue of the eye.

Suitable eyeglasses are prescribed nowadays for vision that is deficient or for the correction of curves in the eyeball, resulting in astigmatism.

When eyeglasses first became popular, they were frequently prescribed when they were not necessary. Everybody who had his eyes examined felt that he had to have glasses in order to justify the examination. Today the reaction against this results in fakers who try to get people to throw away their glasses.

There are three chief reasons for wearing glasses: to protect the eyes, to see well, and to see without fatigue. An eyeglass is a crutch to aid a deficient or weakened eye exactly as an ordinary crutch aids a weakened limb. A crutch lends support until the limb is capable of working for itself. A permanently deformed limb or an eye of which the structure is anatomically wrong demands permanent use of a crutch or eyeglasses. Proper glasses can relieve eyestrain; improper glasses may make the condition more severe.

CONTACT LENSES—The theory of invisible eyeglasses was first suggested as far back as the early part of the nineteenth century, but the first experiments were not made before the late 1880s. Today it is quite possible for people who find them necessary to have eyeglasses that fit directly over the eyeball and which serve fully the purpose of aiding the vision.

One of the first steps is to make a mold of the eye with an especially developed substance, exactly as one makes a cast of the inside of the mouth when it is necessary to have false teeth on plates. From this fragile mold a permanent mold is made with dental plastic; then the glass is modeled to fit the mold. The inner surface of the contact glass must fit the eyeball so that it will not injure the sensitive tissues or interfere with the circulation of the blood. Before the mold has been prepared, it is necessary to fit the contact glasses. This means that the eye must be studied by all of the usual methods in order to determine the difficulties in vision so that the lens prepared for the eye will meet the needs.

In fitting the contact lens after it has been made, the eye is anesthetized; then the contact lens shell is filled with a salt solution of the same density as the blood. The lids of the eye are then separated by the thumb and forefinger of the left hand, and the contact lens is inserted first beneath the lower eyelid and then beneath the upper eyelid. The contact lens is held with a little rubber suction bulb. This is released from the glass before any attempt is made to remove it; otherwise the fluid will be lost from underneath the contact lens. If there are any bubbles under the lens, they must be removed and the procedure repeated until the lens fits closely without any bubbles in the fluid.

At first patients wear these lenses only an hour or two at a time, but many who become well accustomed to them may wear their lenses six to eight hours in a single stretch. Once the lens is well fitted, the patient is instructed as to how to place and remove the glass from the eye for himself. He practices seated by a low, cloth-covered table with a mirror.

Formerly such lenses were made only in Europe, but methods were soon developed to manufacture them in this country, and there are now several places in most of our large cities where contact glasses may be prepared and fitted. In their appearance these contact lenses resemble artificial eyes of the "shell" type. The portion over the eyeball in general is made of clear glass or plastic. The rest of the eyeglass is made to resemble the eye itself.

About half the people who first try contact lenses complain of blurring of the vision for a few hours. Experiments with different types of fluids indicate that some people do better with one type of fluid and others do better with another type. Indeed it has been suggested that the patient's own tears are probably the best fluid to be used if they can be collected in sufficient amounts, or at least a solution may be developed resembling the patient's tears.

A manufacturer states that the final correcting lenses can be supplied within two or three days after the temporary lenses have first been fitted. Producers also make permanent molds and keep permanent records of the finished lenses so that duplicates may be supplied in case there is breakage or loss. Contact lenses are quite expensive. To the fee of the doctor who fits the glasses must be added a cost of anywhere from a hundred to a hundred and fifty dollars and upward for a pair of glasses.

From experiments it has been found that it takes the average patient about nine minutes to learn to insert the lenses. Several months may be required, however, before the patient becomes sufficiently used to them to be able to wear them over long periods of time without taking them out and refilling with fluid and resting the eye between fittings.

STYES—A sty of the eye usually represents an invasion by one of the common pus-forming germs into the glands on the eyelid, most often near a hair follicle. Styes often appear in crops. In many instances they are associated with uncorrected errors of vision. The eye under such circumstances does not protect itself as well against outside substances.

A sty acts like a pimple or a small boil. After a day or two it gets soft and bursts, the infectious material is discharged from it, and recovery follows. Before the sty has softened, its progress can sometimes be stopped by pulling out the hair that runs through it and by treating the spot with some antiseptic that is not dangerous to the eye itself. Usually it is well to apply hot compresses to styes to hasten the development of the inflammation. As soon as a yellow spot is seen, the infectious material should be released.

When styes form repeatedly, physicians collect the germs which cause them, make a vaccine of killed germs, and reinject this into the patient. This may help the patient to develop specific resistance against the germs that caused the styes.

CONJUNCTIVITIS (See also *Conjunctivitis*)—The tissue which lines the eyelids and runs out over the eyeball is called the conjunctiva. An inflammation of this tissue is known as conjunctivitis. When the conjunctiva becomes inflamed, there is burning and smarting of the eyelids, formation of pus, and reddened eyelids. Usually the eye, when inflamed, becomes exceedingly sensitive to light, and tears flood it constantly. In the morning the eyelids will be found crusted together. Doctors treat this condition according to the character of the germ that causes the inflammation and according to the severity of the infection.

PINKEYE—Pinkeye is a common type of conjunctivitis. Shortly after this special type of germ gets into the eyes, they become reddened and the lids are swollen and puffy, and usually glued together in the morning. Pinkeye is usually spread by the use of a common towel, and sometimes by soiled hands.

SWIMMING-POOL EYE INFECTIONS—In some instances the eyes become inflamed by germs which get in from contaminated swimming pools. Physicians are able to prescribe much more powerful germicides than boric acid and in that way bring dangerous infections under control. It is easy to transfer germs of this character from one person to another. The safe step is for people with infected eyes to use individual towels and to make certain that the hands are always thoroughly washed with soap and water whenever any contact is made with the eye.

BORIC ACID WASH PREVENTS INFECTION—Occasionally symptoms are produced by overexposure to ultraviolet rays, to the electric arc used in welding, or to the arc lights employed in motion picture studios. Comfort can be had early by the use of cold compresses, and infection may be prevented by the use of solutions of boric acid. Do not take such conditions lightly because they may progress and seriously threaten eyesight itself. The only way to be certain of the exact character of such a condition is to have the eyes examined by a competent doctor.

IRITIS—The iris is the colored portion of the eye. It becomes infected and inflamed due to various causes. When it is infected it becomes swollen, dull, and discolored. The pupil gets small, gray, and sluggish. There is pain, which is worse at night, radiating to the forehead and to the temple, and there is much disturbance of vision. In most infections of the eye the person who has an inflammation of the iris cannot stand to look at the light, and there is constant watering of the eye.

One of the most common causes of this condition is syphilis. However, the iris may also become infected by other germs and may be involved in rheumatic conditions. It is of the utmost importance to take care of this condition immediately because the inflammation and infection may result in scarring which will either block the pupil entirely or bind the iris down in such a manner as to prevent its motion. Obviously this will cause a permanent disturbance of vision.

When a doctor takes care of this condition, he applies drugs which relieve the congestion and put the part at rest. Dilatation of the pupil will prevent the scarring and tend to break up the small scars that have already formed. Various preparations of atropine are useful for this purpose. There are other drugs which are anesthetic in character and which prevent pain. The doctor may prescribe also moist, hot compresses for several hours, which will tend to diminish the pain and the inflammation.

Of particular importance, however, is the treatment of this, as of other conditions, through the body as a whole. Syphilis affecting the eye means syphilis elsewhere in the body and demands the kind of consistent and persistent treatment that is necessary for this condition. The rheumatic condition with which iritis is associated must be treated for the general rheumatic disturbance, with the detection, if possible, of the focus of infection of the body and with the elimination of that focus when it is found. Other types of septic infection must also be controlled. When there is diabetes, the treatment of the condition by diet and insulin so as to control the diabetes throughout the body generally is even more important than the treatment of the condition as it affects the eyes.

Once the condition is healed, surgical operations of various kinds, including plastic operations, may be necessary to bring about normal restoration of the iris and thus aid vision.

CROSS-EYES—For a long time any attempt to control cross-eyes in children was prevented because people thought that cross-eyes were due to fright, shock, prenatal impressions, or similar superstitious reasons. A squint or walleye may develop from excessive strains placed on the external muscle of the eye by the extra effort in seeing which is required when there is an extreme degree of nearsightedness. Any straining of the eye or imbalance of the muscles may result in cross-eyes or squint.

Many people believe that children outgrow cross-eyes. This may happen, but in other instances the sight of a crossed eye may never develop and in many instances the squint or crossed eye becomes worse as time goes on. Early diagnosis and treatment are essential for the best results in this condition. As soon as you notice that a child is cross-eyed, a specialist in diseases of the eye should be consulted. He will make a sufficiently thorough examination to evaluate the factors in the case and decide on the proper treatment.

In at least half the cases of cross-eyes there seems to be some hereditary anatomical weakness in the eye because there will be a record of other cases somewhere in the family. Most people have some minor muscle out of balance in their eyes. One muscle will pull harder than the other, and the strong one will overcome the weak one. When both eyes are open, the stimulus coming from the brain can supply enough extra effort through the weak muscle to keep the eyes lined up. With both eyes open and seeing, we will see double if one eye turns out of line with the other. In the case of cross-eyes the person affected may avoid seeing double by using only one eye at a time. This happens also in people who have one eye farsighted and the other nearsighted. If they are not balanced suitably with proper eyeglasses, they will use only one eye at a time for seeing. If this is not corrected, the good eye will be used and the weak one will turn. Sometimes good results are secured merely by prescribing eyeglasses which will tend to hold the two eyes in position. Children have been found quite able to tolerate eyeglasses at the age of fifteen months. The earlier the glasses are used, the more valuable will be their effect.

It has also been suggested that the weak eye be exercised by various training devices to overcome the habit of suppressing the image of one eye. In certain types of cases, when the deficiency is very slight, this so-called orthoptic training is successful. Many types of apparatus have been developed by specialists in diseases of the eye for giving training of this character. The most favorable age for training is between three years and six years of age. After the age of seven years the results are rarely satisfactory.

The surgical procedure for overcoming cross-eyes is most certain. Proper placement of the eye muscles will tend to bring the eye back into proper relationship to the other eye and will permit binocular vision. The operation will not improve the vision of the eye but will prevent the vision from being lost from failure to use the eye successfully. Moreover, the correction of cross-eyes is very important for establishing a proper mental attitude in the child. Children with cross-eyes may become so shy and sensitive to laughter that they will become "shut-in" personalities and their lives are thereby ruined.

GLAUCOMA—Glaucoma causes 15 per cent of all blindness in this country and about one half of the blindness in adults. In this condition pressure within the eyeball brings about loss of sight. Interference occurs with the circulation of the fluid that comes into the eye. The accumulation of this fluid causes pressure. As the pressure increases, there is pain, the eye gets hard and reddened, and the pupil gets gray and cloudy. This is the acute form of glaucoma.

There is, however, a second and much more serious form, in which there is gradual obstruction of the drainage system, so that the pressure increases very slowly. In this case the loss of sight takes place gradually.

With the ophthalmoscope and the tonometer the physician determines the extent and effect of the pressure. A new drug called Diamox eliminates fluid and lowers the pressure within the eye.

As the glaucoma develops, the person finds that he can see in front of him as well as he ever could but not so well to the sides. Then the vision in front also becomes narrowed, so that finally there is complete loss of sight.

In the treatment of early glaucoma drugs alone may be sufficient. In later stages drugs prepare the tissues of the eye so that the operation is more easily and successfully performed.

Another device used in disturbances of the eye is the perimeter. The purpose of the perimeter is to measure the width of the field of vision. If it is found to be steadily narrowing, the doctor suspects the presence of glaucoma.

Obviously a correct diagnosis early in this condition means a great deal for the saving of sight. It is also necessary to prevent the pain and the pressure and the general symptoms.

Women who are getting on in years should be particularly careful with their eyes. They are more likely to suffer with glaucoma than men.

Excitement is often a factor in producing an attack because during excitement there is increased flow of blood to the eyes.

Drugs like Diamox lower the pressure in the eye.

All too frequently people who are more interested in selling glasses than in taking suitable care of the eyes will temporize with the condition by providing glasses. In many instances control by drugs is impossible. For cases of this type surgical procedures have been developed which are frequently quite successful in saving eyesight and in controlling the glaucoma. The drugs, when used, help to prepare the eye for operation and enable the surgery to be done under much more favorable conditions.

PREVENTION OF EYE INJURIES IN INDUSTRY—Blindness or impairment of vision is one of the most serious and costly of all non-fatal accidents to which workers may be subjected. For that very reason the speeded war industries have caused special attention to be given to the problem of the care of the eyes of the worker.

Some conditions are known to be definitely associated with processes involving intense light and heat. For instance a cataract occurs in the eyes of glass workers who are exposed to the heat and glare of a furnace for many hours each week. All sorts of devices have been developed to prevent exposure of the eyes of glass workers. Fortunately the introduction of machinery for making glass bottles and the introduction of other machinery to take the place of hand operations has minimized this hazard. All workers regularly exposed to glare from furnaces should, of course, wear appropriate glasses to shut out the light.

Workers in electric arc welding sometimes have inflammation of the eyes, including pain and headache, and similar troubles occur in actors and workers in studios where photography, including motion picture photography, is the chief occupation. Here again careful attention to prevention and planning for very brief exposures to the powerful lights will overcome the hazard.

Certain industrial poisons are dangerous to the eyes, including ammonia, phosphorus, derivatives of lead, benzene, and methyl alcohol. Indeed there are fifty-two different poisons used in industrial processes which may affect the eyes. Sometimes the results follow inhalation of the poison in the form of a vapor, sometimes inhalation of poisonous dusts. There is the possibility of direct action of the poison through or on the skin, and also the contamination of food and drinking materials through handling by workers who have not thoroughly cleaned their hands.

The prevention of such hazards includes chiefly adequate provision for frequent washing of the hands by workers in the industry, also the use of exhaust fans for getting rid of dusts and gases in the air. The prevention of accidents to the eye involves primarily the overcoming of the hazard from flying fragments of metal, stone, and grit. Perforating wounds or lacerations of the eyeball may occur, and there may be secondary infection. Acids or strong caustics may burn the surface of the eyes and thus destroy sight.

In Great Britain a combination of agencies, including the National Industrial Research Council and the Ministry of Labor, has given special consideration to these problems. Many workers object to wearing goggles. A properly prepared protector for the eyes should be made of hardened glass and should have protecting side shields to block fragments coming from the sides. The goggles must fit comfortably and must interfere as little as possible with the worker's capacity. Where the workers are exposed as in arc welding, the goggles should be designed to eliminate infrared and ultraviolet rays and be sufficiently colored to prevent glare. Some workers may find it necessary to wear helmets which protect the entire head, into which the goggles are integrated, rather than goggles alone.

BLOCKED TEAR DUCTS—Tears keep the eyes moist, so that the delicate tissues of which they are made are preserved. If the eyes are not constantly kept moist the tissues dry and are much more easily attacked by bacteria.

In a little bony notch on the inner side of the eye there is a gland called the tear gland, or lacrimal gland. From this six or more little tubes carry the tears to the eyes. There is another tube, which is known as the nasal duct, which carries fluid from the eyes to the nose. Hence, whenever a person cries or his eyes water, his nose is also affected. When the amount of moisture is so great as to overflow, the excess comes down through the nasal duct until there is so much that it falls on the cheeks. Most of the time there is just enough moisture to keep the eye in the proper state of softness and luster.

Occasionally a tear duct becomes blocked because of the presence in it of a cinder or a hair. Under such circumstances it is necessary to open it up. This requires special instruments and the care of a physician who knows how to do the unblocking correctly.

In other instances the gland and the duct become infected. Then there is a reddened swelling in the inner corner of the eye and the discharge of a small amount of pus. Pressure over the swelling will force out most of the pus. It is sometimes possible to get relief by treatment, but in other instances it may be necessary to cut into the gland, and there are instances in which it has to be removed surgically.

Tears have always had a special interest. In 1481 a Latin writer described a girl sixteen years old whose tears resembled blood. More recently a similar case was described in Pennsylvania. Apparently in such cases there has been a leaking of red blood cells out of the blood vessels into the tear gland.

BURNS OF THE EYE—Another fairly common type of injury to the eye is the burn by caustics of one type or another, such as lime or acids. In industry it is well to follow certain rules for all workmen who happen to suffer injuries to the eye:

1. Under no circumstances should an untrained or inexperienced employee attempt to remove any foreign body from the eye.

2. Immediately after an accident, the eye may be bathed with suitable mild aseptic or sterilized solutions, preferably a weak solution of boric acid made with sterilized water.

3. The eye should be covered with a sterile bandage moistened with this solution.

4. The person whose eye is involved should be sent immediately to the physician who is in charge of such cases.

This brings up the question of removing foreign bodies from the surface of the eye. There are hundreds of superstitions as to how this is best done. They concern sneezing, rubbing the other eye, and similar methods. It is much safer to rub the other eye than to rub the one in which the foreign body has lodged. In most instances rubbing tends to push the foreign substance farther into the eye.

People who understand how to remove foreign bodies are exceedingly careful to make certain that their own hands are clean and that every instrument or other material used in the process is clean or sterilized. The eye itself must be handled with the utmost delicacy. The person first looks upward so that the lower lid of the eye may be pulled down and carefully studied. He then looks downward while the upper lid is turned back. It is impossible to turn the upper lid back safely while the person is looking up or moving the eyeball constantly. With practice, skill can be developed in turning back the upper lid. This is then carefully studied.

If the foreign substance is not seen, the physician then looks at the surface of the eyeball, changing the light so as to catch the reflection of any foreign substance which may be imbedded in the cornea.

Of course the competent physician has means of anesthetizing the surface of the eye and of avoiding injury to it in the removal of foreign substances. He is careful not to introduce infection, and to follow up the removal by later inspection to make sure that no untoward results are occurring. Secondary infections may bring about ulcers which will destroy the sight of the eye.

FALLOPIAN TUBES The fallopian tubes are organs possessed only by women. They pass from the neighborhood of the ovary to the uterus, or womb, and they serve to carry the female ovum, or egg, each month from the ovary to the uterus. Hence a normal condition of the fallopian tubes is necessary for pregnancy to occur. These tubes, however, become subject to various conditions which may interfere with their normal state of health. When these tubes are inflamed after infection the condition is called salpingitis.

Sometimes the fallopian tubes become twisted and blocked. This causes serious pain and may be followed by a secondary infection. The most frequent infection of the fallopian tubes, however, is gonorrhea. Indeed, infection with the organism called the gonococcus is said to be responsible for 70 per cent of all of the cases of infection of the fallopian tubes. The symptoms of such infection are much like those of acute appendicitis, including tenderness in the abdomen, a rise in the number of white blood cells, and a fever. In many instances the infection does not become acute but develops a chronic form, so that there is continued ill health and sterility.

Occasionally the fallopian tubes may become infected with the germs of tuberculosis or with other organisms.

The physician in every instance will make a study to determine exactly the cause of the infection and will treat it accordingly.

The discovery of the sulfa drugs and of penicillin and the use of the heat method now make it possible to bring about complete cure in cases of gonococcal infection of the fallopian tubes without a surgical procedure. In very severe cases, however, surgical removal of the tubes seems to be the only successful method.

Occasionally an ovum, or female egg cell, will be caught in the tube and become pregnant. This produces a condition know as ectopic, or tubal, pregnancy. Once this condition is produced, surgical operation is needed immediately to prevent continued growth and ultimate rupture of the tube and the possibility of fatal hemorrhage into the abdominal cavity.

FATIGUE (See also *Exhaustion*) Fatigue is one of the most serious menaces to health and life. Nevertheless, fatigue is also a protection for the body. The human body is built with factors of safety. The tissue cells have remarkable power to recover from ordinary fatigue. Excessive, prolonged, and accumulated fatigue is dangerous for the body because it results in the accumulation of waste products, such as lactic acid and carbonic acid, which are toxic.

The tired feeling called fatigue may be associated with infection and disease, with bad hygiene, with overwork, with too much mental effort, or with undernutrition.

Muscles use sugar in their work. Many vitamins are necessary to proper functioning of the nerves. Iron is required for a good state of the blood. A deficiency of any of these substances may produce fatigue much sooner than it occurs with a balanced or proper diet.

If fatigue is the result of overuse of certain muscles, those muscles will be more tired than others and will probably also develop soreness.

A lack of a sufficient amount of rest and sleep will increase the tendency to fatigue and exhaustion. Some of the signs of fatigue include a tendency to yawn, a feeling of exhaustion on movement, drowsiness, profuse sweating without previous exertion, a tendency to close the eyes, to misplace commonly used articles, difficulty in remembering what has just been said, and an effort to talk more than is usual.

There may also be distraction from work, irritation from slight annoyances, depression, and slowness in getting up and moving around.

If fatigue becomes chronic or long-standing, the person who suffers will have a loss of appetite and weight and increased irritability. Anyone who has reached this state of fatigue should have a careful study to determine what is wrong and to control all of the factors that have been mentioned.

There are certain rules which everyone should remember:

1. The best treatment of fatigue is rest.

2. Stop physical activity before exhaustion.

3. Do not try to overcome fatigue by taking coffee or other stimulants or by taking "pep" pills. This is like whipping a tired horse.

4. If you have exhaustion, that is a condition demanding medical investigation, including a special study of the glands.

FECES   This is a scientific term used to describe the excrement discharged from the bowels. Feces consist chiefly of the undigested residue from food, bacteria, and the materials secreted by the intestinal walls.

FEEBLE-MINDEDNESS   Whenever intelligence fails to develop normally, the person is called mentally defective or feeble-minded. The symptoms of this condition vary according to the amount of mental defect that is present.

The legal profession says that an idiot is a person so deeply defective in mind from birth or from an early age as to be unable to guard himself against common physical dangers. An imbecile is one in whom there exists from birth mental defectiveness not amounting to idiocy but yet so pronounced that the person is incapable of managing his affairs or, in the case of a child, of being taught to do so. Morons are feeble-minded persons in whom there exists from birth or from an early age mental defectiveness not amounting to imbecility, yet so pronounced that they require care, supervision, and control for their own protection or for the protection of others. Furthermore, by reason of such defectiveness the child appears to be permanently incapable of receiving proper benefit from instruction in ordinary schools, so that it becomes necessary to send the child to a special school.

The morons are thus not really the feeble-minded children of lowest intelligence. The moron is next to normal in the amount of intelligence that he possesses. A normal small baby will follow sounds or bright lights. He will smile and grasp objects with his fingers. He learns to walk as he develops and learns to control the actions of his bowels and his bladder. The baby who is mentally defective may be extremely late in developing these normal reactions and remain a baby for a long time.

Statisticians calculate that feeble-mindedness is so fully bred into the race that approximately 10,000,000 normal people in the United States are carriers of some feeble-mindedness. This means that there exists the possibility of such a birth in almost any stock. However, it should be possible through proper practices to minimize greatly the tendency. People must realize the potential danger of marriage when one or more of the ancestors of either one of the persons to be married is feeble-minded, or mentally defective. Licenses to marry should not be issued to anyone who is feeble-minded, or mentally diseased.

Much can be done to help a feeble-minded child to make a reasonably satisfactory adjustment to life. The available special schools often teach even the most difficult cases to take care of themselves and to perform some common tasks which can be developed as a routine. Sometimes the lack of mental power causes the mentally defective child to get into mischief. In evaluating the child's conduct these factors should certainly be taken into consideration.

Class handling of children who are feeble-minded is not likely to get as good results as the kind of care which individualizes the child. The treatment or attention that will work with one child may fail completely with another. Every case must be handled as a special problem.

FEET Among the greatest annoyances of human beings are such simple conditions as painful feet, sweating feet, and itching feet. Many people are born with deformed feet.

When a doctor examines feet that are giving trouble he first looks for signs of pain or swelling. He looks to see if there is discoloration such as results from bruising or hemorrhage. He wants to know if the feet ache during the night or if the pain begins early in the morning. It is important for him to know whether or not the swelling disappears after a night's rest.

In many instances feet are exceedingly painful because of a condition affecting the main bone of the foot known as the astragalus. This is particularly the case in a condition known as fallen arch, which occurs more often in women than in men. People who stand long hours, such as motormen or saleswomen, are especially likely to be disturbed by painful feet due to continuous strain on the arch of the foot. In such cases the pain is the result of rigidity of the tissues and of spasms of the muscles in their effort to overcome the strain. Relief frequently comes when the person concerned stays off the feet. This, however, interferes with occupation and earning power. In such cases hot applications and massage of the feet are helpful. Proper padding of the shoes to change the strains may be comforting if carried out by a specialist who understands the condition. The shoes must be fitted so as to support the arch with a rigid shank of medium width.

HYGIENE OF THE FEET—The feet should be bathed once daily, preferably with soap. After being dried, the feet may be dusted with a simple talcum powder.

Especially helpful to aid the circulation in the feet and thus to relieve pain at night is the contrast bath. Two large buckets big enough to hold both feet and perhaps to reach up halfway to the knee are needed for the purpose. In one bucket is placed hot water sufficiently high in temperature to feel distinctly hot. Warm water is added from time to time to keep the temperature up. The other bucket is filled two-thirds full of cold water. The person who is taking the contrast baths sits between the two buckets. First he puts both feet in the warm water for one minute, then removes the feet and puts them in the cold water for one minute. This procedure is followed for ten minutes. The alternating dilation and contraction of the blood vessels helps the circulation in the feet. Also helpful is light massage, including rotary movement with the fingers. If the skin is delicate, cold cream, olive oil, or some similar ointment may be used to lessen the irritation from rubbing during massage.

All sorts of troubles can happen to a foot, including strains, sprains, dislocations, fractures, excessive sweating, corns, calluses, warts, chilblains, ringworm, bunions, hammertoes, painful heels, ingrown toenails, cracked toes, blisters, bruises, and disturbances of the circulation. Many of these disturbances result from accidents during games like football or basketball or tennis. This applies particularly to sprains and strains and fractures. Others may be the result of malformation of the feet at birth. Still others may result from faulty shoes and stockings.

Most important is the use of a shoe that has the shape of the foot and which fits the foot. The most important shoe measurement is from the tip of the heel to the middle of the big toe joint. The latter point should come opposite that part of the shoe where the shank goes into the sole. Shoes should not be so tight that it is necessary to break them in. When shoes are too tight, and particularly when they are too short, the toes are likely to be forced back into the right-angle position that is called hammertoe. Frequently hammertoe may become so inconvenient that it becomes necessary to amputate.

The best types of shoes have round toes, medium-width shanks, and are made over a last with a straight inner border. Extremes in the heights of heels are undesirable. A good heel is neither too low nor too high; neither is it set too far forward or too far backward.

The feet are built like arches and, therefore, tend to push forward and back. Tight stockings tend to cause the toes to turn in, the toenails to become ingrowing toenails, and in other ways interfere with the proper circulation of the blood in the foot.

Incidentally few people understand how to take care of shoes properly. Shoes will last longer and give better service from the point of view of protecting the feet if they are changed at least once daily and if the pair that is not in action is kept on a shoe tree or shoe form.

The rubber heel has proven so well its advantage in minimizing shock to the feet and body that it is no longer necessary to emphasize its value.

CORNS, BUNIONS, AND CALLUSES— When the skin on any portion of the body is repeatedly rubbed, it responds by thickening. This thickening is called a callus. When such a thickening occurs on the toes or between the toes, it is called a corn. Corns appear, however, not only on the feet but occasionally on the hands of mechanics or golfers or others who subject some portion of the hands to repeated rubbing.

The most common corn is the one that occurs on the outside of the little toe, where the bone or cartilage under the thickened skin compresses the soft part of the toe in the shoe. Such corns may be removed by cutting them away

with a sharp knife or razor blade, but usually the corn occurs again. The only way to get permanent relief is to cut away the bone under the skin. However, this is not a mild procedure and apparently most people prefer to keep on working on the corn rather than to have the operation.

Soft corns usually occur on the inside of the little toe where the joint projects against the inside of the fourth toe. This condition is usually started by a tight shoe causing the tissues to rub against each other. Moreover, the moisture of the skin between the toes helps to macerate the skin, which is then promptly infected—in many cases with ringworm. Soft corns may also be removed by cutting them away. If, however, the conditions remain that produced the corn or the ringworm infection, the condition is quite certain to return.

Most people go on for years and years using ointments or surgery to remove or damage the corn, which, however, continues to recur. There are so many remedies for corns that almost everyone has his own particular cure. The ordinary commercial corn cure is a mixture of salicylic acid with some other substance that will hold the salicylic acid in solution or suspension so that it can act over a long time on the skin. The salicylic acid will soften the skin so that it will come away.

Bunions usually occur on the outer side of the large toe. Sometimes bunions occur on the middle of the foot due to the modern practice of lacing shoes tightly. Sometimes the middle bunion on top of the foot can be relieved by padding the tongue of the shoe or by wearing straps instead of the tight lacings. Complete relief can, however, usually be obtained by a surgical operation.

Calluses most frequently occur on the bottom of the foot where there is continued pressure. Golfers have calluses on the ball of the foot associated with pivoting when driving the ball. Calluses are best removed also by cutting them away with a sharp knife or razor blade. They can be prevented by wearing pads to change the point of pressure on the foot.

FELONS Paronychia is the scientific name for what people commonly call a felon. The condition is also known as a whitlow, and another name for it is a "run-around."

The distinguishing mark of this condition is an infection at the bottom of one or more of the nails. Usually the organism involved is a pus-forming germ called the staphylococcus, but it is quite possible for other germs to be involved. Occasionally there are several types of germs involved as well as the parasites that cause ringworm. Obviously any kind of a germ may be inoculated into a wound near the base of the nail. Thus in a recent group of cases the first felon was the result of penetration of the thumb by a piece of wire; the second, penetration of the skin at the bottom of the nail on the index finger by a safety pin; and the third, a puncture of the skin at the bottom of the nail on the index finger with a needle.

Usually when a felon is found, people are likely to begin treating it with home remedies and antiseptics. It is customary to try painting with iodine, tincture of metaphen or some similar antiseptic, the application of hot, wet packs of saturated boric acid solution, and similar treatment. Sometimes, notwithstanding anything that is tried, the condition becomes worse. If the infection goes deep, so as to penetrate muscular tissue or bone or the covering of the bone, a serious condition indeed prevails.

One of the most important steps is to apply measures which will prevent the pus and infectious material from going deeper. The doctor can take care of this by the following process: he soaks the finger in hot water for a while to soften the tissues, then puts the pointed end of a sharp knife directly into the infected area and painlessly releases the pus from the pocket. As soon as this is done, the pain is relieved, and then the application of hot packs and iodine will bring about a cure.

If the condition is not controlled, there may even be spread of the infection up the lymphatic ducts and tissues, so as to produce a generalized infection of the whole body. The sign of such spread is the appearance of red inflammatory lines upward through the hand and wrist.

Most of us like to think that we are big enough and strong enough to disregard minor scratches or punctures of the skin in different parts of the body. It is never safe to disregard any penetrating injury because of the serious possibilities associated with the spread of an infection. Above all, it is important in manicuring to make certain that every instrument used to cut or push back the cuticle has been properly sterilized either in boiling water or by some other technic before its application to the skin.

FERTILITY The birth of various quadruplets and of quintuplets calls attention to the frequency of multiple births at a single birth and also to large families. A nationwide search for the largest family in the United States made a few years ago revealed the Latorra family with twenty-one members. There is also a record of a woman who had twenty-two children in twenty-six years, giving birth to one child at a time, whereas Mrs. Latorra had two sets of twins. Another medical record reveals a woman who was married at the age of sixteen and died when she was sixty-four, after having given birth to thirty-nine children, one at a time and with the same husband.

Fecundity seems to be an inherited trait, as is also the tendency to have multiple births. Pregnancy has been reported frequently in girls as young as eight years of age, particularly in tropical countries and among the Eskimos. Records are also available of a case of twins in a girl of thirteen. At the end of the life span there are plenty of records of women who have had children when they were between fifty-five and sixty years of age.

Boys may become fertile as early as fourteen, and many men are reported who have retained their power to reproduce until well advanced in years. In the latter case the evidence is sometimes difficult to evaluate.

A study was once made as to the relationship between success and large families. Studies made of the British peerage and of the Harvard graduates both showed that there is a tendency among people who have been successful in life to have families slightly larger than the average. However, the total offspring for college graduates is in general lower than it ought to be to keep up the type.

The chances of multiple births have been estimated by the obstetricians, who report that the chance for twins is once in 88 births; triplets, once in 7500; quadruplets, about once in 600,000. There have been fairly authentic reports of over thirty sets of quintuplets, so that the chance would be about once in 42,-000,000 births. Apparently there have been about a half dozen cases of six babies born at once, one of which, reported in 1888, is probably authentic.

Nowadays with the use of the X ray it is possible to determine that there is going to be a multiple birth fairly early and to be prepared for it. In the old days Josh Billings wrote, "There is one thing for which no man is ever prepared and that thing is twins."

FEVER Fever is generally considered to mean any condition of the human body in which the temperature recorded is above the normal. Normal, as indicated by the little red arrow on the thermometer, is 98.6 degrees Fahrenheit or 37 degrees centigrade. Thermometers are generally graded from 92 to 108 but occasionally from 90 to 110.

It is best to keep the thermometer in the mouth at least three minutes when taking the temperature, since few thermometers reach a definite point in less time. Incidentally, human beings seldom reach a temperature lower than 90 or higher than 110—and survive. A thermometer placed under the arm is likely to record about a degree lower than one placed in the mouth, and a thermometer placed in the rectum is likely to record about a degree higher.

In certain diseases the form of the fever is distinctive. In many infections such as pneumonia and typhoid fever, the temperature becomes high and stays high. In other conditions, as for instance tuberculosis, the fever may be low in the morning and high in the afternoon. In some forms of malaria a fever occurs which lasts about eight hours and develops every other day. In other forms of malaria the fever lasts about eight hours but occurs only every third day. Physicians who have studied the various forms of disease can learn a great deal from a case record of the temperature made every four hours.

Fever may result not only from a disturbance of the heat-regulating mechanism of the body but also through disturbances of the blood or the rate of breathing. Indeed, there are records of a rise of the temperature of the body in which the fever is the sole manifestation of some mental disturbance, which in turn causes tissue changes that bring about an increased temperature.

When the body is invaded by germs, an infectious fever results. This is due to the fact that the mechanisms which in health prevent a fall in temperature when the body is exposed to cold are affected by the poisons produced by the infecting germs. The loss of heat from the body is prevented by constriction of the blood vessels, as seen in the fact that the skin is cold, pale, and slightly blue. There is also a feeling of chilling and shivering, which in turn is due to the fact that the tissues in the skin which provide a feeling of warmth are not stimulated by the warm blood which ordinarily would be coming to them. The chills of fever are due to the spasm of the vessels in the skin and the exclusion from these blood vessels of the warm blood that comes from deeper in the body. In fever, the blood volume being reduced, there are also changes in the concentration of the blood and in its content of salts and other materials.

Drugs which produce a fall in temperature are those that increase elimination of heat from the body through drawing water from the tissues into the blood vessels, increasing the blood sugar, and dilating the blood vessels.

A fever is, therefore, not necessarily detrimental to the human body. It may be an important aid in combating disease. In fact there are some germs which cannot live in the presence of a temperature above that of the normal temperature of the human body.

The first man to measure the temperature was an Italian named Sanctorius, who developed an exceedingly bulky instrument for the purpose. About 1714 a scientist named Fahrenheit invented the mercury thermometer with the Fahrenheit scale. As late as 1870 the thermometers used in measuring fever were about ten inches long, took about five minutes to register, and were placed under the arm because they were hardly of a size to be held in the mouth. The modern compact fever thermometer was developed twenty years later.

In measuring the temperature, the mercury in the thermometer should always be well shaken down before the thermometer is put into the body. The temperature of babies is always taken by putting the thermometer in the rectum rather than in the mouth. A special thermometer with a blunt tip is used. The child is placed face downward, preferably on the mother's lap or on the bed. The thermometer, well greased with vaseline, cold cream, or petrolatum, is then placed in the rectum and held in position until the temperature is recorded. The thermometer is then taken out of the rectum, and the amount of temperature is read.

The mother should never go away and leave the child with the thermometer in place; the child may turn and break the thermometer or seriously injure himself. Neither should the thermometer ever be placed in the rectum with the child lying on his back.

After the rectal thermometer is used, it should be washed thoroughly with soap and water, then placed in alcohol for five minutes, dried, and returned to its case. Never wash a fever thermometer in hot water.

The thermometer that is used in the mouth is likely to have a longer and sharper tip than the one used for recording rectal temperatures. It should be cared for as is any other thermometer; that is, it should be carefully washed with soap and water and placed in alcohol after each use, and then put in its case. The thermometer for the mouth, as previously mentioned, should be held in the mouth at least three minutes to make certain of getting a correct recording.

There used to be a saying, "Feed a cold and starve a fever." Nowadays that saying has been discarded. Fever causes a definite increase in the speed of the chemical changes that go on within the human body. For every rise of 1 degree Fahrenheit in the temperature of the body, there will be an increase of about 7 per cent in the speed of the chemical changes. The excretion of nitrogen in the urine is greatly increased in most fevers. The nitrogen comes from the protein of the human body, so that from 300 to 400 grams or almost a pound of protein may be destroyed daily by a fever. Therefore it has now become customary to feed a fever by increasing the total amount of calories taken into the body and also by increasing particularly the amount of protein that is given. In order to reduce the waste of the body tissue in fevers, a liberal diet is given containing foods that are not contra-indicated by any special feature of the disease. The sugar and fat are also drawn on during starvation as well as in fever. The amount of calories taken by a patient with a fever may be twice the amount normally required to maintain the person at his normal weight. Because people sometimes find themselves unable to take food during a fever, sick people usually lose weight.

There is a section in the brain that is known as the heat-regulating center. A hemorrhage or a tumor in the brain at this point may be accompanied with an exceedingly high fever. Such cases are, however, extremely unusual.

The extent to which a fever is to be prevented or controlled, therefore, depends on the physician's judgment as to just how much control he wishes to exercise. He is likely to provide plenty of water to the patient because the body will evaporate more water from its surface. Frequently the best technic for lowering an ordinary fever is a simple sponge bath with warm water, 85 or 90 degrees or even slightly warmer. The sponge bath should never be given in a cold room. Any of the drugs used to control fever, including aspirin, sodium salicylate, phenacetin, as well as the more dangerous acetanilid, are to be used only when the doctor prescribes them and only in the amount prescribed.

FEVER BLISTERS See *Herpes Simplex.*

FIBRILLATION Whenever a muscle develops a shivering or tremor, the condition is called fibrillation. The term is applied particularly to the heart muscles whenever the individual fibers of the muscles take up independent action and thus produce inco-ordination in the action of the heart. Whenever fibrillation begins in the heart, the heartbeats and the pulse beats become irregular in relationship to each other. This, of course, weakens the force of the heartbeat. A drug called quinidine is now chiefly relied on in the treatment of fibrillation of the heart.

FIBROMA A fibroma is a tumor composed of fibrous tissue. Most fibromas are not malignant as are cancers. There are, however, mixed tumors in which there is fibrous tissue and cancer tissue.

FIBROSITIS One of the forms of rheumatic disease is called fibrositis, a medical term meaning inflammation of the fibrous tissue anywhere in the body.

The cause of fibrositis is not known. The condition is frequently related to exposure to damp or cold weather, fatigue and overexertion, sometimes to infections in the various portions of the body, and occasionally to colds or influenza. At one hospital for rheumatic diseases it was reported that 25 per cent of the patients had fibrositis.

Since there is fibrous tissue in many different portions of the body, the fibrositis may be largely in the muscles, occasionally in the tendons, or sometimes in the bursas, which are sacs of fluid at points where there may be friction in tissues. When the fibrositis is chiefly in the fibers around the muscles, it is likely to affect certain groups of muscles rather than all of them. The muscles most frequently affected are those in the back, the scalp and neck, the buttocks and less frequently those between the ribs.

This kind of fibrositis usually begins with pains which increase in intensity and last from a few days to a few weeks. The condition tends to become chronic, being worse after periods of inactivity. People usually get temporary relief by moderate exercise or massage, by taking aspirin, or by the application of heat. Those who practice regular limbering-up exercises in the morning or keep moderately active are less likely to suffer with recurrences of the pain. If, however, the fibrositis is accompanied by fatigue or exhaustion, movement becomes increasingly difficult, particularly toward the end of the day. There may also be attacks of fibrositis around nerves.

In all such cases an attempt should be made to find some specific cause in the form of an infection, errors of diet, or exposure, and control of this cause will bring about relief of the condition. In general the application of heat with massage is helpful. Firm massage causes a transitory increase in pain for a few hours after treatment, but definite improvement is likely to follow continued care.

People with fibrositis should certainly be protected against catching cold, against chilling, dampness, or sudden changes in temperature.

For fibrositis in which bursas are involved, it is customary to recommend treatment of the bursa by exposure to the X ray. In other instances it may be necessary to inject anesthetic substances directly into the area concerned.

Investigations indicate that small pieces of fat caught in fibrous tissue may be responsible for some of the symptoms of fibrositis.

FILARIASIS American soldiers and sailors in the tropics have become aware of the possibility of invasion of the human body by threadlike worms known as filaria. The female worm, getting into the human body, gives birth to embryos which migrate through the blood vessels and to the skin. Here they may be taken up by any of the blood-sucking flies that are frequent. Inside the fly these embryos migrate into the tissues, where they grow into larvae. These larvae grow further and eventually become motile and pass down the proboscis sheath of the fly or the nose, or combined nose and mouth, so that at the time of the fly's next meal of human blood they are introduced into the person who is bitten.

One form of filaria gets into the lymph vessels or lymphatic tissues, particularly in the groin, and blocks them. The result of this kind of filariasis is the condition called elephantiasis. This kind of filaria is carried particularly by mosquitoes.

It is an interesting fact about this form of filaria that they become active in the circulation typically between midnight and two o'clock in the morning, so that the doctor who is studying these cases examines the blood at that time. They are not seen during the daytime when the patient is active.

A specific method of treatment for this kind of filarial infection has not yet been found. To prevent the secondary infections, the sulfa drugs are used. For the control of elephantiasis, operative procedures are employed.

The prevention of filariasis involves the same kind of control that is used to prevent malaria, including the clearance of mosquito-breeding sites, the use of screening, and particularly the use of insect repellents such as the especially effective DDT repellent that is one of the great discoveries of recent years.

Another form of filaria is the loa loa worm, or eye worm, that is found in Africa. It has the propensity to wander across the front of the eye during its continual migrations through the tissues of the body. As it crawls, it has a raised serpentine track. Thus they are known to reach the temporal region, pass under the surface of one eye, across the bridge of the nose, then the surface of the other eye, and finally out to the other temple and down the neck. As the worm passes, it sets up swelling and irritation. This worm is carried particularly by a fly called the mango fly. The condition is controlled by picking the worm out with a sharp hooked needle when its track of migration is discovered.

FINGERNAILS Just why the human being still has fingernails is not clear in the story of the evolution of present-day man. Animals have more use for nails on their paws than do human beings on their hands and feet. An animal uses his nails to support the body in walking and in climbing and also for defense and attack. Since the invention of gunpowder, man has had little use for fingernails and toenails.

Some authorities believe that the human being continues to have fingernails and toenails as protection of the fingers and toes from harmful external agents and also as a protection to the sense of touch.

Fingernails and toenails are composed of keratin, which is an albuminoid substance containing sulfur. The nails also contain some cholesterin, which is the substance that helps to keep them elastic. There are tiny amounts of calcium phosphate, carbonates, and arsenic, and about 14 per cent water.

Fingernails grow faster in children than in adults. Fingernails grow faster than toenails. The fingernail will grow about 3 millimeters (.12 of an inch) per month. Nails grow faster in summer than in winter. The nail of the middle finger grows more rapidly than the rest of the nails, and the nail on the little finger grows the slowest. The nails on the right side of a right-handed person grow faster than on the left; and of a left-handed person on the left side.

Since the development of manicuring and pedicuring, the care of the fingernails and toenails has been given much more attention than was formerly the custom. Nowadays people look at the hands to see if they are properly cared for. When dirt accumulates under the nails so that the hands seem to be in mourning with a black border, people believe that the person concerned is careless.

For most boys and men, the daily use of a handbrush to cleanse the skin under the nails is desirable, also the use of an orangewood stick for cleansing after washing, and a weekly filing or trimming to keep the nails reasonably short.

Young women are likely to give their fingernails much more attention. They scrub the hands and nails, push back the cuticle, and file the nails at least once each week. Quite recently custom has seemed to indicate the use of polish of a bright color. Nail polish must be renewed frequently, particularly when it chips or cracks.

Any slight injury that separates the skin from the fingernails will permit germs to get into the broken skin and set up a secondary infection. Such infections are associated with painful throbbing and swelling. Finally yellow pus will appear. The swelling may need to be opened so that the infectious material is released. However, the infection may become more severe and spread by way of the lymph channels up the hands and arms. Thorough cleaning with soap and water and the application of any of the mild antiseptics will effect a cure in most cases. In severe cases when the "run-around" spreads to the point where it involves both sides and base of

the fingernail, it may be necessary for the surgeon to cut into the area and permit the infected material to escape.

Brittle fingernails are a constant annoyance to many people. It is not a sign of any infection but is most frequently seen when there are chronic diseases of the body affecting the glands, the heart, or the blood vessels. Improper circulation to the nail plate will produce brittleness of the nails. A shortage of iron in the diet is frequently associated with disturbance of the growth of the nails.

Cutting the toenails with a clipper is preferable to either a curved or straight scissors. With the clipper it is possible to remove the exact amount of tissue required. This also prevents the leaving of a roughened edge.

FISH Most people believe that a diet of fish is not really so valuable for building human health as the meat of animals. However, many nations subsist almost wholly on fish and do very well at it. Among people of low income herring is a frequent article of diet and provides good food at low cost.

The flesh of most of the fish commonly used in the diet, such as halibut, cod, whitefish, salmon, trout, pickerel, and perch, will average from 15 to 18 per cent protein, as contrasted with approximately 21 per cent protein for mutton, beefsteak, and pork.

The flesh of fish generally contains protein, fat, mineral salts, particularly iodine and phosphorus, and vitamins. Most of the fat in the flesh of the fish is stored in the liver, except for the salmon, mackerel, sardines, and herrings, which have from 10 to 15 per cent in the flesh generally.

Whitefish generally is more easily and rapidly digested than most meats. Meats that are rich in fats are digested with greater difficulty than those that have less fat.

The flesh of fish is also particularly valuable as a source of vitamin A, which is associated with growth and general increase in resistance to disease; and with vitamin D, which is important in the relationship to the use of calcium and phosphorus by the body.

Cod-liver oil and other fish-liver oils, notably the halibut and salmon oils, are rich in vitamins A and D. Moreover, the roe of fish also contains vitamins B and E. Careful studies have been made as to the vitamin content of various edible parts of the fish. These indicate that oysters give the most complete vitamin value, followed by salmon and herring as good seconds.

As contrasted with meat, fish has more waste including bones, skin, head, and similar parts. Fish has a high water content and lacks frequently in flavor so that sauces must be added. In lean fish the calories are low. While fish supplies much phosphorus, it lacks calcium.

FISTULA A fistula is a passage that leads from the surface of the body into some cavity or organ beneath the surface. Fistulas are extremely frequent near the anus or rectum. They are sometimes treated by the use of caustic substances which cause the passage to disappear. When they are more severe, it is customary to remove the fistula with surgery.

FLAT FOOT See article on *Feet*.

FLATULENCE (See *Aerophagia; Swallowing Air* under *Child Care;* also *Constipation, Colitis,* et cetera.) Distention of the stomach or intestines with air or gas.

FOOD POISONING (See also *Botulism* and *Dysentery*) Whenever illness follows the taking of any food or drink and is definitely related to the content of the substance taken, the condition is called food poisoning. The expression "ptomaine poisoning" used to be used for this condition because it was thought that bacteria acting on food produced poisons called ptomaines. Now it is known that this view was wrong, and "ptomaine poisoning" is no longer used for food poisoning.

Obviously food may sometimes contain actual poisons like arsenic or lead. This happened once when a banquet was given in Chicago and a cook poisoned the soup, so that three hundred people became ill. Food poisoning may result from the presence of poisonous plants, such as the hemlock or deadly nightshade. Occasionally poisonous parasites get into food.

However, the commonest form of food poisoning is that due to invasion of food by bacteria like the staphylococci or the *Salmonella* organisms. Bacteria may produce poisons or may be poisonous in themselves. They gain access to human food and drink either from animals which suffer with infections or from the excretions from animals which may contaminate human food or from conditions arising in other human beings.

The staphylococci may get into food from any infected wound. One of the most serious outbreaks that ever occurred resulted from an infection of a finger in a boy who was helper to a baker. The boy was squeezing cream from a bag into cream puffs, and the material from the infected finger got into the cream. Incidentally, such creams and custards form an excellent medium in which the germs may grow and develop their poisons. In addition to creams and custards, the foods most frequently affected are preserved meat and fish.

When a person has food poisoning, he suddenly develops abdominal pain, nausea, vomiting, and diarrhea anywhere from four to thirty hours after having eaten. Along with these symptoms come headache, cold sweats, shivering, and occasionally double vision. There may often be prostration or collapse. If death results, it is usually from the shock or from the great loss of water and salt associated with the vomiting and diarrhea. There are, however, outbreaks of severe food poisoning by *Salmonella* in which the death rate has been as high as one tenth of those affected; these are exceptonal. The death rate is seldom more than 1 per cent.

The treatment given by the physician is aimed to remove the infectious material from the stomach and intestines as soon as possible and to overcome the dehydration by giving water, the salt starvation by giving salt, and the exhaustion by the treatment usually used by physicians to support the heart and blood pressure.

FOOD SENSITIVITY See *Allergy*.

FOREIGN BODIES (See also *Nose, Ear*, et cetera) Any strange substance that does not belong in the human body but gets in and stays there for a length of time is known as a foreign body. All sorts of substances can get into the body accidentally or purposely. Children are always swallowing substances that should not be swallowed, and poking them into the nose or ear. Sometimes adults push foreign substances into the openings of the body, such as the genitals or the rectum.

Needles, nails, toothpicks, bullets, shell fragments, and pieces of glass have been found in the heart. Out of 109 cases which one doctor collected, needles were present in 18 and bullets and shrapnel in 85. A nine-months-old girl swallowed a piece of wire with some food because her mother used an old wire strainer for sieving vegetables. She had noticed that several small pieces broke off but she continued to use it. Eventually it was found by the use of the X ray that the child had a piece of the wire in the heart. Still later this passed out of the body. Two years after the X ray showed the wire to be in the heart, the child suddenly coughed up an old blood clot in which was a piece of corroded wire. The X ray was used again and showed that the wire had passed out of the heart.

Surgeons group foreign bodies found in the gastrointestinal tract or elsewhere in the body as hardware, jewelry, pins, seeds, bones, buttons, dental and surgical objects, ammunition, toys, or coins. All sorts of means have been developed for retrieving such bodies. Magnets are used to retrieve steel or iron foreign bodies. Tubes have been invented that can be passed down the throat or into other openings and are thus available for reaching into the farthest corners of the esophagus, the windpipe, the bronchial tubes, and even into the lungs.

When foreign substances get into the nose, more harm is usually done by attempting to dislodge them with improper instruments than by letting them alone until a doctor can be called. If blowing the nose will not remove a foreign substance, sneezing will usually accomplish this. The doctor usually washes out foreign substances or removes them with special forceps.

The toothpick is almost wholly an American institution. There are many cases on record, however, in which people chew toothpicks and swallow portions, subsequently requiring a surgical operation for their removal.

Most important in detecting a foreign body in any portion of the body is the X ray. By the use of the X ray all kinds of materials have been found in the stomach and in the intestines, including hair balls, collections of seeds, or pieces of glass.

A foreign body in the ear is best removed by turning the head to one side and filling the ear with warm oil by means of a spoon. This will help to float the body out of the ear. If an insect is in the ear, the warm oil will suffocate the insect and permit it to float out. After the use of the warm oil, the ear can be syringed with warm water. The water is sprayed against the side of the entrance to the ear rather than against the eardrum. No one should ever attempt to remove a foreign body from the eye or the ear or the nose or any portion of the body without being certain what he is doing and that he is likely to do more good than harm.

FORMALDEHYDE Formaldehyde is a germicidal solution with a pungent odor. It is powerful against germs but is also damaging to human tissues. Weak solutions are sometimes applied to the skin to prevent excessive sweating.

FRACTURES The breaking of a bone is usually called a fracture. There are innumerable types of fractures, depending on the bone that is involved and the way in which the fracture appears when examined by the X ray. Certain fractures are associated with certain occupations or with special types of accident. For instance march fracture occurs particularly to men in the military service. It is a fracture of the small bones of the foot associated with long marches. A chauffeur's fracture is one which used to be quite frequent. It was a fracture of the small bones of the wrist or of the arm due to sudden and violent reversing of the starting crank of an automobile engine during the cranking process. A greenstick fracture is one in which one side of a bone is broken and the other bent. This was also frequently called a hickory-stick fracture. Whenever the bone is splintered or crushed, the condition is known as a comminuted fracture. Whenever the fractured bone penetrates through the skin, the condition is called a compound fracture. This has also been called an open fracture.

FRECKLES People who are sensitive about their appearance seem to worry more about changes in the color or pigmentation of the skin than about other serious conditions affecting the body as a whole.

Among the most frequent changes in the pigmentation of the skin are freckles, liver spots, colorless spots or vitiligo, and pigmented areas produced by powder marks, silver deposits, or similar foreign substances.

About freckles there are many notions and beliefs. Some people think that freckles will disappear if rubbed with dew that is on clover, if bathed with buttermilk, or if rubbed with grass, grapevine sap, or lemon juice, with melon rind or water from an oak stump. This rubbing notion includes also use of the excretions of human beings, cows, horses, and other animals found on the farm. None of these procedures will cure freckles. The belief is dependent on the idea of magic by transference or substitution.

Freckles are merely pigmented spots on the skin; usually more likely to be present in the spring and summer than in the winter. They represent a reaction of the skin to the sun and will not appear if the skin is protected from the sun.

Recently ointments have become available which may be rubbed on the skin to keep away the ultraviolet rays of the sun. In such cases the freckles will not appear.

Freckles are sometimes removed by using substances on the skin that will peel off the superficial layers. All of these substances are dangerous because they contain poisons and because they may produce such serious irritation of the skin that the irritation will be much worse than the freckles. There are also ointments of the same color as the skin which can be used to conceal freckles.

FROSTBITE Whenever the temperature of the air falls below 8 degrees, frostbite menaces health. If the temperature is above 8 degrees, reaching as high as 15 degrees, frostbite occurs only when there is a strong wind. Frostbite seldom occurs with a temperature of from 20 to 30 degrees, no matter how strong the wind may be.

Modern aviation demands that aviators fly at heights above 20,000 or 30,000 feet, where the temperature may fall to 25 or 30 degrees below zero. Aviators have been known to suffer seriously with freezing or frostbite in the short time necessary to come down from a height with a parachute. Hence modern aviation provides the flier with proper clothing to be worn not only at high altitudes when flying but also when coming down with a parachute.

The first sign of the danger of frostbite is contraction of the blood vessels in the skin so that it becomes pale. If the skin is warmed immediately, the color returns. If, however, the frostbite has been exceedingly severe, the blood will not come back to the skin, and it will remain white even after it has been warmed. Gradually the blood will be able to seep back into the tissues; however, they now appear purplish or black. After twenty-four to forty-eight hours the fluid in the skin comes through the lower layers, and then the blisters that are characteristic of frostbite appear.

For the prevention of frostbite the following suggestions have been made:

1. Outdoor work should be postponed when the temperature is below 8 degrees, particularly when there is a strong wind.

2. Clothing, shoes, socks, and gloves should be well fitted. Particularly they should not be too tight, because tight clothing encourages restriction of the circulation and frostbite.

People who are compelled to be outdoors in cold weather should not stay out longer than two hours at a time and should have intervening rest periods of at least one half hour between the two-hour work periods. People with diabetes or any disease of the heart or circulation are more likely to suffer serious damage from frostbite than those who are in good physical condition.

The blisters that occur in frostbite are treated by protection with ointments after they have been opened. They are then covered with a dry dressing that has been sterilized so as to be free from germs. After the first damage has occurred, circulation of the blood in the frostbitten area may be encouraged by the use of mild warmth.

After freezing, there is nothing to be gained by rubbing the frozen part with snow or ice. The parts affected may be massaged very gently for a few minutes to encourage the circulation and then wrapped in several layers of wool. If the warming is too sudden or too vigorous, the return of the extra blood to the part may produce severe pain; then cold may be necessary to cause the blood to withdraw from the frozen area.

In exceedingly serious cases of freezing, tissues may be so damaged that the circulation of the blood cannot return to normal. The result is gangrene, so that in some cases it becomes necessary to amputate fingers or even an entire limb.

FURUNCLE The word "furuncle" is another name for a boil (which see).

GALL BLADDER The gall bladder is a pear-shaped sac usually located on the lower side of the liver. From this sac go tubes which carry the bile from the gall bladder to the intestines. There is also a tube coming from the liver into the gall bladder which brings the bile from the liver to the gall bladder. The function of the gall bladder is to store and concentrate the bile so that it will be ready to aid in digestion.

When anything occurs to block the tubes that carry the bile, symptoms of obstruction occur. The gall bladder may also become infected like any other organ of the body. One of the most frequent disturbances is the occurrence of gallstones. It has been estimated that from 5 to 10 per cent of all adults have gallstones and that women have them about five times as often as men. The woman who is subject to gall-bladder attacks and gallstones is usually said to be the one who is fair, fat, and forty.

No one knows exactly why gallstones form, but they probably result from blocking of the flow of the bile from infections and from changes in digestion. Whereas gallstones may not cause symptoms in a considerable number of cases, the sudden stopping of the passing of the bile resulting from the blocking of a gall duct by a gallstone brings on an attack of gallstone colic. Such an attack may come in the midst of excellent health. There is a severe pain which comes on often just as the person is going to bed. It lasts for a few hours, then passes, and may not occur again for months or years. The great danger is that the blocking may on occasion be persistent. Repeated attacks leave a sense of constant fullness in the stomach, pains under the ribs, especially after eating fatty foods, pains in the upper part of the back, and attacks of flatulence. When infection and inflammation of the gall bladder follow blocking of the flow of bile, the situation is much more serious. This is called cholecystitis. It is accompanied with severe pain and rigidity of the upper part of the abdomen on the right side, there may be some jaundice, and the tongue is coated. There may also be some fever. Gas forms, and there is distention of the abdomen.

Severe attacks demand surgical operation with removal of the gall bladder, preferably carried out in a period between attacks. If, however, an acute infection of the gall bladder goes on to repeated vomiting and increased tenderness, with a rapid pulse and signs of toxemia or poisoning, it may be necessary to operate immediately. The decision is one of the most difficult that the surgeon may have to make.

CHRONIC INFLAMMATION—When a gall bladder is constantly infected, associated with the presence of stones and swelling of the gall ducts, symptoms are practically constant. In most cases these symptoms are like those of chronic indigestion.

When a gall bladder is infected, there is a tendency for the formation of many gallstones. For the detection of gallstones, medicine has developed a special technic which represents one of the greatest advances of medical science. A substance called iodophthalein has been discovered which, when taken into the body either by mouth or by injection into the veins, goes to the liver and is passed with the bile into the gall bladder. Then an X-ray picture is taken; the presence of the iodophthalein permits the gall bladder to be seen in the X-ray picture. If there is no sign of the gall bladder in the X-ray picture, the doctor knows that the bile duct which carries the bile from the liver to the gall bladder is blocked. If, however, the bile has passed into the gall bladder, stones will be seen in most instances if they are present; also an outline of the gall bladder will be visible. Subsequent pictures can be taken so that the doctor can determine the extent to which the gall bladder empties itself and the time

required for that purpose. There are some gallstones which are visible in the X-ray film even without making the dye test. Such stones represent in most cases materials like calcium bicarbonate, which will give a dense shadow. The majority of gallstones consist, however, of a substance called cholesterol and do not give a shadow with an ordinary X-ray film.

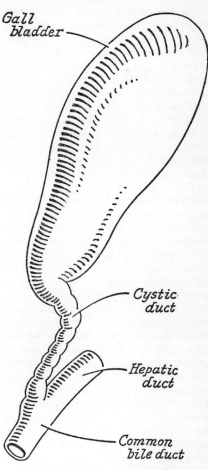

Anatomy of the gall bladder

When there is chronic infection of the gall bladder, the sense of fullness comes on usually after eating and is worse when greasy and fatty foods are eaten. Associated with this sense of fullness, there may be below the right margin of the ribs a dull aching pain which is aggravated on stooping or bending over. Heartburn is quite common in these conditions; in many cases the doctor finds, when he examines the secretions of the stomach, that an extra amount of acid is present.

A person may go along with a chronic infection of the gall bladder for a long time without ever showing signs of jaundice. There are, however, cases in which blocking of the flow of the bile may produce much jaundice. Indeed an infection of the gall bladder may produce such a variety of symptoms, like a sense of tightness in the chest, palpitation of the heart and breathlessness, as to cause the person affected to concentrate most of the attention on organs other than the gall bladder. For that very reason the presence of such symptoms is an indication that a careful examination by a competent doctor is necessary and that such an examination should include all of the modern technics, like X-ray study, which will prove with certainty whether or not a chronic infection of the gall bladder is present. Once the condition is determined, the doctor will have to decide what is to be done.

While it is true that people can live for years in rather good health with a chronic inflammation in the wall of the gall bladder, particularly if they will avoid eating large meals and avoid also heavy and fatty foods, the threat of a serious complication is always present. The gall bladder lies close to other important organs in the abdomen which may get infected from the gall bladder. There may be a sudden blocking with the serious symptoms that have been described. Occasionally also there are more serious complications.

The operation on the gall bladder is a fairly serious one, but when performed by experts it leads to recovery in the vast majority of cases. Usually after the gall bladder has been removed, most of the symptoms promptly disappear, although it is desirable for the diet to be carefully controlled for some months thereafter.

GANGRENE When the blood supply to any part of the body is stopped, the tissues die—sometimes becoming infected in the process. Gangrene may, for instance, be due to obstruction of the blood supply by inflammations of the blood vessels, occasionally by damage done by solutions that are too caustic. Gangrene has also followed too long an application of a tourniquet. Certain organisms produce gangrene as a secondary effect. This, for instance, is the result of infection of a wound with some of the germs that cause gas gangrene. Very old people sometimes develop gangrene, particularly of the toes, because of interference with the blood supply. This happens also to people with diabetes.

Gas Gangrene—Several different types of germs may invade injured tissues of the human body and cause gas gangrene. When these germs act on the tissue, they produce gas because they contain ferments which break up sugars in the tissues. This gas tends to spread through the muscles, so that when the tissues are touched there is a crackling sound.

The appearance is like that of an angry inflammation; indeed, it has been called the "red death." Later, as the damage continues, the color of the tissue changes to yellow, and toward the end the muscles become black and soft like fluid.

No one knows exactly why gas gangrene goes on rapidly in some cases and not in others. Apparently much depends on the extent to which the tissue has been damaged and the blood supply injured.

Gas gangrene can be prevented in wounds, particularly those due to missiles which have carried bits of clothing or soil into the wound, if the surgeon promptly opens the wound, cleans it, and drains it. During World War I, when the incidence of gas gangrene became common, a technic called débridement was developed. War wounds were treated by removal of all of the damaged tissue from the body. During the civil war in Spain gas gangrene came to be one of the most feared of all the menaces to the soldier.

Fortunately in World War II the condition was not so threatening as previously because of new developments in medical science. One of these involves the use of a serum against gas gangrene which can be injected into any patient in whom there is the possibility that this condition may develop. Drug manufacturers are providing more than a million doses of this serum. The new drugs of the sulfonamide type, including sulfanilamide, sulfathiazole, and sulfadiazine, have special virtues in the control of gas gangrene. British surgeons who have had extended experience recommend immediate administration of a dose of antitoxin which contains the substances that are specific against three different types of germs associated with gas gangrene. The patient is given a large dose of the sulfonamide drug that is chosen, and this medication is continued and repeated as needed, so that the level of the drug in the blood is kept constant.

The patient with gas gangrene is taken as soon as possible to a hospital, where he is supplied with all that modern medicine offers for giving him resistance, including blood transfusions and similar supportive measures. If, however, the gas gangrene under all of this treatment does not yield, amputation of a limb may be necessary. Under these circumstances the surgeon does not hesitate to amputate in order to save life.

GAS POISONING See *Carbon Monoxide Poisoning.*

GASTRIC The Greek word "gastro" means stomach. There are in medicine a great many words which begin with "gastro" and which relate to medical conditions affecting the stomach. Thus gastritis is an inflammation of the stomach; gastroenteritis is an inflammation of the stomach and the intestines; gastrectomy is the cutting out or removal of all or a part of the stomach; gastroscope is a device for looking inside the stomach.

GASTRIC ULCER See discussion under *Stomach Ulcers.*

GASTRITIS The stomach, like any other organ of the body, may become infected and inflamed. An inflammation of the stomach is called gastritis. The germs which infect other organs of the body may also infect the stomach.

When the wall of the stomach is infected, it becomes, as do other tissues of the body, red and swollen; if the infection is sufficiently severe, hemorrhages into the wall may occur. The lining of the stomach may also become seriously inflamed following the taking of irritating substances or poisons which have a caustic action on the lining of the stomach. Alcohol, taken in excess, will produce a severe irritation followed by inflammation. Coarse foods, if sufficiently coarse and taken in excess, can inflame the lining of the stomach. Some people are much more sensitive to such irritants than are others. Poisons like iodine, carbolic acid, or strong mustard can also produce an inflammation and irritation.

In the absence of certain vitamins from the diet, the tendency to irritation and inflammation is much greater. Occasionally also there may be disorders of the secretion of the gastric juice, the digestive fluid that comes from the wall of the stomach. Associated with such disturbances, inflammations may occur.

One of the new inventions in medicine in recent years is a device called the gastroscope, a tube through which it is possible to see the lining of the stomach with reflected light and indeed also to photograph it. The use of this device has done a great deal to make clear the nature of gastritis.

Following an inflammation of the stomach, there may be repeated swelling and overgrowth of the tissue. There may also be areas in which the lining cells are lost, leaving irritated or dead patches. When there is an ulcer in the wall of the stomach, there is obviously inflammation and gastritis around the ulcer. Some investigators believe that there is always inflammation and swelling before the formation of an ulcer. Regardless of the way in which the ulcer is formed, inflammation is a definite part of the development.

As in inflammation elsewhere in the body, an infection and an inflammation of the wall of the stomach are likely to be associated with pain, tenderness, and vomiting. Examination of the material that comes from the stomach enables the doctor to determine in many instances the nature of the inflammation and its severity.

If the inflammation is due to some irritant substance recently taken, elimination of that substance and carefulness in the taking of food and other materials usually results in relief. The difficult case is the one in which the irritation goes on constantly, producing irritation called chronic gastritis. There are so many different conditions that may produce repeated irritations of the stomach that the most careful type of investigation that the doctor can make is demanded. Moreover, the treatment of chronic gastritis requires control over the patient for a long time. The doctor usually suggests that small meals of easily digested food be given at fairly frequent intervals rather than large meals at any time. There are many drugs which the doctor can prescribe which serve to overcome excess acidity. Certainly he will recommend the avoidance of such irritating substances as alcohol, mustard, pepper, vinegar, spices, and other irritants. The excessive use of tobacco has also been known to be associated with chronic inflammation of the stomach.

Since the material developed by the stomach is definitely needed for the proper growth of red blood cells, the doctor will have to determine whether or not anemia has occurred, so that actually the study of gastritis becomes a study of the whole constitution and health of the person affected.

GASTROPTOSIS Whenever the stomach is displaced downward as shown by an X-ray picture, the condition is called gastroptosis, meaning simply "dropping of the stomach."

GELATIN Gelatin is a colorless, transparent substance which is hard when dried but jellylike when moistened. It is mostly protein derived from various animal tissues such as the skin, the ligaments, and the bones. Most of the gelatin used as desserts is artificially sweetened with sugar. Pure gelatin does not have a sweet taste. Gelatin is not a complete protein, since it lacks some of the ten protein substances considered to be essential for life and growth.

GENIUS Persons who achieve distinction in life usually reveal in childhood some signs in their behavior that they are of unusually high intelligence or that they are possessed of special mental qualities.

Psychologists at Stanford University who studied the records of three hundred eminent men and women of history to determine the factors that make for success concluded that those who achieve eminence are characterized not only by high intellectual traits but also by persistence of motive and effort, confidence in their abilities, and great strength or force of character. A genius usually appears in a superior family, in which he has superior possibilities for education and other inspirational factors in his environment.

Milton had written an ode pronounced by an eminent critic as perhaps the most beautiful in the English language before he was twenty-one years old. Raphael had painted the Gran Duca Madonna at twenty-one, Beethoven was appointed chamber musician to the king at eighteen, Bacon wrote a book on philosophy before he was twenty, and Jenner thought out the processes that led to the development of vaccination even before he was twenty years old.

Conceivably the Quiz Kids of today have in them the spark of genius.

John Stuart Mill, famous as a philosopher and economist, began to learn Greek at three, was reading Plato at seven, and by the age of nine had mastered conic sections. Goethe had an intelligence quotient of around 180, so that at five years of age he was as far advanced as the average child of ten. When he was twelve years old, he amused himself by planning and sketching out a novel in seven languages. The poet Coleridge could read a chapter from the Bible at the age of three.

Frequently the question is asked as to whether or not certain diseases stimulate those who suffer from them to extraordinary mental or physical activity. Sir Walter Scott early in childhood had infantile paralysis; Lord Byron was crippled, as was Steinmetz, one of America's greatest inventors. Such great authors as Robert Louis Stevenson, John Addington Symonds, and John Keats had serious tuberculosis, as did also Aubrey Beardsley, the artist, the writer De Quincey, and John Ruskin, the author. Often it has been said that the stimulus of starvation is needed to bring out the most in genius. We know today, however, that great ability thrives in cultured atmosphere. While hardship and resistance may stimulate intensive effort, the capacity must be present or genius will never appear.

GERIATRICS A great increase in our population of aged people has developed a new specialty in medicine called geriatrics—a word that is made from two Greek words meaning "old age" and "the doctor." In 1890 less than 3 per cent of the people in the United States were over sixty-five years of age. In 1953 about 10 per cent were over sixty-five years of age. It is predicted that by 1970 more than 20 per cent will be over sixty-five years of age. The problem relating to the care of the aged is, therefore, so important as to make a new specialty for medical practice.

GERMICIDES Any substance that kills germs is a germicide. Germicides are different from antiseptics, which destroy any poisonous materials, not necessarily only germs.

GIANTISM See *Acromegaly.*

GINGIVITIS Any inflammation of the gums is called gingivitis. Pyorrhea is a form of gingivitis, also the common condition called Vincent's disease, or trench mouth.

GLANDERS Occasionally there is transmitted to man from horses, mules, or donkeys a germ—known by a highly technical name—which gives rise to the disease called glanders. When horses were the common mode of transportation and traction, glanders was much more frequent than now. Since the coming of the motorcar, the disease has practically disappeared.

In the United States and Canada glanders was fairly frequent until 1905. During World War I, Germany destroyed almost 6000 horses and at least 21,000 were slaughtered in France because of this disease.

Occasionally human beings who carry glanders have been found. It is known that the discharges from the infected mucous membranes or the skin and the mucus that comes from the nose and throat of the person with this disease may carry the infecting germ.

In the United States only one case of glanders was recorded in the month of July 1939, but the Bureau of Census reports one or two deaths from this cause each year. Mostly glanders affects people like grooms, coachmen, veterinary surgeons, soldiers, and farmers, who are in rather frequent contact with the equine species.

In the attack on this disease medicine has discovered a test which is like the Wassermann test and which can determine the existence of glanders.

When the condition first appears, from a few hours to a few weeks after the germ has gained entrance to the body, there is a high fever, vomiting, diarrhea, swelling of the spot where the germs are located, and the rapid appearance of large ulcers and abscesses of the lymph glands. These appear first as nodules under the skin and are called farcy buds. The disease is sometimes called farcy. Occasionally the condition becomes chronic and will gradually involve the joints and bones and various portions of the body, producing continuous fever and emaciation.

Few cases of acute glanders ever recover, but the curability of chronic glanders is recognized.

There has not yet been opportunity to test the value against this disease of some of the modern remedies like the sulfonamide drugs and penicillin. However, it is quite likely that these will be tried, if cases of glanders come to light, because of the known seriousness of this type of infection.

Whenever glanders is diagnosed, the person affected is isolated from all others. Any discharges that come from the body are received on materials that can be burned. Usually the abscesses are opened and the infected tissues removed.

Because of the great danger of this disease, its spread is controlled by the destruction of animals that are found to be infected, as is done also in the case of hoof and mouth disease.

GLANDS (See also *Pituitary, Thyroid, Goiter, Addison's Disease, Thymus, Pineal,* et cetera) The internal glandular system of the human body develops substances which are secreted into the blood and serve to control the actions of various organs. They initiate the functions associated with childbirth. They determine the rate and character of the body's growth.

Other glands which secrete materials elsewhere than into the blood are concerned with digestion and sex activities. The glands of external secretion include the liver, the pancreas, the salivary glands, and the sex organs. Moreover, some of these organs also manufacture materials which go directly into the blood as internal secretions. The glands which secrete internal secretions exclusively include the thymus, the pineal gland, the thyroid and parathyroid glands, the pituitary, the suprarenal glands, and the sex glands.

A gland is any portion of the body that develops a secretion. The breasts,

for example, secrete milk; the salivary glands secrete saliva, which moistens the mouth and contains ferments which help to digest starches. The stomach secretes hydrochloric acid and pepsin, and these help digestion. The pancreas secretes both an internal secretion known as insulin, which is concerned with the control of sugars, and an external secretion known as trypsin, which is concerned with the digestion of proteins. These external secretions are involved in many functions.

The internal secretions which go directly into the blood act frequently at points in the body remote from the gland by which they are secreted. Indeed the glands of internal secretion have been considered to be an interlocking chain which governs all of the actions of the human organism. Overgrowth of some of the glands may result in the appearance of giants; underactivity by these glands results in the development of dwarfs. Changes in the sex glands may make women look like men or men look like women. Some charlatans have claimed that the glands regulate our personalities. Others have capitalized on public interest by stating that injections of various glandular substances will bring about youthfulness.

The life of the human being may be divided into three well-defined periods: the first, from birth to maturity; the second, up to the time when degeneration of the tissues begins; and the third, from the end of most human activity through the time of senescence and old age up to death. The glandular mechanism of mankind varies in its activity during these periods. Unquestionably in the first period—that of growth up to maturity—the glands which control growth are of the greatest importance. During the time of maturity other glands exercise their functions. In the period of old age the glands begin to break down and degenerate and discontinue their activities.

GLAUCOMA See discussion under *Eye.*

GLEET Chronic gonorrhea used to be called gleet. Modern treatment of gonorrhea with the sulfa drugs and with penicillin is likely to make chronic gonorrhea a rather rare disease. Indeed few cases are seen now by the physicians who specialize in such conditions.

GLIOMA Tumors of nervous tissue are called gliomas. Glioma is also applied to a cancer of the brain. The treatment of gliomas is by the X ray or by surgical operation.

GLUCOSE Another term for dextrose.

GOITER Goiter is the term applied to an enlargement of the thyroid gland, which lies in the neck. The thyroid gland has two lobes and a little connecting portion which crosses the windpipe. Inside the thyroid gland are little spaces containing a yellow material called colloid. This colloid contains iodine. The normal human body of 150 pounds contains about 1/10th of a gram, which is about 1/4000th of a pound of iodine. Most of the iodine in the human body comes in by way of eggs, milk, bread, wine, shellfish, and salt containing iodine. The iodine is deposited in the thyroid gland.

There are several different kinds of goiters, classified according to the nature of the growth and its activities. The ordinary goiter is a simple enlargement of the gland which starts just after the age of adolescence begins. This type of goiter is especially common in certain areas of the world where there is a deficiency of iodine in the water and the food. Studies have shown that goiters may affect as many as half the people in parts of our country where the water and local vegetables contain little iodine. Indeed, it may also affect the animals in such areas. Near the seacoast, where there is some iodine in the water and the plants, goiter is rather uncommon.

Since it has been shown that this enlargement of the neck in growing girls and boys is definitely associated with a deficiency of iodine, it has been customary to prevent the condition by giving iodine to growing boys and girls—especially to girls—since this kind of goiter is about five times more common in women than in men.

Incidentally it has also become necessary to give the iodine to pregnant women so as to prevent the occurrence of changes in the thyroid gland in the children.

In the prevention of simple goiter iodine may be added to the drinking water or to the table salt in the proportion of 10 milligrams of potassium iodide for each 1000 grams of table salt. This is not, of course, a large amount of iodine. Iodine can also be obtained in the form of tablets in this dosage. Doctors prescribe iodine in various forms which can be used for this purpose.

If the enlargement of the gland is so great as to produce deformity, it is customary to remove the gland by surgical operation, even though it does not produce the serious symptoms associated with excessive activity of the thyroid gland in the conditions called hyperthyroidism and exophthalmic goiter.

EXOPHTHALMIC GOITER—When the thyroid gland enlarges and its activity becomes excessive, an abnormal amount of the secretion of the thyroid gland gets into the body. This secretion is an active substance called thyroxine.

Exophthalmic goiter occurs most frequently among young adults in cities where life is strenuous. Women are affected much oftener than men.

Apparently nerve strain occurs with the development of excess activity of the thyroid gland. An overdosage of the extract of the thyroid gland can produce symptoms much like those of exophthalmic goiter. Moreover, a complete removal of the gland can cause symptoms which are due to an absence of thyroid material, producing another condition called myxedema.

When a person has exophthalmic goiter, he suffers with symptoms which include a rapid heart rate, an increase in the rate of chemical changes going on in the body as measured by the basal metabolism, nervous irritability, and occasionally bulging of the eyes. The nervousness, excitability, and loss of weight are often associated with abnormal fatigue. However, even though the person concerned is tired and weak, the drive due to the excessive action of the thyroid gland makes the condition worse. Associated with this excess activity may be an increased appetite, a sense of warmth, and an increase in perspiration. Occasionally the condition may proceed to the point where the hands tremble. Whereas the normal basal metabolism rate is anywhere from plus 7 to minus 7, it may increase with excessive action of the thyroid gland to plus 15 or even to plus 30 or beyond. With this increase the heart rate may become rapid and, indeed, be seriously damaged by being pushed far beyond its ability to work.

In testing for the presence of excessive action of the thyroid gland, the doctor is likely to put the person to bed and carefully watch the basal metabolism and the pulse rate. Under these conditions the giving of extra iodine sometimes helps to slow the heart rate and to improve the symptoms. However, while the iodine is useful as a test, it is not the complete treatment and should never be taken by a person without proper advice of the doctor and the understanding that it be discontinued as directed.

The most important part of treatment is physical and mental rest. Permanent treatment involves removal of the excess glandular material by surgical operation. Operations on the thyroid gland are not particularly dangerous provided the patient is in good condition when the operation is performed. The purpose of the rest in bed for several weeks before operation is to make certain that the patient will be in good condition.

Recently it has been found that certain drugs, known as thiocyanates, have a definite effect in lowering the blood pressure and also in inhibiting the action of the thyroid gland. A drug known as thiouracil has also been found which can control the serious symptoms of excessive action of the thyroid.

When the surgeon operates on the patient, he and the doctor determine the proper care of the patient in order to get him in suitable condition for the operation. At the time of the operation the surgeon determines how much of the thyroid gland is to be removed in order to give an effective result. Following the operation on the gland, it is sometimes necessary to give extra thyroid material until the patient's body can adjust itself to new levels.

Occasionally the thyroid gland, like other tissues of the human body, may become subject to tumor growth. When this occurs, the extra material secreted by the tumor cells may also bring about symptoms like those of hyperthyroidism, or excessive action of the thyroid gland.

A new technic for controlling excessive action of the thyroid involves injection of radioactive iodine which goes directly to the thyroid and diminishes activity of its cells. Cases of cancer of the thyroid have been reported cured by this method.

The range of radioactivity can be measured by the Geiger counter, guiding the doctor in determining the proper amount of the injection.

GONORRHEA Gonorrhea is a venereal disease brought about through an infection with a germ commonly known as the gonococcus and called by the scientists *Neisseria gonorrhoeae*. Usually people are infected with gonorrhea by sexual contact with those who have the disease. Occasionally children are infected by contact of the sexual portions of the body with the contaminated fingers of attendants, towels, baths, or other materials. Babies used to suffer frequently with gonorrhea affecting the eyes sustained at birth, but the modern technic for preventing this condition has been successful in controlling the danger in the vast majority of cases.

When a person becomes infected with the germ of gonorrhea, the symptoms appear in about three days, although occasionally as late as three weeks after exposure. The symptoms in the male are usually first a slight feeling of irritation and a slight amount of discharge from the sex organs but thereafter an increased amount of infection and an increased amount of discharge of infectious material.

Secondary to the original infection there may be damage to other portions of the sexual tract such as the sex glands, and to other parts of the body, including the bones, the eyes, the joints, the heart, or, indeed, any other portion of the body.

Textbooks about gonorrhea written in 1942 are, however, already out of date because of the new discoveries for the control of this disease developed in association with World War II. Formerly an infection with gonorrhea would incapacitate men for periods from a week to months. Nowadays proper use of the sulfonamide drugs under the direction of a physician, with the application occasionally of heat and other remedies that the doctor can prescribe, may bring about cure of the condition within one or two days. Indeed soldiers, when put to bed and properly treated, frequently recover in forty-eight hours. It has been found that some people develop resistance to the sulfonamide drugs—this number representing anywhere from 2 to 10 per cent of all of the cases. In these cases treatment with penicillin brings about a prompt cure in most instances.

Infection with the gonococcus in women has in the past been treated with much more difficulty than infection in men, the reason being that the nature of the construction of the body of the woman tended to make the organs of women who were attacked much more difficult to reach than those of the male body. Nowadays, again, the combination of the sulfonamide drugs and heat and the use of penicillin in the resistant cases has tended to make possible complete cure in a relatively short time. Indeed there is every reason to believe that the application of new methods of treatment will so decrease the incidence of this disease as perhaps to permit within the next score of years its complete elimination.

The great danger in the continued spread of this disease is the stupid idea that such conditions must never be written about or discussed. As a part of the war effort men were taught to undertake suitable preventive measures. Indeed in some of the camps the procedure was adopted of giving the men extra doses of the sulfonamide drugs even before they left the camp and underwent the possibility of exposure to infection with gonorrhea. Now, however, penicillin has practically replaced the sulfonamides for the prevention and treatment of gonorrhea.

GOUT Gout used to be called "the rich man's disease." Now we know that anybody can have gout. The chief manifestations of gout include an inflammation of the joints and the deposit in and around the joints of a substance known as sodium urate. This arises from the digestion of proteins. In gout the uric acid, which is one of the end products of digestion and which is ordinarily excreted from the body, accumulates in the blood. Then, by a combination with sodium or salt, the sodium urate is formed and deposited in the joints.

An English physician named Sydenham, who himself suffered with gout for thirty-four years, graphically described a typical attack:

The victim goes to bed and sleeps in good health. About two o'clock in the morning he is awakened by a severe pain in the great toe; more rarely in the heel, ankle or instep. This pain is like that of a dislocation, and yet the parts feel as if cold water were poured over them. Then follow chills and shivers, and a little fever. The pain, which was at first moderate, becomes more intense. With its intensity the chills and shivers increase. After a time this comes to its height, accommodating itself to the bones and ligaments of the tarsus and metatarsus. Now it is a violent stretching and tearing of the ligaments—now it is a gnawing pain and now a pressure and tightening. So exquisite and lively meanwhile is the feeling of the part affected, that it cannot bear the weight of bedclothes or the jar of a person walking in the room. The night is passed in torture, sleeplessness, turning of the part affected, and perpetual change of posture; the tossing about of the body being as incessant as the pain of the tortured joint, being worse as the fit comes on. Hence the vain effort, by change of posture, both in the body and the limb affected, to obtain an abatement of the pain. This comes on only towards the morning of the next day. . . . The patient has a sudden and slight respite, which he falsely attributes to the last change of position. A general perspiration is succeeded by sleep. He wakes freer from pain and finds the part recently swollen.

Gout has not disappeared. In one large clinic 5 per cent of all of the people who came with disturbances of the joints were found to have gout. Although this is largely a masculine disease, about 5 per cent of the patients are women.

The symptoms of gout usually come on at around thirty-five years of age but occasionally do not occur until people get to be sixty or seventy years old. The symptom of gout called podagra, or painful large toe, and the little accumulations known as tophi, which are found in the ear, are considered of great value in diagnosing the presence of gout. These tophi may occur, however, not only in the ear but elsewhere in the body. These little deposits are found in at least one half of all of the cases.

The doctor also has laboratory tests which can be performed to aid him in diagnosing the disease.

Incidentally the rheumatic symptoms associated with gout are often provoked by the overeating and overdrinking associated with birthdays, weddings, Thanksgiving, Passover, as well as conferences, conventions, lodge nights, and hunting and fishing trips. Excessive intake of purines, or protein substances, and of alcohol is not the cause of gout but the attempt of the body to handle these matters may produce the attack. Indeed the attacks are precipitated by all sorts of excesses such as long walks, motoring, bicycling, boating, golfing, or even mowing the lawn.

In the treatment of gout a substance called colchicine is known to have special value, also other drugs of the salicylate type. Modern treatment may use Cortisone, ACTH, or a new drug called butazolidin. All of these drugs, however, have side effects which are toxic and should be taken only as prescribed by the doctor. Much comfort is given by rest, warmth applied to the affected parts, and protection from the bed clothing by a cradle.

People with gout should also observe a diet which is low in fats and rather rich in sugars and in proteins that are free from the purine substances. These include milk, eggs, and cheese, and exclude liver, sweetbread, anchovies, beef kidneys, brains, meat extracts, and heavy gravies. The cereals, cheese, gelatin, fruits of all kinds, and most vegetables are relatively low in purine substances. Coffee and tea are permissible but, in general, all alcoholic drinks should be avoided.

GRANULOCYTOPENIA The formation of an excessive amount of white blood cells is exceedingly serious. Even more serious may be a sudden lessening of the number of white blood cells or their disappearance from the blood. The white blood cells are the chief line of defense of the human body against infection. A sudden lessening of their number or their disappearance from the blood may lead promptly to an overwhelming attack by dangerous germs, which may produce death in a day or occasionally even in a few hours.

In granulocytopenia the number of red blood cells is normal in amount, but the white blood cells may drop from 7500 per cubic millimeter to 1000, to 140, or even fewer per cubic millimeter of blood. Since the white blood cells in any event are much fewer in number than the red blood cells, the examination of one specimen after another may fail to yield the presence of even a few white blood cells.

The exact cause of this condition is not definitely known, although recently it has become apparent that reaction of the body to various drugs or sensitivity to certain toxic agents may result in this condition. Many cases have been reported after taking a drug called amidopyrine, also in association with various coal-tar remedies, and in some cases after the sulfonamide drugs.

Apparently the bone marrow of the body is attacked, so that it becomes unable to form the white blood cells in the usual manner. There are, moreover, cases in which the condition develops a cyclic character, so that at regular intervals the number of white blood cells tends to become less and then gradually increases.

The condition is still, fortunately, infrequent. Most of the cases seem to occur in women and rarely in children.

Because of the failure of the white blood cells to protect the body against infection, one of the first signs is a severe ulceration of the throat with destruction of the tissue of the gums and tonsils. Other portions of the body may be attacked, and infections of the kidneys, the heart, or even of the skin become apparent.

Because of the severe character of this condition, about 75 per cent of those affected die. In the remaining 25 per cent recovery occurs, usually, however, after a long time and with a great deal of careful treatment. This includes, above everything else, immediate rest in bed, the giving of fluids, cleaning of the infected areas, and the giving of antibiotics like penicillin and terramycin which have the power to control infection, which develops easily in the absence of white blood cells. Those remedies must, of course, be injected by the doctor and only in association with regular examination of the blood, by which the doctor is able to trace the progress or remission of the disease.

GYNECOLOGY Gynecology is a specialty of medicine which is concerned with the diseases of women. A gynecologist is a specialist in diseases of women.

GYNECOMASTIA This is a word derived from two words meaning "women" and "breasts." It is applied, however, to any enlargement of the breasts that takes place in men, so that the breasts of men resemble those of women. The condition is usually related to some glandular disturbance and is most often treated by surgical removal.

HAIR GROWTH—Hair grows in the average person at a regular rate, taking about six weeks to grow an inch. Then the follicle from which the hair grows must have a rest. The resting period varies from a few weeks to ten or eleven weeks. The hair of the head, except in cases of baldness, has an almost continuous activity of the follicles, each hair being replaced nearly as soon as it reaches its full length.

There are many superstitions about the growth of hair. One belief is that continual cutting of the hair will cause it to grow coarse and stiff. It is true that the beard of a young man is soft and fine when he begins to shave and after a few years is coarse and stiff. However, people who never shave still have a beard that becomes coarse and stiff. Two men were compared, one of whom had shaved regularly for twenty years and the other never at all. The facial hairs of both were, as far as could be determined, of the same diameter.

The effect of shaving has been tested on hairs of various parts of the body in both sexes. Apparently shaving the hair does not affect it in any way. Three women shaved one leg from the knee to the ankle twice a week for eight months without being able to produce any change in the growth of the hair on that leg as compared with the other leg.

Tests have also been made of the effects of various external applications on hair growth. Oils have been used; the application of oil to the leg twice a week for eight months did not produce any effect on the hair that could be detected on comparing the treated side and the untreated side. Likewise the frequent application of oil to one eyebrow for some months did not produce any changes in the hair on that eyebrow from the other eyebrow.

It has been claimed that both heat and cold favor the production of hair. Actual investigations have failed to indicate any positive effects. It has also been claimed that the ultraviolet rays of the sun can cause the growth of hair or that the tanning of the skin can stop the growth of hair. Tests have been made which fail to reveal that ultraviolet produces an increased growth of hair or that tanning will either produce an increased growth or cause the hair to fall out. There seems to be some evidence that an increased flow of blood to the skin, brought about by the heat associated with the rays of the sun, may cause a temporary increase in the rate of growth of the hair.

The one physical force which quite definitely can affect the growth of hair is the X ray. It is possible with the X ray to cause the hair to fall out. However, controlled use of the X ray for this purpose is exceedingly dangerous.

Finally there is a belief that the glands of internal secretion may affect the growth of the hair. Unquestionably the hairiness of the man is due to stimulation of secretions from the male sex glands. In the absence of such secretions the hair of the body remains undeveloped. Recently scientific evidence has shown that men who are strongly sexed become bald earlier and more frequently than those who have less testicular activity.

It is known that secretions of the various glands may affect the hair of the different portions of the body. The chief factor in growth of the hair is the kind of cells that exist in the follicles from which the hair grows in the individual person, and that seems to be a part of his constitution which is inherited from his ancestors.

BALDNESS—Alopecia is the word used by doctors to describe baldness. Several different forms are recognized, including the hereditary type and also transient forms of baldness. Cases occur also in which the falling of the hair is due to an infection, and in some instances falling of the hair is associated with excessive activity of the oil glands associated with the hair.

According to Dr. C. H. Danforth, who made a special study of the growth of hair, the fact that baldness is generally confined to certain areas and may be associated with luxuriant growth of the hair on other parts of the scalp does not support the popular notion that cutting the hair, wearing a hat, or even dandruff is significant in baldness. The experts are inclined to believe that the nature of the structure of the scalp and, to some extent, the quality of the tissues underneath the skin determine largely, first, whether or not the hair falls out, and, second, the area over which it falls out.

Experts in heredity assert that baldness is definitely a hereditary, sex-limited trait. That is to say, baldness is inherited principally through the male, in whom it is inherited as a dominant characteristic, and that it is recessive in the female, tending to disappear if it occurs. Just why this is the case no one knows.

Baldness is probably hereditary in some families and not in others. Incidentally, of course, it has already been shown by studies of great numbers of people in various families that not only the baldness but the type of baldness is inherited. Instances are known in which only the eyebrows or eyelashes happen to be affected. Cases are known in which families are entirely hairless. Quite recently an eminent anthropologist predicted that the whole tendency of mankind is toward a complete disappearance of hair from the body and that a hundred thousand years from today, if human beings are still on this earth, they will be entirely without hair. The only satisfaction this gives the average bald-headed man is to enable him to reply to the fun poked at him by his persecutors by saying that he is a hundred thousand years ahead of his time.

Thus there is no cure for baldness. Possibly one may delay somewhat the falling of the hair in a member of a family in which baldness is hereditary, but even that is not certain.

CARE OF THE HAIR—Innumerable articles have been written about the care of the hair with a view to making it look better and last longer. Rapid falling of the hair that follows sickness is a toxic disturbance due to the presence in the body of the poisons caused by bacteria. This type of baldness is usually temporary, and the hair will grow out again in a few months. Cutting the hair short or shaving the head will not make it grow in any faster. About the only thing we know that helps under these circumstances is slight rubbing of the scalp frequently with the fingers to encourage the circulation. A fairly stiff brush can be used for the same purpose.

Dandruff, which means scurf on the scalp and that means most often on the coat collar, represents an excess of secretion, in many instances, from the oil glands. Men are affected more often than women. Cleanliness is especially recommended as a help in cases of dandruff.

Specialists in conditions affecting the skin and hair propose the following outline for its care:

The hair should be washed often enough to keep it clean. That means for short hair at least once in two weeks and for long hair at least once in three weeks. For most hair any good toilet soap that will lather freely will serve the purpose. The use of an egg in a shampoo is of little more value than throwing the egg in an electric fan would be. It helps to disseminate the egg but does nothing to help the scalp.

After the hair has been washed with soap and water it should be rinsed thoroughly and dried fairly slowly, rather than by the use of a hot blower. If the hair is too dry, a small amount of oil may be rubbed into it after it has been washed and dried.

Singeing the hair accomplishes nothing except for the pocketbook of the barber. The hair is not a hollow tube, and singeing it does nothing except to put a charred tip on it. It does not help to prevent the escape from the hair shaft of any vital substance.

When the body in general is in ill-health, the hair is likely to be ill also. Therefore good health is frequently associated with a good state of the skin and hair.

The question is often asked as to what to do about gray or white hair. The philosopher's answer is "Admire it." We do not know of any vitamin or any substance taken internally that will prevent or delay the appearance of gray hair in families in whom the hair tends to become gray early. Gray hair, however, can be dyed successfully by experts in the field. Some people are especially sensitive to paraphenylendiamine, which is an ingredient of many hair dyes. A careful hairdresser will test the surface of the skin to the reaction of this substance before using a dye containing it.

As far as growth of the hair is concerned, hope springs eternal in the masculine breast. Many a charlatan has earned an excellent living because of the credulity of mankind in this regard.

SUPERFLUOUS HAIR—For what is commonly called superfluous hair the specialists in diseases of the skin (called dermatologists) have a scientific term—namely, hypertrichosis. The word "hypertrichosis" means excessive hairiness. Men seldom worry overmuch about excessive growth of hair but for women it may be a serious problem.

Modern opinion inclines to the view that the glands of internal secretion have a definite relationship to excessive growth of the hair, particularly on the upper lip and chin in women. It is known that certain forms of overgrowth of glands can be associated with excessive growth of hair.

Nobody knows whether or not the dog-face boy whose entire face and neck grew a thick coat of hair worried much about his condition. The bearded woman in the circus makes a living by exhibition of her superfluous hair. Apparently there are considerable numbers of people who grow hair at the base of the spine, like the tail of an animal. This, however, is usually out of sight. Apparently such hairiness tends to occur in families.

In women excessive growth of hair is more likely to occur after they have passed the menopause. A young girl with a fine mustache can treat the matter lightly if her appearance otherwise is attractive. However, if the mustache is dark in color, it can so affect her life as to become a major psychologic problem.

It has been urged that overexposure to wind or sun may be responsible for excessive growth of hair, also that cutting the hair, shaving, or otherwise removing it makes it come in worse. There is not the slightest evidence to support the belief that any of these actions in any way influence the excessive growth of hair. The hairs are generally permanent unless they are completely destroyed, including the hair follicle.

Three different agents are known by which removal of superfluous hair can be accomplished. By far the safest and the only one generally recommended is the use of the electric needle. This requires patience and endurance. The pain is usually slight. The woman who is anxious to have excessive hair removed will endure the treatments quietly and patiently, so that in most instances the doctor is exhausted long before the patient is tired. When the electric needle is used, a needle or wire carrying the current is inserted into the hair follicle and a weak electric current is turned on for a brief time. Seldom is it possible to remove more than 10 to 15 hairs in a single sitting. Since there may be 1200 to 1500 hairs on a single upper lip, the scope of the problem becomes apparent. However, even with the best operators from 10 to 50 per cent of the hairs that are removed recur, depending on the extent to which the hair follicle is damaged by the electric current.

Practically all experts warn against removal of superfluous hair by X ray.

One of the most experienced has said that the results are so uncertain and the possibilities of harm so great that treatment by this method should not be undertaken except in extreme cases. A dosage of X ray sufficient to cause the hair to fall out is likely also to produce permanent damage to the skin.

A third technic is the use of heat. However, this method also is most delicate and most dangerous.

This means, therefore, that for the majority of cases temporary relief from excess hair is to be obtained by shaving, by rubbing with pumice stone, by the application of waxes which harden and which can then be pulled off, bringing the hair with them.

Hydrogen peroxide is sometimes used to bleach the hair so that it is not so easily visible.

HAIR OF THE HUMAN BODY—The production of hair differentiates those animals that nurse their young from other classes of animals that have spines. Birds have feathers, and fish have scales.

All kinds of hair, mainly that of man and of the other animals, have a certain similarity. Essentially the hair is an outgrowth from the skin. The tip of the hair commonly points backward or downward. The shaft of the hair is not hollow, but the central portion is less dense and solid than the outer portion. The hair contains pigment, which gives it its color. Closely associated with the hair is a gland which develops an oily secretion; this is known as the sebaceous gland.

The hair in some portions of the body of animals has the ability to become erect, so that when people say their hair stands on end, they are referring to something that actually has taken place in the bodies of animals. Not all the hair of the body has this ability. The hair of animals, particularly the whiskers and feelers, is especially endowed with such ability, since it is related to certain activities of the animal concerned. The hair that does not have this special ability is also classified into that which is coarse and that which is fine.

Animals differ as to the amount and distribution of the hair on the body, and, in fact, various human beings differ in this regard. Animals in warm regions are likely to have less hair than those in cold regions. This may not, however, be any special differentiation that has occurred in response to the climate. It must be remembered that an animal insufficiently protected against cold cannot live in a cold climate. Animals differ also in the amount of fat in the tissue under the skin from which the hair grows.

Man is unique among other animals with hair in the fact that he does not have tactile hairs. These are the hairs that have the ability to convey sensation to the body in relation to its surroundings.

The human being has, in general, less hair than other animals, but he is not the most nearly hairless animal. Certain areas of the human body are usually without hair, including particularly portions of the hand and foot. A newborn baby may have a very fine hair called lanugo. Most of this hair is shed before birth. By the time of birth the hair of the eyelashes, eyebrows, and scalp has shown a more vigorous growth than that elsewhere on the body.

The hair in different portions of the body has different characteristics. The hair on the scalp varies considerably both as to the number of hairs and the length to which they grow. The rate of growth of the hair per day is .4 of a millimeter. The average length to which a hair will grow in a woman is 60 to 70 centimeters, or about 25 inches; it takes about four years to reach that length.

Hair that is cylindrical hangs straight from the head. Hair that is oval becomes curly.

The total number of hairs in each eyebrow is around 600, and such a hair lasts about 112 days. As people become older, the eyebrows tend to curl and grow longer, so that they have to be trimmed. The hair of the eyelashes is practically identical with that of the eyebrows except that it is slightly more curved.

The average diameter of the hair of the beard increases throughout life, so that these hairs become coarser and more bristling in advanced years. The beard is scanty among the more darkly pigmented races.

Women generally have little hair on the face, but the number of women who shave or use other means of removing superfluous hair from the face is much greater than is popularly supposed.

There are also sexual differences in the distribution of hair on the rest of the body.

HALITOSIS Most doctors are convinced that a bad odor of the breath arises principally from the mouth, teeth, and throat and is usually due to either decay of the teeth or infection of the tissues.

The word "halitosis," a scientific term for bad breath, was popularized through the promotion of a mouth wash. No mouth wash known has the power to prevent a bad odor arising from a decayed tooth or from an infection. All that it can do is temporarily wash away the infectious material. Only scientific treatment with removal of the source of the infection or decay can prevent the odor permanently.

Decay of the teeth can be determined only by regular dental inspection. Cleanliness of the teeth is controlled only by proper use of the toothbrush and associated therewith such a toothpaste, tooth powder, or solution, as preferred by the individual.

Occasionally an odor comes from an infection in the tonsils. The little crypts or pockets in the tonsils become filled with infectious material, even with decaying particles of food. This material will give off a bad odor with each breath. The physician may squeeze out these crypts and cleanse the surfaces that are left with antiseptic solutions. Gargles occasionally will wash off the surfaces, but few people can get a gargle down to the points that are involved. If the tonsils are seriously infected and if there is an unpleasant odor from an infected throat, surgical removal of the tonsils is necessary to produce a cure.

Infections in the nose with crusting may be associated with a foul breath. The diagnosis and treatment of such a condition is a problem for the specialist. Washing the nose and the cavity behind the nose is a procedure for which special training is required.

Occasionally the lungs or the stomach develop materials which give a bad odor to the breath. Garlic can be eliminated from the blood through the lungs and thus contaminate the breath. In one experiment people swallowed raw chopped garlic in double gelatin capsules, so that none of the garlic could possibly come in contact with the mouth or the teeth. The odor of garlic appeared on the breath just as soon as it was released in the stomach and continued even when the garlic had passed from the stomach into the intestines.

The only way to overcome such an odor is to use flavored oils, which will cover it up with a nice odor. Some mouth washes accomplish this result by substituting for the odor that is to be removed the odor of the mouth wash. Masking of an odor is not in any sense a cure for halitosis.

Recently, preparations of chlorophyll have been urged as efficient in halitosis. The evidence is not good and there is proof that chlorophyll will not prevent mouth odors.

HARELIP See *Cleft Palate* and *Lips*.

HAY FEVER Hay fever, caused by the giant ragweed, is also called ragweed fever and autumnal catarrh. Seldom is scientific advice needed nowadays to make the diagnosis; the sneezing, watering of the eyes, running of the nose, itching of the nose, throat, and palate that come on coincident with the development of the ragweed pollen have been widely recognized. Occasionally, however, there are still people who feel that the early symptoms of hay fever represent a common cold. Anyone who has these attacks regularly will do well to be tested for

sensitivity to make certain that the condition is really hay fever and not some other chronic disturbance.

We endeavor now to prevent hay fever rather than to treat it. Some people can go away from home to areas in which the pollens to which they are sensitive are infrequent. For those who stay at home all sorts of protective glasses for the eyes, filters for the nose, and nose masks have been advised. However, the best preventive is a modern air filtration machine which conditions the room in which the patient works or sleeps.

Good general advice for the hay-fever sufferer is to keep out of drafts, avoid automobile trips in the country, stay on the fairway instead of in the rough while golfing, thus avoiding possible contact with the ragweed pollens.

Each section of the United States contains about thirty pollens which are important causes of hay fever. It therefore becomes possible for a physician to test the patient for his sensitivity to these pollens. After having determined the particular pollens to which the patient is sensitive, it is then possible to attempt desensitization. It is unwise for the person with hay fever to wait until the attack begins before he is desensitized. Much better is regular treatment each year with desensitization at regular intervals, so that the patient is protected against the sensitivity up to the time when the pollens begin to fill the air.

There are many methods of treatment by which the person with hay fever may be made more comfortable. Some of the remedies sold in drugstores are of this type. They do not cure hay fever; they merely help to relieve the worst of the symptoms. However, the physician can prescribe or apply remedies which cannot be sold in the form of ready-made drugs and which are known to be much more effective than the type of remedy that is sold without any control.

Such remedies as adrenalin and ephedrine and some of the treatments that are derived from narcotic drugs are immensely important in controlling symptoms but, obviously, cannot be sold or applied without suitable control.

HEADACHE At least one half of all the people who come into the doctor's office complain that they have headaches. The men who have charge of the employees in our large industries say that about one fourth of all of the absences of employees are credited to headaches. Thus this symptom—because headache is not truly a disease—is responsible for much human disability.

Headaches are due to a great variety of causes—indeed a variety so great that the determination of the single cause or multiple causes of any one headache may require the highest art and technic of the doctor. Innumerable classifications have been developed so as to group the causes in various ways and thus to guide the technic of study. One of the simplest methods groups some 203 different causes under three classifications—mechanical, toxic, and functional. Thus the mechanical headaches would be those associated with conditions related to the head itself. For instance, when the sinuses become blocked, changes in pressure will produce headache. When the membranes of the nose swell, this in turn blocks the sinuses and produces headache. When the frontal sinus is involved, the headache is likely to be worse in the morning and to improve during the day as the sinus drains.

The brain lies in a fluid known as the cerebrospinal fluid, which in turn is enclosed in the membranes that cover the brain. These membranes are sensitive to stretching. Anything that causes an increase in the cerebrospinal fluid or that produces pressure inside the membranes can produce headache. There are a number of different actions that could thus raise the intracranial pressure, or the pressure inside the skull.

Some people rarely have headaches; others have them all the time. Headache that comes on occasionally may be definitely related to some action that occurs occasionally, such as overindulgence in alcohol, tobacco, or drugs, excessive eating, exposure to gases or other toxic substances. The accumulation of toxic substances may so alter the pressure inside the skull as to produce headache. Certain headaches are known to be due to overuse of the eyes or to strain brought about by the fact that defects of vision have not been properly corrected. Some people are more sensitive than others to headache of this type. This form of headache is more easily cured than some that are less simple in their causation. If an error in vision can be determined and suitably corrected, if exposure to glare can be controlled, if excessive use of the eyes can be lessened, headaches related to the eyes promptly disappear.

Some headaches are related to high blood pressure. If the blood pressure falls during rest, the headache disappears. A tumor growing in the skull, once it becomes sufficiently large to cause pressure, can be a permanent cause of headache. Infectious diseases which produce inflammation and, associated with this inflammation, an outpouring of fluid, can also produce serious headache. For that very reason headaches are frequently among the earliest of symptoms of infectious diseases.

The migraine, or sick headache, is attributed to a variety of causes. One of the most frequent points of view has it that the sick headache is the result of sensitivity to some protein substance and that the changes brought about by this allergy in the form of swelling and fluid inside the skull cause the headache. Sick headaches vary, however, in various persons and also in the same person. The associated factors of mental and physical state have a great deal to do with the intensity and duration of sick headaches.

Especially disturbing to the physician are headaches for which no definite cause can be assigned. These are commonly called functional headaches, and in many instances a psychologic cause related to the emotions may be determined. The modern approach to such conditions is called psychosomatic medicine. Even the most careful studies will not detect any changes in the tissues that can be measured. Yet a severe emotional reaction may be followed by a most severe headache. The pain of such a headache can be just as real as that produced by some toxic substance.

Interestingly enough, some of the most frequent causes of headache produce the least serious symptoms outside of the pain itself. Fatigue, hunger, constipation, indigestion, menstruation, kidney diseases, mild infections in the sinuses, and similar causes are frequently detected in people who have repeated headaches.

The number of remedies offered for headaches is almost as great as the variety of causes. Yet the vast preponderance of these remedies are simple sedative drugs which in no way get at the cause of the disease. The great majority of people take aspirin, which is no doubt among the least harmful of the sedative drugs available—certainly much less harmful than the dangerous pyramidon or aminopyrine, which has been shown to bring about in many cases serious damage to the blood. The barbituric acid sedatives, of which there are dozens available in the drugstores, help to relieve pain but also produce sleepiness and in many instances can produce toxic effects. The simple remedies, such as rest, change in eating habits, moderation in the use of tobacco and alcohol, should all be given a trial before resorting to drugs with dangerous possibilities. The establishment of a good hygiene of the body relating to the taking of food and the elimination of waste material often brings about great benefit in the case of chronic headache.

If a person who has never had headaches suddenly begins suffering repeated attacks, the need of careful study by a physician is much greater. If the physician can determine the relationship of the headache to some physical or mental factor and can control that factor, relief is likely.

HEAD BANGING AND HEAD ROLLING Sometimes an otherwise apparently normal and healthy infant, when put to bed, rolls his head from side to side on the pillow, occasionally bangs the head up and down or against the sides of the crib. In many instances actual bruises result from this action. Some infants will roll the head so hard and so persistently that they will rub the hair away from the back of the head. Sometimes the child will keep up this banging for two or three hours at a time.

Children tend to imitate each other, so that the head rolling and banging will spread through a hospital ward or a dormitory. Seldom does it continue after the fourth year, although a child who has once rolled the head or banged it about may during semisleeping states or in sleep again reproduce this habit.

Parents are likely to become greatly frightened by head rolling or head banging, but they need not be alarmed because rarely indeed is it associated with any organic disease of the brain or any other portion of the body. Some parents are likely to be especially disturbed for fear that it represents a vicious habit or some mental or emotional disturbance. Actually it seems to be a fundamental reaction related to the child's craving for rhythmical activities. Many psychologists are inclined to believe that it is in some way a pleasure-seeking device. One physician felt that it represents a response to some obstruction to breathing, as might be caused by adenoids, and that the rolling of the head is an attempt to obtain relief. When the adenoids are removed, the symptoms clear up, but the rolling and banging of the head, he says, may continue if there is chronic congestion of the nose. Certainly it is worth while to remove enlarged or inflamed adenoids, but there is no certainty that the condition is really related to head rolling or head banging. It has been found that the use of sedatives which cause the child to sleep more deeply will stop the head rolling and head banging.

One observer thought that head rolling was due to the fact that children had been rocked to sleep in an old-fashioned rocking chair or in a crib and that later, when they were put to sleep in a stationary bed, they missed the rocking and therefore rocked themselves. Conceivably the escape from emotional tension brought about by rolling and rocking, that the child may have secured when being artificially rocked, is automatically reproduced when the artificial rocking is discontinued.

Children develop strange habits, many of which are exceedingly difficult to explain by any simple mechanism. Fortunately head rolling and head banging so certainly disappear in the vast majority of cases, as the child gets older, that the matter need not give too great concern to the parent.

HEARING, HARDNESS OF See *Deafness* and *Otosclerosis.*

HEART The heart is essentially a pump that circulates the blood through the body. At birth the heart weighs less than an ounce. In a grown person, if the heart is normal, it weighs about a half pound and is somewhat larger than a fist.

At birth the heart beats about 130 times a minute; at six years it beats 100 times a minute; at ten years about 90, and at fifteen years about 85. Among grownups rates of anywhere from 65 to 80 per minute may well be within the normal. During a lifetime the heart beats 2,500,000,000 times and pumps a total of nearly 15,000,000 gallons.

The impulse which causes the heart to contract develops in some nerve tissue which is called the pacemaker of the heart. An attempt to measure this impulse indicates that its energy is the equivalent of one thousandth of a volt.

The blood comes into the heart after having been collected from the veins of the body and passed through the lungs, where new oxygen is taken up. When the heart muscle contracts, the blood is forced out of the heart and then goes by way of the large arteries and blood vessels to the farthest extremes of the body.

The heart moves a total of 500 gallons of blood a day. Since there are about 6 quarts of blood in the whole body, the heart moves the same fluid, slightly modified chemically as it travels about, over and over again.

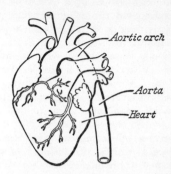

The aorta is the large blood vessel that carries the arterial blood from the left ventricle of the heart. From the aorta come all the arteries that carry blood to various portions of the body

The heart never gets a complete rest until we die; then of course the rest is too late. It begins working before the child is born and is never quiet until death. The only rest it gets is when its beat is slowed a little or decreased somewhat in its force.

The heart is one of the involuntary muscles of the body. A few instances are recorded in medicine in which people have been able voluntarily to control their heartbeat. Most people, perhaps fortunately for them, do not have this power. If they did, they might want to try it once too often.

NATURE PROTECTS THE HEART—The vital organ must, therefore, be protected in every way possible against overstrain and damage. By its situation in the body the heart is reasonably well protected against most ordinary dangers. The heart lies just below and to the left of the lower two thirds of the chest bone. Its shape is like that of a large pear with the broad end upward and under the chest bone, and the pointed end downward and to the left. If you put your finger in the space just below the fifth rib and slightly to the left of the breastbone, you can feel the impulse of the heartbeats.

The heart lies inside a sac which is called the pericardium. This serves to separate the heart from the other organs in the chest and to hold it in position. Sometimes the strain and pressure on the heart may be so great that it would swell like a balloon if it did not have this sac around it to keep it from stretching too far. The outside of the heart, too, is enclosed in a membranous sac. A thin layer of fluid keeps these two layers of tissue from being rubbed together when the heart beats.

The heart is a muscle. This muscle is called the myocardium. The interior of the heart is lined with another membrane which is called the endocardium.

CORONARY ARTERIES—The heart gets its own nourishment from small blood vessels which pass into the muscle tissue from the large blood vessels that carry the blood away from the heart. These small blood vessels which nourish the heart itself are known as the coronary arteries. Remember this name. Today trouble with these coronary arteries is responsible for a good many cases of sudden death in people past middle age.

All of the openings leading into the heart and passing out of it are controlled by valves which open and shut as the blood comes in and passes out. There are similar valves governing the passing of the blood from one portion of the heart into another.

HEART FAILURE—Heart disease and failure of the heart to carry on its work are among the commonest and most serious conditions that affect human beings. This is particularly the case since man has increased his life expectancy. When human beings died young of infectious diseases, the number of cases of breakdown and degeneration of important organs was not nearly so great as now.

The human body is built ordinarily to run about seventy years. If it is used to excess or if it is attacked by infections or in other ways damaged, it sometimes fails to last that long. Even when the human being lives much longer, however, the tissues begin to break down somewhat past middle life and, having broken down, fail in their capacity to carry on their functions.

The failure of the heart to do its work is especially serious because the

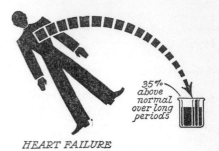

35% above normal over long periods

HEART FAILURE

3½ quarts of blood each minute through the arteries

3½ quarts

EMOTIONALLY CALM MAN

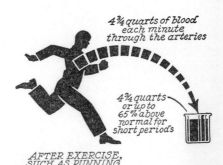

4¾ quarts of blood each minute through the arteries

4¾ quarts or up to 65% above normal for short periods

AFTER EXERCISE, SUCH AS RUNNING

Indication of manner in which extra work is thrown on the heart by exercise, forcing unusual amount of blood through the heart and giving the heart increased work

whole body depends on the blood as a means of sustaining its life. When the heart fails to get blood out to the cells, they cannot function satisfactorily. Failure of the heart to do its work may be due to inability of the muscle to pump, failure of the pump to force out a sufficient amount of blood at each beat, or failure of the pump to force the blood all the way around and back again, since the blood must circulate continuously. When the heart is insufficient to force the circulation completely around, there is a tendency for blood to remain in various portions of the body, particularly in the feet; fluid collects in the abdomen, and there occurs finally what is known as congestive heart failure. Sometimes when the heart has become weakened, rest of the patient and aid given to the body by other means of modern medicine will permit the heart to carry on its work satisfactorily. With time, the muscle of the heart may increase in amount, so that the heart, though enlarged, is able to do its work. This is known as compensation.

Some of the ordinary signs of failure of the heart to do its work are shortness of breath, collection of fluid in various portions of the body, and swelling of the tissues. Shortness of breath is particularly a sign of the failure of the heart to push the blood into the large blood vessels. The tendency is, therefore, for the blood to back up, and the first signs of congestion are seen in the lungs, from which the blood comes to the heart. The result is a distressful, rapid, shallow breathing which demands again the most careful consideration by the doctor in order to overcome the disturbance before permanent changes in the structure of the tissues occur. Sometimes these patients have trouble when they lie down because of the increased amount of fluid that moves promptly into the circulation.

All of the difficulties that have been described are so serious and so definitely progressive unless properly cared for that physicians have never hesitated to advise again and again a regular examination of the human body at least once each year, or, better perhaps, once every six months, after middle age. With such an examination serious breakdowns are detected early, and proper treatment can stop progress in the early stages.

THE PROBLEMS OF HEART DISEASE— Today heart disease is the outstanding cause of death. The attack on heart disease is directed primarily against those forms of infection and overstrain of the human body which primarily affect the heart.

Rheumatic fever is one of the foremost foes of health in children.

The second great problem in heart disease is the deaths of people of advanced years from breakdown of this vital organ. This is associated with the fact that more people are living longer than people used to live. The diseases involving breakdown of the heart, and especially blocking of the coronary arteries, affect men far more than they do women. Certainly this should indicate that many of these deaths may be prevented by taking from the male workers, and particularly people occupying positions of stress and strain, much of the demand that is now placed on them.

The third group of heart conditions to which attention should be given is the group of old people who have gotten so old that their hearts are in constant danger of breakdown. Here the necessity is for additional facilities for examination and diagnosis of such cases, facilities for home care, including adequate nursing, and, finally, institutions where such people may be given hospital attention.

Primary in the treatment of all types of conditions affecting the heart is the provision of adequate rest. This means not only relaxation, but in many instances long-continued actual rest in bed. The number of beds available in hospitals and institutions in the United States for patients with heart disease is far below the number actually required. This applies to beds in hospitals for all types of convalescents from disease and for all types of chronic disease.

RHEUMATIC FEVER (See also *Rheumatic Fever*)—Today rheumatic fever is among the foremost health problems of youth. Most of the cases occur in the months from March to June, with the smallest number of cases in the months from August up to December.

In most instances the condition appears following infections of the nose and throat. It may also, however, be associated with an infection of the ear, with scarlet fever, St. Vitus' dance, or other similar conditions. In at least one fifth of all the cases of rheumatic fever the most serious associated condition is the attack on the heart.

The child who is likely to have rheumatic fever is one who has frequent illnesses, especially sore throat, tonsillitis, and infections of the nose and throat. Such children seldom gain weight as they should, they become easily tired, and frequently they have deficiencies in the blood. Whenever there are frequent fevers of unknown cause, with fleeting pains in the joints, special attention should be given to the possibility that the child is getting rheumatic fever. The so-called growing pains so commonly talked about in a previous generation are now recognized to be, in the vast majority of cases, early attacks of this disease.

Rheumatic fever is dangerous because it comes on insidiously. Often the family does not suspect that the child is ill until so much damage has already been done to the heart that recovery is impossible. A child acutely ill with rheumatic fever will have a high fever, a rapid heart, difficulty in breathing, drowsiness, weakness, profuse perspiration, and prostration.

Sometimes the joint involvement is serious; other times it is absent. The joints when involved are swollen, red, and tender. Sometimes a child who seems to be recovering from the disease suddenly seems to be reinfected with an acute period as bad as or worse than the initial attack.

Most difficult are the smoldering forms of the disease in which the child never seems to be seriously sick but at the same time is constantly suffering from an infected heart. Such children may appear fretful and indisposed with poor appetite and restless sleep. A careful examination may show, however, that the heart is already subject to murmurs and difficulty in its functions.

Some years ago it was discovered that a sudden and severe abdominal pain might be the only sign of an acutely inflamed heart. Such cases have been mistaken for appendicitis. In the absence of the other positive signs of appendicitis, the doctor nowadays always suspects the possibility of rheumatic fever.

Seven years of age is the time when most children are attacked but many are attacked even as early as five years of age. Since children of school age are the ones chiefly affected, many communities have been trying to develop suitable plans to meet the situation.

In New York City classes for children with heart disease have been developed in the public schools. Such children have to be continuously under medical supervision. Moreover, their instruction must be conducted by teachers who have had special interest in heart disease and who know how to watch developments in such patients. In most instances special transportation has to be provided to get the children to schools. There must also be definite rest periods for them in order to relieve them of the possibility of strain.

Prevention of Rheumatic Fever—In the prevention of rheumatic fever, attention must be given to many details which are important for improving general health. The whole life should be quiet and restful. There must be particularly plenty of periods of rest and recreation. If a child becomes fatigued and exhausted, his digestion is interfered with and he becomes easily subject to infection. For children who are exceedingly nervous and who tire easily, a rest period of a half hour before and after meals is useful.

Damp, wet clothing should always be

removed from the child when he comes indoors. Research has proved that attacks of rheumatic fever can be prevented by giving sulfadiazine or penicillin at the first indication that a child has a sore throat. This controls the streptococcus.

A new form of penicillin has been found called depot penicillin which when injected will keep up the level of penicillin in the body for a month.

Wholesome Diet—The child requires a diet with plenty of milk, butter, eggs, leafy green vegetables, fruits, cod-liver oil, and other foods. These give adequate amounts of protein, carbohydrate, fat, mineral salts, and vitamins for satisfactory nutrition. If there is a tendency to persistent underweight, if the child eats without appetite, and if his digestion is constantly disturbed, he will become more easily a victim to heart disease.

Particularly important is prompt attention to every cold and sore throat and avoidance of cold and sore throats as far as possible. Children who suffer constantly from sore throats or infections of the nose and sinuses should be carefully watched by a physician and should be given, if possible, the benefit of a warm climate in order to permit opportunity for complete recovery.

There is no certain cure for rheumatic fever, no drug or serum that has specific effect on which dependence may be placed. The child, as has already been said, must be put to bed promptly if this condition occurs. He must be constantly under the care of a doctor who understands heart disease. He should be allowed out of bed only gradually, remaining in bed for at least two weeks or even longer after the fever has completely disappeared.

Many cities now have hospitals and sanitariums specifically designated for care of patients with rheumatic fever. Clinics are being established to provide sulfadiazine or antibiotics to children with possible rheumatic fever and to control relapses.

Convalescence (See also discussion under *Rheumatic Fever*)—The doctor can determine, after the child has recovered, how much damage has been done to the heart. He will have to regulate the amount of exercise and the amount of work that the child may do day by day, in order to see that strain and overwork are not put upon this vital organ. If a heart has been damaged by rheumatic fever, it will not do its duty adequately as a pump. This will be shown by discomfort after exertion, shortness of breath, swelling of the feet, blueness of the complexion, and other symptoms which indicate that the tissues of the body are not receiving adequate amounts of oxygenized blood. Such cases demand constant, careful watching.

ENDOCARDITIS—Among the most fatal of all diseases affecting the heart is bacterial endocarditis. In this condition the germs which have infected the heart will frequently be found circulating in the blood. This form of heart disease is most often seen after the patient has had rheumatic fever or some other form of heart disturbance. If the valves of the heart have been damaged by any previous disease, the bacteria which get into the blood may adhere to the valves of the heart, survive, and grow.

As a result of this infection, blood clots accumulate and form a material in which the germs may grow and multiply with facility. Sometimes this form of infection of the valves of the heart may occur without the germs being found in the blood. But it must be remembered that the streptococcus, which is the germ most frequently responsible, is found in almost all noses and throats throughout life.

The condition has been produced experimentally in animals by injecting the germ into the blood of the animal. The germs settle on the heart valves and begin to destroy the tissue. One of the great difficulties in attacking this disease is the fact that the germs penetrate into the tissues of the heart and into the accumulation of fibrous tissues on the valves of the heart, so that it is difficult for remedies to reach the germs. Several suggestions have been made for the prevention of the formation of these fibrous deposits. One of them was the use of a new substance called heparin, which prevents the formation of clots, with the idea that this substance would loosen the clots. Another substance with similar effects is known as dicumarol. Sulfanilamide, or one of the new derivatives, or penicillin may be given to attack the germs.

The patient who recovers from infection of the heart valves may die subsequently as the result of damage which has been done by this condition to the kidneys, the blood, or the brain. Unfortunately, when clots or fibrous formations occur on the heart valves, they sometimes break off and circulate in the blood, coming eventually to an artery through which they cannot pass, thus blocking that artery. This condition is called an embolism with thrombosis. Should the artery that is blocked be an artery in the brain or one associated with any other vital organ, that in itself may cause death.

CORONARY THROMBOSIS (See also *Angina Pectoris*)—Thrombosis means blocking by a clot of blood. The coronary arteries are the blood vessels which furnish blood to the heart. The term "coronary thrombosis" therefore means blocking of the blood vessels to the heart by a clot of blood.

If the person has been well previously, or if the person has had previous attacks of pain referred to the heart, the diagnosis is usually justified. If the blocking occurs gradually, the symptoms may have developed over a period of weeks.

Far too often the symptoms suggest a disturbance of digestion. There is a sense of fullness in the abdomen relieved by the belching of gas.

There may be nausea and vomiting; discomfort associated with the stomach often follows a meal, and there may be other symptoms of indigestion, so that far too often the condition is passed over with a diagnosis of acute indigestion.

Most people with this disease are past fifty years of age, but occasionally there are cases between forty and fifty.

If the attack takes place gradually, the other blood vessels which supply blood to the heart may take over the function of the one which is blocked. There may be slight changes in the heart with symptoms during this process, but under such circumstances the condition is not necessarily fatal.

In an acute attack of coronary thrombosis there is pain—sudden, severe, and persisting. There is also a feeling of impending death, so that the person becomes pale and is in a cold sweat.

Most often the pain, which is described as deep-seated, cutting, or tearing, is referred to the heart. It may persist for minutes or even hours. As the pain lessens into a dull ache, there is still a feeling of apprehension.

A physician is able to make examinations which will verify the diagnosis. This he does by studying the pulse, the blood pressure, the breathing, and sometimes by using an electrocardiographic device, which gives him an indication of the action of the heart.

There are, however, some cases in which even such methods fail to show definitely the nature of the change. An experienced physician, particularly someone who has studied heart disease, is able to make the diagnosis by the use of observation, by listening to the heart, and by the type of study called physical as contrasted with laboratory diagnosis.

No doubt many patients die almost with the onset of the attack. However, an equal number of patients recover and remain free from attacks for several years or even longer.

Dr. Paul D. White records several instances in which patients have survived seven or eight years or more. Dr. Arthur D. Master found 50 per cent of his patients surviving more than ten years.

One man had his first attack at the age of sixty-three, passed a life-insurance examination two years later, and at the age of seventy-two climbed mountains without symptoms. He died at the age of eighty of brain hemorrhage, without any sign of heart disease except the healed scar in the heart.

The post-mortem examination showed

definitely the scar associated with the attack of coronary thrombosis seventeen years previously.

This case serves to illustrate the wonderful recuperative power of the seriously injured heart muscle, and indicates that the occurrence of one attack may not necessarily mean permanent crippling.

The moment an attack of coronary thrombosis occurs, the person affected should be put immediately at complete rest in bed. Then a competent physician will be able to prescribe drugs according to the symptoms, relieving the pain, making sure that the patient stays quiet until the condition of the heart warrants slight exertion, then controlling bodily exertions so that activity is gradually resumed.

Some patients die immediately, regardless of what the physician can do, because the heart is mortally wounded with the first blocking that occurs. Others have such a small area of heart tissue involved that they incline to recover. There is a large group in whom control of the condition and treatment mean the difference between life and death.

Most important of all, however, is the advice to persons past forty-five years of age that what seems to be an attack of acute indigestion should never be disregarded, particularly when the pain is referred largely to the heart.

Most patients who feel the first symptoms of this disease do not feel themselves sick enough to call a doctor. If they do not recover by good luck, they make their first medical contact with the coroner.

Every means of publicity available ought to be used, even at the risk of creating some unnecessary fears, to teach middle-aged and older people that diagnoses of ptomaine poisoning and acute indigestion are usually serious cases of mistaken identity, and that every case of pleuritic pain and neuritis of the chest, neck, jaw, or arms demands the most prompt and painstaking diagnostic scrutiny possible.

The only advice that can be given for prevention is that best advice of medical science—moderation in all things. The avoidance of overeating and of over-strenuous life are the two main points to be considered.

Here are ten heart commandments which you should keep to prolong your life:

1. Do not subject your heart to sudden, strenuous, or prolonged physical exertion.

2. Eat regularly, slowly, and temperately.

3. If you are excessively overweight, seek sound counsel as to how best to dispense with this form of heart handicap.

4. Try to avoid physical activity for at least thirty minutes after eating, particularly after the heaviest meal of the day.

5. Avoid emotional stress and strain. Worry is an important factor in its relation to heart strain.

6. By appropriate measures, keep your body as free as possible from so-called foci of infection.

7. Regular intestinal elimination is highly important.

8. Average not less than eight hours of sleep in a room abundantly supplied with fresh air.

9. Perennial health demands a proper balance between work, play, and rest.

10. A periodic examination may often reveal defects of which you are totally unaware. A stitch in time saves nine!

HEART BLOCK When the heart is damaged by disease so that the muscular interconnection between the auricles and ventricles (the upper and lower portions of the heart) is interrupted they will beat independently of each other, and the condition is called heart block. As a result the beat of the heart becomes slowed and occurs in paroxysms or spasms.

HEAT SICKNESS (See also *Sun-* and *Heat Stroke*) Workers at glass and metal furnaces, rolling mills and open pit mines, women in laundries, and bakers may be overcome by heat, owing not only to the summer season but also to fatigue.

A few salt tablets taken during the day help to prevent heat stroke. These tablets replenish the salt lost from the body by excessive sweating. Loss of salt is not, however, the only factor in heat stroke.

In summer, workers need a diet low in fat. They should take plenty of water. If they wish, they may take fresh fruit juices, milk, or carbonated drinks to keep up the water supply. Although beer and ale are permissible in small quantities, drinks high in alcohol content are likely to increase the possibility of heat stroke. Small amounts of fluid taken frequently are better than a large amount taken at one time. Ice-cold drinks should always be consumed slowly.

Among foods not easily digested in hot weather are fried foods, heavily spiced foods, and material that is thick with fiber.

Short periods of recreation between the hours of work are especially important during the hot season. A cool shower or tub bath before going to work and after coming home will do much to minimize effects of a job in an overheated plant.

Most plants provide workers with salt tablets of five grains each, which they may take as needed. Two tablets every two hours are plenty for the purpose.

Here are good rules for health during the hot season:

Wear cool clothes—loose and lightweight.

Eat "light" food—fruits, vegetables, and milk. Do not overeat.

Drink cool water—iced drinks in moderation.

Avoid exposure to the sun in the middle of a hot summer day.

Avoid strenuous exercise on a hot day.

Wear a helmet or hat of a porous material when working in the sun.

HEIGHT The impression is increasingly prevalent that boys and girls are growing taller than they used to be. Nevertheless, the records of the Selective Service indicate that the average height of the American boy over twenty-one years of age was just about the same during the Civil War, World War I, and during World War II.

Children do not grow constantly from birth to maturity at an even rate. Like plants, they grow more during some seasons and less during others. The rate of growth of a child is influenced by the weather, sunlight, exercise, diet, and particularly by the actions of his glands.

There is in the pituitary gland a secretion known as the growth hormone, which definitely controls growth. There are also glandular materials coming from the parathyroid glands which are related to this activity.

For years there has been a belief that the boys in California grow bigger than boys elsewhere in the nation. Coaches of football and track athletics, and particularly of basketball teams, assert that the boys who come from California with the teams are much taller and stronger. However, in 1944 the tallest boys on basketball teams came from Oklahoma. Nevertheless, a study made on children in California revealed the fact that the Los Angeles children are on an average over an inch taller than children from San Francisco and from Oakland. In attempting to account for a superiority in height of children from one section of the country as compared with those from another, the environment is given chief credit. The items in environment especially emphasized are increased sunshine, greater variety in diet, including many fresh vegetables and fruits, and more hours of outside play. Incidentally, however, there has also been for some time consistent drill in posture of children who attend the Los Angeles schools. To some extent the improvement in posture is reflected in the increased height.

When there is overactivity of the pituitary gland, there is a tendency to acromegaly and giantism. When there is underactivity of the anterior lobe of the pituitary gland, dwarfism results.

The glandular principles, given sufficiently early in life, can definitely affect height. Unfortunately, once a person has attained adult age, there is nothing that can be done to increase height. Occasionally advertisements appear of strange devices which are supposed to bring about stretching or in other ways extend the length of the human body. There is no scientific evidence to indicate that any of these can accomplish the purpose for which they are sold. About all that can be done is to practice good posture and then to supplement the height by raised heels and similar means.

HELIOTHERAPY The use of the sun's rays to treat disease is called heliotherapy. This may be either by the natural sun or by the use of artificial ultraviolet rays. Treatment with light generally is called phototherapy. One form of this can be the infrared therapy which is the use of the heat rays from the sun or artificial heat rays.

HEMATURIA Abnormally the urine contains blood. In a small percentage of cases the source of this blood cannot be determined, but in the majority the doctor is able, by a careful examination, to find out the source of the bleeding.

For about 2 per cent of all cases bleeding in the urine is said to be of unknown origin. In such cases the blood appears spontaneously and without any pain. Seldom is it sufficient in amount to lead to a state of anemia or to faintness. In many instances such blood appears to have oozed from a varicose vein somewhere along the urinary tract. The condition is usually found in people less than thirty years old.

Other causes of blood in the urine are related to the portion of the urinary tract through which the urine passes. Urine is developed in the kidney and passes down a long tube known as the ureter to the bladder. Here it is collected and at intervals passes out of the body along another tube that is known as the urethra. A severe infection, in-

flammation, or congestion of the kidneys can cause some red blood cells to escape into the urine. A tumor that breaks through the blood vessels can do this. Certain chemicals like turpentine, cantharides, and carbonic acid can so damage the tissues that blood will appear in the urine. Occasionally the sulfonamide drugs act on the kidneys of some people and cause blood to appear in the urine.

Not infrequently a stone, by its irritation and damage to the walls of the tissues in the urinary tract, can cause the appearance of blood. A rupture or breaking of the kidney, the bladder, or the tubes that have been mentioned, due to any cause, is followed by the appearance of blood in the urine.

Instances are known in which exhausting physical exercise or exposure to cold have been followed by the temporary appearance of a few red blood cells in the urine without any evidence of great damage to the kidney.

There are cases of blood diseases like hemophilia and thrombocytopenia or purpura—easy bruising—in which blood passing from the body by way of the urine is not an infrequent sign.

When the doctor is called on to determine the nature of such disturbances, he is likely to make certain, first, that blood actually is present, and, second, the spot from which the blood is coming. This he can do by a number of observations, including the nature of the coloring material and the state in which it appears. Certainty, however, is brought about by those methods which involve the passing of a tube into the bladder and from the bladder into the ureter so as to determine exactly the point from which the blood emanates.

Incidentally, children occasionally pass urine which is bright red because of eating too many beets containing red pigment.

Whenever blood is found in the urine in any amount, it is desirable that the person get to bed at once and that the physician determine as soon as possible what is wrong. Uncontrolled or continuous bleeding invariably threatens life itself.

HEMOGLOBIN The portion of the red blood corpuscles that carries oxygen is the red pigment. This is called hemoglobin. The amount of hemoglobin is measured in order to determine whether or not the blood is normal as relates to this constituent. Usually normal is called 100 per cent. Modern scientific measurements determine the hemoglobin by weight in relationship to a definite volume of blood. Various devices have been invented for measuring the hemoglobin. When the red blood coloring matter appears in the urine, the condition is called hemoglobinuria.

HEMOPHILIA Among the most dramatic of the diseases that affect mankind is hemophilia. This is the disease that affects the royal families of Spain and of Russia—a condition with a peculiar hereditary basis, limited to the males of the family but transmitted by the females.

In hemophilia the clotting time of the blood is much prolonged; the person with this condition may bleed to death because means have not been found to cause the blood to clot successfully. In these cases the number of red blood cells and white blood cells is usually normal at the beginning of the bleeding. The condition is distinguished from purpura by the fact that the blood platelets are not diminished as they are in purpura. In fact they are sometimes increased over the normal in response to the bleeding that occurs. Hence in hemophilia some other element in the blood-clotting process is missing rather than the platelets.

Innumerable investigations have been made in the attempt to find out what happens in the blood of a person who is hemophilic. The defective coagulation in some cases may be due to difficulty in the formation of the blood-clotting element called thrombin, but the cause for the deficiency in this element has not yet been determined. Another element in the blood called anti-thrombin may interfere with the clotting, and an excessive amount of this substance may be responsible.

The chief symptom in hemophilia is the bleeding. Bleeding frequently follows an injury which would not cause bleeding in a normal person. Cases are known in which the pulling of a tooth, a scratch with a needle, or a slight nosebleed has progressed to a hemorrhage which resulted in death.

The person with hemophilia will have bruises under the skin, with the formation of large masses of blood, but will not have spots of the type that occur in purpura. Occasionally bleeding from a slight injury will occur into a joint— a severe symptom that will cause much distress.

Because of the severe character of this condition and the inability of medical science to control it, children with hemophilia seldom live to adult age. It is almost impossible for the average person to avoid slight bruises or accidents; the hemophiliac is therefore in constant danger of some accident that will cause death.

The most important measure of treatment in cases of hemophilia is to stop the bleeding when it occurs. Many different procedures have been used for this purpose. It is possible to pack a wound with gauze or cotton or to sew it together tightly. Various substances have been discovered which the doctor may apply to the wound in an effort to aid clotting by supplying the missing elements. It is also possible to supply these elements by the transfusion of blood directly into the veins. New research suggests that the missing principle in the blood, responsible for hemophilia, has now been determined. Investigators have found the specific substance lacking in the blood of hemophiliacs and such preparations can now be injected and will control the bleeding.

HEMORRHAGE Bleeding at any time and under any circumstances is a serious symptom. Some people bleed more easily than others. Some people bleed longer than others because the blood does not clot easily. When bleeding is difficult to stop, the condition menaces life itself.

Many factors are concerned in bleeding. The cutting of a blood vessel will result in bleeding that is not easy to stop, particularly if it is a large blood vessel. For the formation of a blood clot, calcium is necessary and also certain materials from the fluid portion of the blood which, with the calcium and with a substance called fibrinogen, make up the product called fibrin. Fibrin is the material of a blood clot.

The blood of a normal person contains materials necessary for forming a blood clot. In abnormal instances some of these materials are absent. This is particularly the case in a condition called hemophilia, also in another condition called thrombocytopenia. People with thrombocytopenia have an insufficient number of blood platelets. They tend to bleed easily and to bruise easily. They bleed particularly from the gums, from the sockets of extracted teeth, from the nose, and occasionally from the internal organs. Hemorrhage into a vital organ, such as the brain, may cause death.

When a doctor finds that a patient bleeds too often and too easily, he will try first to determine the cause. The normal blood contains as many as 200,000 or more blood platelets for every cubic millimeter. However, a fairly good blood clot can occur with as little as 50,000 platelets in each cubic millimeter of blood. When the number is below 50,000, the formation of a good blood clot is less likely to occur.

Every person who bruises easily, who bleeds a long time without forming a blood clot, or who tends to have an insufficient amount of the red blood cells or of the red coloring matter of the blood should have a careful examination to determine the deficiencies that exist and should have treatment to bring the amounts of the deficient materials up to the normal.

When bleeding occurs, regardless of the cause, it is important to stop the hemorrhage. One of the simplest ways to stop bleeding is to put on a pack of sterile gauze and to cover this with a tight bandage. This will control the flow of blood in the majority of wounds. If a large artery of an arm or a leg is cut, a tourniquet may be necessary to stop the flow of blood. When there is bleeding from the socket of a tooth after a tooth has been pulled, the hemorrhage can easily be controlled by plugging the socket with sterile gauze or applying hot water. If the bleeding continues, a doctor or dentist should be called immediately. He will have available various drugs which he can apply directly to the bleeding spot and thus stop the hemorrhage.

In persistent nosebleed the person should be put flat, preferably with the face down. Ice water or hot water may be applied to the nose or the nose may be temporarily packed with sterile gauze. If nosebleeds occur frequently, proper study of the blood and the tissues generally should be made to determine the cause.

Hemorrhage from the skin or from wounds may be prevented by avoiding the sources of injuries that produce hemorrhage. All broken glass, razor blades, or sharp instruments should be carefully put away so that children particularly cannot get at them. Tools with sharp edges should be used with the greatest of care. All sharp knives and other sharp utensils should be kept in a special drawer with the handles pointing in one direction. Among the most frequent causes of cuts on the hands is carelessness in opening cans. The use of a proper can opener will prevent a jagged edge on the can.

HEMORRHOIDS Hemorrhoids, or piles, are actually varicose veins that occur at the lower end of the bowel. Doctors estimate that at least one third of all grown people have hemorrhoids.

Hemorrhoids can be classified into two kinds—external and internal, depending on whether they are inside or outside the muscular ring that closes the lower end of the bowel.

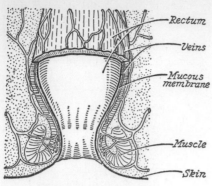

Fig. 1—The structure of the rectum and anus

Among the many causes of hemorrhoids are any kind of condition which interferes with the proper flow of blood in these blood vessels. Therefore an extremely sedentary life, the development of overweight, pregnancy, constipation, or the excess use of cathartics may be associated with the appearance of such varicose veins. The most that can be done to prevent the occurrence is the opposite of the things that are associated with the cause. People who are sedentary must get more exercise. Those in whom the circulation is poor should do what can be done to improve the circulation. Overweight is benefited

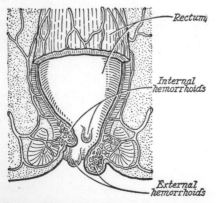

Fig. 2—Distinction between internal and external hemorrhoids

by weight reduction. It is known, however, that many irritant substances, such as vinegar, spices, coffee, and tobacco, help to increase congestion in the blood vessels at the end of the bowel. Also much can be done to prevent the blocking that comes from hardened material in the rectum. The bowel movements may be made regular by practicing good habits, and softness may be encouraged by the use of small amounts of mineral oil.

Hemorrhoids become painful when the blood in a dilated vein becomes clotted. This occurs when the person concerned has been sitting for a long time or when he has been using violent cathartics. There may also be secondary infections in the area where the hemorrhoids are present. Secondary infection with the fungi of the type that cause athlete's foot will produce severe itching. Indeed this itching may become of such torment that people actually scratch and tear their tissues to get relief. The more damage that is done in this way, the more likelihood is there for spread of the infection.

Occasionally hemorrhoids inside the circular muscular ring will be pushed through at the time when the bowels have an action. They are then called protruding hemorrhoids. If these blood vessels are scratched or broken by straining, the dilated veins will bleed until the blood clots. Then the hemorrhoids are called bleeding hemorrhoids. The quacks and the people who sell remedies for treating these conditions have a great deal to say about itching, bleeding, and protruding hemorrhoids. When hemorrhoids get to the point where they are simply intolerable, most people are willing to have them treated by surgical care. There are innumerable ointments, suppositories, and other preparations that can be applied to hemorrhoids to relieve the symptoms that have been mentioned; such relief is, however, frequently only temporary rather than permanent. Surgical control, whether done by the kind of injection that is used for varicose veins elsewhere in the body or by electric coagulation or by removal with the knife, is a matter for special consideration.

HEPATITIS, INFECTIOUS A virus infection of the liver, formerly called catarrhal jaundice. Treated with rest, protein diet, and gamma globulin.

HEREDITY Our bodies are a reflection of our inheritance from our ancestors. A special branch of science, which deals with the origins of man, the kind of material from which he is constructed, and the effects of his constitution on his life, is known as the science of genetics.

The belief that thoughts held by a prospective mother may induce changes in the body of her child is not borne out by any facts. There is good evidence, however, that the color of the hair and its form—whether curly or straight—the pigmentation of the skin and color of the eyes are characteristics that are inherited to a considerable extent by the child through his father and mother. Tall parents are likely to have tall children, and short parents to have short children. However, each of us is the accumulated result not only of factors coming from the mother and father but also from their mothers and fathers and even further back. Occasionally a child will represent apparently far more of some ancestor two or three generations previous than of the immediate ancestors.

We inherit a type of constitution which seems to make some of us more susceptible than others to certain diseases. People do not inherit tuberculosis. The germ of the disease must be present before it can occur in the human body. Inheritance in cancer is of the same type. Conditions of marriage among human beings are such, however, that the control of cancer by the control of marriage is hardly feasible. Many an old-time novelist and dramatist created an absorbing plot by presupposing that every family that shamefacedly admitted it included a drunkard had in it a hereditary strain of drunkenness.

Modern students of heredity say that there is no proof of the inheritance of a strain of drunkenness. It has been said that fat parents are likely to have fat children because the parents eat too much and the children imitate the parents. Conceivably the tendency to drink alcohol can be begun in much the same manner.

Certain mental characteristics may be inherited, as for example musical memory or memory in general.

What the child inherits is not a series of fixed traits or characteristics but a multitude of substances called genes which interact with each other to produce certain characteristics in the organism. When it is realized that a great variety of such genes enter into combination, it is not at all surprising that several children in one family will differ greatly from one another. The chances in the combinations are tremendous.

Among the constitutional diseases in which heredity seems to play a part, the tendency to allergies or sensitivities to various protein substances should be mentioned. The condition called hemophilia, the tendency to bleed, which was inherited in the royal families of Russia and Spain, is transmitted to the sons of the families by the mothers, who did not themselves suffer from the disease. Some forms of mental defect may be inherited because of the inheritance of the wrong structure of the brain, exactly as high qualities of brain tissue may be inherited. Many a state now has laws which control the propagation of persons who are insane, mentally defective, or possessed of other characteristics which might be passed on to their children.

HERMAPHRODITISM A hermaphrodite is a person who has or appears to have both male and female characteristics. Modern research shows that these cases vary from cases in which the organs of one side are male and the other female to those in which the sexual organs are predominantly female with some of the characteristics of the male and vice versa. Sometimes the external organs are female and the outer male, and vice versa. Such cases are treated successfully with glandular products, surgery, and psychotherapy combined.

HERNIA The examination of millions for entrance into the United States armed forces has focused attention particularly on rupture as a cause for rejection. A rupture is merely the protrusion of the contents of the abdomen through a weak place in the abdominal wall. There may, however, also be ruptures at other portions of the body, as in the groin or even in the back.

When the tissues underneath the surface force their way through an opening in the body wall a lump appears. Certain portions of the wall of the body are weaker than others. One of the weak spots is in the midline between the large muscles that pass between the breastbone downward toward the groin. Another common spot for a rupture is in the groin itself at the bottom of the abdominal cavity. Still another place for a rupture is in the sex organs.

There are many different causes for ruptures. Sometimes they are present at birth. Frequently the pressure inside the abdominal cavity is increased in an attempt to lift a heavy object. Occasionally an athlete will strain in competition and a rupture will apear. Occasionally ruptures are associated with excessive fat. Sometimes also they occur from failure of the tissues to heal properly after a surgical operation.

Many people who have small ruptures obtain relief by wearing a truss or a support which holds the tissues in place and, if the person concerned is young enough, may give opportunity for healing. However, a hernia or rupture that has been present for a long time is more likely to increase in size, if it is not properly controlled, rather than to heal. As the tissues inside push out more and more, the opening is enlarged, so that eventually the tissues may completely fill the opening. Then the walls of the opening may so constrict or press upon the tissues inside that the blood

flow stops. When this occurs, the hernia is said to be strangulated. The stopping of the blood supply to any tissue is exceedingly serious because the tissues will die without a blood supply. Therefore the tissue that is pushed through may become gangrenous or secondarily infected, at which time, of course, the condition threatens life itself.

The treatment of hernia naturally depends on the place where the hernia is located and on the technic decided upon by the doctor. He may wish, although this is rare, merely to push back the material and to apply a support. Such treatment is tried only in very small babies and is seldom recommended in older people. In older people the methods of treatment usually include the permanent wearing of a support, the injection method, or surgery. The decision as to the method to be employed must obviously be made on the basis of the condition that exists in each case.

The injection method aims to produce irritation of the separated tissues so that they will heal together. This method does not have the certainty that is associated with surgical care.

In the surgical method the tissues are observed during operation and the stitching is placed in such a way as to bring about healing. The operative method for the treatment of hernia is exact. The risk is relatively slight, particularly since the operation is often done nowadays without a general anesthetic. If the patient will consent to remain in bed for anywhere from ten to fifteen days so that healing occurs completely, there is little if any chance that the operation will not be completely successful.

Improvement in surgical procedures involves the use of metallic woven material which integrates with the tissues.

An unusual form of hernia is diaphragmatic, with a weak spot in the muscle between the chest and the abdomen.

HERPES SIMPLEX The common name for ordinary herpes is cold sores or fever blisters. Everybody knows what a cold sore looks like. It is usually just an accumulation of blisters, most frequently around the lips. However, any part of the skin may be affected. Frequently cold sores are associated with infectious diseases like pneumonia, malaria, and meningitis. Indeed 40 per cent of all such cases develop fever blisters.

Often a sensation of heat and burning will be followed by the development of a lot of small blisters containing clear serum. Later the small blisters may run together. Then the large blister breaks and a crust forms, followed by healing in a few days.

Another favorite site for fever blisters is the genital area. The possibility of secondary infection in this area is more common and occasionally the blisters may be filled with infected material or blood.

Most experts today believe that cold sores represent a reaction which comes primarily through the nervous system but which may be induced by a variety of causes. Sometimes these causes are physical changes like the rays of the sun, a draft of cold air, or simple rubbing. In other instances an infection may be concerned, as has already been mentioned. The simple cold sores frequently occur in women at the time of menstruation.

Obviously there is little that can be done to prevent cold sores. Fortunately, however, they tend to be self-limited and in most instances should disappear, recurring at intervals. Such danger as they represent is associated with the possibility of secondary infection. There is also, of course, the chance that women particularly will become much too seriously concerned about them and overtreat them, using all sorts of astringent lotions, covering ointments and, even worse, constantly picking off the crusts. The ordinary camphorated ointment or other similar care that the dermatologist prescribes is sufficient in most instances to keep the condition under control until it disappears.

HERPES ZOSTER See *Shingles.*

HICCUPS Way back in the days of Plato, who lived about four hundred years before the Christian Era, a Greek was talking to another Greek who was suffering with hiccups. He said, "Let me advise you to hold your breath, and if this fails, then to gargle with a little water, and if the hiccups still continue, tickle your nose with something and sneeze, and if you sneeze once or twice even the most violent hiccup is sure to go."

Now more than two thousand years have passed and people still treat hiccups first with these measures.

Hiccups are due to a spasm or constriction of the diaphragm, the large muscle that separates the abdominal cavity from the chest cavity. When the diaphragm constricts, the nerve that shuts off the breathing tube from the throat (called the glottis) is closed. Ordinarily the motions of the glottis opening and closing are co-ordinated with the activities of breathing, so that breathing takes place noiselessly. Anything that disturbs the co-ordination can cause a hiccup.

The causes of hiccups include naturally anything that can bring about a failure of co-ordination in the action of the nerves and muscles involved in breathing. A sudden distention of the stomach will disturb the action of the diaphragm and bring on hiccups. An irritation of the center in the brain which is connected by a nerve with the diaphragm can set up a contraction of the diaphragm and hiccups. Trouble along the nerve which controls the diaphragm can also produce hiccups. Finally, hiccups may be associated with nervousness, worry, anxiety, shock, or accidents, since we now recognize the close relationship between the mind and the body and realize the possibility that an emotional cause can be reflected in a physical reaction.

Among the popular treatments for hiccups in addition to coughing, sneezing, swallowing ice, vinegar, or cold water, we include pulling on the tongue, pressing the upper lip with the finger, and breathing into a paper bag so that the breath is reinhaled. The reinhaling of the breath fills the body with carbon dioxide and thus stimulates breathing.

When, however, hiccups persist to the point of exhaustion, more serious remedies must be used. In such cases it may be necessary to try narcotic drugs, to inject potent remedies, to anesthetize the patient, or even to operate.

A new drug called chlorpromazine or Thorazene has been used successfully in treating persistent hiccups.

Since hiccups may have both physical and mental factors study is required to determine just which causes are concerned and to treat the patient accordingly.

Among other technics that occasionally work doctors mention the use of an icebag on the neck, the spraying of ethyl chloride as a refrigerant on the front of the abdomen, slight pressure on the eyeballs, and pressure on the ribs near the place where the diaphragm is fastened.

HIVES The hive is also called a wheal and is a manifestation of a condition that is known technically as urticaria. Abscesses sometimes develop by secondary infection, however. Wheals develop after insect bites, and conditions like hives are associated with poison ivy. A common name for the hives is nettle rash.

Usually hives follow the eating of certain foods to which people are sensitive, like shellfish, pork, nuts, mushrooms, cucumbers, or indeed any one of a variety of foods. Sometimes hives are caused by reactions to light, heat, cold, or scratching, to which a person may be sensitive, the common belief being that these physical conditions bring about changes in the chemistry of the skin so that absorption of certain substances produces the reaction of hives.

Some people have a much more sensitive skin than others. The sensitivity of the skin may be indicated by a phenomenon that the doctors call dermographism, which means simply that it is possible to write on the skin with pressure. Thus the drawing of a pencil point or a fingernail along the skin will be followed by the appearance of an elevated area which, if sufficiently severe, is actually like a hive.

There are many different varieties of urticaria, so that doctors call them acute, chronic, recurrent, or persistent. Sometimes a crop of hives appears and goes away within three or four days, only to be followed by the appearance of new crops. Fortunately most hives tend to disappear in time, but people will scratch them, irritate them, or infect them, so that they may be much more serious than they would be if merely palliated or let alone. If the doctor can find out, with the aid of the person who is affected, the special substance to which the person responds with hives and then eliminate that from the diet, the hives are kept under control. A new technic is to desensitize the person with gradually increasing doses of the extract of the protein concerned. Particularly useful for hives are the new antihistaminic drugs like pyribenzamine and benadryl. In the treatment of intractable urticaria, Cortisone and ACTH have proved successful.

In very serious cases of hives the symptoms are aided by stopping foods, cleansing the intestinal tract, and using applications directly on the skin of lotions which contain substances that help to control the itching. Most specialists in diseases of the skin prefer lotions to ointments. Some, however, like powders rather than lotions. The advantage of the powder is the part that it plays in keeping the area dry, while allaying the itching.

Garments that produce much warmth of the skin and perspiration are certainly to be avoided in the presence of hives, since they will tend to increase the amount of the eruption and irritation of the broken blisters.

HOARSENESS (See also *Laryngitis*) When the human voice suddenly assumes a pitch well below that to which its user has become accustomed, the condition is called hoarseness. Usually such a sign means that the cords in the larynx, or voice box, which vibrate during speaking, have become inflamed. In most instances mere rest and discontinuance of the use of the voice will bring about improvement. However, hoarseness occasionally persists. Continuous hoarseness demands an immediate, direct examination of the vocal cords and of the larynx by a physician who specializes in such conditions. There should, moreover, be a complete physical examination to determine the presence of any constitutional disease.

The vocal cords must come together properly or the voice will not be normal. They must be under proper tension and they must vibrate properly. Therefore any factor that produces swelling and inflammation of the vocal cords may so damage them that they will not work as they should.

Among the dangerous conditions that may interefere with the proper use of the vocal cords are tuberculosis, cancer, and syphilis. However, the most frequent causes are simple infections with the kind of germs that cause sore throat and colds.

Singers who use the voice too freely for long periods of time sometimes develop small nodules on the cords. The result is hoarseness. Means have been found for controlling the development of such singers' nodes. Businessmen frequently complain of hoarseness after long conversations associated with excessive eating, drinking, and smoking. The throats and vocal cords of some people are especially sensitive to various ingredients of tobacco smoking. People with intelligence soon learn to associate attacks of hoarseness with excessive smoking or with other determinable factors. Then if they are really intelligent, they discontinue the exposures.

The voice is also modified by infection in the nose and in the sinuses. Under such circumstances it develops a nasal twang or tone. Frequently treatment of the nose will take care of the condition and at the same time elimi-

nate the continued infection in the vocal cords.

Fortunately the venereal diseases are now being controlled by new remedies like penicillin and terramycin.

Tuberculosis of the throat, if seen early, may be treated not only as tuberculosis elsewhere in the body but also by direct application of ultraviolet rays.

If a cancer of the larynx is seen early, it may be removed early and in many instances may be treated successfully with radium. Already there are many reports of the saving of life when it was threatened by cancer of the larynx. However, the most important single step is early diagnosis so that proper treatment may be administered before the condition can spread too freely.

HODGKIN'S DISEASE In 1852 an English doctor named Thomas Hodgkin first described a disease in which the lymph glands of the throat, the spleen, and the tonsils become swollen and remain swollen, thus differing from the kind of inflammation that occurs when there is an infection by the ordinary types of germs. Because there are so many other conditions that may cause swelling of the lymph glands, the condition called Hodgkin's disease is sometimes overlooked in its early stages. The cause of Hodgkin's disease is still unknown. The only way that the doctor can be certain that the disease is actually Hodgkin's disease is to take out a piece of the lymph gland and examine it under the microscope. This is not too difficult when the glands are near the surface of the body.

Hodgkin's disease occurs about twice as often in men as in women. Whereas it may develop at any age, the largest number of patients are young adults between the ages of twenty and thirty.

The first symptom of Hodgkin's disease is frequently just a painless enlargement of the gland on one side of the neck. However, this spreads to the other side of the neck and to glands elsewhere in the body. Persistence of the swelling is the vital factor that differentiates Hodgkin's disease from other glandular enlargements.

The average person with Hodgkin's disease lives two or three years after the earliest symptoms are noted, since it is a form of malignant swelling of the lymph glands. In rare cases people have survived for ten to fifteen years. Instances are on record of patients who have lived for seven years and of one patient who lived fifteen years after a positive diagnosis of Hodgkin's disease had been made.

Unfortunately a specific method for treating Hodgkin's disease has not yet been discovered. However, experimentation goes on and new technics are being developed which offer encouragement. At present the methods of treatment most in use include radium and X ray. The irradiation is applied to the enlarged glands, particularly those in the neck. The use of X ray or radium reduces the size of the tumor masses and thus controls much of the discomfort as well as the pain that comes from pressure of the swellings on the nerves. From time to time experiments have been made in the use of vaccines, arsenic, iron, liver extracts, and blood transfusions. Experiments are now being made with the use of what are called radioactive isotopes, and with chemical substances derived from war gases. Aminopterin, which is an anti-folic acid, is also being tried.

HOMOSEXUALITY Homosexuality is a condition in which sexual attraction is toward persons of the same sex rather than the opposite sex. Female homosexuality is known as lesbianism.

HORMONES Hormones are chemical substances which are produced in some of the organs of the body and then transported by the blood to other areas where they produce specific effects. Hormones are secreted by most of the glands of the body.

HYDROCEPHALUS (See *Spina Bifida*) Water on the brain.

HYGIENE, PERSONAL (See also discussion under *Clothing*) Doctors are often asked to supply a simple set of rules for health. Many years ago at Salerno, Italy, there was a medical school which published a list of rules for health known as the regimen of the school of Salerno. One of the most important lines in that regimen was one which said that three doctors were necessary for health—namely, Dr. Diet, Dr. Merryman, and Dr. Quiet. In other words, proper understanding of food, a good mental attitude, and plenty of rest are the very basis of good hygiene.

One set of rules, developed by Irving Fisher and E. L. Fisk in their book called *How to Live,* gives sixteen important recommendations. They are:

AIR

1. Ventilate every room you occupy.
2. Wear light, loose, and porous clothes.
3. Seek outdoor occupations and recreation.
4. Sleep outdoors if you can.

FOOD

5. Avoid overeating and overweight.
6. Avoid excess of high-protein foods, such as flesh foods, eggs; also excess of salt and highly seasoned foods.
7. Eat some hard, some bulky, some raw foods daily.
8. Eat slowly and taste your food.
9. Use sufficient water internally and externally.

POISONS

10. Secure thorough intestinal elimination more than once daily.
11. Stand, sit, and walk erect.
12. Do not allow poisons and infections to enter the body.
13. Keep the teeth, gums, and tongue clean.

ACTIVITY

14. Work, play, rest, and sleep in moderation.

15. Take deep-breathing exercises several times a day.

16. Keep serene and wholehearted.

Concerning two of these there might be some doubt. Most competent observers of the human body would disagree with No. 10. They would say that the majority of people get along rather well with only one elimination of the bowel daily or perhaps at most two. It was the concept of Fisher and Fisk that repeated eliminations were desirable.

Rule No. 15 suggests that deep-breathing exercises be practiced several times each day. Most experts would consider this a health fad. There is no doubt that thorough ventilation of the lungs is desirable, but ordinary breathing does well for thorough ventilation. Careful studies that have been made on marathon runners have not shown that excessive breathing, in which they must indulge in practice, improves their ability to breathe or improves their "wind" beyond that of people generally.

Dr. Alfred Worcester of the Harvard Medical School emphasized four factors as most important for the health of the aged. These are more warmth, more rest, less strenuous work, and less food.

Finally, the one word on which most emphasis must be placed in personal hygiene is cleanliness. Frequent washing of the hands and a bath at least once daily are now recognized as essential to good health.

Assume that you are in good physical condition and that your doctor has made a complete physical examination and found nothing that needs to be corrected. You probably want to know how to conduct yourself so as to avoid disease in the future. Certain health habits are conducive to the maintenance of good health.

As I have observed people over a good many years, I have found that most of them incline to pick some single point on which to put emphasis in relation to the maintenance of health— exercise, rest, bathing, or diet. From the point of view of good general health

with relation to the prevention of infections, most doctors would emphasize cleanliness as the number one point for maintaining health. Cleanliness means more than just bathing. Everyone ought to take a bath, if possible, at least once each day. There are great varieties of baths—hot, cold, warm, steam, carbonated water, and other baths. The moderately warm bath cleanses the body, draws the blood to the surface, increases perspiration, and has a soothing effect. Bathing in very hot water may be dangerous, particularly to persons not in the best of health. A cold bath taken in the morning stimulates the nerve endings in the skin and drives the blood from the surface, to which it returns with a rush when the person emerges from the bath and has a rubdown with a towel. Cold-bath fanatics who submit themselves to exposure unduly with the notion that they will in this manner harden themselves against catching cold are simply indulging in a notion. There is no good evidence that the taking of a cold bath every morning is an effective protection against colds. One way to take a cold bath with a reasonable amount of safety is to fill the tub with water, step in, sit down, immerse the body completely and promptly step out again. A cold bath is preferably taken under a shower.

Baths in which all sorts of materials are placed have little effect, since few materials are absorbed through the skin. The chief value of salt-water bathing is credited to the air, the breeze, the sunlight, and the buffeting of the waves. Sea salt in bags thrown into a tub does not carry with it the sunlight, the buffeting of the waves, the brisk ocean breezes, running and playing on the beach, or the pleasures of conversation with the surrounding company.

Hot vapor baths stimulate excretion of material through the pores of the skin. They are not especially health-inducing for the normal person and should be considered a special bath to be taken only when recommended by the doctor.

All human society may be divided

into classes according to bathing habits. The hygienic person bathes daily and sometimes includes a cold bath in the morning and a cleansing warm bath at night. The average person seems to be one who bathes every three days whether he needs it or not. Finally, there are the Saturday-night bathers, who are limited in their conveniences to a galvanized iron tub and the water they can carry in a bucket.

In addition to bathing the body as a whole, good personal hygiene demands some attention to the cleanliness of various special portions of the human body.

Hand-to-mouth infection is one of the most common causes of illness. Many of the early religious bodies incorporated washing of the hands into religious ritual in order to make certain that people would thus protect themselves against the danger of infection. Thorough washing of the hands before eating and after attending to excretion of material from the body is recognized as the most important step in all hygienic practice. Washing of the hands can, of course, be made a fetish, so that people rush to the washroom on the slightest appearance of soiling. More important is the decision, however, to keep the fingers out of the nose, mouth, ears, or other openings into the body. With the minimum amount of washing of the hands, there would be the following: On arising, before and after meals, before and after attending to the excretions of the body, before going to bed and whenever there is exceptional soiling. Finally, the hands should always be washed thoroughly whenever one has been in contact with infection of any kind.

It is customary also to clean the teeth with a brush and a suitable paste, powder, or other material at least twice a day—on arising and before going to bed. Some people, however, find it necessary to give more attention to the teeth than this minimum, particularly those who have artificial dentures or plates. They may find it necessary to practice washing of the teeth and of the artificial dentures on more frequent occasions.

The use of a mouth wash or gargle accomplishes little beyond the actual washing that takes place, so that most physicians are inclined to attach little value to using medicated mouth washes or gargles. Strong solutions should be used on the advice of the physician or dentist only.

The third type of cleanliness to which attention often is called is internal washing of the body such as is brought about through the taking of cathartic substances that cause fluid to be poured into the bowel—the so-called saline cathartics or salts—and the use of enemas for washing out the bowel from below. The routine use of enemas is unnecessary for a person in a healthful state. Such enemas should never be used unless prescribed for a special purpose by the doctor. Neither should saline cathartics be taken except with the advice of the doctor, since the harm that they may do by establishing habits is greater than the good that they may accomplish through sweeping waste material out of the body.

Finally, there is the cleaning of the fingernails, which all intelligent persons practice regularly. Nothing gives greater indication of body carelessness than the mourning bands carried at the tips of the fingers. This does not mean that everyone must have a professional manicure at frequent intervals. The cuticle may be pressed back, perhaps twice weekly, with an orangewood stick and may be softened by the application of some bland oil or vaseline. In all manicuring cleanliness is of the utmost importance. Before receiving the manicure, the person should wash the hands thoroughly with soap with a good deal of lather, using hot water and a nail brush. The manicurist who has just finished a manicure of some other person should treat her hands to the same process. All instruments used in manicuring should be suitably sterilized. When the manicurist cuts too deeply and bleeding occurs, it should be controlled by pressure with dry sterilized gauze and not by the application of a styptic pencil or surgical powder. Suitable antiseptics should be applied under these circumstances.

The nose, eyes, and ears do not demand routine washing with medicated solutions or indeed in any other way except when they are giving trouble. In such cases the attention should be regulated by the doctor.

Cleaning of the ear should never be practiced with a rigid instrument of any kind. Doctors prefer syringing with lukewarm water, directing the stream toward the side of the opening, so that pressure will not be directly against the eardrum.

The care of the eyes is largely automatic, since the eye is self-adjusting and self-lubricating. There is no need for the constant use of eyewashes, eyedrops, eye salves, or any other medicines. The use of such preparations is likely to do more harm than good. Nothing should ever be put into the eye except on the advice of a competent oculist. The popular eyewashes that are advertised, applied in barbershops and beauty shops, represent merely a solution of borax, costing about five cents a gallon to prepare and retailing at one dollar an ounce. Occasionally a few drops of some other medication are added, without, however, producing any effect whose specific virtue is required by the eye.

WORRY—Assuming that a person is in good physical health as shown by a suitable examination, one of the most important suggestions that can be made from the point of view of general health is to keep calm. Without being able to measure exactly the amount of damage that may be done to the human body by worry, high tension, or irritation, the experience of centuries has shown that these factors play a definite part in the onset of disease. Nowadays that branch of medicine which gives special attention to such relationships is known as psychosomatic medicine. Many years ago, however, worry was listed as a contributing cause to high blood pressure, hardening of the arteries, diabetes, and many degenerative diseases. Worry plays a part in the causation of such diseases by the secondary effects that it exerts on the circulation of the blood and on the other tissues of the body.

The expert in the treatment of mental diseases attempts to find out the primary cause of the worry or mental distress, to inform the person about it, and to make him realize its relation to his physical condition. Healers of various faith-healing systems rid the patient of worry by providing him with a substitute or by concentrating his attention on a system. Coué did it by having the person say over and over, "Every day, in every way, I am becoming better and better." The intelligent person, realizing his troubles, will do better to say to himself that he has realized and that he will no longer fear his trouble or avoid it. Nothing is gained by telling a person who worries that he must not worry. Emphasis on the situation serves only to cause such a person to concentrate still more on the problem. In fact a person can get to the point where he worries as much about worrying as he worries about the original cause of the worrying.

As a result of the war people have suffered more mental anxiety than ordinarily. From the point of view of mental health war brings both dangers and comforts. The American people's reaction to war has always been one of confidence and of union and of faith in the future of the nation. The fellowship of a common objective binds people together in courage and resolution. Mental wounds, however, tend to be repressed and to be buried under the surface. Experts in psychiatry are of the firm belief that repression and burying of mental problems do not relieve them but intensify them.

HYGIENE OF CLOTHING (See also *Clothing*)—Few people are enough disturbed about their health to select clothing primarily with a view to its healthful features. Style plays a greater part than any other factor in the selection of wearing apparel. Many of the styles are at times detrimental to health, but people wear them just the same.

From the hygienic point of view clothing should protect against cold and permit diffusion of heat by circulation of air in warm weather. Moisture must not be permitted to collect on the body surface, where it may macerate the skin and open the way for infection. Accumulated perspiration tends to produce a disagreeable odor.

Woolen clothing has the value of warmth and takes up perspiration. Woolens are especially desirable as wear for winter.

Modern women workers seem to make little provision for changes from the hot season to the cold. Hence offices are customarily overheated to meet the needs of women, with the result that men workers, who wear heavier clothing, are more likely to suffer unduly with the heat and the dryness of the atmosphere.

Most unhygienic in relationship to clothing of all types are constrictions of various portions of the body. The garment of primitive man was usually a simple robe that covered the body and was suspended from the shoulders. The garments of modern man are suspended from any point of protuberance on the human body, and this means women too.

There was a time when men wore suspenders regularly to hold their trousers in a position both comfortable and modest. Nowadays belts have largely displaced suspenders, although many a conservative man indulges in both belt and suspenders. Presumably constrictions at the waist are undesirable, although good scientific evidence as to any harm being done by wearing a belt that is tight enough to hold up the trousers is not yet available.

Collars that are worn tight enough to constrict the neck may cause pounding noises in the ear and be associated with headache. Garters worn tight enough to constrict the blood vessels of the leg may be associated with varicose veins, pains in the feet, and swelling of the ankles. Healthful garters are worn loose and are made of a wide web; hence they are not likely to produce any serious harm.

Women have discarded the corsets that used to produce wasp waists. The modern girdle is made of an elastic material and is not unduly constrictive.

Constriction is especially not advisable during the childbearing period. Rubber garments of any type which do not permit satisfactory ventilation of the skin may cause maceration and infection.

Especially important also is the wearing of proper shoes and stockings. Stockings which do not fit well cause ingrown toenails, hammertoes, and bunions. Stockings that are too long form wrinkles, an uneven pressure, and irritate the skin. Stockings should always be changed daily. Shoes should fit well because cramping of the feet results in corns, calluses, and bunions.

PUBLIC AND PERSONAL HYGIENE—The hygienic functions that each of us must carry on for himself, such as washing the body and the teeth, using clean cooking utensils, and securing regular action of the bowels, are supplemented by other functions of hygiene that must be carried out by the community as a whole. These include the provision of pure water and food supplies, sewage disposal, education of the public in health, destruction of insect menaces to man, and of rats and other rodents, and the provision of pure air, good light, and safety during working hours. Every person can help the public health agencies in achieving these objectives.

Most of these activities are related to the prevention of the growth and spread of germs. Nobody's germs are his exclusive property. A cough, a sneeze, or a touch of the hand may transfer germs that will initiate epidemics. Each of us must be responsible for keeping his own germs within reasonable bounds.

Several authorities have from time to time outlined for the average person the routine of a healthful day. Here is a schedule which may be followed without developing overemphasis on any single aspect of healthful living.

1. Simple setting-up exercises upon

arising to loosen up muscles. Simply bending over eight or ten times or stretching the arms and legs will be sufficient for people of middle age.

2. Attention to activity of the bowels, which should be without laxatives.

3. Thorough washing of at least the hands and face in the morning, cleansing the teeth at the same time.

4. A breakfast, to be followed by at least two other meals during the day which will provide altogether the essentials of a balanced diet. Meals should be eaten with sufficient leisure in a quiet, restful place to provide the maximum of nutrition with relaxation.

5. Enough relaxation at various times during the day to relieve accumulated fatigue.

6. Some daily exercise, at least walking, in the open air.

7. Attention to some hobby or avocation that provides mental relaxation.

8. At least eight hours of sleep or rest in a well-ventilated room.

9. Full use of the week end and other holidays for relaxation rather than work.

10. A semiannual visit to a dentist for attention to the teeth.

11. A physical examination by a competent physician at least once a year.

HYMEN The hymen is a membrane, commonly called maidenhead, at the entrance to the female sex organs. The presence of this tissue is usually considered synonymous with virginity, although it may not be; likewise its absence is not to be considered certain evidence of loss of chastity.

HYPERHIDROSIS (See discussion under *Perspiration*) This is the scientific name for excessive sweating.

HYPERTENSION See *Blood Pressure, High.*

HYPERTHYROIDISM See *Goiter.*

HYPOCHONDRIASIS People who enjoy ill-health are unfortunate for themselves and for those around them. Even doctors, unfortunately, like to avoid them. Hypochondriasis, which is the term used for the condition in which people get pleasure out of ill-health, has been called the most foolish and at the same time the saddest of all diseases.

Seldom, if ever, is a human being perfectly healthy. Even those whose pictures are printed in the physical culture magazines, swelling their muscles, when carefully investigated, are found to have aches and pains. The vast majority of people have thresholds of irritation—that is to say, minor pains and aches do not too much disturb them. They pay little attention to these as long as they can do their daily work and be unaware of their bodies during both work and recreation. The hypochondriac is aware of his body at a threshold much lower than that of the average man. To the hypochondriac every cough is the threat of consumption. To a person who knows, a cough is just a symptom of some irritation in the breathing tract, and the vast majority of coughs, he knows, are not too serious.

Symptoms are the means by which nature warns us that something is wrong. The reaction of a normal person to any kind of symptom is not a reaction of alarm but merely the awareness of a signal for investigation. The intelligent person who hears a noise in the house at night knows in the vast majority of cases it is just the effect of the wind or the weather or the expansion or contraction of the furniture. The alarmist takes every sound as an invasion by burglars or the beginning of an explosion. The nervous system is, therefore, constantly subjected to a series of unhealthful shocks.

Most serious for the hypochondriac is fixation on some one or another organ of the human body. Thus there is a tendency for the person with hypochondriasis to fix the attention on the organs associated with childbirth, on the intestines, on the brain, or on the vision, and to begin to develop symptoms especially related to some one or another organ. The result is likely to be constant consultation with specialists and repeated trials of all sorts of unnecessary treatments. Because the mind is so definitely related to the functions of the organs, the hypochondriac who begins to fix his attention on his gastrointestinal tract can promptly develop such symptoms as loss of appetite, nausea, belching, fullness in the stomach, and distress after meals.

One of the greatest assets in overcoming fear is knowledge. Familiarity breeds contempt. The person who knows and can judge the relative importance of various signs and symptoms is not likely to be too easily alarmed.

HYPOTENSION See *Blood Pressure, Low.*

HYSTERECTOMY The five-syllable word "his-ter-ec'-tome-y" is a technical term that is used by the doctor for removal of the womb. The operation is performed by the gynecologist (a surgeon specializing in conditions affecting women) when he believes that the operation is desirable for the health of the woman or for the relief of conditions which may incapacitate her for her daily life. The operation may be done because of the presence of fibroid tumors, which may be responsible for irregular bleeding or for a variety of other disturbances.

Sometimes the physician at the time of removal of the uterus will also wish to remove either or both of the fallopian tubes, which carry the egg from the ovary to the uterus, and perhaps either or both of the ovaries, depending on their physical condition. If they do not show evidence of disease, the surgeon is not likely to remove them. Certainly he will not interfere with the function of the female sex glands, known as the ovaries, unless they are diseased by infection or by cysts, which are collections of fluid, or by tumors. The ovaries are one of the most important parts of the female glandular chain. Complete removal of the ovaries is followed by an artificial menopause. The symptoms associated with that may make it necessary for the surgeon to give female sex gland hormones for a long time until the body of the woman has become adjusted to the new conditions.

Several different surgical procedures are used by surgeons for removal of the uterus. Occasionally the operation is done through the lower opening of the body rather than through the abdomen. The decision as to the type of surgery to be done must rest with the gynecologist, who makes his decision on the basis of the conditions that exist in the individual woman.

Removal of the uterus alone will not bring about an artificial menopause, since the uterus is simply the organ in which the child lies before childbirth and is not concerned with supplying materials. Of course removal of the uterus does bring an end to the periodic flow, since the material comes from the uterus.

While many thousands of hysterectomies are now done each year in the United States, the operation is considered a major one in which anesthesia as well as residence in the hospital are necessary. Following the operation, time must be allowed for the tissues to grow together. The convalescence should include plenty of rest, avoidance of fatigue, avoidance of heavy lifting or climbing, and only moderate, light exercise.

Many women ask whether or not removal of the uterus will interfere in any way with the ordinary marital relations. The answer is that it will not interfere in the slightest, once healing has occurred.

HYSTERIA For hundreds of years doctors have recognized the nature of the condition commonly called hysteria. The average person believes that an individual is hysterical when he screams, tosses his arms and legs about, or, if it is a woman, breaks into a crying fit. This is not necessarily hysteria but may be simply what is better described as a tantrum. A child who has been frustrated will throw himself on the floor, kicking, hitting, and screaming. While this is not hysteria, it may be the preliminary step to a hysterical attack.

During hysterical conditions various functions of the human body are disordered. Many of the usual activities of everyday life are disturbed. Queer actions take place related to eating, sleeping, working, remembering, listening, or talking. In most cases the basis of hysteria is an emotional situation in which an illness or the imitation of illness is the only way in which the person concerned can get out of his trouble. So-called "shell shock" is a condition in which hysteria may develop. A soldier may, for instance, develop a paralysis that does not actually indicate a disease of the nerves to avoid going back to the front line. This is not deliberate malingering, it is actual mental disturbance. Disappointment in love affairs is frequently the form of emotional upset that brings about an attack of hysteria.

There is hardly any disease that hysteria may not imitate. The degree to which hysteria imitates a disease depends on the knowledge that the person affected has of that disease. Thus friends of the patient or even the doctor himself may suggest that certain symptoms are characteristic of a disease, whereupon the person concerned will promptly imitate those symptoms. Incidentally, a person who has hysteria often fails to go the complete limit in the performance. He may stumble and appear dizzy but will manage to save himself from a fall. A person who actually has dizziness or stumbles because of a tumor of the brain or a real physical condition will not be able to save himself from a fall.

The most important step in the cure of hysteria is the certainty of the diagnosis. Failure to detect a real physical condition and to call it hysterical is exceedingly serious for the patient. By psychologic study, by the use of persuasion and the power of suggestion, the physician is able in most instances to bring about relief from the symptoms of hysteria. Once the patient understands the basis of his disturbance, there is likely to be a sudden and what has sometimes been called a miraculous cure. The physician understands that the cure of a psychologic disturbance in this manner is just as scientific as the cure of a physical condition. He is unlikely to claim a miracle. However, many a charlatan has made a reputation on the sudden cure of blindness, paralysis, loss of hearing, inability to swallow, or some other unusual symptom that was wholly hysterical.

ICHTHYOL This is the proprietary name for sulfonated coal tar. It has been used particularly in the treatment of conditions affecting the skin. Nowadays it is little used in medicine because of the development of remedies known to have specific action.

ICHTHYOSIS Babies are sometimes born with a skin that is dry, rough, and scaly like that of a fish. The condition is also called fishskin disease. The exact cause is not known. There is a tendency nowadays to believe that it is due to deficiencies in the diet.

ICTERUS See *Jaundice.*

IMMUNIZATION During the first six months of his life a child usually has in his blood, derived from his mother, substances which aid him to resist certain infections. After the sixth month, however, the infant stops nursing in most cases. Until this age the baby comes little into contact with other people. After this age he begins to be exposed to the infections that other people have. Therefore, as a means of protecting children against the infectious diseases to which they are so regularly exposed, modern medical science has developed a routine of immunization.

At about nine months of age children should be vaccinated against smallpox. The vaccination is usually made in the upper part of the left arm or on the outer side of the left leg above the knee. Most physicians still prefer to vaccinate on the arm. Occasionally, however, mothers feel that a girl baby is bound to be sooner or later an actress or an opera star and therefore prefer to have the vaccination done where it will not show. In view of the nature of modern swimming and ballroom costumes, there is no certainty that the vaccination will not show except in an exceedingly restricted area of the human epidermis.

By the twelfth month children should be protected against diphtheria. Such protection is achieved by inoculating the child with a substance called diphtheria toxoid. This is usually injected into the loose tissue of the arms or legs, occasionally into the buttocks or the abdominal wall. Most doctors nowadays use a two-dose toxoid, giving the two injections about ten days apart. Usually a child begins to develop within his blood resistance against diphtheria almost immediately after the injection and after a period of four months will have developed enough of such materials to protect him against diphtheria for some time.

Inoculations are also available against lockjaw, or tetanus. All of the soldiers in the United States Army are inoculated against tetanus and smallpox. Tetanus is so serious that doctors generally recommend the use of inoculation against this condition whenever a child has had a cutting injury or been in some way damaged by fireworks or explosives, or indeed whenever there is the possibility that a cut has been contaminated with soil, clothing, or other materials.

Scarlet fever is another disease against which it is possible to immunize the child. Physicians for the most part, however, do not immunize against scarlet fever unless there happens to be an epidemic in the community or in an institution where the child is exposed to the disease.

Many physicians use blood from persons who have recovered from whooping cough to immunize babies against whooping cough. The most modern approved technic includes the use of vaccines.

A technic has been developed for inoculation against measles, using a substance called gamma globulin. The gamma globulin is derived from the blood, which is made available through the vast amounts of blood now being contributed for blood transfusions. Antisubstances against measles, poliomyelitis, and hepatitis are carried by this gamma globulin.

Immunization against typhoid and the paratyphoid infections can be had whenever there is an outbreak of this condition in any community.

The Salk vaccine is an efficient preparation for raising resistance to infantile paralysis and for maintaining it at a high level.

New technics are also available by which a child can be immunized at one time against several infectious conditions. The decision as to when to use the individual or the combined immunization must be left to the physician who has the responsibility for the care of the child.

IMPETIGO Among the contagious conditions that affect the skin impetigo is frequent. In this condition the skin is covered with blisters, often filled with infectious material or pus, intermingled with the dry crusts or other blisters that have broken. Should these crusts be removed, a reddened, moist surface is found below. Occasionally the impetigo spreads from the face, where it is most frequent, to the hands or other portions of the body.

Usually impetigo is transferred from one person to another by the fingernails or hands, which carry the streptococci and staphylococci, both pus-forming germs. The condition is frequently transferred from one child to another during playtime. Women occasionally get the disease from children, but in men the most frequent source of infection is the barbershop. Not infrequently also men get their skin contaminated on wrestling mats or from boxing gloves or other athletic apparatus.

Sometimes the infected spots dry up quickly, but in other instances they become secondarily infected and result in boils or abscesses. After impetigo becomes established, it is much more difficult to treat than when the condition has first appeared.

With proper treatment the average case will clear up in one or two weeks.

For the prevention of this infection it is necessary to avoid the possibility of contamination with infectious material from people who have the disease. People who are infected should always use a separate washcloth, towel, and similar personal articles. If a case occurs in a school child, the child should be excluded from contact with other children until he has recovered. Those who have the condition should always be warned against scratching themselves; they contaminate their fingers. Thus infection is spread from one person to another.

Incidentally, children who happen to be infested with lice or with the itch mite sometimes get impetigo on top of the other condition. This means that both conditions must be treated simultaneously, since the combination causes both conditions to persist.

Formerly impetigo was treated with various antiseptic substances. Nowadays it has been found that the sulfonamide drugs are especially useful in controlling infections with the germs that cause impetigo. Moreover, the latest information indicates that ointments containing penicillin also have an almost specific effect against infections with impetigo. Such materials as the sulfonamides and penicillin must, of course, be prescribed by the physician before they are used.

INDIGESTION Among the most common of human complaints is indigestion. It is also a relative term because often symptoms called indigestion represent ulcers of the stomach or duodenum or occasionally disturbances of the gall bladder and in some cases actually difficulty in digesting food. The old term "dyspepsia" really means pain accompanying functioning of the digestive processes regardless of the cause. Of course there may be pain due to arthritis, gall-bladder disease, or other conditions not directly related to the digestion of food. This must be differentiated from dyspepsia.

What happens when food is swallowed? It passes down the esophagus or gullet into the stomach. The stomach was characterized long ago as a mixing vat. Actually digestion begins in the stomach. The saliva that is secreted helps to stimulate digestion. The pepsin and hydrochloric acid of the stomach help to soften the food and then the stomach passes it along into the first portion of the intestines. This is called the duodenum. The name comes from the Latin word for twelve. The duodenum is about twelve finger-breadths long. In the duodenum the food is mixed with bile from the liver and with another digestive juice that is produced by the pancreas. The pancreas also produces insulin which digests sugars. The insulin, however, goes directly from the pancreas into the blood. As the food passes along, digestion is completed and the digested material is picked up by the blood and carried through the body. People wonder why the stomach does not digest itself but there are means by which the glandular tissues on the inside of the stomach are protected against the acid and the pepsin. In cases of ulcers of the stomach, when the living tissues in the inside of the stomach have been damaged the acid can produce constant irritation and burning.

Symptoms of Indigestion—The chief symptoms of indigestion are pain in the neighborhood of the stomach or in the lower part of the chest and sometimes in the back. There may be belching and even vomiting of food. These symptoms are not due to the fact that the food is failing to be digested. They are actually due to irritation of the lining of the stomach by the acid in the stomach juice. This acid, as has already been explained, will not hurt a healthy stomach. It may seriously damage a stomach in which the lining has been injured. People with indigestion take alkaline substances like bicarbonate of soda. These neutralize the acid and thus help to relieve the pain. The stomach may be emptied by vomiting, thus relieving the stomach of the acid and stopping the pain.

Ulcers of the stomach are exceedingly serious since they may perforate. When an ulcer perforates, a hole is formed in the stomach or duodenum and the material gets out into the abdominal cavity. For perforation of the stomach or duodenum there is just one proper treatment and that is surgical operation to sew up the hole and stop the leakage. Occasionally an ulcer will eat its way into a blood vessel. Then a hemorrhage occurs. The blood may be vomited from the stomach or may pass along through the bowel. Then the material excreted from the bowel appears black and shiny like tar.

Experts in conditions affecting the stomach and intestines recommend that every symptom of indigestion be treated promptly. This is one way to prevent the formation of ulcers. The treatment includes methods that soothe the injured lining and permit the living tissues of the body to heal themselves. If such methods of treatment do not bring about healing of the ulcer, various surgical operations have been developed which permit removal of the ulcer and repair of the tissue. One operation involves the cutting of the nerves that control the movements of the stomach and its activity. This operation is known as vagotomy, since it is the vagus nerve that is cut.

TREATMENT OF INDIGESTION—Recently Dr. C. M. Fletcher, a distinguished British physician who specializes in disturbances of the stomach and intestines, has offered a number of suggestions regarding the diet of persons who have digestive disturbances, frequently called dyspepsia.

These suggestions follow:

1. Have regular meals. The stomach is affected by habit. It likes regular hours. It gets ready for food at the time when the meal is expected. This it does by producing digestive juice and acid. If the meal is delayed, these substances have contact in concentration with the walls of the stomach and may cause harm.

2. Have frequent "snacks." Food, and particularly milk, helps to neutralize the acid in the stomach. That is why the pains of indigestion are lessened by taking a snack. Some people have thought that it is better to avoid food when there is indigestion. A light meal or snack taken at fairly frequent intervals helps to overcome the excess acid in the stomach. Indeed this has become routine advice for digestive disturbances.

3. Avoid big meals. Big meals overfill the stomach and by stretching the tissues may do harm. In general six small meals a day are better than three big ones.

4. Eat slowly and chew thoroughly. Meals that are hurried are not properly chewed. A large mass of unchewed food means that the food will remain a long time in the stomach because it has to be penetrated and softened by the digestive juice. Again there is the danger that lumps may irritate the walls of the stomach. If your teeth are not good enough to enable you to chew your food sufficiently, you will do well to see a dentist, who will be able to correct the condition. Some foods are hard to chew even with good teeth. A certain amount of hard foods is necessary for health but this can be taken in the form of finely macerated fiber.

5. Avoid irritating stimulants. Physicians are now convinced that tobacco, strong tea, coffee, or alcohol may irritate the stomach. Smoking after a meal is less likely to irritate than before a meal. Alcoholic drinks taken before a meal increase appetite because of the irritation to the wall of the stomach. The investigators are convinced that tea and coffee taken with plenty of milk or cream are less irritating than black coffee or strong tea. Most people have sense enough to realize that a certain food is irritating to them. Certainly one

should avoid foods that are known by experience to be irritating.

THE MIND AND THE STOMACH—Research of recent years has shown that the stomach and the digestion of food are greatly influenced by mental factors. People talk of being sick with fright. They say that the stomach turned over. Some people are easily nauseated and vomit when affected by odors or sudden shocks. A sudden shock of fright does not do serious harm. When, however, a person is subjected to repeated nagging, mental strain, anxiety, frustration, or resentment, he is likely to react with a continuous irritation in the stomach area and eventually symptoms of either indigestion or ulcers. The people who get indigestion are often people who worry a lot or who are especially sensitive to criticism. Dr. C. M. Fletcher suggests that such people ask themselves the following questions:

Do you turn little worries over and over in your mind, although you try to appear calm and unconcerned?

Do you brood over bad luck, or when you feel you have been "done"?

Do you resent criticism or worry about what people think of you?

Do people "get on your nerves" easily?

Do you have to drive yourself all day because you have really got too much to do, so that you are always "on the go" and cannot relax?

Are you usually dissatisfied with yourself so that you are always striving to do "one better"?

Do you feel people do not understand or appreciate you enough?

Dr. Fletcher says that if you must honestly answer yes to more than one of these questions, mental strain is playing a considerable part in upsetting your stomach.

People can learn to worry less. Indeed people can learn to take things less seriously simply by constantly reminding themselves that irritation and anger are bad. Someday perhaps we will learn to teach little children early in life that worry and anger and sensitivity are unhealthful. Long ago people learned that it is a relaxation of tension to talk over your problems with somebody else. You may talk about your problems to a religious counselor or with friends whom you can trust or even with members of your family unless they are the cause of your trouble. Of course the doctor is a specialist in listening to people's troubles and worries. He can, moreover, give not only advice but medicines that help to dull the sharp edge of sensitivity and lower the threshold of irritation.

THE HYGIENE OF INDIGESTION—Rest has always been a fundamental remedy for human illness. Nowadays people learn to get up fairly early after surgical operations or after childbirth, but for fatigue and particularly for mental irritation, rest and relaxation are still most important.

Dr. C. M. Fletcher suggests that people avoid exercise either just before or just after a meal because the exercise places a strain on the blood supply and thus takes away from the stomach materials needed to aid digestion. Indeed he suggests that people sit still for at least a quarter of an hour before and after each meal so that the stomach can do its job in peace. For people with serious indigestion or ulcers, a long stay in bed is helpful not only because it gives complete rest but also because it offers an opportunity for control of eating habits. Most restful of all of the procedures in which the human being can indulge is a really sound sleep. A restless night is worse on the stomach than a day full of anxiety. The doctor can always help to overcome restless nights.

People who have serious mental strains at regular intervals should learn particularly to practice good mental hygiene and good physical habits before, during, and after such periods of strain. Among the worst of these periods is the quarterly income tax payment, the period immediately following return from vacation, the rush before Christmas to get the Christmas gift shopping done, and, for many people, any fall in the stock market. Just how to anticipate a fall in the stock market is not yet clear but physicians have noticed for years that any sudden drop in the stock market is immediately followed by an increase or rise in the cases of ulcers of the stomach, diabetes, arthritis, and even colds. Thus the proper hygiene for overcoming digestive disturbances and the onset of ulcers includes, first, a suitable diet with regular, frequent, small, unhurried meals; second, avoidance of all stimulants or other substances that experience has shown will irritate the stomach; third, a calm mind and time to relax; and, fourth, sound sleep. With these practices, Dr. Fletcher says, anyone's stomach will get well and stay well.

The following is the smooth diet that is recommended to people who have nervous indigestion. It is taken directly from the recommendations of Dr. Walter Alvarez.

If you are to give this diet a fair trial, eat no coarse foods with fiber, skins, seeds, or gristle. Avoid particularly salads with celery, tomatoes, cucumbers, and pineapple, many of the green vegetables, raisins, berries, jams full of seeds, nuts, and many of the raw fruits. Beans, cabbage, onions, green or red peppers, melons, cucumbers, and peanuts are notoriously gassy. If you are living in a boardinghouse you can stick to this diet by simply avoiding the forbidden foods and eating more of the digestible ones which are put before you.

Avoid sugar in concentrated form and take no candy or other food between meals. Hot cakes and waffles might not be bad if they were not eaten with so much syrup. Fried foods are not bad if they are properly fried—that is, totally immersed in fat at the right temperature. Avoid eating when in a rush and when mentally upset. Family rows should be held away from the table. Chewing gum may cause distress, as much air is swallowed with the saliva. Digestion is greatly helped by a good chewing surface. If there are any gaps in your teeth, have your dentist fill

them with bridges. Purgatives often cause flatulence and distress in the abdomen.

The following are suggestions for breakfast: Orange juice, grapefruit (avoid the fiber in the compartments); cantaloupe and melons are inadvisable. Coffee, if desired, is allowed in moderation; it sometimes causes flatulence. If you are sensitive to caffeine, try Kaffee Hag or Instant Postum. Chocolate, cocoa, or tea, one or two eggs with ham or bacon (avoid the tougher part of the bacon), white bread, toast, or zwieback with butter, any smooth mush such as farina, germea, cream of wheat, corn meal, or rolled oats (a fine oatmeal can be obtained by calling for Robinson's Scotch Groats), puffed cereals and cornflakes are also allowed. Shredded-wheat biscuits and other coarse breakfast foods are not allowed. Bran is particularly harmful. Graham bread is permitted but not the coarser whole-wheat bread.

Suggestions for lunch and dinner: In fruit cocktails avoid the pieces of orange and pineapple. Broths, bouillon, cream soups, and chowder are allowed, also meat, fish, or chicken, squab, or game, excepting duck (avoid the fibrous parts and gristle). Veal may be tried; it is not digested well by many persons. Eat no smoked fish or pork. Crab and lobster had better be left alone. Oysters and sausage may be tried later.

Bread and butter are allowed, and hot biscuits if they are made small so as to consist mainly of crust. Rice, potatoes—mashed, hashed brown, or French fried—are allowed; and later may be added sweet potatoes, hominy, tomatoes stewed, strained, and thickened with cracker or bread crumbs, well-cooked cauliflower tops with cream sauce, asparagus tips, Brussels sprouts, squash, beets, turnips, creamed spinach, Italian pastes, noodles, macaroni, and spaghetti cooked soft, purées of peas, beans, lentils, lima beans, or artichoke hearts. All skins or fiber should be removed by passing the food through a ricer. Sweet corn may be used if passed through a colander. There are practically no other vegetables that can be puréed to advantage. String beans (large tender string beans which can be used as a vegetable or salad can now be obtained in cans) are allowed if they are young and tender.

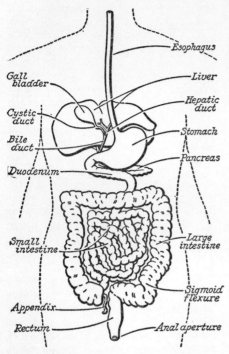

Gall bladder

Cystic duct

Bile duct

Duodenum

Small intestine

Appendix

Rectum

Esophagus

Liver

Hepatic duct

Stomach

Pancreas

Large intestine

Sigmoid flexure

Anal aperture

The anatomy of the digestive system

No salad should be taken at first. Later you may try a little tender lettuce with apples or bananas, tomato jelly, or boiled eggs. Mayonnaise and French dressing are allowed. Potato salad without much onion may be tried.

Suggestions for dessert are: Simple puddings, custards, ice cream, jello, plain cake, and canned or stewed fruits, particularly pears and peaches. Cottage cheese is permissible; other cheeses often cause trouble. Apple, peach, apricot, custard, and lemon-cream pie may be tried if only the filling is eaten.

In case of constipation stewed fruit may be taken once or twice a day. In winter the dried pared fruit may be used for stewing. Prunes are probably the most laxative of fruits and if eaten every other morning they will relieve the average case of constipation. They should be cooked slowly, until they almost go to pieces. If the skins are still tough, they should be discarded. Applesauce is much more palatable if made from unpared and uncored apples. The sauce is strained later. It may be mixed with a little tapioca or sago. The apples may be baked. Apples, even when cooked, often cause distress. Blackberries and loganberries can be stewed and strained and the sweetened juice thickened with cornstarch. This makes a delicious dish with the full flavor of the berries. Later you may try fully ripe pears and peaches.

Make no effort to drink water. Be guided by your thirst. Avoid excessive use of salt or other seasoning. If you wish to gain in weight, eat as much cream, butter, fat, and starch as you can. If you wish to lose or to stay thin, live largely on vegetables, fruits, and salads, with a moderate amount of lean meat.

INDUSTRIAL ABSENTEEISM

The disabilities that keep employees from their work include the common cold as the most significant; second are the disturbances which occur in women simply because they are women. Third are disturbances of digestion and, fourth, mental problems.

No one has yet found a method for lessening absenteeism due to colds. Routine inoculation of people against colds with vaccines made from germs or from the influenza viruses does not do the job. Some people still believe that exposure to cold while hot and sudden changes of temperature are important. Therefore, avoidance of exposure and elimination of drafts may be attempted.

Physicians in some large industries report that employees who take shower baths before going outdoors tend to fight off colds. This is believed to be part of a hardening process. In some industries it is believed that prompt attention to colds in the factory dispensary will lessen the number. Measures instituted include such treatments as the use of alkaline powder and, in other places, drugs like aspirin.

Most important probably is a study of the industrial plant with relation to the departments in which colds are most prevalent and an attempt to find out why colds spread more rapidly and more frequently in those departments. Certainly overcrowding of personnel aids transmission of infectious germs. Moreover, it has been proved that germs may float for an hour in the air, held by drops of moisture due to coughing and sneezing.

In plants where great numbers of women are employed, investigators divide women into those who work through their periodic disturbance without complaint, those who begin work but sooner or later show up in the rest room, and those who invariably stay home a full day or longer.

Disturbances of digestion are more likely in men than in women in industry. They occur more often in the summer months. In plants where employees lose much time because of digestive disturbances an investigation will frequently show that the disturbances are associated with hurried eating, use of eating places that are not quite suitable, and complete failure to understand the simplest facts about nutrition.

INDUSTRIAL HEALTH Sickness causes approximately twenty times more cases of absenteeism in industry than are caused by accidents and about seven times the total loss of working days. The sicknesses which are mostly responsible include the common cold, diseases of the stomach, pharyngitis and tonsillitis, functional nervous diseases, menstrual disorders in women, rheumatism, arthritis, and gout. While colds are responsible for more absences than other diseases, the severity of this type of absenteeism is low. Functional diseases of the nervous system actually cause the highest average working days lost per case.

There are very few strictly occupational diseases, although some industries give rise to certain kinds of disability.

Examples are exposure to silica dusts, which produce silicosis, or to the inhalation of lead, which produces lead poisoning, or the breathing of carbon monoxide gas, which produces carbon monoxide poisoning.

Especially frequent nowadays are inflammations of the skin due to irritation from various chemicals to which the worker may be exposed. The experts have listed hundreds of different types of chemical substances which may cause inflammations of the skin. Certain industries by the nature of the work produce constant pressure against various portions of the body, so that calluses form or swellings of protective oil sacs take place. Such swellings are called bursitis. Housemaid's knee is an example of this kind of occupational disease. Fatigue or strain from certain movements that are often repeated, as in sewing, writing, holding a pneumatic hammer, operating a telegraph key, can also produce conditions which are classified as occupational disorders.

Some occupations expose the worker to certain kinds of infections. The worker with infected cattle may get undulant fever. Anthrax is contracted from contact with infected hides or wools. Machinists get serious inflammations and infections due to irritations from oil and cutting compounds. In other industries the worker may be exposed to such hazards as ultraviolet light or constant glare, so that conditions occur like electric ophthalmia, glassworker's cataract, nystagmus of coal miners (which is a shifting of the pupils due to working under irregular light). There is also the kind of inflammation of the eye called conjunctivitis which happens to movie stars who are not protected against the light. Laundry and kitchen workers may suffer from severe heat exhaustion from abnormally high temperatures, and workers in cold storage plants suffer with disturbances due to exposure to cold. Boilermakers have disturbances of hearing associated with noise, and workers in tunnels and those who fly at high altitudes develop conditions like caisson disease and altitude sickness. Certain monotonous jobs expose the worker to the double danger of fatigue and functional nervous disturbances.

INFANTILE PARALYSIS Most terrifying of all the diseases which attack children is infantile paralysis, sometimes called poliomyelitis. There are other diseases that constitute a double threat to mankind—the threat of crippling and the threat of death—but infantile paralysis is the most visibly crippling.

In the schools for crippled children and in the hospitals and institutions that care for them, the great majority of children with paralyzed legs are there as a result of what infection with the virus of infantile paralysis can do to the human body.

Infantile paralysis is caused by a virus. A virus is living material, previously characterized by the fact that it is so small that it can pass through the pores of a clay filter. However, we now know that there are germs that pass through such filters. Viruses differ from germs mainly by the fact that germs can multiply in cultures or tubes outside the human body, or outside of any living host, but viruses cannot. Viruses cannot move by themselves; they cannot reproduce themselves. Therefore the investigators who study viruses in the laboratories grow them in the bodies of animals or on the embryo chicken in the shell. The viruses of infantile paralysis have been grown best outside the body on the tissue of the kidneys of monkeys.

The virus of infantile paralysis is one of the smallest of the known viruses. It does not seem to affect many animals. Man is the favored host for this agent of disease. A few of the monkeys can be infected. Quite recently some rats have been found which can be inoculated successfully with this virus. In the United States the virus of poliomyelitis occurs in three types known as Lansing, Brunhilde, and Leon types.

Simply because of its dramatic and terrifying character, scientists have concentrated greatly on this disease in recent years; we have learned much about it and its method of spread. Each year in the United States since 1940 some 25,000 to 30,000 cases are reported annually. Non-paralytic poliomyelitis is now more frequent than the paralytic form.

The development of a successful method of vaccination against infantile paralysis means that eventually this condition will occur infrequently. The inoculation of some 30,000,000 children may require ten years or more. By early 1956 20 million doses of the vaccine were ready but priorities had to be maintained for children up to the age of 15 years and for pregnant women. The first two doses were given two to four weeks apart and the booster dose ten months later.

Quite possibly, however, far more people have infantile paralysis than are recognized as cases of the disease. The reason is, of course, that many people who become infected do not get paralyzed. Perhaps the vast majority of those who get infected do not get paralyzed. There are some who think that just as many people have infantile paralysis as get measles. Few of the people who get measles—speaking proportionately—get an earache and a running ear. If we could recognize measles only by an earache or a running ear, we would probably miss many of the cases. If there were a rash on the skin in infantile paralysis, we would probably recognize many more cases. It is fortunate for mankind that everyone who becomes infected with infantile paralysis is not paralyzed. If he were, the crippling might constitute an intolerable burden to a weary world.

These facts indicate some of the lines of study that are still needed in order to bring about complete control of this infection. We need a test like the Wassermann test for syphilis or like the examination of the throat in diphtheria, which would make possible the identification of infantile paralysis in every instance. We need a method of determining how the infection actually passes from one person to another. We need to know why some people do not get the disease and others fall ill. We need to know why some people who get the disease become paralyzed and others do not.

All of these questions are now being investigated by workers in clinics and laboratories throughout the world. We have actually made great progress. No doubt more progress will be made as time goes by. When an outbreak of crippling infantile paralysis strikes fear in a community, mothers ask first of all what they can do to help their children escape the disease. Dr. Philip M. Stimson summarized a few suggestions which everyone should keep in mind. Here they are with my explanations:

1. We do not know that infantile paralysis is spread by water. We do know, however, that the virus is found in sewage and that sewage can carry the virus for considerable distances and for a long time. Therefore avoid the use of water that may possibly be contaminated with sewage either for drinking, for swimming, or for washing dishes.

2. Experience in a number of epidemics has shown overexertion and chilling during the period when the virus is in the body and before the person becomes paralyzed seem to augment the effects of the virus on the body. The time that passes between entrance of the virus into the body and the development of the first symptoms may be as short as four or five days; it may be as long as ten days or two weeks. Therefore, in times when there is an outbreak in the community, do not permit children to become exhausted from exertion. Do not permit them to become chilled from swimming too long in pools, rivers, or lakes.

3. There are records of cases of infantile paralysis following removal of the tonsils during the period of an epidemic. Apparently the removal of the tonsils leaves open pathways in the throat whereby the virus may get into the nervous system and pass perhaps to the higher areas of the nervous system,

which are those that control the vital activities of the body. This produces the bulbar type of infantile paralysis, in which paralysis of the breathing comes early. In several outbreaks there has been a relatively high percentage of bulbar cases; therefore avoid injury to the membranes of the nose and throat. Unless necessary because of serious infection, operations on the tonsils and adenoids should not be performed during the time of the outbreak.

4. The earliest symptoms of infantile paralysis are like those of many other infectious diseases. During the time of an outbreak every minor illness should be considered as a possible case of infantile paralysis, and particularly if there is fever, headache, or spasms of the muscles of the neck, the spine, or the thighs.

Any child suspected even slightly of having been infected should be kept quiet for several days in bed and should not get up until the doctor says that he may do so.

5. Flies and other insects may carry the virus of infantile paralysis and thus contaminate food or water used. The insect, in contact with sewage or filth, picks up the virus and perhaps deposits it on food, milk, or water that is going to be taken by a child. Therefore screening of the house against flies and mosquitoes may be important in keeping away infection. The best evidence shows that insect transmission is not the common method of spreading infantile paralysis. In any case it is good sanitation to destroy flies and their breeding places. Even though it has not yet been proved in any single place that flies actually carry enough virus from infected sewage to produce the disease definitely in any human being, the path of safety is to avoid the danger.

6. Most infectious diseases are spread from one person to another. Therefore in times of outbreaks of infectious disease unnecessary physical contacts with other people should be avoided. Wash the hands carefully before eating. Do not put unclean objects in the mouth.

Certainly it has been proved that people who have been infected with the virus of infantile paralysis can continue to pass it from their bodies by way of the bowel for several months although they themselves are well. Proof seems available also that the usual way for the virus to get into the human body is by way of the throat and stomach.

7. We now have gamma globulin and a vaccine that have been shown experimentally to be able to protect a child against infantile paralysis. Controlled studies have been made on thousands of children in many different states with gamma globulin. This affords about thirteen weeks of protection. The vaccine as now prepared uses the three types of virus which are grown artificially outside the body. All the results were achieved through research supported by the National Foundation for Infantile Paralysis. Most experts believe that abolition of poliomyelitis as a crippling disease is now possible.

Usually when the child gets infantile paralysis there is a period called the preparalytic stage. Such children have fever, sometimes a sore throat, a cough, or a cold, a headache, nausea, or vomiting. These symptoms occur in practically all infectious diseases. Many times there is diarrhea. In some instances there may be pain or distress in the abdomen so severe that the parents fear appendicitis. Some children seem to be fatigued to the point of exhaustion and so apathetic that they have apparently lost interest in what is going on, yet others are nervous and irritable, indeed frightened out of all proportion to the severity of their symptoms.

Important and alarming symptoms include trembling of the hands or other parts of the body and pain or stiffness in the neck and back. Difficulty in moving the back, such as would be involved in putting the chin on the chest or the head between the knees, is an indication that something is wrong. The child may perspire a great deal and his face may flush with a minimum amount of exer-

cise. These symptoms are, however, still such that the diagnosis of infantile paralysis cannot be made with certainty even when all of them are present.

Sometimes the symptoms are so mild that the first one noted is actual paralysis. This, however, is unusual. Most commonly for anywhere from a few hours to several days the early signs of the illness are detected. If any of these signs appear, call a doctor at once. Another serious symptom of the early stages of this disease is pain. The muscles are sore, the pain gets worse when the legs and arms are moved, the muscles are tender if anyone touches them. In many instances even when these symptoms are present paralysis does not follow and recovery is rapid and complete. Some patients—the exact percentage varying, however, from one epidemic to another—proceed and develop definite paralysis. This early stage of the disease is the time when the services of the doctor and the trained nurse may be most important. The extent of the permanent paralysis may depend a great deal on what is done at this time.

The detection of the muscles that are involved at this time demands a careful kind of study that only a physician trained in observation of infantile paralysis can give. As everyone knows, the number of muscles that may be involved vary from case to case and from epidemic to epidemic. Seldom are all of the muscles of a leg or an arm incapacitated. However, groups of muscles in various portions of the body may become paralyzed. Usually from two to three days after the first signs of paralysis appear all of the damage that is going to be done will have occurred.

Thus far, particular mention has been made of the muscles. However, infantile paralysis is not a disease of muscles, but a disease of the nervous system. The virus gets into the nervous system and attacks the cells in the front part of the spinal cord that are responsible for carrying the impulses to movement along the nerves to the muscles. If the nerve cells are damaged but slightly or if only a few nerve cells are destroyed, the muscle weakness will be temporary. If many nerve cells are killed by the infection, the paralysis may be extensive and it may be permanent. Nerve cells, unlike many of the other tissues of the human body, do not easily grow back again after they have been destroyed. In fact nerve cells are so delicate that they are more easily destroyed than other cells of the body. These are just some of the reasons why early competent attention may be so vital in the control of infantile paralysis.

Frequently there are changes in the spinal fluid which bathes the spinal cord and the nerve cells as an early sign of this disease. Hence the doctor may want to put a needle into the spinal column in order to get out some of the fluid for examination. If this can help him diagnose the disease earlier and thus be helpful in controlling it, the measure is more than warranted. Once infantile paralysis is diagnosed, the case should be reported immediately to the health official. The family should be willing to keep the infected child absolutely quarantined so as to prevent as much as possible spread of the condition to other children.

During the early stages of infantile paralysis, when the muscles are tender and painful, the doctor, the orthopedic surgeon, and the nurse must co-operate in doing the utmost possible to prevent extensive paralysis. A few simple suggestions have been prepared for nurses by the National Foundation for Infantile Paralysis. It is well that every mother should be familiar with these suggestions given to nurses.

1. Keep patient in a quiet room out of drafts.

2. Handle the patient as little as possible. Touching and moving the patient aggravate spasm.

3. Always be sure hands are warm before touching patient.

4. Warm bedpan or urinal before giving to patient.

5. Omit baths during stage of painful spasm. When baths are given, handle patient gently. Blot up moisture with towel. Don't rub.

6. Omit alcohol rubs.

7. Allow patient to assume any position which is comfortable but, as painful spasm is relieved, gradually bring the body into normal alignment.

8. Use an air ring instead of a pillow under the head during the time there is difficulty in breathing and swallowing.

9. In turning the patient, give support to joints and avoid touching muscle bellies.

10. Never tire the patient by care being given. Stop care before patient shows signs of fatigue.

11. Observe and report promptly to physician any of the following symptoms:

a. Retention of urine.

b. Constipation.

c. Difficulty in breathing, swallowing, talking.

d. Accumulation of mucus.

e. Increase or recurrence of spasm. Some of the signs which indicate presence of spasm are shortening of muscles, causing the body to be pulled from its normal position, presence of abnormal skin creases, sulci, or bony prominences, absence or diminution of skin folds, prominence of muscle tendons, and flatness of muscle bellies, pain.

The following list of rules is especially directed to parents:

1. Keep the covers from touching the patient's body by draping them over the footboard or using a bed cradle or other support.

2. Allow patient to lie in the position which is most comfortable for him. As the pain is relieved, the nurse will teach you how to place him in the normal position.

3. Scrub your hands thoroughly after giving any care to the patient. The nurse will show you how to protect the patient, your family, and yourself in giving care. This instruction will include method of disinfection of stools and disposal of stools and nasal discharges in accordance with directions given by your physician.

During the acute stage of infantile paralysis many parents become alarmed and are willing to try any kind of massage, manipulation, pulling, heating, freezing, or any other treatment that almost anybody will suggest. Actually there is no disease in which so much harm can be done in the early stage by the wrong application or the unnecessary application of such methods.

Modern investigations and particularly the Kenny method have shown that control of the pain, the tenderness, and the spasm by that technic do much to relieve pain and spasm, maintain the function of the tissues, and save life. However, even these methods demand application by persons who have been trained in the technic. Long before Sister Kenny, some doctors advocated warm baths for this stage of the disease. Others had developed other technics. However, as Dr. Frank R. Ober points out, Sister Kenny's treatment combines good nursing and common sense.

The problem in the early stage is expert nursing, expert application of the hot packs, gradual controlled movement within the range of discomfort in order to prevent stiffness of the muscles and joints, and controlled active exercises of groups of muscles as soon as the spasm and soreness have disappeared.

We do not know of any drug or serum that will cure infantile paralysis. Already the sulfa drugs and penicillin have been tried and have not seemed to be more promising than other drugs in their attack on this virus condition.

This means, therefore, that the doctor who treats the patient with infantile paralysis will be responsible for the methods that are used to control the pain, the tenderness, the fever, and the other symptoms. He will want the advice of an orthopedic surgeon who specializes in nerves and muscles, bones and joints, who will use all that that special branch of medicine provides to prevent deformities and disabling injuries.

The use of splints, frames, and plaster casts in the care of early cases of infantile paralysis has been largely replaced by the so-called Kenny method. Not all patients recover completely even with this method. Apparently many more recover completely with the Kenny method than used to recover when the affected parts of the body were kept almost wholly under the control of splints, frames, or plaster casts early in the disease.

The National Foundation for Infantile Paralysis, 120 Broadway, New York, N.Y., has up-to-date books and pamphlets for doctors, nurses, and the public generally that they gladly send on request.

Under the auspices and with the assistance of the National Foundation for Infantile Paralysis, research on infantile paralysis has been intensified throughout the world. Under grants made by the Foundation the care of the patient with acute infantile paralysis has been greatly improved. Several drugs are now known that control muscle spasm. Physical therapy technics have been introduced that maintain the tone of the tissues until the greatest possible recovery of the nervous tissues has occurred.

The latest development is the recognition of the need for scientific rehabilitation of the handicapped patient. Many special services are integrated around the patient including orthopedics, physical medicine, psychiatry, nursing, occupational and recreational treatment, and resettlement. Departments of rehabilitation and centers are being established.

Usually the patient with infantile paralysis is seen first by the family doctor. Then he calls as a specialist the pediatrician, who takes care of children, the specialist in nerve conditions, or the orthopedic surgeon. Since the attention of all of these may be helpful or most desirable in most cases, it is probably best for the infected child to be taken promptly to a hospital. In the hospital the toxic symptoms of infection may be overcome. Frequently the child will be found depressed because of a lack of fluid in the body. Doctors may inject a 10 per cent solution of dextrose directly into the veins in order to overcome these conditions. Remember, however, that all these children should be subjected to a minimum amount of handling until the initial painfulness and tenderness have disappeared.

Naturally such troubles as difficulty in swallowing, breathing, or urinating must be given the immediate attention of the doctor. Anyone with infantile paralysis who has trouble with breathing is likely to be put immediately in a respirator or breathing device. The National Foundation for Infantile Paralysis has established twelve centers in the United States where patients who require treatment in a respirator may be given care by trained teams. New types of respirators which fit like a jacket are now available.

Most important in the control of infantile paralysis is the maintenance of the morale, not only of the patient but of the patient's parents. There are few illnesses which so greatly shake the courage of parents as does this disease. The use of the Kenny method helps morale because it gives visible evidence that a great deal is being done.

The final steps in the care of a patient with infantile paralysis are usually carried out by the physical therapist and the surgeon. It is in these stages of the disease that the underwater treatment or swimming-pool technic is particularly valuable. A pool itself is useless unless there are available competent teachers who encourage the use of weakened tissues, control the amounts of exercise and rest, and aid in developing properly those muscles that are capable of being developed. The surgeon can transplant muscles so that parts of healthy muscles will take the place of those that are not able to carry on their work. By the use of braces and supports the weakened tissues may be helped in carrying the weight of the body. Joints can be made to bear weight, and walking power can be restored. These braces and supports are used, however, only until healthy muscles can be made to take over the functions of those that have been damaged or destroyed by disease.

Certain patients in spite of everything that can be done remain crippled. For these patients modern civilization provides schools which can help to improve the physical condition and help to readjust the mental state. Many a child who has had infantile paralysis recovers and goes on to lead a successful life. Wherever patients crippled by infantile paralysis assemble, one sees the great boost to their morale that has come from the notable example of famous persons who have been crippled and who made successful careers despite their handicap. As was said by Violet Storey in her beautiful poem:

> Milton, the blind, who looked on Paradise!
> Beethoven, deaf, who heard vast harmonies!
> Byron, the lame, who climbed toward Alpine skies!
> Who pleads a handicap remembering these?

Most notable was, of course, the example set by President Franklin Delano Roosevelt.

INFANTILISM Sometimes because of the failure of development of certain glands the characteristics of childhood persist into adult life. The condition is called infantilism and is marked by mental retardation, underdevelopment of the sexual organs, and sometimes diminished stature.

INFLUENZA Differentiation between the common cold and influenza is a job for an expert and even many an expert has some trouble making this fine distinction. However, influenza is likely to occur in epidemics whereas the common cold goes on all the time. Influenza spreads rapidly, usually beginning with a sudden fever, marked prostration, pains in the back and legs, redness of the eyes, and some inflammation in the throat.

The first epidemic of influenza carefully recorded was in 1510, and there have been at least eight instances when influenza spread throughout the world. At first these outbreaks seemed to come about fifty years apart, then forty years apart, and nowadays about twenty-five years apart. However, there is no exact regularity in this matter. Frequently small waves of recurrence will follow a great epidemic.

Several viruses have now been isolated when epidemics of influenza have occurred recently. Viruses, it must be remembered, were only discovered and seen in recent years. Two of the forms of virus associated with epidemics recently are called influenza A virus and influenza B virus. However, when influenza occurs, many other germs are likely to invade the infected and swollen tissues. These others include the germ of pneumonia and several different forms of streptococci and staphylococci. The combination of an influenzal infection with a streptococcal infection may be particularly deadly.

Usually from one to three days after a person has been exposed he comes down with the disease. The fever lasts from one to five days, in the majority of cases about three days. The symptoms related to the nose and throat are worse at the end of twenty-four hours and then in general get better. Most serious is a secondary inflammation of the lungs, so that there is a constant harassing cough.

Following influenza there is usually a period of depression and weakness which, for many people, is far more serious than the acute disease itself. In fact it is the secondary depression and weakness and the complications which make influenza a serious disease. The majority of people with influenza get well promptly but a considerable percentage develop the secondary complications (particularly pneumonia) which are responsible for death.

Recently vaccines have been developed which are known to be especially useful in preventing influenza. They have been tried in some outbreaks in colleges and universities. The influenza virus is classified as virus A, A^1, and B.

If an influenza outbreak is exceedingly serious, it is now customary to try the antibiotic drugs as a means of preventing secondary complications, including the invasion of the pneumococcus and the streptococcus.

The best advice of the doctors for the person with influenza is to go to bed until convalescence is well established and the danger of complications is passed. Take plenty of fluids, including citrus drinks, which have a tendency to alkalinity. The diet is usually light. Various remedies are prescribed to relieve any pains or headaches or symptoms that might cause sleeplessness.

INSECT PESTS The number of insects that disturb human beings is legion. Most common of those that attack the body directly are the lice and the itch mites. Less frequent are bedbugs and spiders. In the woods and in tropical areas chiggers and mosquitoes, ticks and the biting flies annoy mankind.

Among soldiers in the armed forces insects are so serious a menace that special divisions of the department of preventive medicine are concerned with the control of insects.

Chiggers are known scientifically as *Trombicula irritans.* They hook themselves onto the skin; the skin becomes irritated, and an intolerable itching begins. Red blotches appear, and blisters form. The chiggers do not burrow into the skin, but they inject a substance which dissolves and softens the tissue, and this causes the itching.

Infestation with chiggers can be prevented by putting flour of sulfur on the stockings or underclothing when going into tall grass or weeds. Soldiers are protected by wearing leggings and closing off the bottom of the trousers.

If one has been seriously bitten by chiggers, it is customary to wash the skin thoroughly with soap and water and allow the lather to remain on the skin ten minutes before removing. Then any of the anti-itch preparations can be applied to keep the itching under control until healing has occurred.

Recently insecticide and insect-repellent mixtures have been developed, based on the use of freon, containing pyrethrum, and there is also the new insect repellent called DDT. These are efficient in controlling not only chiggers but mosquitoes, moths, and many other types of insects.

The louse is an annoying inhabitant of the human body. In the armed forces and wherever great numbers of people are assembled, delousing technics have been developed for ridding the body of this unwelcome visitor and also for removing both the lice and their eggs from clothing. Usually live steam is used for disinsectization.

Following is the advice circulated by the health department of the city of Chicago:

Articles Needed—Kerosene oil; olive oil (sweet oil), half pint of each.

To Kill Vermin—Mix the kerosene and sweet oil and rub this mixture well into the scalp. Then with a piece of muslin cover the hair for at least two hours or, better, overnight. Do not bring the head in contact with a lighted gas jet or flame of any kind. When the muslin cover is removed, wash the hair and scalp with soap and hot water and rinse well with clear water. Repeat this procedure as often as live vermin are found in the hair.

To Remove Nits—Wet the hair thoroughly with hot vinegar, and comb with a fine-toothed comb. Repeat this daily until all nits are gone. Always dry the hair thoroughly before going out.

A product called Kwell is efficient and not as disagreeable to use as kerosene.

Scabies is a disease caused by the itch mite, which burrows under the skin. It causes what is called the seven-year itch. Usually it is controlled by sulfur preparations or Eurax.

The only venomous spider in the Western Hemisphere is the black widow. When a person it bitten by a spider, the first step is to prevent absorption of the poison into the circulation. The wound can be disinfected with tincture of iodine or any other good antiseptic.

Finally, the housefly is under suspicion not only of being an annoying insect but also one capable of menacing health by carrying filth and germs from one person to another. The common housefly spreads disease as do also the tropical flies and fleas.

In Africa the tsetse fly spreads African sleeping sickness. Texas fever and Rocky Mountain spotted fever are spread by ticks. Indeed any insect that sucks blood or that injects poison into the body is a menace in relation to the spread of disease.

INSOMNIA Failure to sleep at any time when sleep is ordinarily expected is called insomnia. Very few, if any, people have complete insomnia. That ocurrs only when pain is continuous and unrelieved or when there is mental disease. However, partial inability to sleep is a frequent condition and may be due to a variety of causes.

Sleep may be so disturbed as to be inadequate, so that when one awakens he is not refreshed but tired.

Regardless of the vast amount of study that has been conducted in laboratories of physiology all over the world, the exact mechanism of sleep is not yet fully understood. Since certain forms of disorder in the brain may produce inability to sleep, there seems to be reason to believe that some portion of the brain is involved in the mechanism by which sleep is induced. However, there are many contributing factors which have to be considered in insomnia, and allowance must be made for people's peculiarities and habits.

People who are especially sensitive to noises will awaken much more easily than others. There are light sleepers and heavy sleepers. Some people get along with just a little sleep—say, six hours a night—whereas others require from eight to ten hours each night.

When a doctor treats a person with insomnia, he tries to determine whether or not the insomnia is associated with any mental or physical condition in the brain, whether or not it is associated with high blood pressure, hardening of the arteries, whether or not there are infectious conditions or poisoning due to various drugs. He will try particularly to find out whether or not the person has anxieties about his family relationships, his money, or his career.

If the insomnia is due to anxiety, sleep is likely to be disturbed and fitful. The person with insomnia goes to sleep but shortly thereafter awakens and is often unable to get back to sleep. As a result he gets up in the morning tired and with the feeling that his brain has been working all night. Sometimes indulgence in hard mental work just before going to sleep will keep the mind so active that it is difficult to go to sleep in the first place.

Physical discomforts of all kinds, such as coughing, difficulty in breathing, indigestion, overactivity of the bladder, or ringing in the ears, may also produce sleeplessness. The treatment of insomnia is obviously directed in such cases to the physical condition that is responsible. Insomnia is not a disease but a symptom. The treatment is directed to the cause when that is found.

Today there are innumerable drugs which tend to depress the activity of the brain. These drugs are known as hypnotics, and very strong ones as narcotics. People can very easily get into the habit of taking some hypnotic drug just before going to bed. However, preparation for sleep without the taking of a hypnotic often enables one to do without the drug. A walk outdoors for fifteen to twenty minutes may be good preparation. A light massage with a genial masseur often produces both a physical and mental frame of mind conducive to sleep. A heavy meal should not be taken within four hours of the time of going to bed, but a snack including hot milk, cocoa, or any similar drink just before going to sleep is sometimes helpful. Difficult study should not be practiced within an hour of going to sleep, but reading of a relaxing book—that is, one which does not induce mental tension— also aids sleep when the habit of reading before going to sleep has been formed.

INTELLIGENCE Probably there are in the United States about 500,000 people who are mentally defective. These have been classified as including 30,000 idiots, 100,000 imbeciles, and the remainder morons.

Among the factors related to the failure of a human being to develop intelligence are injury to the brain at birth, infections or inflammations of the brain like meningitis and encephalitis, severe injury to the brain resulting from accident and defective actions of the glands, as well as the effects of heredity.

Intelligence is described as the total capacity of anyone to think rationally, to act with a definite purpose, and to be able to deal effectively with the situation in which he lives. Other factors also are related to intelligence or the intellect, but there is also the possibility of confusing intelligence with education and knowledge. Some people know a great deal about many things and still cannot meet the standards for intelligence. The only way by which we can measure intelligence is to test a large number of different factors which measure the power to reason, the memory, the knowledge, and the experience of the person who is being tested.

Intelligence tests are simpler for children than they are for adults because the amount that a child has experienced or learned during the short time of his existence is not so great as that of an older person. With very old people, experts who make these tests must take into account the possibility of mental deterioration.

Some of the technics by which we distinguish various grades of intelligence are relatively simple. An idiot will not protect himself against common physical dangers because his instinct of self-preservation is not strong. An imbecile cannot manage his own affairs and cannot be taught to do so. Morons cannot compete with others in earning a livelihood or in protecting themselves from those who would exploit them. Therefore morons require constant supervision and care.

The scientists distinguish between

mental defects and mental retardation. A mental defect cannot be corrected beyond the limitations of the brain in the person concerned, no matter how skillful or persistent the treatment may be. If, on the other hand, a child has merely been retarded in his mental development, the possibility for bringing him up to a proper age level in intellect exists. A child may be retarded, for example, because of impaired vision or hearing, or because the people around the child speak a language which is not the common language of the community, so that the child does not get beyond the language and mentality of those who care for him. Finally, anxieties and fears will hold back development, and removal of such anxieties will permit the child to develop rapidly.

Out of a sampling of almost 46,000 registrants examined for Selective Service, 1.9 per cent of white boys had to be rejected because of educational deficiencies, and 12.2 per cent of Negro boys had to be rejected for this cause. Careful analysis has not yet been made as to the causative factors chiefly responsible.

INTERMITTENT CLAUDICATION See *Buerger's Disease* and *Limping, Intermittent.*

INTERTRIGO What the mother usually calls "diaper rash" the doctor describes under the scientific name of intertrigo. The term really refers to any irritation of the skin which develops where two moist surfaces are in contact. This roughness and irritation are usually seen in the folds of the groin, between the thighs, between the buttocks, under the arms, under the neck, or behind the ears.

Not often is there a determinable infection. In many instances the roughness and irritation are merely the result of the combination of moisture, rubbing of the surfaces, and want of cleanliness. Crusting and itching are seldom observed.

About the worst form of this condition is ordinary diaper rash, which affects babies. Sometimes the irritation is due to the use of laundry soap with an excess amount of alkali, which is left on the diaper when the latter is not properly rinsed after washing. In other instances it seems to be associated with the action of germs on the ammonia in the urine. For a while doctors thought that the ammonia was caused by having the baby drink an insufficient amount of water. Now it is recognized that the ammonia results only from bacterial action on the components of the urine.

When the redness occurs outside the diaper area, it can usually be controlled by the use of a good dusting powder. The combination of dryness and cleanliness will usually take care of the condition. When, however, the inflammation extends into the urinary passages, so that there is burning and irritation, the mother as well as the baby is likely to be seriously disturbed. The strong smell of ammonia makes her more frightened. Under these circumstances she will do well to consult a doctor and to follow some simple precautions in relationship to the handling of the diapers. Burning and irritation on urination or in the area of the buttocks is so uncomfortable for the baby that it should have prompt attention.

In such cases the constant wearing of rubber or rubberized silk diapers may have to be discontinued until the condition is brought under control. Zinc oxide ointment is frequently used to protect the skin. The washing of the diapers with mild soap, rinsing at least three times to remove all the soap, soaking of the diapers overnight or for at least three hours in water containing three tablespoonfuls of boric acid powder to each gallon of water, and, finally, the wringing of the diapers lightly and hanging in the sun for drying will overcome the infection in the diaper. If the diapers are lightly wrung out, so that when they dry enough boric acid is left to prevent bacterial decomposition of the urine, the condition is rather certainly controlled.

INTESTINES The intestines of the human being are a long tubular apparatus which includes the small intestine (23 feet long), the large intestine (5 feet long), and the rectum (about 6 inches long). This tube is lined with tissues which have the power in some places to secrete materials used in digestion and in other places to take up material.

The small intestines will hold about 3 quarts. In the small intestines digestion goes on actively in the upper part but absorption takes place throughout the entire length. The small intestines include the duodenum, the jejunum, and the ileum. Usually it takes about four hours for food to get through the small intestines from the time when the food leaves the lower end of the stomach to the time when the food enters the cecum. The food thereafter moves at the rate of about an inch a minute. The walls of the intestines have muscles, and the food is passed along by waves of muscular action.

The large intestine handles the indigestible material that is left after the food has given to the body what it requires. The food will stay in the large intestine from ten to twelve to forty-eight hours. The large intestine includes various portions: the ascending, transverse, and descending colons. The cells of the large intestine can take up water and sugar solutions.

When the contents of the bowel pass into the rectum, a mechanism is set up which indicates to the person that material is ready to be expelled from the body.

Any obstruction of action of the large or small intestines is a serious matter. Such obstructions may occur from an intussusception in which one portion of the bowel is drawn inside the other like the drawing in of the toe of a sock. This is occasionally due to a tumor, sometimes to the fact that the indigestible material becomes hardened and impacted. Occasionally the bowel is obstructed by a pushing of the portion of the bowel into a rupture.

When such obstruction occurs, the pain is severe and demands immediate attention of a doctor. Since almost any acute condition inside the abdomen may simulate intestinal obstruction by producing pain and vomiting, the doctor must make a most careful diagnosis. If actual obstruction is found, operation is usually necessary. There are instances in which the bowel becomes paralyzed. This also would constitute a most serious condition.

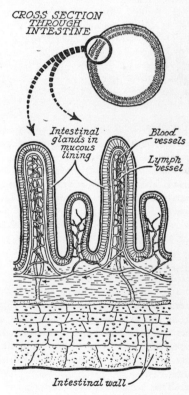

CROSS SECTION THROUGH INTESTINE

Intestinal glands in mucous lining

Blood vessels

Lymph vessel

Intestinal wall

Structure of the intestinal wall

IODINE Iodine is a medical substance. Usually iodine is applied to the body in the form of the tincture, which is a mixture of iodine with alcohol. There is also a solution of iodine made up with water. When iodine is extremely concentrated, it may blister the skin. Surgeons use iodine to disinfect the skin. It is also employed in various skin diseases to destroy germs. It can induce an acute inflammation of the skin and thus help to overcome disease. Iodine taken internally has a corrosive effect on the mucous membranes and is, therefore, poisonous if taken in concentrated solutions. An antidote in cases of iodine poisoning is a solution of starch.

IRITIS See discussion under *Eye.*

IRON Iron is used in medicine chiefly for its effect on the formation of the coloring matter of the red blood cells. When iron is prescribed properly, it produces an improvement in the red blood cells and the red coloring matter in them. Its chief value is, therefore, in anemias.

ITCHING Two hundred years ago a philosopher defined itching by saying, "Itching is an unpleasant sensation in the skin provoking the desire to scratch." Scientifically itching is a combination of the senses of touch and pain, since both these sensations must be active or itching will not occur. Incidentally, people can itch while they are asleep or while they are unconscious, so that involvement of the brain in this activity is not absolutely necessary.

Some people itch more easily than others because their threshold for feeling in the skin is lower than that of other people. The more you itch, the more easily you itch. Old people itch more often and more easily than young people.

Itching occurs in many different diseases of the skin. It follows sensitivity to food or drugs when there are eruptions on the skin. Some people itch particularly after they have had a bath. Housewives who are sensitive to heat will develop itching while cooking. Some parts of the body itch more frequently than others.

Itching is usually associated with infection by fungi of the type of ringworm. The bites of many insects produce itching.

Rarely the whole body will itch at one time. This is usually due to sensitivity to heat or to cold or to various chemicals such as may occur in soaps or bath salts or such as are now used in the treatment of underclothing.

The sensation of itching is, moreover, not a single sensation but the blending of several sensations. In some instances, for example, the sensation is the same as that of something crawling on the skin.

Winter itch is about the same in type as bath itch. This is apparently associated with the drying of the skin. It disappears in warm weather because perspiration helps to keep the skin moist and soft.

The control of itching depends on finding the specific cause, as for instance of sensitivity, and removing that cause. If the skin is dry and thin and without moisture, the use of ointments to keep it flexible will be helpful. Solutions containing such substances as menthol and camphor, as well as witch hazel, water, and alcohol, help to control itching. Plain hot water or ice water will relieve the symptoms. Ointments containing tar are frequently prescribed by doctors as especially useful in conditions that itch. The new ointments containing antihistamines are helpful in many cases of itching. There is no routine treatment for pruritus. Itching is no more a single condition than is eczema. Proper diagnosis and treatment related to the cause are the scientific method for control.

ITCH MITE See discussion under *Insect Pests.*

JAUNDICE Whenever bile circulates in the blood, a condition develops that is called jaundice or icterus. Formerly jaundice was never diagnosed until the skin and the other tissues turned yellow. Nowadays a condition of jaundice is diagnosed by finding excess of bile salts in the blood. After the amount of bile in the blood is reduced to normal, the skin may still remain yellow, requiring some time to return to its natural color.

When red blood corpuscles break down in the blood, that portion which contains iron is used again to produce new red blood cells. The remaining portion is apparently useless in the body and passes through the liver to become a part of the bile.

Whenever the elimination of the bile through the bile ducts is disturbed or whenever the liver fails to carry out its part of the process satisfactorily, jaundice occurs. Sometimes jaundice develops because the destruction of red blood cells is excessive, so that more material is developed than can be eliminated through the liver. If for any reason the liver fails to excrete the bile, it gets into the blood. There are also instances in which the bile ducts are blocked, so that the bile is dammed back. This can be the result of tumors, hardening of the liver, enlarged glands, or similar conditions. Under these circumstances the material excreted through the bowels has a China clay color, is bulky, and has an especially offensive odor. The pale color is due to the absence of the pigment from the bile. The bulkiness and the odor are due to the presence of fats and materials derived from fat which cannot be properly digested because of the absence of the bile acids from the intestines. Under these circumstances the urine becomes dark-colored due to the presence of bile pigments.

There are a number of infectious conditions which so seriously damage the blood as to produce an excessive destruction of blood cells. These include poisonings by various toxic substances including mineral poisons, snake venoms, and the effects of various parasites. Damage to the liver cells may also occur from infectious poisoning with poisons of various kinds including arsenic, phosphorus, and cinchophen. There are also the poisons of eclampsia and similar conditions. There are certain infections with spirochetal organisms which damage the liver and the blood and which are associated with severe jaundice.

The most common type of jaundice is called catarrhal jaundice. This is apparently due to infections by viruses which occur in small epidemics. Such outbreaks are fairly frequent in times of war.

Jaundice is a symptom and not essentially a disease. It is a symptom of damage to the liver in most instances. In order to prevent extension of such damage it is customary for physicians to inject glucose into the body as one of the main portions of the treatment. Because of the damage to the body it is necessary to watch carefully the progress of the condition.

Any patient with severe jaundice should be in bed and all of the necessary tests that can be carried out by the doctor are desirable to determine exactly the nature of the condition and the procedures to be followed in each case.

JOINT DISTURBANCES (See also *Arthritis, Backache, Gout,* et cetera) For purposes of action the human body is made with joints which represent the tissues holding together the bones at different points and permitting them to work in relationship to each other. The number of joints in the body is tremendous because there are so many bones. Many people pay little attention to the small joints between the individual fingers and toes or the many bones of the spine, but joint disturbances may affect these joints as well as the very large ones like the knee, the hip, or the shoulder.

A common disturbance of the joints is the accumulation of fluid due to internal irritation. For instance water on the knee is the common name for the flowing of serous fluid into the knee joint following an injury. Sometimes such an accumulation of fluid occurs without any detectable cause. Cases are known in which the knee joint or another joint has filled with fluid which has disappeared within a few days. The scientific name for this condition is intermittent hydrarthrosis, which merely means a collection of fluid in the joint which comes and goes.

People who bleed easily sometimes have sudden pouring of blood into a joint following either an injury or some other disturbance. This condition is called hemarthrosis, which merely means blood in the joint.

Another condition affecting joints that is fairly frequent is the loose body in a joint to which the slang name "joint mouse" is given. Occasionally small pieces of cartilage or bone will break off and get into a joint. Occasionally also such substances as bullets, pieces of glass, or needles will get into a joint, but these are known as foreign bodies and not as loose bodies or "joint mice." The chief disturbance caused by a loose body in a joint is a locking of the joint. The loose substance gets into a place where the bones should come together and acts as a wedge so that they cannot get together. Sometimes pulling the leg will extend it and open the area between the bones so that the joint mouse drops down and out of the way. This will relieve the locking. The joint in which this occurs most often is again the knee joint. Usually one of the semilunar cartilages (which means a half-moon-shaped piece of tissue) will be subjected to an injury by a sudden twist of the leg and a portion of the cartilage will get caught between the bones. This results in locking the knee joint. The injury is seen frequently in football, baseball, basketball, and tennis players. The condition can be relieved by extending the leg and turning it inward. When, however, a locking of the joint occurs so frequently as to interfere with ordinary activities of life, it is customary by surgical operation to remove the torn piece of cartilage and thus to bring about permanent relief.

Another rather common injury to a joint is a pulling away of the ligament which passes from the kneecap to the large bone of the lower leg. When this pulls away, as occurs sometimes when a boy kicks a heavy, wet football,

he will be temporarily disabled. The special name of Schlatter's disease has been given to this condition, from the physician who first described it.

Whenever a joint is subjected to severe or sudden strain, the ligaments and the muscles associated with the joint may give way or, as has been mentioned, the cartilage may break or tear loose. Usually muscle tissue will tear first and the ligaments afterward because the ligaments are stronger. The amount of tearing may vary from the splitting of a few fibers to a complete pulling away of the ligament from the bone, sometimes a part of the bone coming with the ligament. This is the condition that occurs particularly around the kneecap and the elbow joints.

The first step to take following any injury to a joint is to make certain that there has been no breaking of bones. An X-ray picture—particularly several pictures taken from different angles—should show whether or not the bone has been broken. Sometimes the X-ray specialist will take an X-ray picture of the joint on the opposite side of the body for comparison with the one that has been injured. If it is found that a bone has not been broken but that the joint has been strained or a ligament torn, it is customary to apply a bandage to make certain that the joint will be protected and properly supported. Sometimes a local anesthetic is injected directly into the joint to relieve pain.

Healing can occasionally be hastened by bathing the affected joint in hot water or by applying heat in some other manner. Occasionally light massage at first and then gradually heavier helps to develop circulation and motion in the joint. As the joint improves, it is moved more definitely.

Sometimes people suffer from what might be called a chronic or frequent spraining of a joint. The accident occurs so frequently and repair takes place so slowly that the joint is constantly in a condition of swelling, inflammation, and irritation. Under such circumstances adhesions and scar tissue may form in the joint. Then it becomes necessary for a specialist in orthopedic surgery to manipulate the joint so as to break up these adhesions and finally to secure healing of the joint with sufficient looseness of movement to enable it to do its work satisfactorily. Adhesions will limit movement and give a feeling of unsteadiness and pain. Many new types of bandages have been developed which are elastic and adhesive and which will aid to hold the tissues in place, at the same time permitting motion of the joint. These have been helpful in treating sprains, strains, and dislocations of joints.

KNEECAP—The kneecap is called by the doctor the patella. If the kneecap breaks following an injury, straightening the leg is difficult. The kneecap will break occasionally from a fall. Many cases have been reported in which the kneecap has been broken following a motorcar accident in which the kneecap has been struck suddenly against the dashboard.

As with other injuries affecting bones and joints, the first step following injury to a kneecap is to have an X-ray picture, so that the doctor will know exactly what the conditions are underneath the skin. If the swelling and pain are not too great, the condition can be determined by feeling with the fingers. However, the X-ray picture taken from several different angles will show exactly how the fragments of the kneecap are distributed. This will guide the surgeon in knowing just what to do.

If the kneecap is broken without wide separation of the parts, the condition is frequently helped by simply holding the leg quiet by a cast or a splint and thus permitting the parts to grow together. If there is a great deal of blood or fluid in the kneecap, the surgeon may wish to withdraw some of the fluid with a sterile needle and syringe.

If the doctor puts on a cast, it may be necessary for the patient to remain in bed for from four to eight weeks, after which the cast is removed. After a cast is removed, it becomes necessary to aid in bending the joint involved. This is helped by the use of hot, wet packs or the application of dry heat two or three times daily and by gradual manipulation or forced movement of the joint.

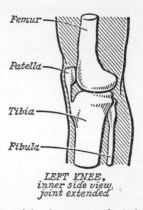

LEFT KNEE,
inner side view,
joint extended

The knee joint is composed of the large bone of the thigh, called the femur, and two smaller bones of the leg, known as the tibia and fibula. The patella is the scientific name for the kneecap

Sometimes when the fragments of the kneecap are widely separated after a fracture because of the pull of the muscles and the ligaments, a surgical operation is necessary. This is done with an anesthetic. The fragments are drawn together and kept together with stainless steel wire or some similar material which the surgeon may select. At this operation any soft tissues that have been torn are also sewed together by the surgeon. Following such an operation, it is usually necessary to put on a plaster of Paris cast for four or five weeks. When the cast is removed, the patient is permitted to exercise the knee and to bear weight on it with the knee in a straight position. From eight to twelve weeks may be required before the weight can be put on the bent knee. Sometimes six months may have to pass before a knee joint is returned to normal following a severe fracture.

ELBOW (See also discussion under *Elbow*)—The elbow joint moves in two ways: by flexion, in which motion the hand is drawn toward the shoulder, and by extension, in which the hand is drawn away from the shoulder. Two other motions are called pronation and supination. These occur by rotating the elbow joint, moving the palm of the hand toward the body or away from the body.

The elbow joint is often the seat of trouble because it may break following a fall in which the elbow is struck against the ground. It is sometimes injured in throwing a baseball or a football or in playing tennis. Tennis elbow occurs not only as a result of sports which require the use of a racquet such as tennis and squash, it may occur also in golf, baseball, or any occupation which demands lifting and sudden pulling and extending of the elbow joint. These occupations include, for instance, those of the violinist, telephone operators, pressers of clothing, and salesmen who carry heavy sample cases.

In the majority of instances the injury that occurs to the elbow joint is a pulling of the muscles or ligaments with the tearing of some fibers. Occasionally, however, a portion of bone may be broken off from the tip and there is always some pain and swelling.

A small sac of fluid that rests over the nodule at the end of the bone may become inflamed. Such sacs of fluid are called bursas. When these sacs become inflamed, the condition is known as bursitis. The pain may be relieved by permitting the excess of fluid to escape. The physician may sometimes press on the point where such a sac of fluid occurs and break it, so that the fluid will escape into the surrounding tissues. Sometimes he will try with a needle and syringe to remove excess fluid. Frequently the application of rest and heat will cause absorption of the fluid. In severe injuries to the elbow it may be necessary to put on a cast and to hold the elbow quiet for a long period of time. Following removal of the cast or sling in which it has been carried, exercise is necessary to restore motion to the injured joint.

KALA AZAR Along the shores of the Mediterranean, in West Africa, and in southern Russia, also in India, China, and Brazil there appears a tropical disease with fever, progressive anemia, enlargement of the spleen and liver, and filling of the tissues with fluid. This tropical disease is transmitted to human beings by the bite of the sand fly, possibly also by bedbugs and mosquitoes. Some cases have occurred in American soldiers who were stationed in these areas. The condition has also been called Dumdum fever, black fever, and Mediterranean fever.

KELOID Whenever the skin heals with a scar that overgrows considerably, the condition is called keloid. The keloid is actually a fibrous tumor. Usually a keloid develops after a surgical operation but overgrowth of scar tissue has followed even a pinprick, a broken pimple, or a fleabite. Keloids occur to people of all ages but most frequently among young adults.

The exact cause of keloids has never been determined. Some people are particularly liable to develop such growths; others never have them. A morphine addict had over two hundred keloids because he developed an overgrowth of scar tissue every time he punctured himself with a needle. Negroes have keloids apparently more often than people of other races.

Keloids may appear anywhere on the body but are most frequently found on the chest and the neck. When a scar overgrows into a keloid, there is first a rather bandlike mass that rises above the level of the skin. The surface is hard and shiny. The edges at first may be sharp but gradually will extend out into projections into the skin.

Occasionally keloids disappear spontaneously, leaving a depressed scar. However, this is a rare rather than common occurrence.

Usually keloids are quite painless but because of their size or the areas into which they infiltrate, they may become tender or painful. Occasionally people will complain of burning, itching, or pricking sensations. However, there is a tendency, particularly in women, to fix the attention on the scar and to worry about it a great deal, so that the sensations may be exaggerated.

Injection of hyaluronidase directly into keloids and the surrounding area seems to be the first really effective method found for controlling this condition. Attempts have been made to cause the keloids to disappear by electrolysis or by electric injection of drugs into the scar. These methods have also failed to meet with general approval. In some instances very careful plastic surgery, by which the scar is cut away and the tissue sewed together again, has been successful but in most instances surgical treatment is unsuccessful because new keloids form where the skin has been cut and in the stitch tracks.

In old, hard, and stationary keloids which have not changed for a good many years and which fail to respond to treatment with radium or X ray, the surgical removal is sometimes successful. In general physicians today feel that they have discovered the best method of treating keloids by the use of radium or the X ray. Radium is used on small keloids—the amount of the exposure depending on the experience and decision of the specialist in radium treatment. Great care is always taken under such circumstances to protect all of the skin that is normal and to apply the radium or X ray only to the keloid itself. Another technic involves the insertion of radium seeds directly into the keloid.

KIDNEYS Most of the elimination of substances from the blood that are to go out of the body is accomplished by the two kidneys. They help to keep the material in the blood constant. The kidneys are made of great numbers of little tubes associated with the blood vessels. A complete tubule is about two inches long. Since each kidney contains about 1,200,000 tubules, the total length of these tubules in an adult man is about seventy-five miles. They are so

tiny that they are difficult to see without a microscope. At the end of each of these little tubes is a cup in which the urine to be excreted from the body is collected.

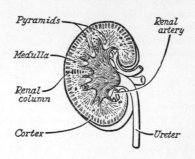

Here is a view of the kidney cut lengthwise to show its structure. An artery enters the kidney and a vein comes out. The ureter carries the urine from the kidney to the urinary bladder. Each kidney is a compact area of collecting tubules and wonderfully small filters. These are found in the cortex of the kidney, from which the fluid passes through tiny tubules to reach the ureter

All of the blood in the body passes through the kidneys repeatedly. It has been estimated that more than sixty quarts of blood pass through the kidneys in order to eliminate one and a half quarts of fluid. Fortunately the human being has two kidneys, one of which is sufficient to carry on the work of the body if the other happens to be completely incapacitated.

Various conditions may so damage the kidney that it will not do its work well. An infection of the kidney is called pyelitis. In most instances the germs are brought to the kidneys from other parts of the body and localize there, setting up a secondary infection. When such an infection occurs in the kidneys, the symptoms include fever, nausea, vomiting, occasional pain in the abdomen, and the other changes that are associated with infection anywhere in the body. People with long-standing infections of the kidney show the results by damage to the blood, loss of appetite, headache, loss of weight, and general illness.

Fortunately modern medicine has developed technics for controlling infections in the kidney that are better than previous methods. There are, for instance, the sulfonamide drugs and penicillin, also mandelic acid and furadantin. The drug to be used, however, depends on the nature of the infection, its scope, and the physician who is handling the individual case.

Whenever there is disease of the kidney, determination of the cause is of first importance. The kidneys when damaged may be rested exactly as the heart may be rested when it is damaged. Rest in bed will stop the kidneys from doing much of the work that they generally do. The tissues will form fewer waste products for the kidneys to eliminate. Some of the strain may be taken off the kidney by aiding elimination from the body by the bowels or by perspiration. The diet may be so controlled as to eliminate the substances to be excreted by the kidney.

Some people are born with kidneys of extraordinary shape or size or kidneys that may in some manner have been damaged. Occasionally the two kidneys are joined together, so that they form a horseshoe in shape. This is called horseshoe kidney. Sometimes the tubules are blocked, so that the kidney becomes full of little cavities containing fluid. This is called a cystic kidney. Occasionally people are born with only one kidney. Frequently people with abnormalities of the kidney do not know about them until trouble begins. The doctor can determine the nature of the trouble by injecting into the body fluids which tend to pass through the kidney and which are opaque to the X ray. An X-ray picture taken under these circumstances will show definitely the shape, size, and other structural conditions in the kidney. It is also possible for the doctor to obtain from the bladder specimens of the urine coming from

each kidney separately. It is also possible for the doctor to look at the ureters, which are the tubes that carry fluid from the kidneys to the bladder.

KNEECAP See discussion under *Joint Disturbances.*

LARYNGITIS (See also *Hoarseness*) Inflammation of the vocal cords may follow overuse of the voice, irritation by chemical substances, or infection.

Men, who are more frequently subjected to exposure to irritant substances in their occupations and who indulge more than women in deleterious habits, suffer more from laryngitis than do women. Contributing causes to inflammation of the larynx include the swallowing of hot or spicy foods, the abuse of alcohol and tobacco and similar irritants. Occasionally the larynx becomes inflamed because there is an infection in the throat or the lungs. In fact any condition that blocks breathing through the nose helps to cause laryngitis because large amounts of air then pass directly to the larynx without having been modified, as is usual, in passing through the nasal tract.

Often laryngitis occurs in such infectious diseases as scarlet fever, measles, chicken pox, and diphtheria as a secondary complication. Eruptions on the skin and mucous membranes may also affect the larynx. Sensitivity to foods which will produce blisters in the mouth and gastro-intestinal tract may also produce swelling and blisters in the larynx. Finally, hemorrhagic diseases, with exudation of blood into the skin or mucous membranes, may cause blood to flow into the tissues of the larynx and thus produce hoarseness.

In serious cases of laryngitis it is customary to go to bed and keep quiet. Nothing helps the vocal cords under such circumstances like continuous rest, speaking only in a whisper. The application of an icebag or ice collar to the throat or of moist compresses is soothing. Some people prefer warmth. This does not seem to make a great deal of difference. A measure which comes down from ancient history is the inhaling of steam to which various aromatic oils can be added. Apparently the chief benefit is derived, however, not from the aromatic oils but from the moisture and the warmth. Nowadays many special devices have been developed, using electrical heat in order to produce such steam for inhaling. These devices are usually much safer than the old-fashioned dish or kettle of hot water. Many instances have been known of severe burns from accidents with open kettles of exceedingly hot water used in this way.

With serious laryngitis, particularly that complicated by inflammation or infection, the physician may prescribe many drugs that are helpful in securing rest and in soothing the area concerned.

LARYNX The larynx, commonly called the voice box, consists of a number of cartilages held together by muscles and ligaments so as to make a tubular structure holding the vocal cords. At its upper end is a structure called the epiglottis, which serves to keep food from going down the larynx and windpipe and causes it to pass instead from the pharynx into the esophagus and stomach.

The chief purpose of the larynx is to aid speech. However, it also is capable of helping with expectoration. When a moving column of air strikes the vocal bands, it is set in vibration. Speech includes, however, not only the vibration of this column of air but the molding of the column with the help of the tongue, the teeth, the palate, and the lips. If any of these structures does not function properly, the voice can be greatly changed. The adult male possesses a deep voice because of the action of the long vocal cord during its relaxed state. A low-pitched voice is produced by a slow-moving cord and a high-pitched voice is produced by a vocal cord that vibrates with an increased frequency.

The doctor looks at the larynx with several different technics. For the usual examination he wears a head mirror which casts light into the mouth. The person who is going to be examined puts out his tongue, which is held out with a piece of sterile gauze. While the tongue is held gently, the patient breathes through the mouth with short gasps of breath. Then the doctor puts a mirror, which has been slightly

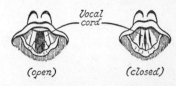

(open) *(closed)*

The larynx is the organ of the voice. The vocal cords in the larynx, by stretching and shortening, open and close and give rise to sounds of various pitches

warmed to prevent condensation of air on its surface, into the back of the throat and requests the patient to say "Ah." This raises the palate, and the mirror may be passed a little farther into the throat. By regulating the angle of the mirror the doctor can see the vocal cords. If the patient makes various sounds, the doctor can determine whether or not the vocal cords vibrate properly. He can also see whether or not they have been modified by inflammation or swelling or the growth of nodes. For some people who are very sensitive, the use of a local anesthetic may be necessary to permit passing the mirror into the back of the throat. Technics have also been developed which permit the doctor to look directly at the vocal cords with instruments especially designed for the purpose.

One of the first signs of inflammation of the larynx and of the vocal cords is hoarseness, so that hoarseness and laryngitis have become almost synonymous. There are, however, many causes for inflammation.

LAUGHTER When a human being laughs, he exercises a number of muscles that are not usually put into action. Laughter serves also to stimulate the circulation and for that reason it is a healthy performance. Animals do not laugh but they have other methods of expressing joy.

When a person laughs, his diaphragm moves up and down and the outgoing air stimulates his larynx and produces the sounds that are known as chuckles. Babies laugh very early in life. They respond to tickling by laughter. Women as a rule do not laugh as heartily or easily as men. Experts in etiquette are inclined to rate loud laughter as vulgar. Therefore exuberant laughter by women is not considered refined.

There are still some differences of opinion as to the age at which the baby first laughs. Even tiny babies smile but most scientists are convinced that this is a reaction of some internal mechanism, even "gas on the stomach." Real laughter occurs in babies after they are one month old.

Laughter is seldom followed by any harmful reaction to the body except that occasionally hiccups follow due to the stimulation of the diaphragm. Cases are also known in which excessive laughter resulted in a sudden revulsion of the stomach or contraction of the diaphragm resulting in vomiting. Excessive laughter may also cause loss of control over some of the voluntary muscles of the body so that those which control the bladder and the rectum suddenly relax. This happens particularly to children who soil themselves following excessive laughter. Tickling to excess may produce this kind of reaction.

The chief value of laughter in health is the fact that it is associated with relaxation of the mind and the body, which means a lessening of nerve tension.

While it is true that laughter will exercise the spaces of the lungs that are not easily ventilated, the practice of laughter as a means of ventilation is not helpful. There are other ways of ventilating the lungs. Laughter is then, like every other function of the body, a mechanism that should be used enough but never too much. Overexercise or overuse of any function of the human body is not conducive to its best development.

LAXATIVES See *Cathartics and Laxatives.*

LEFT-HANDEDNESS From the beginning of time left-handedness has had associated with it the idea of evil and right-handedness of good. Man was probably in the first place ambidextrous —that is, he could use both hands with equal facility. The celebrated artist, sculptor, painter, and anatomist, Leonardo da Vinci, according to reports, had equal facility with both hands. It is said that he used to draw with his left hand and paint with the right. It has also been argued that the ancient Semitic peoples were left-handed because they read and wrote from right to left. However, the Bible mentions specifically the fact that David received a company of men who could use both the right and left hands in hurling stones and shooting arrows out of a bow.

Our knowledge of the development of human beings indicates that they gradually tended to become more and more right-handed down to modern times. One suggestion is that man had to face new hazards as civilization developed and that these hazards involved exposure of his vital organs to his enemies. He therefore protected his left side (the side on which his heart lies) and turned his right side toward the foe. Death probably removed those who could not make this adjustment, so that the right hand became dominant. In the modern prize ring it is the custom of good boxers to lead with the left hand so that the left side is the one turned toward the foe.

Attempts have been made to correlate left-handedness with the sizes of various sections of the brain or with various psychological traits. Left-handed pitchers and baseball players generally are supposed to be somewhat bizarre as compared with right-handed pitchers.

Most important about left-handedness is recent evidence to the effect that attempts to cause the right hand to dominate in the child who is normally left-handed are likely to lead to difficulties of mental hygiene. The change from normal left-handedness to right-handedness has been associated with the development of stuttering and awkwardness.

Few people realize that those who are left-handed are also likely to give the preference to the left eye, the left ear, and the left foot exactly as those who are right-handed give preference to the right eye in aiming a gun, turn the right ear when they wish to listen best, and always step first with the right foot. Beyond these facts the normally left-handed child does not differ in any particular of importance from those who are right-handed, so that there would seem to be no good reason to force a normally left-handed child to change to a right-handed one.

LEPROSY Known to the world since biblical times, leprosy is a chronic transmissible disease due to a specific germ. Characteristic of the disease is the gradual development of areas of tissues without feeling which eventually die and become gangrenous, mutilating the body. In the United States persons with leprosy are kept in colonies—most important of which is at Carville, Louisiana. The condition is directly transmissible and is not nearly so fearsome as its repute would indicate. The condition was without any serious harm to our troops stationed in various portions of the world where leprosy has been more frequent than in the United States.

LEUKEMIA Leukemia is one of the most fatal of all diseases of the blood. For this condition medicine has not yet established a specific cure. Nevertheless, technics have been developed which are helpful in many cases; anyone who has the disease or the family of a person who has the disease should not despair, since cases are now known of people who have lived a good many years following the first appearance of the symptoms of leukemia.

Normally a human being has about 7500 white blood cells in every cubic millimeter of blood. In leukemia the white blood cells increase rapidly and may reach figures of from 100,000 to 1,000,000 white blood cells for every cubic millimeter of blood. As the white blood cells increase, the red blood cells and the red coloring matter of the red blood cells break down. This produces a severe condition of anemia and bleeding. The white blood cells are manufactured in the marrow of the bones and in the lymphatic tissues like the spleen, the tonsils, and similar organs. The cells that are made in the bone marrow differ from those made in other places. The white blood cells that are made in the bones have the job of fighting infection whenever germs invade the body.

The sudden tremendous increase of white blood cells which occurs in leukemia has been characterized as a cancer of the blood. The condition occurs not only in human beings but also in horses, dogs, cattle, and other animals. When leukemia develops, the spleen (which is involved in all activities related to the blood) begins to enlarge, and the bone marrow also changes greatly. The doctor makes the diagnosis of leukemia by counting and examining the white blood cells, using a microscope.

A new technic which has given some hope in the treatment of leukemia involves injection into the blood of phosphorus which has been made radioactive with the cyclotron. In twelve cases treated with combined aminopterin and Cortisone benefit was definitely established. New methods of treatment have proved that the life of the patient can be lengthened.

Previously it has been customary to treat leukemia by exposing the spleen and the bones to the X ray. Much depends on the time when the X-ray treatments are given and the extent to which they are capable of lowering the total number of white blood cells. It is also important during the treatment of the patient with leukemia to keep the red blood cells at a proper level by the use of blood transfusions and similar methods.

LEUKOCYTES The white blood cells are known technically as leukocytes. They are masses of material seen under the microscope as collections of granular tissue. There are many different kinds of leukocytes, which are classified according to the number and nature of the cells that they contain. In certain diseases, such as granulocytopenia, they may be found almost totally absent from the blood. In other diseases, like leukemia, their number is tremendously increased. Sensitivity to certain toxic drugs like pyramidon may cause a complete disappearance of the white blood cells. Since these cells are necessary in resistance to infection, absence of the cells may result in death.

LEUKOPLAKIA Sometimes great white patches develop on the tongue, the cheeks, and the gums. These patches are separated by little fissures or paths, so that the condition looks like a relief map. Because it has been believed to be related to smoking, it has also been called smoker's tongue and smoker's patches. The exact cause of the condition has not been determined but it is advisable to discontinue smoking. Continuous irritation is sometimes followed by cancer.

LEUKORRHEA The word "leukorrhea" comes from two Greek words meaning a white flow. The condition is called in slang "the whites." Usually it represents the excessive formation of mucus and secretion from the cells of the female sex organs. Continued excessive flow means that the physician should be consulted to determine whether or not there is any infection or continued irritation. The repeated use of douches, sometimes containing irritating substances, may make the condition worse rather than better.

LIBIDO This term, popularized by the writings of Sigmund Freud, refers to the sexual desire and to the energy that is developed by primitive impulses. The term "libido" thus may be used to describe the motivation that derives from sex life or psychic energy in general.

LICE See discussions under *Insect Pests* and *Typhus*.

LIGAMENTS Ligaments are the tough fibrous bands that connect bones at the joints and also serve in various portions of the body to support the organs of the body. Ligaments are usually fibrous tissues. They can be torn from the bones at the points where they are joined or otherwise damaged. They may heal by fixation of the part that has been injured. Sometimes a surgical operation is necessary to bring together the torn ends of ligaments. In modern orthopedic surgery motion may be restored when it has been lost by paralysis through the transfer of ligaments from one place to another.

LIMPING, INTERMITTENT Whenever the blood vessels in the legs become obstructed or obliterated by inflammation, by hardening, or by other diseases, there occur symptoms like numbness, tingling, and burning sensations in the toes. Other sensations of deficiency in the circulation include a feeling of heaviness and pain, cramps in the legs, and weakness of the legs and feet.

Before the signs of complete blocking of the blood vessels are apparent, the condition called intermittent claudication, or intermittent limping, may occur. This begins with severe cramping pains in the calf muscles during walking. The pains subside with rest. The symptom is apparently due to narrowing of the blood vessels in the area concerned together with the loss of ability of the body to develop increased blood circulation. People with intermittent limping can regulate the appearance of the symptom by stopping activity of the legs as soon as the sensation appears.

Intermittent limping is particularly associated with a condition called Buerger's disease which is due to an inflammation that blocks the blood vessels. There are other conditions which are much like intermittent limping and which need to be differentiated from Buerger's disease when this symptom occurs. Spasms of the muscles due to difficulties with the nerves that supply the muscles may cause cramplike pains. Lack of suitable balance because of the wearing of the wrong kind of shoes, particularly the wearing of exceedingly high heels by women, may produce trouble in the muscles of the legs and, associated with such trouble, the symptom of limping.

In one case an actor who had been tap-dancing as a job for many years developed a shortening of the tendon which goes to the heel. When he was out of work, he walked a great deal, seeking employment. This overstretched the large muscle at the back of the leg and threw it into spasms so that limping followed. Proper attention to the condition of the muscles and the tendons brought about a cure.

When a doctor is confronted with this condition, his first step is to study the circulation to find out whether or not it is being carried on adequately. The color of the skin is dependent on an adequate supply of blood. In one simple test the leg is raised and then the foot is flexed several times—that is to say, it is bent toward the knee. This will cause the skin to become colorless because of an absence of circulation. When the leg is lowered the color will return if there is adequate circulation. Additional studies are made of the circulation of the blood in the leg. Of course cold will cause the skin to become pale. Therefore it is preferable that the leg be warm and that the air in which the test is performed be warm to prevent disturbance of the test by this factor.

Occasionally limping develops because of damage to the nervous system.

In other instances it is associated with dislocations of the hips and still other cases are associated with diseases like infantile paralysis. A child may limp because the foot has been bruised. Adults sometimes limp because of the breaking down of the arch of the foot. A proper study, however, by someone who thoroughly understands the muscles and their functions will reveal the cause of the limping and the steps to be taken to bring about a cure.

LINIMENTS   Liniments are usually oily preparations containing irritating substances that are rubbed into the skin with a view to affording relief from pain and to bringing about increased circulation of the blood and thus promoting cure. While liniments are themselves helpful, they are not specifically curative of any condition.

LIPOMA   Tumors made of fat are called lipomas. They are usually not malignant and are usually painless. Because of the appearance that they create, they are usually best removed by surgical procedures.

LIPS   Lips are essentially muscles covered by mucous membrane.

When the human body is formed before birth, the lips sometimes fail to grow together as they should. The result of such a failure is called harelip. In the more severe cases the palate also fails to grow together, so that harelip is combined with cleft palate. Fortunately modern plastic surgery is able to repair these conditions, frequently with such a high degree of success that the previous existence of the condition is not recognized. Usually the operation is done in early infancy, as it is more easily performed at such time and the possibility of cure is greater.

Another change which occurs in the lips is the development of overgrowth of some of the glandular tissue, so that a gradual painless enlargement (usually of the upper lip) takes place. This condition is also treated surgically with success.

Inflammation of the lips is not infrequently due to irritation or infection. Action of wind, the cold, the sun, or sensitivity to the chemical ingredients of lipsticks may bring about inflammation of the lip with crusting and cracking. Removal of exposure to the cause and application of a protective ointment usually will bring about a cure of such mild inflammations.

More recently there has been recognized a condition in which the corners of the mouth crack with the appearance of blisters. This has been associated with a deficiency of riboflavin. The taking of an adequate amount of this vitamin, together with the practice of scrupulous cleanliness and the application of an ointment to protect the irritated area, usually results in a cure.

Not infrequent also are serious infections of the upper lip of the type of the carbuncle. These are exceedingly serious because the profuse blood supply of the upper lip may cause the infection to extend rapidly to some of the vital areas of the body. Cases are known in which a carbuncle or abscess of the upper lip resulted in death. Infection with the organism called the streptococcus is especially dangerous. Fortunately modern medicine has developed specifics like the sulfonamide drugs and penicillin for infections of this type, so that the danger of death nowadays is much less than previously.

About the most serious condition that can affect the lip is cancer. For years doctors have warned against chronic irritation of the lip. An irritated spot on the lip is much more serious than one elsewhere on the body because cancer of the lip grows more rapidly and spreads faster than does cancer elsewhere. Fortunately there are now excellent methods of treatment, so that early attention to such an irritated area will prevent cancer and bring about a cure. Cancer of the lip is treated by removal with surgery, by irradiation with radium or X ray, by electric coagulation, or by combinations of these methods.

Fever blisters or herpes of the lip are common, particularly in women. They are usually associated with nerve strain, menstruation, or with the eating of substances to which people may be sensitive.

LIVER (See also *Hepatitis, Jaundice*) One of the largest single organs of the human body is the liver. It develops at least a pint of bile each day. Every vein that leaves any part of the digestive tract in the abdomen goes to the liver; these veins carry to the liver in the form of blood the protein, the sweet, and the starchy foods absorbed by the blood vessels of the stomach, the small intestines, the pancreas, and the large intestines. They carry the products of meats, sugars, and starches. The sugar is stored in the liver until it is needed, in the form of a substance called glycogen, which is then used in the muscles when they act.

The liver also acts to break down poisons coming from the stomach and intestines as well as other parts of the body. It helps to remove various foreign substances from the blood. Probably it helps also in regulating the concentration of the fluid material in the blood and in regulating the heat of the body.

So important are the functions of the liver for health that several tests have been developed to measure the scope of its activities. These tests are based largely on determinations of the amount of bile salts regularly developed by the liver, carried in the blood, and excreted in the urine. There are also tests for measuring the ability of the liver to take care of sugar that is put into the body. Tests have also been devised for determining the ability of the liver to get rid of various toxic substances.

When the liver becomes infected or inflamed for any reason, therefore, a serious condition may develop. This is largely dependent on the difficulty in maintaining enough sugar in the circulation to carry on the work of the body. In any instance in which the liver cells have been greatly damaged, the cells react by pouring out their glycogen. Under such circumstances physicians inject extra glucose into the body to meet its needs for sugar and often give insulin as well to help the body take care of the extra glucose. Symptoms indicating a shortage of sugar sometimes brought about by an excess of insulin are abnormal fatigue, sleepiness, apathy, and confusion. There are, of course, many other conditions in which somewhat similar symptoms occur. The diagnosis is made by the physician through actually testing the amount of sugar in the circulating blood.

Fortunately the human being has great factors of safety in relation to the liver. It has been estimated that each of us has about seven times as much liver as is required to carry on the necessary functions of the body. The normal liver weighs three or four pounds.

Among the most serious of the diseases that may affect the liver are cirrhosis, or hardening, and atrophy, or wasting, as well as infection by a wide variety of bacteria and parasites which may cause abscesses. Recent research indicates that vitamin deficiencies, particularly a deficiency of thiamin, or vitamin B_1, may be related to hardening of the liver.

The liver reacts to poisons of various sorts by the disappearance of its functioning cells and their replacement by fat. A high excess of fat in the diet may also tend to produce actual storage of fat in the liver. Drugs particularly harmful to the liver are chloroform, carbon tetrachloride (which is used in dry cleaning), arsenic, and phosphorus.

Most important in relation to the liver is the fact that it can almost completely regenerate itself, if given a chance, after it has been damaged.

LIVER EXTRACTS Liver extracts are used in the treatment of pernicious anemia. It has been found that the liver contains a substance which stimulates the formation of red blood corpuscles in the blood of people suffering from pernicious anemia.

LIVER SPOTS Liver spots, scientifically called chloasma, frequently ap-

pear without any definite cause. They also represent a deposit of color pigments from the blood in the skin. Liver spots seem to be associated with glandular disturbances. They appear where there is pressure from a pad or belt; sometimes they are associated with the application of light, heat, or perfume. Often they disappear spontaneously.

It is not safe for anyone to attempt to peel away these liver spots by selftreatment because of the dangerous character of the substances that are used.

LOCKJAW See *Tetanus.*

LOCOMOTOR ATAXIA When syphilis gets into the nervous system, it produces serious changes. By modern scientific technics it has been determined with certainty that two diseases —namely, locomotor ataxia (also called tabes, paresis) and paralytic dementia —are definitely related to syphilitic infection. Locomotor ataxia is the result of infection of the spinal column. Frequently it comes on five to fifteen years after the person was first infected with syphilis.

In locomotor ataxia the tissues of the spine are so damaged that reflexes like the knee jerk disappear. Changes take place in the ability of the pupil of the eye to react as it should. In a typical case of locomotor ataxia the eye will react to looking at a distance and then at a near object with the opening and closing of the pupil. The eye will not, however, in the presence of locomotor ataxia react to dark by closing and opening the pupil. In many cases the pupils are irregular in size and slow to react.

Other disturbances associated with locomotor ataxia are knifelike pains in the abdomen, legs, or face and all sorts of abnormal sensations related to cold and warmth and numbness. Sometimes there is a feeling of tingling and often a sensation that bugs are running on the skin.

One of the most serious symptoms of locomotor ataxia is inability to co-ordinate actions of the muscles. The affected person may not be able to touch the tip of his nose with his finger. His legs get out of order, so that he finds it hard to walk in the dark. His gait may change so that in the late stages his foot seems to be thrown up and then brought down unsteadily as if it were being slapped on the floor. The cast of the legs is somewhat like that in a horse called "string halt."

The sudden severe pains in the internal organs have on occasion been mistaken for appendicitis or inflammation of the intestines.

Without suitable treatment cases of locomotor ataxia get worse but the progress of the disease may be slow, requiring years before the case terminates in death.

New methods of treatment are now being studied with a view to determining whether or not they can control syphilis as it affects the nervous system and thus stop the progress and bring about cure in cases of locomotor ataxia. In some of these studies the drug called penicillin is being injected directly into the spine.

LONGEVITY In Sweden in 1755 the average age at death was 34.5 years. In the United States in 1789 life expectancy at birth was about 35 years; in 1955 a child born in the United States can reasonably expect to live more than 68 years. The will to live is deeply rooted in all mankind. From the beginning of time man has sought not only increasing years but increasing years of usefulness. Apparently the older we get, the more anxious we are to keep on living. The person of 85 wants to reach for 90. Those who pass 90 begin to think about reaching 100.

In some families most of the people live to a ripe old age; in others this is the exception. Oliver Wendell Holmes suggested to those who wanted to live long that they select parents and grandparents who live long. In other words, the tendency to live long is to some extent an inherited tendency.

The gag that life in the country is not really longer than life in the city is not based on truth. Of course life in the country may seem longer but the figures show that people who live in the rural districts actually do live four to five years longer than those who live in the cities.

Some jobs are associated with longer life than others. Aviators have a high death rate in contrast even to chauffeurs. The death rate among school teachers is low. Apparently the occupation that is about as safe as any with a view to living longer is that of college professor or president.

Women generally have a better chance of living through to a ripe old age than men. Indeed the largest banks and the insurance companies insist that this tendency is resulting in the gradual concentration of most of the wealth of the nation in the hands of women. It has long been known that retirement not infrequently hastens the death of the aged. A successful businessman when relieved of his usual life tends to degenerate rapidly. Every trifling ailment begins to receive his undivided attention. Dignitaries of the church, chief justices on the Supreme Court benches, prime ministers, and others whose activities may be prolonged to advanced years seem to live much longer than other people.

The common idea that the person who lives long is one of exemplary habits, particularly as relates to the use of tobacco, alcohol, and similar substances, is a false one. An actual study of a considerable number of men who have reached the age of 100 showed that 54 per cent had used alcohol as a beverage during their lives and 46 per cent had been abstainers. Of 26 men over 90 years of age 6 smoked, 5 chewed, and 2 both smoked and chewed tobacco. The remaining 13 (or 50 per cent) had never used tobacco in any form.

Recent figures from the life insurance companies show that a good environment, which means healthy surroundings, is more important in living long than having long-lived parents. One of the reasons why people whose parents have died young also tend to die young is the fact that such people do not have the protection as they grow up which comes to those whose parents live. The child who is an orphan has much less chance of being healthy and of living long than the child whose parents are alive. Children from broken families are more poorly housed, fed, and clothed, and receive less medical care than children of families living together with both parents present.

LUNGS Primarily the function of the lungs is the provision of oxygen to the red blood cells and the elimination of waste carbon dioxide. The lungs are made of tiny spaces, on the surface of which the smallest blood vessels are exposed to the inhaled air. This surface by actual measurement is fifty times larger than the skin of the whole body. In the rest of the body the capillary or tiny blood vessels give up oxygen and take up carbon dioxide. In the lungs the capillary blood vessels take up oxygen and throw away carbon dioxide.

In a period of twenty-four hours an active man can absorb more than twenty cubic feet of oxygen, and the blood will give up more than twenty cubic feet of carbon dioxide. The lungs work like an automatically self-regulating bellows. Seventeen times a minute the bellows take in air and expel waste products. Automatically the bellows will speed up to seventy or eighty times a minute if the need for air is exceedingly great, as during severe muscular effort or in pneumonia.

When we take a full breath, we use every possible means for enlarging the cavity of the thorax, or chest. We lift our shoulders by action of the muscles; we lift the ribs and breastbone. The diaphragm, which is a large muscle between the chest and abdominal cavity, helps lift the ribs and shoves down the abdominal contents. In this way the capacity of the chest cavity can be enlarged more than two quarts above its resting capacity and more than three quarts above its capacity at the end of a forced outbreathing or expiration.

The mechanism is so complete and so elastic that breathing can go on when the body is in almost any position.

The right lung is larger than the left. It contains three parts, or lobes, whereas the left lung contains two. Sometimes in pneumonia only one lobe will be affected.

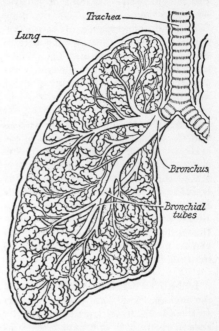

The anatomy of the lung

Among the diseases which affect the lungs, the most serious are tuberculosis and pneumonia. However, other infections may cause bronchitis or bronchiectasis. All sorts of parasites may affect the lung besides the pneumococcus and the tubercle bacillus. Moreover, the lungs on occasion become subject to cancer. Formerly surgical operations on the lung were impossible. More recently new developments in anesthesia and new methods of surgery have made it possible to operate on the lung. In a period of ten years the surgeons in one hospital did 218 operations on the lungs, removing either an entire lobe or an entire lung, with a total death rate of only 30 deaths out of 218 operations. In a previous century every one of these patients would have died. In 172 cases one lobe was removed, and in this group there were only 9 deaths. In 46 cases an entire lung was removed, and in this group there were 21 deaths. In another hospital an entire lung was removed in 19 cases, and 10 of the patients recovered. Fifty-five per cent of patients who had an operation on the lung because of the presence of cancer recovered. Of course not all cases of cancer can be operated on. The cancer must be localized and accessible, without the possibility of harming other vital organs like the heart.

LYMPH In addition to the arteries and the veins, most of the tissues of the body are connected with the lymphatic system. The lymphatic vessels contain a transparent, slightly yellow fluid that is called lymph. When red blood cells get into the lymph, it may have a light rose color. The lymph helps to maintain the fluid state of the tissues. The lymph channels serve to carry away infected material from the tissues.

LYMPHOPATHIA   VENEREUM Among the conditions that can affect man and which are spread widely by sexual relations is one called scientifically lymphopathia venereum but known also throughout the world by a wide variety of other names, including climatic bubo and tropical ulcer. It has also been called the fourth venereal disease, the other three being gonorrhea, syphilis, and chancroid.

This venereal disease is caused by a filtrable virus—one of those agents so small that it cannot be seen with an ordinary microscope. Most significant of its symptoms, as suggested by the name, is the swelling of the glands following infection by sex contact. Usually a few days after contact with a person who is infected, a small ulcer will appear on the organs. Often this heals without very much trouble, but occasionally it becomes secondarily infected and becomes a large ulcer. The infec-

tion spreads, however, along the lymph channels and reaches one of the large lymph glands after ten to thirty days.

The first symptoms are stiffness and aching in the groin, followed by swelling. After the swelling has been large and hard for a while, it breaks down, frequently leaving an opening with an abscess. The breaking down and gradual healing may take anywhere from two months to two years. In very severe cases the infection may spread from the original gland to other glands, may cause a secondary infection of the veins of the leg with great swelling of the tissues, and may, in fact, involve the whole body in a general disease.

About twenty years ago a diagnostic test for this disease, like the skin tests that are used in other diseases, was discovered, and vaccines have been developed which are used in the treatment.

At first it was thought that this condition affected only males because those who suffered from it were chiefly sailors, but more recently the condition has been found also among women all over the world. The condition can be spread from one person to another by the use of nozzles of syringes and in other ways when strict sanitation is not properly practiced.

Usually the first spot of infection will disappear if simply treated with alcohol and antiseptic dressings, but when the glands swell and are infected, other treatments are tried, some of which seem to have yielded success. A vaccine made from the material taken from an infected gland has been reported by many physicians to be especially useful in controlling the duration of the disease.

LYSOL Lysol is the proprietary name for the compound solution of cresol, an antiseptic solution which is also caustic and poisonous in high concentrations.

MADURA FOOT In 1898 a Boston physician reported the occurrence in the United States of a peculiar disease usually found only in the tropics.

Another case was reported from Galveston in 1921, and a third from Cleveland in 1925.

In this condition a parasitic type of organism gets into the tissue through an opening in the skin, usually an open wound, and there sets up an inflammation which is associated with granulation and overgrowth of the tissues.

The growth slowly progresses, ulcerates sometimes, and eventually may cause serious disability, if not death. The organisms usually enter through wounds in the feet, so that the condition has also been called Madura foot.

In the most recently reported case a Negro meat packer was involved. He had first injured his foot in 1914 and had suffered intermittently with trouble with the foot for twelve years. He was a common laborer during most of that time, and had never attempted to get good medical treatment but had constantly attempted to manipulate and treat the swelling with simple methods of his own.

As a result the granulation had grown until the lump on his foot was about the size of a hen's egg. Scientific investigation revealed the presence in the wound of the organism associated with maduro-mycosis.

The lump was removed by surgical methods and the resulting wound was treated with special antiseptic solutions which have the power to attack the organism that causes Madura foot. In six weeks the condition from which the patient had suffered for more than twelve years was cured.

Other conditions somewhat similar to Madura foot occasionally occur in the United States, among them being a granulation called actinomycosis, which is caused by an organism similar to the one that causes the tropical disease. However, even actinomycosis is a relatively rare condition.

MAGNESIUM CITRATE This is among the most popular of the mild saline purgatives. It is usually bought by the bottle and taken in the morning on arising in the amounts prescribed by the doctor.

MAIDENHEAD See *Hymen.*

MALARIA Malaria is the number one menace in the world. This disease was known in the fifth century B.C., and its various types were classified at least three hundred years B.C. Scientific control began, however, around 1880, when a French army surgeon named Laveran found that there were parasites in the red blood cells which seemed to be responsible for the condition. Since that time the nature of the disease has been more thoroughly studied. It has been shown that the disease is carried from one human being to another by the anopheline mosquito. More recently means have been found for preventing the disease through the control of the mosquito and also by the use of preventive drugs.

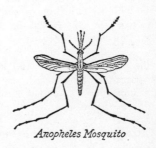

Anopheles Mosquito

The Anopheles mosquito, which carries malaria

In the United States there are at least 1,000,000 cases of malaria at all times and about 5,000 deaths occur each year from this cause. Great numbers of our soldiers were infected with the parasite that causes this disease.

The mosquito does not carry the parasite directly from one person to another. Actually the mosquito gets the parasite into its body at one stage of its existence; this parasite must develop into another stage, which then produces the disease in the second person who is bitten. For the infection to be transmitted, the female Anopheles mosquito must first bite a person who has male and female malaria parasites in the circulating blood. Inside the stomach of the mosquito these parasites undergo fertilization. The male parasite pushes out little filaments which break loose and come into contact with the female form. Exactly as the sperm cell of the male human being penetrates the ovum of the female, so does one of these male parasites penetrate the female and fertilize it. The fertilized forms then push their way out of the stomach cells and gradually enlarge, so that they rupture into the body cavity of the mosquito and make their way to the salivary glands of the mosquito, where they lie. When the mosquito bites an individual, these parasites pass with the saliva and start the development of the parasite in the person who has been bitten. About ten days after the infection has been acquired in this way, the first parasites will be observed in the red blood cells of the person who has been infected. This parasite devours the red pigment and iron-containing material. Then the red cell ruptures and about sixteen parasites are released, each of which attaches itself to a new red cell.

There are various other forms of the parasite which produce different forms of malaria in man. The chief symptoms vary according to the form of the parasite.

The condition begins with backache, muscle soreness, and fever, with paroxysms and chills, about the fourteenth day. When paroxysms occur on alternate days, it is due to the fact that there are two broods of the same parasite developing in the blood. This gives the condition a cold, a hot, and a sweating stage. In the cold stage there are chills with chattering of the teeth, the skin becoming blue and cold, and, associated with this, an uncontrollable shaking. Then comes a high fever, and after that a sweating stage, when the temperature drops to normal.

In quartan malaria four days intervene between the sets of symptoms, the paroxysms occurring usually every seventy-two hours. In falciparum malaria the temperature is high, the incubation period is about twelve days, the fever is irregular, and bleeding (including blood in the urine) is a frequent complication.

The doctor diagnoses the form of the malaria from the symptoms and the order in which they occur and also, of course, by a study of the blood. Another test involves the giving of quinine, which will control malaria.

Among new drugs are chloraquine, which has advantages over atabrine or quinacrine. For radical cure primaquine is favored. Camoquin is much used for prevention and Daraprim in the treatment of malaria.

Fortunately we have been able to control malaria by the use of quinine and of another form of cinchona known as totaquine, all of which are useful in the prevention and treatment of malaria. About twice as much totaquine as quinine must be given for both prevention and treatment.

One of the most important steps in relation to malaria is the prevention of the spread of the disease through control of the mosquito. This involves cleaning up swamps, removal of excess rain water, and the spraying of areas with oils or insecticides that destroy the mosquito in various stages. People who are constantly exposed to malaria in tropical areas take quinine every day one hour before sunset. They also screen their beds at night and keep the air moving, if possible, by the use of an electric fan. They wear suitable clothing, including leg coverings of soft leather, double stockings, and face nets.

Whereas the mosquito repellents of the past were somewhat ineffective aromatic oils, there are now available powerful insect repellents which are most effective in preventing the bite of the mosquito, the louse, and various other insects.

MAMMARY GLANDS The scientific name for the breasts.

MARASMUS Infants are sometimes attacked by an inability to utilize food which produces progessive wasting and emaciation. This condition has been called marasmus.

MASSAGE The word "massage" is applied to any manipulation of the tissue of the body, using the hands or certain special devices that have been invented. Several different movements are used in massage for special purposes.

The simplest form of massage is the superficial stroking movement designed to have a sedative effect. These movements were, no doubt, discovered spontaneously thousands of years ago. Everybody knows that slow, rhythmical stroking will help to relieve pain in various portions of the body and to induce sleep. The chief rules for sedative movement are that it be superficial and rhythmical and that it be done in a manner that is acceptable and not irritating to the person who is receiving the massage. Indeed it is customary to begin over an area that is not sensitive and to continue the massage until it takes in the painful or sensitive area, because only in this way is it possible to find out whether or not the stroking is acceptable to the patient.

A second form of stroking movement used in massage is the deep movement, which is designed to assist the flow of the blood and the lymph through the veins and the lymph channels. Since the flow in these channels is toward the body rather than away from it, it is customary to practice these deep stroking movements toward the center of the body. Such deep stroking tends to relax the muscles and to reduce swelling. Deep stroking over the abdomen will excite the intestines into motion, particularly in a case in which the intestines are sensitive to such stimulation. Actually normal contraction and relaxation of the muscles of the abdominal wall can produce the same effect.

Another movement commonly used in massage is the squeezing movement, in which pressure is applied to the tissues between the fingers or the hands. The tissues may be pulled up and thus pressed between the fingers, or the pressure may be from the outside against the underlying muscles and bones. Such movements help to break up adhesions, to stimulate the circulation, and to induce heat. In these motions there may be friction on the tissues which also increases heat, or there may be vibratory movements which shake and agitate the tissues and thus improve the circulation.

Still another technic used in massage is known as the percussion movement. This is a hammering movement which may be done with the fingers or with various instruments, the effect being, in general, like that of vibration.

Following massage, there should be relief of pain, decrease of swelling, and increase of motion of the parts involved. If, however, the effects are in an opposite direction, it is probable that the massage is not beneficial.

MASTITIS Inflammation of the mammary glands is called mastitis. The condition is usually due to infection with various germs. Infection by the streptococci or the staphylococci produces suppuration. The treatment of mastitis may involve surgical emptying of abscesses and the use of such drugs as the sulfonamides and penicillin, which act specifically against the infecting germs.

MASTOIDITIS Mastoid is the name applied to a portion of the bones of the skull. The cells of the mastoid are behind the ear. When an inflammation occurs in these cells following any infection, the condition is called mastoiditis; this merely means inflammation of the mastoid.

Doctors believe that mastoiditis occurs frequently due to bad habits in blowing the nose. When the little boy with the running nose and sore throat blows his nose vigorously, at the same time keeping both nostrils shut, air is forced from the throat and into the

Eustachian tube which passes from the back of the nose to the ear. With the air go the infecting germs that are in the throat. Soon the little boy hears a clinking sound in his ear. Then there is a dull feeling and the ear begins to ache. The doctor finds that the eardrum is quite red and that the boy cannot hear. There is swelling behind the ear and the point is painful on pressure. Usually the doctor will decide to open the eardrum as soon as possible so as to permit infected material to escape and thus to avoid further damage to the mastoid and to the hearing.

The cells of the mastoid are close to the mechanism of the internal ear with which we hear and with which we maintain our equilibrium. They are also close to the outer covering of the brain and to many important nerves. Obviously everything possible should be done to prevent serious damage to these important organs and tissues.

Infection of the mastoid frequently follows such diseases as measles, scarlet fever, and diphtheria. Mastoiditis is a dangerous disease and not to be trifled with.

Fortunately two recent discoveries have done much to prevent mastoiditis as a complication of infectious diseases and also to cure without an operation. The use of the sulfonamide drugs helps to prevent the infections with the streptococcus, which is the most frequent cause of mastoiditis. Quite recently in the more serious cases penicillin has also been found capable of stopping the progress of infections in the ear before the mastoid has become seriously involved.

MEASLES Measles continues to be one of the most prevalent ailments affecting young children. Studies made in our large cities show no appreciable reduction in the number of cases of measles reported each year for the last twenty-five years. However, the ability to control the disease is now greater than ever before. In 1913 there were 12.4 deaths from measles for every 100,-000 population in Chicago. By 1940 this

figure had dropped to 1 death for every 100,000 persons.

The factors said to be responsible for the decrease in the death rate include improved housing, better medical care, improved nursing, and, above all, the use of drugs which have been found efficient in controlling the complications of measles. It is the complications of measles which primarily cause death in those who are infected.

Today measles is generally considered to be a virus disease caused by an infectious agent too small to be seen with an ordinary microscope. Medicine has developed a number of protective technics which are of great importance in preventing measles.

Among these technics is the injection of serum from the blood of children who have recently recovered from the disease. This is available through so-called serum centers or blood banks which keep such convalescent serum available. The modern technic includes the use of what is called immune globulin. Formerly this immune globulin was developed from the placenta, usually called the afterbirth, the structure by which a newborn child is attached to the body of his mother. More recently it has been found that immune globulin, with all of the virtues for the prevention of disease, can be secured as a by-product of the blood collected through the blood banks. The gamma globulin of the blood contains antisubstances against measles, infectious hepatitis, and poliomyelitis. Globulin is now manufactured by several companies. The amount given depends on the age and weight of the child.

In 1955 John Enders grew the measles virus in pure culture outside the human body. Scientists may soon prepare a vaccine for prevention of measles as effective as that against infantile paralysis.

Following are seven preventive measures recommended in times when an epidemic of measles is prevalent:

1. Don't unnecessarily expose a child to measles. This disease can be very dangerous to young children.

2. Don't permit a child who has been exposed to measles to play with other children for at least two weeks. He may be getting the disease himself, and it might take this long for you to be sure.

3. Don't permit your child to play with another child known to have been exposed to measles within two weeks. You don't want your child to have the disease if you can help it.

4. Don't permit your child to receive repeated exposures to measles. Even if you know he has been exposed, don't let him play with a child sick with the disease or thought to be developing it. Repeated exposures add to the severity of the attack.

5. Don't send your child to school if he is not well. If you think he is sick, call a doctor; if you are not sure, keep him home so you can watch him.

6. Don't let a child who has had measles get out of bed until the doctor says it is all right. Even if he does not appear too sick, the child with measles is very susceptible to such complications as pneumonia and abscessed ears.

7. Don't say, "It's only measles." Measles is a serious disease, and the child with measles requires good medical and nursing care.

The complications of measles are primarily responsible for trouble with that disease. These include infections of the eyes, the nose and throat, the bronchial tubes, and even of the digestive tract. After measles has attacked the body, secondary germs like the streptococcus, pneumococcus, influenza bacillus, and even the organism of meningitis may invade. The complications appear in any stage of measles but are most likely to develop after the eruption has occurred fully.

Once upon a time diphtheria was a frequent complication of measles, but that is no longer the case since we have learned how to prevent the contacts that permit the two diseases at one time. Fortunately the secondary infections of the ear, nose, throat, and glands are controllable nowadays by the use of the new drugs that have been developed, including particularly the sulfonamide drugs and penicillin. These drugs can be given only by the physician, who determines when the drug is to be given and how much is to be administered at any one time.

One of the most serious complications of measles is an inflammation of the brain, which seems to be due, however, not to any secondary organism but actually to the virus of measles itself. We know now that the virus may attack the brain.

Fortunately the secondary inflammation occurs in less than .1 per cent of all cases. Nobody knows just why it occurs in any individual case. It does not seem to be directly related to the severity of the measles.

When death from measles occurs, it is usually among children who are weakened and undernourished. Deaths from measles in children under six months of age are extremely rare because these children carry in their blood the immunity that they derive from their mothers. The maximum death rate occurs among children of preschool age.

Once upon a time tuberculosis was most feared as a complication of measles. Nowadays that also has been greatly decreased because tuberculosis is detected early in children, and with proper care prompt healing is brought about.

The very latest figures show that about .2 per cent of all children infected with measles die, and even this figure is supposed to be too high because it is estimated that at least two or three times the number of children reported as having measles actually have the disease.

MEASLES, GERMAN Among the infectious diseases which appear most often in spring and early summer is German measles. Usually it affects children of grade school and high school age and rather seldom those under five years of age. Although the word "measles" is attached to this condition, it is not at all related to ordinary measles. Apparently German measles is spread as are the other infectious diseases—by material coming from the nose and throat of the person who is infected. Usually about eighteen days pass after a person has been exposed to German measles before he comes down with the disease, although the period seems to vary from nine to twenty-one days. Often the first symptom observed is the rash, although occasionally the usual signs of an infection appear, including headache, runny nose, slight sore throat, and a general feeling of illness. The eruption usually appears on the chest in the form of pale pink spots. It spreads rapidly, however, over the rest of the body, finally producing a distinct scarlet appearance. The fever is not usually high in German measles, nor are the patients so severely ill as they may be with measles or scarlet fever.

One of the special signs of German measles is the swelling of the lymph glands at the back of the head and neck, which most often are about the size of a pea but occasionally may get as large as a hazelnut. Usually the swelling of these glands disappears rapidly, but occasionally it persists for several weeks.

Quite frequently German measles is mistaken for scarlet fever or measles.

Ordinarily a child with German measles is kept at home so as to prevent spreading the infection to other people. The control of the condition, however, is exceedingly difficult because of the long period of time during which it is undergoing development in the body when it is also possible to transmit the disease. Fortunately, however, the disease is not severe and does not last long. In most cases indeed the treatment of German measles simply involves isolating the patient and keeping him in bed with a light diet until the temperature has fallen and the rash has disappeared.

German measles, attacking a pregnant woman during the first four months of pregnancy, may cause a deformed child.

After a child has had German measles, the room is thoroughly cleaned, aired, and sunned, and the linens washed and boiled. No other disinfection is necessary.

MEDICINE CHEST Most Americans, being independent and individualistic, feel themselves competent to fix defects in plumbing and almost equally competent to take care of their own disturbances of health, as well as to prescribe for more complicated disturbances which really ought to have the prompt attention of a physician.

If one looks over the average family medicine chest, he is likely to find it full of strange concoctions and things of all kinds—an array of disorder which actually endangers the family's health and safety. A survey which I made of the contents of the medicine chests of a considerable number of families brought out some exceedingly interesting information.

Among the strange items found in these medicine chests were old cloths to be used as bandages, cracked atomizer bulbs, horehound candy, shoehorns, curling irons, dried sponges, packages of seeds, hair grease, mange cure, face bleach, shoe polish, empty toothpaste and shaving-cream tubes, fifty different remedies for colds, combs and bobby pins, cuff links, nail polish, bath salts, and discarded sets of teeth. The number of antiseptics found, and their efficiency, varied tremendously. One or two antiseptics were found in some cases, and as many as six different antiseptics in others, individual members of the family having their own likes and dislikes in these matters.

Apparently most American housewives need a lot of education concerning the significance of what are actually effective and useful household remedies. A household remedy should be one with a certain definite action, and usually it should contain but one active ingredient. If the thing is worth keeping in the medicine chest, it should be something which is used fairly frequently.

Dangerous poisons have no place in the family medicine chest. A dangerous poison is one which is likely to produce serious symptoms or death if taken in even moderate amounts.

Prescriptions ordered by the family doctor for a certain illness should never be kept for the future. If any of the material remains in the bottle, it should be poured promptly into a safe place of disposal. Since useful bottles are rare around most homes, the bottle may be thoroughly washed with hot water, dried, and stored away. Few people realize that most drugs deteriorate with age and that a prescription for a certain illness is not likely to be useful for the future.

REGULAR CLEANING—The wise person will go over the family medicine chest at least once every three months and discard all materials not constantly in use. It is also well to have the family doctor take a look at the materials to offer his advice on those worth keeping and make suggestions as to what is needed. Unless measures of this kind are taken, the amount of "junk" that accumulates in the average medicine chest becomes something appalling. Used safety-razor blades are dangerous. A good rule is to put the old blade in the package every time a new blade is taken out. Then when the package is filled with old blades, the box can be thrown in the household rubbish.

ITEMS IN MEDICINE CHEST—Most families want to keep on hand a laxative or cathartic. Under certain circumstances any laxative or cathartic may be exceedingly dangerous. The most conspicuous example is appendicitis. This is at first just an infected spot on a little organ which comes off the large bowel and which apparently has no serious function in the human body. If this infection develops the way a boil develops from a pimple, it is in danger of bursting and spreading throughout the body. Therefore no laxative or cathartic should ever be taken when the abdomen is exceedingly painful.

The most common laxatives used in a family medicine chest include liquid petrolatum or mineral oil, which is a mechanical lubricant without possibility of serious harm. Other common prep-arations much used include phenol-phthalein, castor oil, Seidlitz powders, milk of magnesia, psyllium seed, sodium phosphate, aromatic cascara, and mineral oil mixed with agar.

The next most commonly used preparations in a family medicine chest are pain relievers. Most of these are used for headaches, although sometimes they are used for neuritis, neuralgia, toothache, and other pains of unknown origin, as well as to produce sleep. Most headache powders bought under patent trademarks contain phenacetin or acetanilid, sometimes in considerable dosage. It is not well to experiment with acetanilid because it may, in large dosage, have serious effects on the body, including particularly the blood and the heart. Moreover, there is a tendency to form the habit of taking such preparations. Other drugs much used to produce sleep are derivatives of barbituric acid, of which some of the best examples are veronal, trional, and combinations of barbituric acids with other drugs. The family medicine chest is better off without preparations of this character, as the possibilities for harm are sufficiently great to suggest that these preparations should not be used except with medical advice.

The most commonly used general pain reliever is acetylsalicylic acid, commonly called aspirin. So far as is known, aspirin is relatively harmless except for a few people who are especially sensitive to it. Such people cannot take even small doses. One aspirin is as good as another, provided it is up to the standard of the United States Pharmacopoeia.

Among the strongest of medicinal preparations are the narcotics and anesthetics. Narcotics should never be used by anyone without a physician's prescription and, indeed, no drug that has to be administered with a hypodermic syringe should find a place in the average family medicine chest. There are some people with diabetes who have been taught by their doctors to inject themselves with insulin. Even these people should keep their syringe outfit separate from the materials in the family medicine chest.

There are all sorts of antiseptics available for use on the skin, in first aid and also for gargling and for washing various portions of the body.

The most widely known skin antiseptics are tincture of iodine and 2 per cent mercurochrome. The Council on Pharmacy and Chemistry of the American Medical Association permits advertising of recognized antiseptics for first aid, and tincture of iodine and mercurochrome are included among such preparations.

This same Council has concluded that no antiseptic substance is of value when used as a gargle for the destruction of germs in the mouth and throat. If the antiseptic is applied directly on a swab so that the material is held in direct contact with the localized infection, it may have some definite use.

Among the antiseptics approved by the Council on Pharmacy and Chemistry are preparations of hexylresorcinol and preparations of metaphen, also neutral solution of chlorinated soda and hydrogen peroxide. The Council has not approved antiseptics commonly represented as being useful in the relief of all sorts of infections of the throat and also for the prevention of various types of infectious diseases, including colds.

One of the best old-fashioned antiseptic solutions for common use around the home is boric acid solution. Most people prefer to have packages of crystals of boric acid or of the powder and to make up the solution fresh just before use.

FIRST-AID SUPPLIES—Among the materials needed for first aid are adhesive tape of various widths, sterile cotton, sterile gauze bandages, sterile gauze pads, and scissors, which should be kept in the medicine chest exclusively for such purposes. You should also have the ready-made combinations of a piece of adhesive tape with a tiny piece of sterilized bandage that can be used to cover small wounds after they have been treated with iodine or mercurochrome.

People should know that the proper way to stop bleeding of small wounds is simply to press upon them with a sterile piece of gauze. In case of very serious wounds affecting arteries and thereby difficult to control, it may be necessary to put a tourniquet around the limb. The tourniquet should be fastened just tight enough to stop the bleeding. An ordinary piece of rubber tubing or a narrow towel tied and twisted with a stick will serve most purposes satisfactorily.

The family medicine chest may also contain aromatic spirits of ammonia, which is sometimes given when a prompt stimulant is needed following fainting. Half a teaspoonful in water, for a sudden fainting spell, is a fairly safe thing to give in most cases of this emergency.

The widely publicized milk of magnesia and sodium bicarbonate, or baking soda, are two preparations which can safely be kept in the family medicine chest and which are frequently advised by physicians for alkaline purposes.

Some families keep paregoric as a useful preparation in case of cramps that affect women at periodic intervals.

These items constitute practically all the equipment that need be in any average medicine chest because they are the few materials that can be used safely by most people.

SHAVING MATERIALS—Most modern women prefer to keep their cosmetics in their own boudoirs, but the man of the house is very likely to put his into the family medicine cabinet. They should include, in most instances, a razor, which should be kept in its box and not permitted to lie around loosely; also some shaving soap or cream, and some face lotion, which may be either witch hazel or a special lotion which he prefers.

It is not advisable to use a styptic in the form of a stick of alum to stop slight bleeding points after shaving. Much better are any of the astringent surgical powders, of which a small amount may be taken from the box on each occasion and applied directly to the bleeding point. Finally, any good talcum powder may be used after shaving and after bathing, according to the individual preferences of the users.

All such materials should be kept in orderly position and not scattered around the chest helter-skelter, as many men are inclined to do.

ADDITIONAL ITEMS—It is taken for granted that every modern household has a good clinical thermometer, a hot-water bottle, and an ice bag. These are three exceedingly useful devices in any home, and when they are available in an emergency the comfort they give is tremendous.

In addition to the materials used for first aid, most families will have bed-pans for use in cases of illness, glass drinking tubes, syringes for giving enemas, atomizers, and sometimes special devices for creating steam to be medicated with small amounts of tincture of benzoin for relief in various forms of hoarseness or other conditions affecting the larynx and the lungs.

DON'TS—There are certain "don'ts" which should be remembered:

Do not save poisonous preparations of any kind, including particularly bi-chloride of mercury, pills containing strychnine, or solutions containing wood alcohol.

Do not keep samples of patent medi-cines of unknown composition recom-mended beyond their actual virtues.

Never permit any preparation of opium or morphine in the family medi-cine chest.

Never save any prepared prescription after the specific use for which it was ordered by the physician has disap-peared.

MELANCHOLIA Sometimes with advancing years both men and women tend to develop a mental reaction that leads to melancholia. The symptoms usually come on at what women call "the change of life."

There still seems to be some question as to whether or not men also have a change of life. Certainly they do oc-casionally develop symptoms following the passing of middle age much like those that women develop under the same circumstances.

At this time the man or woman may find that life is beginning to be more disturbing, the resistance to pressures becomes less capable of meeting the need, the bounce or resiliency that is associated with youth has disappeared, and mistakes are more difficult to cor-rect.

Under the circumstances here de-scribed, anxiety, apprehension, and in-decision may lead to breakdown. The mental condition that develops repre-sents an attempt to escape from pres-sure that cannot be overcome. Dr. Ed-ward A. Strecker emphasizes the fact that the increasing likelihood of failure to attain successes that have been sought, financial reverses, disappoint-ments, family worries, and the increas-ing number of family and friends that are taken by death tend to increase the internal psychic upset.

Women suffer more frequently from this type of melancholia than men—in fact the ratio is about three women to one man. The age range in women is from forty to fifty-five and in men from fifty to sixty-five.

Of course inspiration from the lives of others is the answer to the problem for many people. Far too many men and women have made great successes of their lives following the climacteric for anyone to believe that this period represents the end of much that is vital in living.

Moreover, advancement in the care of the human body makes the modern woman realize that one past forty years of age need not necessarily be unat-tractive. The aids to beauty are suffi-cient to enable her to be just about as attractive as she wants to be provided she will put in the time and study re-quired.

The chief symptoms, however, are related to the mind and not to the ap-pearance of the body. The woman ap-proaching melancholia tends to blame herself unnecessarily for activities or for lack of action.

Fortunately with the aid of the modern psychiatrist many of these people can be brought to prompt recovery. The treatment includes a study of the mental aspects which can be done only by someone properly trained in this field. The food should be sufficient, and proper sleep must be obtained by the methods that doctors can prescribe.

The glandular preparations which have been developed to replace the hormones (including the estrogenic hormone for women and the testosterone for men) are reported by many to be helpful. Equally important is development of suitable occupations and hobbies so that the mind can be turned to productive purposes.

MELANOSIS Abnormal deposits of pigment in various portions of the body are described as melanosis. Since pigment may be involved in all sorts of tissues, the prefix "melano-" may refer to pigment in sweat, melanidrosis; to the pigment in tumors, melanocarcinoma or melanosarcoma; pigment in the menstrual flow, melanorrhagia.

MEMORY Memory is one of the strangest of all of the functions of the human mind. It has given great concern to the psychologists to determine how it is carried on. Some information has come from experiments on the brain. It is known, for instance, that persons who have tumors of the frontal lobes of the brain complain of loss of memory, particularly for recent events.

Memory is so valuable an attribute to success that its importance cannot be overestimated. We know that hardening of the arteries and diminished circulation of the blood associated with the coming of old age also have an influence on memory.

There are many people who are only apparently unable to remember well. This, however, is the result of absent-mindedness and preoccupation and of the failure to give attention rather than any disorder of memory. Many people have a special faculty for remembering, which can be better developed by training. They are thereby more successful in occupations in which memory is important.

The type of loss of memory that is most serious is that which occurs suddenly and is accompanied by confusion. This may be a sign of disease. However, there is no reason to believe that a gradual failure of the memory indicates the beginning of any disorder of the brain.

Among the most dramatic and impressive disturbances that can affect the human being is the loss of memory called amnesia. This is an inability to remember occurrences that have happened during a certain period of life. Such loss of memory comes on frequently in relationship to a sudden emotional conflict or difficult situation. Usually memory begins to come back when some thread in the past is uncovered. The doctors find it difficult in most of these cases to decide whether or not complete inability to remember anything is actual or simulated. If anyone simply refuses to remember, the diagnosis is difficult. Cases are on record of people who have had as many as five such periods of sudden and complete loss of memory with subsequent recovery.

The psychoanalysts explain this form of loss of memory as a weak attempt of a weak personality to escape conflicts in daily life. Associated with the desire to escape is the fear of punishment, the fear of bodily injury, or the fear of certain human relationships.

MENIÈRE'S DISEASE In 1861 a French physician named Menière described a series of symptoms related to an acute disturbance of a structure in the internal ear called the labyrinth to which the name "Menière's disease" is now given.

Apparently there are several different causes for disturbances of the labyrinth. The chief symptoms are deafness and ringing in the ears associated with dizziness, vomiting, and sudden movements of the eyes from side to side. The attacks come on at regular intervals, and once the condition has started they may return with increasing frequency. Some cases seem to improve without anything special in the way of treatment. Others get better and alternately get worse. Sometimes improvement follows operations on the sinuses, removal of the tonsils and adenoids, treatment of the hearing, the extraction of infected teeth, the blowing out of the Eustachian tubes, and changes in the diet.

It has been thought that possibly the difficulty was associated with a disturbance of the water balance of the body, also that it was associated with a retention of sodium in the body. For this reason diets that are low in sodium and high in protein are sometimes prescribed. Also ammonium chloride is given with a view to preventing salt retention.

More recently a surgical procedure has been evolved. This includes especially operations on the nerve of hearing, also attempts to investigate the area concerned for the presence of infections, tumors, or similar disturbances.

Ménière's disease rarely occurs in young people. Most of those affected are between the ages of thirty and sixty.

Dramamine and Bonamine have aided in controlling the dizziness associated with Ménière's disease.

MENINGES The coverings of the brain and spinal cord are called the meninges. Inflammation of these coverings is meningitis. A tumor in the meninges is a meningioma. The prefix also appears in many other conditions affecting these membranes.

MENINGITIS Meningitis, an infection of the brain and incidentally also of the blood, is caused in most instances by the germ called the meningococcus. It is possible, however, for other germs like the pneumococcus or the streptococcus to cause meningitis and also for viruses to cause inflammation of the coverings of the brain and spinal cord, which are known as meninges.

The doctor diagnoses meningitis not only from the history of the patient, which may indicate that he has been in contact with the infection, and from the symptoms but also by obtaining specimens of the spinal fluid, which are studied for the presence of germs and for other changes which indicate infection and inflammation. In times when epidemics of meningitis are present, doctors examine not only the spinal fluid of those who are sick but also the secretions of the nose and throat of the sick and of those around them to determine whether are not the germs are present. Occasionally examinations are made of the blood to find out whether there is or is not a meningococcemia, which means germs of meningitis in the blood.

The symptoms of meningitis arise from the changes that the germs and their poisons produce in the tissues of the nervous system. During the period of invasion sore throat, dullness, fever, chills, rapid pulse, and a general soreness of the body indicate that an infection is present. Then comes a rash of pin-point-sized red spots or even large spots over the body. In the stage when the infection has spread to the nervous system severe pain is felt, associated with bursting headache, vomiting, and even delirium and convulsions.

Meningitis is particularly a disease associated with overcrowding, so that it appears in wartime when great numbers of men are housed in barracks. Although there had been just a few cases of meningitis in Great Britain up to 1940, the assembling of the army at that time brought about a sudden severe outbreak which affected more than 4000 men in the first six months of 1940.

The way to prevent meningitis is to avoid overcrowding and to avoid contact with sick people. In many of our American camps provision had been made for a cubicle system, so that a curtain or screen comes down at night between the beds of men in barracks. Even without such intervening devices it is possible to decrease the incidence of meningitis by lessening the crowding. In one camp it was found that the carrier rate was 29 per cent when the space between the beds was nine inches, 20 per cent when a foot was allowed between adjacent beds, and only 5 per cent when a three-foot space was allowed.

Before the discovery of a serum which could be used against meningitis, the death rate used to be 80 or 90 out of every 100 cases. There was a severe epidemic in New York in 1904, when there were 2755 cases with 2026 deaths. Following the discovery of the anti-meningitis serum, the rate was greatly reduced. Then came the discovery of the sulfonamide drugs, which were found to have great powers in controlling the germs, and the rate was cut down to much less than 20 per cent. More recently penicillin has been developed. This is injected into the muscles, into the blood, and in fact directly into the spinal fluid. The most recent report on the use of penicillin intensively used in cases of meningitis indicated that there were 75 recoveries out of 76 consecutive cases. Thus the fear formerly associated with this dangerous disease has been lessened. Obviously there are many complications and associated symptoms possible in meningitis which demand the very best of medical attention. Preferably every case of meningitis should be cared for in a good hospital.

MENOPAUSE Between the ages of forty-five and fifty the average woman undergoes certain physical changes which are grouped by the diagnosticians under the single term of menopause. This is also called by women in general the climacteric, the climax, or the change of life. These changes occur in rare instances before the age of forty and sometimes as late as fifty-five. They are definitely associated with the gradual inability of certain glands to provide the secretions which they provide during youth and maturity.

In some women all of the changes take place suddenly and abruptly and without much trouble. Many, however, go through this period in their lives over a duration of three or four years. Most of the serious symptoms that occur involve the nervous system and the blood. The most common symptom is the appearance of what are called hot flashes, during which the entire body becomes warm and there is excessive perspiration followed by chilliness. The flushes come on at any time, sometimes without any apparent cause and at other times associated with slight excitement. The change in the circulation brings about also such symptoms as palpitation, headache, and dizziness. The symptoms related to the nervous system include irritability, occasionally depression, and quite often insomnia.

The active period of the reproductive system of a woman is about twenty-five years. Then the tissues involved in reproduction gradually become unnecessary and deteriorate. Ordinarily a woman develops once each month an egg cell, or ovum, which is released from the ovary so that she may give birth to a child. The ovaries develop internal secretions, or chemical substances, which go directly into the blood and which govern the condition of the uterus in which the ovum, when it is fertilized by the male cell, comes to rest. If the egg is not fertilized, the wall of the uterus is cast off and washed out by bleeding. This is called menstruation because it occurs about once each month. The Latin term for month is *mensis*. There is no special function for menstruation other than getting rid of this cast-off lining from the uterus. Menstruation is not a means of getting rid of body poisons as some women foolishly believe.

Most of the complaints that occur during the menopause are, after all, relatively minor disturbances. In most instances it is possible nowadays to overcome these disturbances by giving the internal secretion that is lacking from the body in the form of a drug. The physician who takes care of a woman under such circumstances is able to determine whether or not the symptoms are the ordinary symptoms of the menopause, also how much of the hormones should be prescribed and when they should be taken. A medical examination at this time is of the greatest importance because there are other conditions which can produce symptoms like those of the menopause. The new drugs that have been developed and the technic of their use represents one of the greatest discoveries of modern times for freeing women from the fear associated with the menopause and for overcoming the disagreeable symptoms.

MENSTRUATION The average age at which girls in the United States mature varies between twelve and sixteen, although normal girls may mature before twelve or after sixteen. The average interval between periods in women is twenty-eight days, although it may be as short as twenty-one or as long as thirty-five days. Moreover, irregularity may be normal with some women. The length of the periods may vary from two to six days. Slight variations should not cause any mental distress. Physicians should be consulted, however, when there is a sudden change in the regularity or a disappearance of the period.

A disappearance of the period is frequently associated with undernutrition, anemia, wasting diseases, or severe infections. These may not only cause a disappearance of the period but interfere seriously with the regularity, the duration, or the intensity of any particular period. Typhoid fever, rheumatic fever, or tuberculosis may bring about irregularity. Disturbances of the thyroid, pituitary, or the ovarian glands also are responsible for difficulties with the menstrual periods.

If the appearance of maturity should be unusually delayed, a young girl should be taken to a physician for a careful examination so that he may determine whether or not the organs involved have developed as they should. If there is too much delay in making an investigation, changes may occur in the organs and tissues which may ultimately make normal childbirth impossible.

Of course the most frequent cause of failure of the period to appear is pregnancy.

Formerly many girls and young women were incapacitated during the time of the period due to pains in the lower part of the abdomen and the thighs and similar symptoms. When pain is not severe, the use of mild doses of the ordinary sedatives frequently brings about relief. Persistent pain demanding more than such relief means that study should be made as to the cause of the disturbance. Some of the pain-relieving drugs are dangerous to health and life. The use of simple pain-relieving drugs is not harmful but persistence may develop the habit of dependence on the drug even if it does not develop addiction.

Ordinarily the young woman need not change her habits greatly during the time of the period. Most doctors believe that strenuous exercise is to be avoided at this time. Generally it is not considered advisable to take a tub bath for at least the first two days of the period and certainly not to go swimming. When it is realized that the period represents merely the throwing off by the organ concerned in childbirth of excess tissue developed in preparation for fertilization of the ovum and that this is not concerned in any way with the maintenance of health or with getting rid of poisons from the body, the importance of considering the period a normal physiological reaction is apparent.

MENTAL DEPRESSION In times of war or of economic disaster there is a tendency for many human beings to be greatly depressed from a mental point of view. This depression is reflected in their attitudes toward other people and in their actions. Depression is a state of mind in which initiative and decision are paralyzed. When people are depressed, they grow too careful. They fear to spend money; they fear to enjoy pleasures and amusements;

they hesitate to meet other people. Eventually the person who is depressed becomes on bad terms not only with the world in general but also with himself. Under these circumstances he thinks too much about himself, both physically and mentally. He tends to live in the past and to evade the future. Quite soon his depression reflects itself in his personal appearance. The person who is depressed is slouchy. He permits his clothing to go without suitable attention; he neglects to shave if he is a man or to tend to her cosmetic appearance and her hair if a woman. For this reason people who are depressed come soon to resemble one another.

During a period of depression a man is likely to change his former judgments of other people. Those whom he formerly liked he now finds unbearable; he may actually begin to seek out those whom he formerly hated. His depression makes him irritable, so that he is rude and hypercritical.

Obviously one of the most important steps in overcoming depression if you have it is to understand your own condition. This at least will serve to prevent constant worry and anxiety. People who insist that they never worry have learned to reason themselves, by rationalization, out of anxiety over situations in which they find themselves. Other people develop mental tranquility or peace of mind by accepting some belief which eliminates from consideration anything that is displeasing. This is not rationalization but may bring about the same effect for a person who is capable of shutting out from his thoughts any problem that disturbs him. Peace of mind is necessary for accomplishment because absence of peace of mind gives a constant feeling of insecurity. Often mental depression is transferred to physical conditions, so that worry may cause a person to have palpitations of the heart or to feel extra beats.

If the nervous condition brings the focus of attention on the stomach and bowels, such symptoms as constipation and diarrhea may occur.

Unfortunately failure to practice good mental hygiene may lead eventually to an attempt to escape from mental disturbance by the use of drinks, drugs, sedatives, or gambling, which in themselves may be worse than the worry that they replace. A restful night's sleep, a vacation, indulgence in outdoor sports, or even frequent use of the radio and the movies are better ways of escape from worry.

MENTAL DISEASE One person out of twenty becomes a patient in a mental hospital at some time during his life. Sooner or later one person out of ten becomes incapacitated by mental disease, at least for a short time. It has been estimated that the national expenditure for hospital care for mental disease approximates at least $200,000,-000 a year.

To the expenditure for mental disease must be added the problem of the feeble-minded. Statistics indicate that over 2 per cent of the total population of the United States is feeble-minded. These people are so deficient mentally that they are not capable of supporting themselves or even of guiding their own conduct.

In addition there are the backward children. Of these, perhaps 850,000 are unable to keep up with the courses in ordinary public schools. Special schools must be developed for them. This is the great burden of mental disturbances carried by the American people.

There is hardly a patient of any kind who does not have something of a mental problem. Disease elsewhere in the body is likely to be reflected in the mind or vice versa. Obviously the problem of mental deficiency comes close to the problem of the national defense. Many of our young men were unable to pass the examination of the Selective Service. Some who passed were later found unable to bear the strain of life under military conditions.

Recent surveys of institutions for the care of the mentally afflicted indicate that many of them are overcrowded. Some of them are very old, and the sanitation has not been kept up to date; some represent serious fire hazards. The deficit is estimated by the National Committee for Mental Hygiene as representing 150,000 beds, with long lists of patients waiting to be admitted. Proper control of mental hygiene would also provide for much-needed research in these fields, with a view to getting patients out of the hospital and back into ordinary life.

Many institutions are now devoting themselves to the study of dementia praecox, or the insanity of adolescence. Insulin and metrazol shock have been used, also electric shock, and more recently surgical treatment of various portions of the brain. Studies are being made as to the extent to which such technics can bring these people back to normalcy and also as to the time they will remain normal after this type of radical treatment.

Special attention is also being given by educators to the problems of the mentally defective. We are moving forward in our control of mental disease, but the field is vast and the conditions of modern life tend to increase the number of persons needing scientific mental hygiene.

MENTAL HYGIENE Health is generally considered to be freedom from disease. However, health also involves a state of mind in which the human being is satisfied with life, in which his mind functions accurately, and in which he possesses enough force, driving power, and impetus to give him confidence in himself and the ability to accomplish his work.

Happiness has been described as a balanced flow of energy and the satisfaction of desires. In other words, you are happy if you get what you want. One of the troubles is that many people do not know what they want and most people differ from other people in the things they want. Everyone who is ordinarily healthful is interested in getting enough to eat, in getting enough rest, and in satisfying the ordinary desire for reproduction. There are, how-

ever, different levels in these fundamental desires. Some people get hungry without really needing food; others require far more rest than the average. The nature of any desire is conditioned by experience and knowledge. A person who has never eaten strawberries is not likely to crave them.

Most of the drives of life are concerned with the fundamental things that have been mentioned. An unsatisfied wish is a driving stimulus until it is satisfied. Good mental hygiene requires a certain amount of rationalization. Rationalization is a term used to describe the ability of a human being to satisfy himself with what he gets rather than constantly to be wanting something that he cannot have. For instance every four years several people want to be President of the United States. For many of them this is quite out of the question. Some of them, therefore, satisfy themselves by becoming governor of the state, senators, or even president of a lodge or a club.

Because it is possible to find happiness with less than a maximum of the desires we possess, mental hygienists suggest that everyone develop as a major interest not only a job but perhaps some hobby or game in which he may achieve the success that is not possible in another field. The basic rule for a happy and contented mind is to cultivate certain standards of living against unexpected changes; then maintain a flexible attitude of mind so as not to be incurably depressed when you fail to achieve something you want.

METABOLISM In the functions of the human body, it uses up oxygen. The tissues use more oxygen during digestion, during exercise, and during exposure to cold than they do when the human body is resting under conditions of warmth. The rate of use of oxygen to carry on the activities of life and in resting gives a figure which is known as the basal metabolism. Standards have been established for human beings of various weight and size. Infants use up more oxygen for the weight of their bodies than adults. Old people use less. Women use less than men.

The kind of work that a person does determines particularly the use of oxygen for the production of energy. For that reason a person who is in a sedentary occupation like a desk worker or a tailor may require only 2300 calories of food per day, a carpenter may require 3300 calories per day, a lumberman as much as 5000 calories per day. A calorie is also merely a measure of energy. It is the amount of heat necessary to raise a certain amount of water 1 degree in temperature. A woman who is doing practically nothing except a little light dusting can get along on 1200 calories per day. If she eats more, she will get big in all the places where she would rather be little.

The human body has a great many standard factors which indicate to the doctor when he makes an examination that the functions of the body are in the range that is called normal. For instance the basal metabolic rate is generally said to be normal when it is somewhere between plus 7 and minus 7 as measured by the basal metabolic machine. In other words, a standard has been established for the basal metabolism.

The human body needs a certain amount of protein every day in order to provide the body with energy and take care of the waste of tissue and the necessity for rebuilding tissue. The body also requires a certain amount of sugar and a certain amount of fat. It is possible to replace the fat by sugar. Sugar can be taken to spare the necessity of burning protein in order to provide energy. These factors are also concerned in the metabolism of the human body. Metabolism, therefore, represents all of the processes involved in changing the food materials, the oxygen, and other substances taken into the body into the tissues of the body or in converting them into energy.

Chemical tests are possible to check the manner in which the body is using the materials that come in. For instance the chemist can determine the amount of protein in the blood plasma. He can determine the amount of materials eliminated from the body by way of the urine or by the bowels or by perspiration. The level of sugar in the blood is now determined by a number of tests. We know, for example, that the amount of sugar in the blood plasma is reduced when there is exhaustion or when the liver is failing to carry on its work satisfactorily. In order for the various tissues of the body to work as they should, hormones or glandular substances, vitamins and ferments are necessary. All of these substances work together in bringing about a normal state of the body. The failure of any one gland to function may throw an extra burden on others. Some glandular activities are in the nature of breaking down materials; others in the way of building them up. The material from the male sex glands favors the storage of protein in the body, increases muscular development and the growth of hair on the body. Insulin, which is the secretion of the pancreas, helps to develop stores of protein and sugar in the body. Other glandular secretions tend to diminish such storage. Thus the body is in a constant state of balance with these various functions working opposite each other. All of these various activities are included under metabolism.

A number of diseases are definitely related to failure of the body to carry out its chemical functions satisfactorily. Included are particularly gout, diabetes, obesity, and acidosis.

METRITIS The prefix "metro-" usually refers to the uterus, so that metritis is an inflammation of the uterus. Metrorrhagia is a hemorrhage from the uterus, and metroscope is an instrument used in looking into the uterus.

MIGRAINE See discussion under *Headache.*

MILK Whereas milk was available in early America only in the form of the fluid taken directly from the cow, modern technology has developed a number of processes for treating milk so that it may be preserved for a long time. In many primitive portions of the world, where such technological developments are not available, American products are shipped.

Dried milk is one of the forms most widely used. When dried milk is shipped, one saves the costs and trouble of handling large amounts of water. Moreover, dried milk by its method of preparation is free from danger of bacterial contamination, since the bacteria are destroyed in the process. One of the difficulties with dried milk is the fact that some people insist that it does not taste like fresh milk when water is added.

Dried milk is prepared by three main technics. By one method the milk is passed in a thin layer over a heated surface. A second method blows air through layers of partially evaporated milk on drying cylinders. The third method sprays partially evaporated milk into warm drying chambers. The last described is the one most frequently used.

In such milk powder less than 2 per cent of moisture remains. The fat, sugar, and protein of the milk are not changed chemically but are merely dried. The food value, when this form of powder is reconstituted into milk, is just about the same as that of fresh milk except for the vitamin C, which is destroyed by oxidation and much of which may be lost in the drying process. However, vitamin C may be made up by a small quantity of orange juice or any of the fresh fruit juices or tomato juice or potatoes or many other foods.

Dried milk is especially useful in cooking and baking. Today in the United States the production of dried milk is somewhere between 400,000,000 and 500,000,000 pounds per year. In addition to dried whole milk, preparations are also made of dried skim milk, in which the butterfat is much less.

Between fresh and dried milk are such products as evaporated, concentrated, and condensed milk. Evaporated milk is simply fresh milk from which the water has been evaporated to such a point that it contains not less than 7.9 per cent of

milk fat and not less than 25.9 per cent of the total milk solids. Concentrated or plain condensed milk is like evaporated milk except that it is not processed by heat, and the container may be unsealed.

Sweetened condensed milk is a liquid made by evaporating a mixture of sweet milk and refined sugar or corn sugar so that the sweetened condensed milk contains not less than 28 per cent of the total milk solids and not less than 8.5 per cent of milk fat. The sugar is used here to prevent spoilage.

When fresh milk is not available, canned milk is obviously preferable to no milk at all. Moreover, in many places the fresh milk that is available is not properly controlled from a sanitary point of view by pasteurizing and sanitary handling. Under such circumstances condensed or evaporated milk is far preferable.

One of the difficulties with the use of sweetened condensed milk is the fact that the large amount of sugar must be considered in calculating the diet. Babies brought up on sweetened condensed milk are likely to be fat babies.

The canned milk industry uses almost 5,000,000,000 pounds of milk a year, which is about 15 pounds of canned milk for every person in the country. About the same amount of canned milk is used by the ice cream industry, and that incidentally is enough to provide 3 gallons of ice cream for each person per year. The chief value of ice cream in the diet lies, of course, in its milk content. Ice cream varies from place to place in quality and in the nature of the ice cream mix. These milk products are exceedingly important, since milk is one of the most nearly perfect foods and should occupy a place particularly in the diets of growing children.

MISCARRIAGE See *Abortion.*

MISCEGENATION When two people of different races marry and have children, the condition is called miscegenation.

MONONUCLEOSIS   As early as 1889 a German named Pfeiffer described a disease which was called glandular fever. It occurred in children, the chief symptoms being the appearance of fever with general sickness, swelling of the glands in the neck, redness of the throat, and often enlargement of the liver and the spleen. After the passing of some years other doctors began investigating this disease much more carefully, making studies particularly of the blood and of the swollen glands. This has enabled them now to recognize a special disease called glandular fever as a common name but infectious mononucleosis as a name which means much more to the doctor. In it he recognizes two important factors: the first, that the condition can occur as an epidemic or an infection; and the second, that the changes in the blood are especially significant.

The causative organism of this condition is not known, but it is now believed to be a virus—one of those toxic agents so small that it cannot be seen under an ordinary microscope, so small indeed that it can be filtered through the pores of a clay filter.

In the United States the persons most affected with infectious mononucleosis are young people between the ages of fifteen and thirty. Outbreaks have occurred among boys in schools. Rarely have epidemics occurred among adults.

Usually about a week after a person has been exposed to the disease he gets the fever, sore throat, and enlargement of the lymph glands that are significant. Sometimes these are so mild that they are overlooked and the study of the disease is not carried far enough to make a positive diagnosis. Often when there is an infection of the throat with a germ like the streptococcus or the staphylococcus, the glands will swell and even suppurate but the glands in infectious mononucleosis do not suppurate.

When the blood of a child with this infection is examined, the red blood cells and the red coloring matter are found to be normal but the white blood cells vary in number and character during the different stages of the disease. Gradually after six to ten days the white blood cells increase greatly in number and the character changes so that there are a majority of cells with a single central staining spot or nucleus in contrast to having the majority of cells with many nuclei. The name applied to a cell with a single nucleus is mononuclear. The name applied to a cell with many nuclei is polynuclear. Other names given to a cell with a single nucleus are lymphocyte or monocyte.

Usually by the end of the third week the number of white blood cells will have gone back to normal and the characteristic percentage and distribution of the different types of cells will also change.

A blood test has been discovered which makes it possible to diagnose this condition in the same way as the Wassermann test is used to diagnose syphilis or the Widal test is used to diagnose typhoid. Usually these patients get well in three or four weeks with proper attention, although occasionally they may feel somewhat "under the weather" for five or six months.

Thus far ACTH is the only drug found beneficial in treating the disease but of course the sulfonamide drugs and penicillin help to prevent secondary complications which may bring about serious results.

Research carried on by the Army and Navy definitely established prolonged wet kissing as the most significant factor in outbreaks of mononucleosis which have occurred among troops. This means that the virus which causes the condition is not spread through the air but by contamination with saliva.

MOTION SICKNESS   See *Seasickness.*

MOUTH, DISEASE OF   See *Pyorrhea, Teeth, Tongue,* et cetera.

MULTIPLE SCLEROSIS   Multiple sclerosis is probably third or fourth in frequency among all of the disorders that affect the nervous system. Usually this condition begins fairly early in life —between the ages of ten and forty. Then it gradually develops and becomes worse over a period of many years. Apparently the condition does not occur in families, nor does there seem to be any hereditary factor involved.

Occasionally the condition begins after childbirth or a surgical operation or some such incident, but apparently this may easily be coincidence and not have any direct relationship.

In multiple sclerosis the nervous system is involved with degenerative changes and secondary scarring as a result of which its functions are interfered with and disappear. This means that all kinds of combinations of symptoms can occur, including paralysis beginning with moderate weakness in the legs and symptoms like sudden jumping of the legs due to a spastic condition of the muscles. The arms are less frequently involved than the legs and usually much later in the condition. Speech changes are somewhat characteristic, the speech becoming slow and monotonous, so that the person talks as if he were spelling out every word. There are tremors of the hands when some definite movement is attempted. Occasionally the head may develop a tremor.

The mental symptoms may include gradual deterioration with depression or instances in which there are serious disturbances of the emotions and the ability to think. Usually, however, patients with multiple sclerosis are optimistic and seem to feel well almost regardless of the extent of the disease.

Ultimately the important organs of the body involved in seeing, hearing, or taking care of the digestive functions become affected, which means that the patient will have to have nursing care.

The duration of these cases varies from a few years to many years, depending on the rapidity of progress of the disease.

Medicine is still investigating to determine whether or not multiple sclerosis is due to an infection with a virus or an inflammatory disease produced by some toxin. So far a specific organism has not been identified as responsible for these cases.

Unfortunately specific methods of treatment that will definitely halt the disease or cure it are not known. Much comfort can be given by proper nursing and by attention to the individual symptoms as they develop. People with long chronic diseases die not so much from the disease as from the secondary complications.

MUMPS When the glands in front of the ear begin to swell rapidly, associated with fever up to 101 degrees Fahrenheit, the condition is probably mumps. The swelling is generally below and in front of the ear but it may extend backward and may also involve other glands. Usually the swelling and the fever are about as bad as they are going to get by the second day, after which the temperature drops and the swelling goes down. Cases are known, however, in which the condition persists even for weeks.

The worst danger of mumps is the well-known complication, which occurs, however, in only 1 out of 100 cases. In serious epidemics as many as 10 per cent of cases have the complication of swelling of the sex glands—the testes in the male, the ovary in the female. This complication means more fever, more sickness, some pain, and in a good many instances destruction of the glands that are infected to the extent of depriving them of their function.

Mumps is caused by the smallest type of infectious agent—namely, the virus. This has been proved by transferring the infection from man to animals. The disease is quite contagious whenever there is close contact. It is not, however, as contagious as measles or chicken pox. The virus is found in the saliva during the disease and can be disseminated by droplets of the saliva or by contaminated hands.

Usually the disease affects children between the ages of five and fifteen. Rarely does it affect any child under ten months of age. Most cases of mumps occur in the early winter and in the spring. Usually a person has mumps only once because the first attack will give the body protective substances against subsequent attacks. Cases are known, however, in which the disease has occurred two or even three times.

Fortunately few people die of mumps and the treatment involves in most cases merely rest in bed as long as the fever and swelling persist, scrupulous cleanliness of the mouth, a diet with plenty of fluids. The doctor may prescribe drugs for the relief of pain if that is considered necessary.

When the complications occur, the physician will want to give the patient his special attention. This is necessary to relieve the pains and to make certain that the amount of damage to the tissues is kept at a minimum.

In time of war mumps becomes epidemic in camps. For instance in World War I one third of the men in one camp were infected during an epidemic of mumps. For that reason it is customary to isolate infected patients immediately when cases are discovered under such circumstances.

MUSCLE CRAMPS Many people suffer with cramps in the muscles which come on during exercise or at night when they turn or stretch or sometimes when an arm or leg is held in an unusual position for a rather long time. The mechanism of the cramp is the occurrence of an involuntary contraction of the fibers imposed on a voluntary movement. The cause of the cramp is, therefore, this spasmodic contraction, which produces pain. Observations indicate that the cramps come on more frequently in the presence of fatigue, lack of sufficient blood supply, and inflammation of the muscle or nerve, a deficiency of thiamin, and a lack of sufficient calcium in the body.

Various technics have been developed for increasing the consumption of oxygen as a means of relieving the cramps, including, for instance, breathing into a paper sack which acts as a stimulus to the intake of oxygen. The suggestion has been made that the taking of extra calcium would be effective but an actual trial showed that it is ineffective. Certain drugs which seem to have the effect of stimulating the chemistry of muscles, among them quinine, have been used with some success. In the vast majority of cases, however, the cramps are hardly of sufficient significance to demand much beyond an encouragement to keep the tissues warm and to use enough exercise to encourage the circulation. If muscle cramps come with great frequency, a careful medical study needs to be made, particularly related to the efficiency of the circulation of the blood in the muscles.

MUSCLE DISEASES Muscles constitute a large portion of the body structure; involvement of the muscles by disease is likely to have a tremendous effect on the body as a whole. In most instances, however, diseases affecting the muscles result from damage to nerves by which the muscles are made to move or to be at rest. There are instances in which muscles are damaged by mechanical activities. There is, for example, tearing of a muscle fiber due to overstretching or a sudden jerk or blow. Sometimes the biceps muscle in the arm is torn. Occasionally the large muscles which manipulate the thumb are pulled away. Many times the tendons or fibrous structures by which the muscles are attached to the bones are torn. Tearing of the muscles in the thighs and in the back of the foot occurs fairly frequently in running and in games like tennis and squash, where there are sudden turns of the foot and leg.

Usually the first sign of such an injury is a sudden severe pain at the point where the breaking of the tendon or muscle has occurred. Then there is weakness. Frequently there is a flow of blood between the fibers of the muscles. As long as clotted blood is present, there may be pain on motion.

When such an injury has occurred, the treatment naturally has to depend on the nature and severity of the injury, on the age of the person involved, and on the general condition. Sometimes it is necessary to repair serious tears of muscles and tendons by surgical operation as soon as the condition is discovered. Modern surgery has technics for sewing the torn parts under strictly sterile conditions and then, by the use of casts, holding them tightly until healing has occurred.

Following healing, it becomes necessary to use physical therapy in the form of heat, massage, and controlled movements to recover completely the function of the muscle. There are also conditions in which muscles become infected and inflamed due to invasion by germs. One inflammation which is localized in muscles is trichinosis, since this parasite localizes and grows in the muscle. There are instances, however, in which infectious germs also get inside muscles, producing pus and abscesses, with subsequent threat to life itself. Here again the diagnosis of the condition must be made by the doctor after careful study, and the treatment depends on what he finds as to the nature and extent of the inflammation.

There is also a group of diseases known as muscular dystrophies, in which the muscles waste away and lose their strength. The causes of these conditions vary. In many instances the causes are not known. In a typical case a child who seems to be normal at birth will begin at the age of four or five to be unable to use his legs properly and to tumble about. The back muscles become weak, so that the child cannot sit erect. Soon he finds difficulty in getting up when lying on the floor. In some cases there is complete wasting of the muscles, whereas in others there is continued progressive weakness without so much destruction of the tissues. As the muscles that are affected become weak, the stronger muscles pull, so that the body may become twisted and distorted.

MUSTARD PLASTERS   Mustard plasters are used as counterirritants with a view to drawing blood to the area where the mustard plaster is applied. They can be so strong that they will blister the skin. They should be milder for women and children than for men.

Mustard plasters should not be left on for more than from fifteen to thirty minutes.

NARCOLEPSY   Among the strange conditions that afflict human beings is narcolepsy, in which recurring attacks of sleep come on suddenly; in a number of cases sleep is continuous. Incidentally, there may be associated with this a condition in which the muscles of the body suddenly seem to lose their strength, so that the knees give way and the person falls to the ground without loss of consciousness. This is called tonelessness.

Cases of narcolepsy have been known to develop following serious injury to the head; some cases have been associated with tumors involving certain portions of the brain; some instances are known in which excessive sleepiness or ease of falling asleep was part of a purely mental condition.

Usually the person who has this condition is not what we would call dynamic—not one of those persons who simply overflows with energy. The person with narcolepsy has a sleepy look on his face and is disinclined to move around much. He will keep awake while working at something that interests him, but when left alone or when lying on a bed, he quickly falls asleep. Sometimes these people fall asleep while standing in a streetcar. One such person fell asleep while walking on the street and wakened only when he stepped off the curb. In most instances, however, the person is likely to fall asleep gradually while sitting. Sometimes these cases are associated also with a condition called bulimia, which means a morbid hunger.

The sudden weakness of the muscles that has been described is often associated with some emotion, such as amusement, laughter, anger, or fright. A woman, aged forty-four, had a tendency to fall asleep in church and at social gatherings but the condition became really serious when she fell asleep while standing at the cookstove.

Fortunately few people die of narcolepsy unless as a result of an accident. It has been found that a remedy called ephedrine sulfate will help to prevent these attacks of sleep. More recently the product called amphetamine or benzedrine has also been found useful in controlling this condition. These remedies are powerful drugs and should never be used unless prescribed by a doctor, who will determine whether the product is to be used, the amount to be taken daily or nightly, and other controls to prevent harm.

NARCOTIC ADDICTION Twenty years ago a survey made by the United States Public Health Service indicated to the experts that there were between 110,000 and 150,000 people in the United States who were addicted to various forms of opium. It was estimated a few years ago that there were between 35,000 and 50,000 addicts in the United States. Obviously all such figures are estimates, since secrecy is the very life of the opium trade.

Women seemed to be much more likely to become addicted to the drug than men. Indeed it was rather well established before the new narcotic laws were passed that about two women were addicted for every one man. The figures now seem to indicate that four men are addicted for every one woman. It is believed that women became addicted in the earlier days because they led a more secluded and sedentary life and that they treated themselves with drug preparations containing dope or opium for all sorts of real or imaginary ills. Once, however, the use of such remedies was brought under control, it was not easily possible for women to obtain drugs; naturally women are much more law-abiding than men and are not as likely to get into bad environments as men.

Investigators of the United States Public Health Service point out that women were treated and cured in great numbers following the passing of the narcotic laws and that thereafter women avoided illegal contacts with opium. Men were still able to make such contacts and thus became addicted to the drugs.

The person who takes drugs and becomes addicted to them does so because he is emotionally unstable and is unable to adjust himself to his environment. He feels restless, discontented, and inferior. The taking of a drug which breaks down his mental processes gives him a sense of ease, contentment, and confidence. This, of course, gives him pleasure.

Some people still become narcotic addicts because they develop serious and painful chronic illnesses in which they obtain relief from pain only through the use of strong drugs. The addiction to narcotic drugs is harmful because it breaks down character.

When the Harrison Narcotic Act was passed, it became apparent that people who were addicted to drugs had to be cared for. In 1929 a law was passed creating two narcotic farms which are now located in Lexington, Kentucky, and Fort Worth, Texas. In these places physicians are investigating the nature of narcotic addiction and are undertaking work to rehabilitate narcotic addicts who are admitted to the farms. The narcotic addict who may be committed to one of these farms is, of course, not free to go as he will, but he is treated as a patient and not as a prisoner.

The method of treatment usually followed is to withdraw the drug rapidly from the patient, taking care of his physical health in the meantime so that he will not suffer unduly or seriously. This process requires from ten days to two weeks, after which measures are begun leading to the rehabilitation of the patient from both the mental and physical points of view.

It is recognized also that there are addictions to marihuana and cocaine, but these addictions are believed to be more of a police problem than addiction to opium.

NAUSEA See *Vomiting*.

NAVEL, DISEASES OF The navel is the scar that is left when the umbilical cord, by which the body of the child is attached to that of its mother before birth, is cut. The scientific name for the navel is the umbilicus. After the cord is cut, there is a gradual shrinkage of the excess tissue. Once the scar has healed, the navel needs little attention unless it becomes involved in an infection or some other disturbance.

The care of the navel in a newborn child is important. The cord must be tied off satisfactorily at a sufficient distance from the body. It is covered with a sterile dressing and it is watched carefully until it is healed. Exceedingly dangerous would be a secondary hemorrhage from the cord or an infection.

Some years ago a distinguished surgeon wrote a two-volume work on diseases of the umbilicus. Most of the conditions which might concern this tissue represent failures to heal satisfactorily, leaving an opening or a fistula or a possible rupture, so that the tissues of the abdomen protrude through the opening. Such conditions demand surgical attention. The surgeon repairs the failure to close by sewing and reconstructing the area.

Because the navel contains creases and folds, it demands attention as far as its cleanliness is concerned. Removal of accumulations of tissue debris or of soap should be a part of the regular hygiene of daily life.

The tissues of the navel are like those of the skin. They become subject to any disease that affects the skin. When there is an ulcer in the umbilicus, the same attention should be given to it as to an ulcer anywhere else. This means removal of infectious material and the application of suitable drugs to control the germs that may be present. Instances have been described in which the tissue around the umbilicus developed a blue appearance. This has been due to an accumulation of blood inside the abdomen following rupture of one of the fallopian tubes of a woman or from a hemorrhage or any other cause.

There is an old story to the effect that the only two people in heaven without an umbilicus were Adam and Eve. Nowadays surgeons find it necessary occasionally to remove the umbilicus while doing a surgical operation, so that there are considerable numbers of people here and there around the world without an umbilicus.

NECK, BROKEN "Broken back" and "broken neck" once meant almost certain death or a lingering disability. With the discovery of the X ray and with the extension of its use, breaks in the bones of the spine are now found to be exceedingly frequent. Studies of 200 consecutive cases in New York showed that the break in the bone of the spine in 117 cases occurred when the person fell from a height; 69 were struck by moving objects, including 31 automobiles; 2 people were thrown; and in 12 instances the cause of the break in the bone of the spine was not determined. In 35 of these 200 cases death occurred, not, however, because of the break in the bone of the spine but because there was an associated serious injury to the head or a secondary pneumonia and in some instances severe shock.

Fractures of the spine may occur in the upper region, in the middle, or, as frequently happens, at the bottom. Most of the serious breaks occur in the region around the neck. A broken neck is much more serious than a break in the bones of the spine lower down. Sometimes the injury to the spine may be so forceful that the bones are twisted away from each other, making a much more serious condition than a mere breaking of one of the portions of one of the bones. The most serious results follow when there is a break directly into the center of the spinal column with the occurrence of hemorrhage around the spinal cord. Serious also are cases in which the material of the spinal cord itself is seriously damaged, or, as occurs in some cases, completely cut through.

When the patient loses all sensation below the level at which the injury occurred and loses complete control of the ordinary actions of the bowels and of the bladder, the symptoms may be taken as an indication that there has been serious damage.

The earliest possible attention of a physician who can do everything possible to remove pressure and to aid restoration of the tissues to their normal positions may save life. First aid, if correct, may save a life. People with an injury to the spine must be moved only when lying on a flat board and with the minimum amount of manipulation. If the injury is in the region of the neck, some technic should be found to hold the neck absolutely still. The shock is treated by the usual methods of application of warmth and the use of proper remedies. For this, of course, a physician is necessary.

As soon as the condition of the person who has been injured warrants, an X-ray picture is taken to show exactly how much damage has occurred. Then the surgeon or orthopedic surgeon arranges the proper supports and braces to hold the tissues in proper position and the physician makes certain that the functions of the body are cared for during the process of recovery.

When the patient recovers, careful study must be made by a specialist in nervous and mental diseases to determine the extent of the damage that has been done and the possibilities for further treatment to bring about complete recovery.

NEPHRITIS Whenever a man goes for a physical examination in relation to taking out life insurance, being inducted into the Army, or playing football with a high school or college team, the examination is likely to include some simple tests of the urine to determine whether or not the urine contains albumin. The presence of albumin in the urine is abnormal; that is to say, most healthy men are free from this condition. The presence of albumin may on occasion be due to a purely temporary condition (for instance, doctors recognize today what is called emotional albuminuria), but in most instances the presence of albumin means that there has been an inflammation of the kidneys sufficient to cause protein to leak through from the blood into the urine or perhaps sufficient to destroy

enough tissue of the kidney itself to cause such waste material to appear in the urine.

The word "nephritis" means simply inflammation of the kidney. However, it includes a number of conditions which may be acute or chronic, all of which are characterized by the appearance of albumin in the urine and, in addition, occasionally by the appearance of blood and of portions of kidney tissue. Nephritis is usually listed as fourth in the list of the causes of death and each year in the United States is responsible for the death of something over 100,000 people, or about 7 per cent of all deaths.

An acute inflammation of the kidneys is so serious that no one is likely to neglect it long. Associated with the disturbance of excretion of urine, there are swellings of the tissues, waterlogging of the circulation, and even enough poisoning of the body in general to cause convulsions or unconsciousness. Chronic inflammation of the kidneys includes a number of different forms depending on the part of the kidney that is involved. Failure of the kidneys to do their work throws much more work on the heart.

For many years chronic inflammation of the kidneys has been known as Bright's disease. It was named after a famous London doctor, Richard Bright, who first demonstrated the association of swelling of the human body due to accumulation of water in the tissues and the presence in the urine of a substance which coagulated when the urine was boiled. These observations were presented to the medical profession in 1827, and Bright's name has been attached to this group of disorders since that time.

The kidneys—to make their nature clear—are two kidney-shaped masses which lie high up in the abdominal region behind the stomach, attached near the spine. Each of them includes millions of tiny grapelike masses of specialized blood vessels called glomeruli. Each little clump empties into a funnellike structure leading to a small coiled tube, and all of these tubes finally empty into a larger collecting space called the pelvis of the kidney. The urine is formed in these grapelike masses. It escapes from the clump of blood vessels through a small funnel that is only one seventh the size of the tube by which the blood entered the glomerulus. The action of the glomerulus is to squeeze out the fluid, like a wine press, so that the waste matter passes out of the body in the urine and the filtered liquid goes back into the blood. The amount of work done by this machinery can be realized from the fact that it handles about 150 quarts a day. Since there are something over 6 quarts of blood in the body, it will be realized that the blood goes round and round, being relieved on each passage through the kidney of the material to be passed out of the body.

Whenever there is an infection elsewhere in the body, the possibility exists that the poisons or germs may be carried into the kidney and set up some trouble in the kidney tissue. This would be called acute nephritis. The poisons that can set up an acute inflammation of the kidney are not always germ poisons, since it is known that poisonous metals and other toxic substances can produce this result. Whenever there is a suspicion that an inflammation of the kidney is present, an immediate examination of the urine should be made. When the urine is heated, the albumin, if present, will coagulate as a solid clot, much like the white part of a boiled egg. When strong acid is added to the urine, the albumin will coagulate. There are, of course, quantitative tests which will show about how much albumin is present in the urine.

The conditions which are likely to cause suspicion would include persistent headache, mental depression, and fatigue. The skin will develop a pale or pasty appearance. There may be puffiness and swelling under the eyes, on the backs of the hands, and around the feet. As the condition progresses, the blood pressure may be raised. The swellings due to accumulation of fluid may become enormous, so that even the abdomen and the space around the lungs and heart become filled and action of the organs impeded by the retained liquid. This may read like the text of some of the old almanacs which used to be freely circulated in selling somebody's kidney pills or kidney remedy. They usually showed a haggard individual, bent over, with his hand on the middle of his back. Usually the hand was not in a place anywhere near the place where the kidneys actually are. Most pain in the back is not due to disturbances of the kidneys. Enough people have symptoms like those that have been mentioned, however, to indicate that the presence of such symptoms should demand an immediate study of the urine.

When the urine of a person with inflammation of the kidneys is examined under the microscope, particularly after a fair amount of the urine has been caused to settle by the use of a centrifuge, the material will be found to contain not only some red blood cells but also molds which resemble casts of the tiny tubes of the kidney. Casts are of many different varieties, depending on the nature of the material that they contain. They are described variously as blood casts, hyaline casts, granular casts, and with other adjectives. In the presence of such kidney conditions the doctor can also learn a great deal by examination of the blood, since failure of the kidneys to function properly will produce chemical changes in the blood.

It used to be thought that acute Bright's disease was a fatal disorder. Now we know that this is far from the truth. It is the tendency of most cases to get well, given a reasonable opportunity. Indeed authorities say that about 90 per cent of all cases will recover completely if recognized early and if properly treated. In the remaining cases the disease tends to persist and eventually to pass over into what is called chronic nephritis. In the period between the acute inflammation of the kidney and the gradual change to the chronic form, there is an intermediary state that is sometimes called nephrosis. The urine in this form of kidney disease is usually decreased in amount, and the amount of albumin in the urine is considerable. The distinction between various stages of inflammation of the kidneys is difficult and depends largely on the experience of the doctor.

People with acute inflammation of the kidney are urged to go to bed and stay in bed until the kidneys function normally. They take a diet that is simple and nutritious, usually keeping the amount of salt and the amount of protein rather low in relation to the average diet. Indeed some physicians limit the patient with acute nephritis to milk and fruit juices for a few days. We know, however, that any fever or inflammation or infection tends to use up the protein of the body, and protein is required for repair of damaged tissue. Hence regulation of the protein in the diet is a delicate matter and one which is best left to the expert who is taking care of the patient. When there are signs of severe suppression of the flow of urine, many doctors choose to cause the patient to perspire freely so as to get some of the waste material out of the body.

There has been a popular belief that meat in any form is harmful to people with Bright's disease. If the blood shows a deficiency in protein, the amount of protein in the diet—and this means meat—may in most instances be increased.

Whenever there is swelling of the tissues due to accumulation of fluid, the intake and elimination of water from the body must be watched carefully. Such people are warned against taking excessive amounts of fluid, but some fluid is absolutely necessary for proper function of the tissues and particularly for the elimination of toxic waste materials. Among the most difficult conditions to overcome is accumulation of the fluid in the tissues. Sometimes the fluid around the eyes is so profuse that they may actually be swollen shut. Sometimes the legs swell so greatly as to make walking difficult if not impossible. If fluid collects in the brain in sufficient amounts, it will disturb thought and action. The diet and the elimination of the patient need to be watched particularly because many of these people will seem to be large, due to accumulation of fluid in the body, whereas actually they are undernourished and even emaciated. In the early stages the heart and blood vessels may not be affected, but later the damage to the heart and blood vessels may be so great that life is maintained with difficulty.

The competent doctor who is caring for a patient with inflammation of the kidneys will make studies of the blood, as has already been mentioned, and will frequently examine the urine and also test the functional ability of the kidney to determine whether or not it is doing its work satisfactorily. Repeated examinations will be made to determine whether or not the condition is getting better or worse. Any diet or fluids taken by the patient will be regulated by the results of the functional tests and in fact may serve to some extent themselves as a means of testing the ability of the kidney to work.

Nephritis is so variable as it occurs in different people that it is simply impossible to say in any given case what the rate of progress is likely to be. Since control of the disease depends on constant observation of its progress, everyone who has had albumin in the urine should have at least one annual survey, including study of the urine and the blood and functional tests of the various vital organs of the body.

NERVOUS BREAKDOWN Nervous breakdown includes a wide range of mental disorders.

With the public interest in mental disturbances a whole new vocabulary of terms has come into common use. Some of these terms have vague meanings. The term "breaking point," which really has a physical meaning, has now been applied to the human mind. Other terms now applied to mental factors are stress, tension, pressure, weight, force, and impact. Even the specialist in disorders of the mind finds it difficult to define exactly what is meant by "nervous breakdown."

Often the person who has what is called a nervous breakdown has begun with emotional instability. Out of his lack of tolerance of a situation in which he finds himself, he begins to develop changes in the secretions of the stomach that may lead eventually to ulcers, difficulties in vision that may finally be called eye strain, or pains in different portions of the body that receive the classification of neuralgia.

What we call morale in a human being appears to be emotional stability. Many men who might break down when left to themselves are able to sustain their morale when they are in a large group through the influence of leadership. They break down when this protective influence is removed.

Not all men have a mental breakdown under severe stress. Some men seem to be able to stand almost any trial or disturbance. But even these men may eventually develop physical changes or organic diseases which alter their mental stability.

Nervous breakdown in children may result in refusal to go to school and similar infractions. These children are different from those who are simply truant and refuse to go to school out of what might be called "meanness." They are neurotic children, and their symptoms may involve the whole family.

Frequently they are depressed and often overly preoccupied with sex questions. The children refuse to obey orders; they become aggressive, which contrasts with their formerly timid behavior. The child who formerly went easily to school now clings to his home and may refuse to leave his mother. Usually if the child is allowed to remain at home the acute symptoms tend to lessen, but they appear again if attempts are made to force the child back to school. In several cases reported this impasse continued for months. Obviously a mother confronted with a problem of this kind in the home becomes anxious and depressed and soon is entirely unable to handle the child.

Truant children may steal and lie, but the neurotic child is of an entirely different character. The latter represents a case of mental difficulty and must be treated from that point of view. The neurotic child is in most instances above average intelligence but is also timid, sensitive, and dependent. Often he is the only child and has been spoiled by parents who have yielded to the child and favored him in every way. These children are finicky about their food. Usually their emotional disturbances are related to the mother.

Attempts to treat these cases have indicated that treatment is difficult and must often be carried on for a long time in order to secure satisfactory results. The complete co-operation of the parents is required. Sometimes the best first step is to remove the child from contact with the parents to a suitable hospital or home where study may be made and proper treatment administered. Thus the child is saved a great deal of anxiety and misery. Moreover, the treatment is much easier if the child is removed from the emotionally high-charged atmosphere of the home. When the child is away from home, he can go to school each day from the hospital and gradually become relieved of the causes of the excessive emotional reactions.

NEURALGIA Pain in a nerve is called neuralgia. Neuralgia may, therefore, be facial neuralgia or sciatic neuralgia or dental neuralgia, depending on the nerve that is involved. In facial neuralgia there is a characteristic pain, stabbing and knifelike, which follows the course of one of the chief nerves which is known as the fifth or trigeminal nerve. This nerve spreads over the face, coming from a spot over the ear. In facial neuralgia the nerve may be so sensitive that even a cold current blowing on the face, or the light touch of a finger or feather to the face, may cause this stabbing pain to pass through the nerve.

Dental neuralgia usually begins with the decay of a tooth or an inflammation of the pulp cavity. At first the tooth is painful but soon the pain will spread from the tooth along the upper or lower jaw but not across the mid-line to the other side.

The typical pain of neuralgia of the facial nerve is called tic douloureux or trifacial neuralgia. This condition occurs usually in people around middle life and most often in those above fifty. Women are more frequently affected than men.

The exact cause of neuralgia has never been determined. Occasionally the condition may be controlled by using inhalations of a drug called trichlorethylene. However, the relief obtained by this method tends to wear off. Alcohol has been injected directly into the nerve area, and this technic gives relief for a certain length of time. It has been suggested that in certain instances the administration of large doses of thiamin has been helpful, these being given by injection, but again it has not been established with certainty that this produces long-continued relief or will prevent the condition.

In the very severe cases of neuralgia it is customary to do a surgical operation which destroys the nerve roots along which the sensation of pain is carried.

Whenever neuralgia affects any nerve, it is customary for the physician first to determine the nerve area involved and then to see what can be done to prevent the passing of the sensation of pain along that nerve. For this purpose sedative drugs are used, local anesthetic substances are injected into the nerve area, alcohol has been injected with a view to destroying the nerve, and X rays have been used, as well as similar technics.

There are instances, of course, in which the sensations of pain limited to certain nerve areas are more mental than physical. That makes such neuralgias a special problem in diagnosis for the doctor.

NEURITIS Any inflammation of the nerves is called a neuritis. The condition appears with pain and tenderness over an area supplied by the nerve. Sometimes there is loss of feeling or disturbances of sensation; sometimes paralysis, so that it is impossible to move a part supplied by the nerve. There are many different causes of neuritis, including alcohol, infections with germs like the diphtheria germ, or infections by malaria, which would supply the diagnosis of alcoholic, diphtheric, or malarial neuritis. When neuritis occurs in diabetes or rheumatism, the condition is known as diabetic or rheumatic neuritis. If more than one nerve is affected, it might be called multiple neuritis. Obviously the treatment of the condition depends on determining the cause and directing the treatment toward the cause. For relief sedative drugs may be used, fixation of the tissues to prevent movement, the application of heat, and other specific measures which the doctor prescribes.

NEUROSIS Any functional disorder of the nervous system is known as a neurosis in contrast to a neuritis, which is an actual inflammation of the tissues. Because a neurosis is more likely to be mental than physical, it is sometimes called a psychoneurosis. A neurosis is sometimes related to certain tissues of the body, so that it can be called a cardiac neurosis as related to the heart, a gastric neurosis as related to the stomach, or a sexual neurosis when it involves the sex functions. Sometimes the neurosis is described in terms of the mental side, such as an anxiety neurosis, in which there are abnormal fears, or a compulsion neurosis, in which the person feels absolutely compelled to say or do certain things. A neurosis may be related to the occupation or profession, in which it is called a professional or occupational neurosis, or to a condition that causes anxiety, such as a war. This gives us the term "war neurosis."

NIGHT TERRORS If it were not for adults, babies would never be afraid, because they would not know the difference between what is dangerous and what is not dangerous. Babies become frightened because older people frighten them. They tell the baby about the "boogeyman" and teach babies to fear the policeman and the doctor and most of the other people on whom they must really depend for protection and health.

Apparently a baby may be born with a fear of a loud, sudden noise and a fear of falling. Those things we call instinctive. The baby learns to be afraid, however, of many things by seeing his parents suddenly draw back in fright. Babies learn from their parents to be afraid of thunder and lightning. A baby can be made afraid of his nursing bottle or his mother's breast if something that burns or tastes bitter happens to come to the baby in that connection.

Certain fears are so completely abnormal that they are reflected in the child's dreams and sleep. These are recognized in medicine under the name of night terror or by the Latin words *pavor nocturnis,* which means the same thing. These night terrors are usually a remnant of something that has happened during the day. The parents are likely to attribute them to something that the baby ate that he should not have eaten or to overstimulation by the radio or moving picture. Scientific investigation by child mental specialists, however, reveals that in most instances these night terrors occur in children whose parents are overanxious and excessively affectionate and also in those who are constantly being threatened with damage or mutilation by parents or nursemaids who know no other way in which to discipline a child.

A common source of the development of night terrors is the threat that the child's hands or his organs will be cut off because the parent or nursemaid is displeased with something the child was doing. Sudden attacks at night in which a child awakens screaming are occasionally associated with nervous disorders, which in turn are precipitated by similar unfortunate experiences.

From time to time the conditions have been blamed on adenoids, worms, or various infectious diseases. Occasionally the child screams at night because he is having a dream that he is being threatened or pursued. In some cases children who have sick headaches are likely to waken screaming at night. Since these headaches have been shown to be due occasionally to sensitivity to various protein substances, that type of investigation should be made so that that kind of stimulus can be avoided if it can be determined. Obviously, however, prevention by education of parents as to the proper attitudes toward the child and by the control of such physical defects as can be found is the ideal way to get rid of night terrors in children.

NOISE Unnecessary noise is a health hazard. The nervous reaction that follows exposure to noise is called echeosis.

Certain sounds are painfully loud and are therefore harmful to the ear or the brain or both. Rhythmical sound has the effect of preventing or postponing fatigue, as for example in soldiers who are marching. Sounds that are not rhythmical may startle, disturb, or irritate.

While the healthy man can stand the ordinary noises of the streets, including even unexpected blowing of motor horns, a hypersensitive man will suffer greatly from such disturbances. In cases of pneumonia infection, heart disease accompanied by insomnia, and in the case of people who are weakened after surgical operations, noise may be a serious menace. For this reason most cities provide for zones of quiet around hospitals and sanitariums.

Experiments have been conducted to determine the results of constant impinging of sound on the nerves. The investigators report that the noise raises the blood pressure and that a degree of noise sufficient to awaken a sleeping person will cause the muscles to contract and remain tense for as long as thirty minutes before they relax.

It has been shown that hardness of hearing, dizziness, and headaches may develop in persons who earn their living in noisy places. It is said that it requires 19 per cent more energy to perform a duty in noisy surroundings than to perform the same duty in a quiet environment. A healthy person can adapt himself to all sorts of peculiar disturbances but invariably adaptation brings about some wear and tear on the nervous system.

Fortunately various methods have been developed for diminishing noise, and modern society recognizes noise as an unnecessary nuisance. For those who are especially sensitive to noise, rubber ear stoppers or defenders serve to reduce the noise or to shut it out. Much better, however, is the prevention of unnecessary noises by careful study to determine the causes and by the elimination of every source of noise that can be eliminated.

NOSE The nose is composed of small bones and cartilages and soft tissues which surround two cavities. Also directly related to the nose are the nasal sinuses.

Most important in the nose from the point of view of health and disease is its mucous membrane, or lining. The mucous membrane of the nose is one of the most sensitive tissues in the body. When it is bruised or hurt in any way, when it becomes infected, the response is prompt and the effect on the general health of the body may be serious.

Minor infections occur particularly in the hair follicles or in the roots of the hairs in the nose. The purpose of these hairs is to filter out dust or infectious material which comes into the nose with the air. Such germs as the streptococcus, the virus of influenza, and similar organisms are widespread. Many germs float in the air. When they get into a tissue which has in any way been damaged or of which the resistance has been lessened, they may set up an infection which eventually may spread throughout the body. The pernicious habit of pulling hairs out of the nose, squeezing pimples, or picking crusts is often the first step in injury leading to secondary infection.

An infection in the lining of the nose manifests itself by redness, swelling, discomfort, and pain, which increases steadily. If the swelling is sufficiently great, the outer aspect of the nose becomes swollen, and the swelling may extend even up to the eyelids. Whenever there is a swelling in the nose, a physician should inspect the area to determine the presence or absence of infection and to provide for a release of infected material so as to obviate the danger of a generalized infection.

The right way to take care of the nose is to remove carefully, by proper use of the handkerchief, such materials as can be reached easily. Those which cannot be reached may be washed out by the use of a mild spray without pressure. There are now generally available all sorts of sprays and materials which can be sprayed into the nose safely. Under no circumstances should materials be put in the nose under high pressure. This applies particularly to oils of various kinds, since it has been found that such oils may get into the lungs, and on occasion pneumonia has resulted from such procedures.

NOSEBLEED—When serious hemorrhage occurs from the nose, the patient should be put flat on the back. Cold may be applied. If the bleeding persists, sterile gauze packs may be used to make pressure.

FOREIGN BODIES IN THE NOSE—Children, particularly infants, are likely to put into their mouths almost anything they happen to pick up. Occasionally also they push things into the nose. A substance of fairly small size taken into the mouth is not likely to be harmful, providing it is clean, even after it is swallowed. The digestive passages are big enough in most instances to let it pass through. Usually after eighteen to twenty-four hours the foreign materials will have disappeared from the body.

The breathing passages are much smaller than the digestive tube. Moreover, the breathing passages are curved and their walls are rigid. A substance forced into the nose is likely to remain there and serve as an obstacle which blocks the passage of air. Even more serious, however, is the fact that it will block the outflow of secretions.

Buttons, beans, pieces of chalk, or erasers that have from time to time been pushed into the nose get lodged there. Occasionally they are inhaled and get into the windpipe. Then an exceedingly serious condition develops. The continuous presence of a foreign substance in the nose results eventually in the damming back of secretions and in the development of secondary infection. Soon there is a bad odor, a secondary swelling, and danger to life itself.

A doctor can utilize some of the special instruments that he has available and get a foreign substance out of the nose without very much trouble. The great danger of trying to get out a hard object like a button or piece of chalk is the damage to the tissues that results from manipulation. In many cases it is necessary to give the child an anesthetic to prevent jerking and moving of the head or interference by the hands and arms.

When a foreign substance is inhaled into the tube that leads to the lungs or into the lung itself, it is an immediate menace to life. Under such circumstances there must be no delay. An X-ray picture is taken as soon as possible, which aids the doctor in localizing the foreign substance. Special instruments have been developed which permit the placing of a tube down into the lung, and forceps and similar devices have been developed by which a foreign substance can be grasped and removed from the body.

PLASTIC SURGERY—When for any reason the nose is lost entirely, the facial expression naturally suffers. When the bridge of the nose disappears, as sometimes occurs in certain infections, the resulting appearance is anything but beautiful.

Automobile accidents which bring about sudden contact of the nose with the windshield often leave an expression on the face which, while not one of continual surprise, is nevertheless one that arrests attention. Falls, industrial accidents, railroad wrecks, and gunshot wounds pick the nose as a special target. Finally, the results of boxing are a constant source of income to specialists in nasal reconstruction.

As if the nose itself were not sufficiently prominent with most people, nature helps the situation by bestowing upon it a hump, a knob at the tip, or a deviation to one side or the other. Forms of the nose have been described as long and short, upturned and downturned, humped, flat, wide, pointed, narrow, and saddle-shaped.

Modern surgery has developed many different technics for changing the shape and appearance of the nose. These operations are done under conditions which insure reasonable success in most cases. Operations are done from inside the nose so that the scars do not appear on the surface. Unfortunately most of the people who want nasal reconstruction have a mental condition, so that the new nose still lacks something of perfection to them. As one expert in plastic surgery said, "They study themselves in the mirror until the mirror itself gets tired of looking at them."

If the loss or destruction of tissue in the nose resulting from an accident is such as to injure the health of the person concerned, surgical attention is desirable. There are many ways of building up a broken-down or absent bridge. Some surgeons transplant bone or cartilage or similar materials. Humps are removed by dissection and scraping or cutting away the excess material. During World War II many a man had been provided with an almost completely new nose by the transplantation from other parts of the body of large amounts of tissue.

Obviously a field of this kind can be made exceedingly lucrative through exploitation of the patient. Hence people who are going to invest in plastic surgery on the nose should make certain that the surgeon who is doing the work is one of recognized skill and established honesty. They will do well also to make certain that the work is to be done in a hospital that is known for proper scientific control over its surgery. They will do well also to have a clear understanding as to the approximate cost of the procedure, the amount of time likely to be lost from work, and their ability to meet the necessary requirements.

NUTRITION See *Weight, Over-* and *Under-*.

NYMPHOMANIA Excessive desire on the part of a woman for sexual activity is called nymphomania.

NYSTAGMUS Nystagmus is an involuntary, rapid movement of the eyeball. It is especially associated with disturbances of the nervous and brain tissues involved in control of eye movements. Sometimes it appears in certain occupations, as in the case of miners.

OBESITY (See also *Weight, Over-* and *Under-*) Of all of the annoyances that affect human beings, overweight is the one likely to receive least sympathy.

There are probably many different causes for overweight, but the main cause is taking in more food than is used up by the work of the body. Therefore the matter of stabilizing the weight at a proper level is simply a matter of physiologic bookkeeping.

The experts say that the "extraordinary thing is that more people do not really become fat." The reason more people do not become overweight without regulating the amount of food they eat is adjustment by the appetite to meet the ordinary needs of the body. In time, however, this adjustment may lose its delicacy, and people will begin to eat for a variety of reasons which have nothing whatever to do with appetite. They may eat purely as a habit. They may eat to overcome states of fear or social maladjustments. Sometimes they eat just to spite other people.

In a few instances overweight is due to some disturbance of the pituitary or thyroid glands, which fail to develop their secretions properly and in suffi-

cient amounts. These are, however, the minor rather than the major number of cases.

The basal metabolic rate of the human being has a great deal to do with the speed and efficiency with which he uses up food for the production of energy. However, two people with the same basal metabolic rate may differ— one gaining weight readily and the other not. This is due to the fact that the total metabolism may be different from the basal metabolism. Extra muscular work and the taking of food will accelerate the metabolism. Emotional disturbances will speed up the metabolism. Total metabolism is the basal metabolism plus all of the other activities of the type mentioned. Probably for this reason people who are placid and calm tend to gain weight more rapidly than those who are excitable and "nervous." The placid person reacts less intensively to stimuli than the one who is excitable. People who gain weight readily are usually phlegmatic, worry less, sleep longer and more soundly, and relax more completely than people who are thin.

When overweight first begins, the fat tends to be deposited in certain portions of the body that are known as fat depots. These are the area of the breasts, the abdominal covering called the omentum, the hips, and similar areas. Later, however, fat can actually invade organs like the heart and the liver.

Ordinary overweight does not produce symptoms. However, excess weight can be associated with shortness of breath on exertion, an increased tendency to fatigue, trouble with the joints, increased danger of failure of the heart, and damage to some of the other vital organs. People with obesity seem to get diabetes more often than those who are of ordinary weight. Fat people with high blood pressure tend to have a lowering of the pressure when they take off weight.

The prevention of obesity is much better than trying to treat it. People who are interested in controlling their weight should weigh themselves every day and watch their waist measure. If the weight is steadily increasing and the waist measure likewise, it is best to begin to restrict the total consumption of food. The will power of the fat person is the fundamental factor in relief. No one can be satisfactorily reduced who does not really wish to reduce. Most fat people, though they may not admit it, simply love to eat, and if they do not eat much at meals, they begin taking extra food in small amounts all through the day and before going to bed at night. These habits must be broken. Women are more likely to reduce their weight successfully than men because with them the desire to have a handsome appearance plays a considerable part.

The rate at which weight can be reduced depends on the amount of weight and on the manner in which the reduction is accomplished. Ordinarily two pounds a week is sufficient. For very heavy people, three or four pounds a week may be necessary. At the beginning the rapid loss of weight is due chiefly to loss of water from the body. In most severe cases of overweight the best results have been accomplished by putting the person in a hospital, where the exact amount of food taken in can be controlled over a long period of time.

Most recent in the control of obesity is the use of certain drugs which control the appetite. These drugs are, however, exceedingly stimulating and have a tendency to produce insomnia. They should never be taken unless prescribed by a doctor and in the amount that the doctor prescribes.

All sorts of special diets have been proposed from time to time for reducing weight. The best diets are those which cut down largely on fats and the concentrated sugars, on bread, and on starchy foods like potatoes. In the diet for those who are overweight the protein must be maintained at about 60 grams of protein per day. A reduction in protein below that amount tends to weaken the patient by using up the protein of the body. Fruits and vegetables which are low in carbohydrates (so-called 5 and 10 per cent vegetables) are invaluable in reducing weight because by their bulk they reduce hunger. They also supply necessary mineral salts and vitamins.

There is no single diet that is desirable for all patients who are reducing weight. The doctor can plan the diet to meet the requirements of the individual patient. For very severe cases of overweight, doctors put patients in hospitals and reduce the diet as low as 300 calories a day. For the average, diets of 600 to 800 calories a day can be prescribed which will take off weight rapidly. All such diets are best supplemented with the necessary vitamins and mineral salts, since it is exceedingly difficult, on diets as low as 600 calories, to get all of these essential substances. Diets have also been developed of about 1200 calories a day which can be continued for long periods of time combined with vitamins and mineral salts and thus hold the weight stable.

Coupled with these diets there should be a program of prolonged gentle exercises which, however, must be taken regularly.

Thyroid extract has frequently been taken by people to speed up the metabolism. Thyroid should never be taken unless prescribed by the doctor and in the amounts that he prescribes. Amphetamine, benzedrine, or dexedrine are prescribed by the doctor to destroy appetite. A sweet taken one half hour before a meal will also allay hunger or kill appetite.

ODORS Among human beings the ability to smell varies greatly. Few, if any, human beings have the power to detect odors and to identify those odors in relation to certain hazards that attaches to many of the lower animals. Moreover, the ability to detect odors by the use of the olfactory nerves and the portion of the brain associated with them may be seriously damaged by such ordinary conditions as the common cold or allergy.

Several devices have been invented for measuring the ability to detect odors, one of them inelegantly named the "stinkometer." This apparatus consists simply of a lot of bottles with chemical solutions which respond to certain chemical substances that are associated with vaporized materials. One stinkometer is used to evaluate the freshness of foods by measuring the odors.

Doctors recognize a condition called anosmia, which means a complete loss of the capacity to smell. This may be permanent or temporary, depending on whether or not it involves damage of the nervous structures or their complete destruction. If a person loses the sense of smell on only one side, it is called hemianosmia. Such defects in smelling may be due to dryness of the mucous membranes in the nose, infection, injuries, the actions of drugs or deterioration of the tissues. The term hyposmia means a partial loss of the ability to detect odors, whereas hyperosmia means that there is an excessive response to odors. This may be associated with hysteria or may result from excessive irritability of the tissues involved in smelling.

Sometimes people think they are smelling something when the reaction is purely mental. Some people complain of constantly smelling fish; others of smelling roses—which is certainly more pleasant. The sensation of smelling an odor that does not exist may be the result of a hallucination.

If the doctor can find something positive in the tissues to account for disturbances of the olfactory sense, the patient is fortunate. Such conditions are frequently correctable. Most difficult of all are the cases in which the disturbances related to odors are mental.

The ordinary healthy person is not subject to offensive odors, provided he keeps himself clean. Some people who work in sewers, stockyards, and chemical works, as well as students in dissecting rooms, carry odors around with them to which they have become quite accustomed but which are immediately detectable by other people. One of the chief advantages of air conditioning in modern industry is the help it gives in getting rid of disturbing smells, some of which may be of human origin.

In many instances people have unpleasant odors on the surface of the body which cannot be controlled by bathing or changing garments. Everyone knows that garlic can produce a smell about the body, which is frequently associated with nationalities that have a great deal of garlic in their diets.

Young people are usually less odorous than older people. Sometimes odors attach to people who suffer with disease conditions such as diabetes or cancer. These represent in most instances disintegration of tissues. The odor frequently associated with feet is due to maceration of the skin between the toes.

Certain drugs are known which can diminish the output of perspiration and thus control unpleasant odors. Furthermore the use of the X ray, which must be done only by experts because of the danger, can destroy sweat glands and thus diminish odors.

OLD AGE See *Senescence*.

OLFACTORY The sense of smell is known as the olfactory sense. This may be disturbed in a variety of conditions. Frequently in examining for disturbances of the brain, tests are made of the ability to smell various odors.

OMENTUM The omentum is a large membrane which is a part of the peritoneum, or lining of the abdominal cavity. It covers various organs of the abdomen and portions of the omentum extend from the stomach to adjacent organs. Like other tissues of the body, it may become inflamed and subject to various infections or tumors requiring surgical procedures.

OPHTHALMIA An inflammation of the eye is called ophthalmia. The term "ophthalmus" refers to the eye and there are a wide variety of conditions with the prefix "ophthal-." Thus ophthalmoplegia is a paralysis of the eye; ophthalmitis, an inflammation of the eye; ophthalmoscope, an instrument for looking into the eye; ophthalmology, the study of diseases of the eye, and a specialist in diseases affecting the eye is known as an ophthalmologist.

ORCHITIS Orchitis is an inflammation of the testicle. The prefix "orchid-" has nothing to do with the flower of the same name but in medicine is used to refer to any condition affecting the testicle. When there is inflammation of the testicles, the symptoms include pain, swelling, and a feeling of weight. Such an inflammation may be due to the organism of gonorrhea or to any other germ such as that of tuberculosis or syphilis. Treatment depends altogether on determining the nature of the disturbance. Sometimes surgery is required.

ORGASM The crisis of sexual excitement is called orgasm. Absence of this phenomenon under the usual circumstances is, in many instances, associated with a mental rather than a physical disturbance.

ORTHO- The prefix "ortho-" in medicine means straight. Thus orthopedics has to do with the correction of deformities of the joints and spine; orthodontia with the straightening of the teeth; orthopsychiatry with the straightening out of behavior and personality.

OSTEOMYELITIS Osteomyelitis is an infection of the bones of the body. Most of these cases are due to the pus-forming organisms like the staphylococcus and the streptococcus but instances are known in which the pneumococcus and the typhoid germ caused osteomyelitis.

In most cases the germs get into the bones by way of the blood stream. Occasionally, however, infections in the tissues near the bones work through into the bony area. This happens particularly when a bone is infected from a joint.

The long bones of the body, like the bones of the legs and arms, are most frequently affected but any bone may be involved. It is known that infections of the jawbone are much more serious than a similar infection in a long bone.

The first sign of osteomyelitis is pain in the infected bone. This comes on suddenly and is associated with fever and rapid pulse and all of the usual signs of infection. Frequently also there are swelling, redness, and the other signs of disturbance at the spot that is infected.

When the doctor makes an examination of the blood, he will find that there has been a great increase in the white blood cells. The child with an infection of the bone will probably refuse to have the arm or leg examined and will be apprehensive about having it touched.

Because the bones are associated with the production of blood for the body and because the blood may carry the infection from a bone throughout the body, osteomyelitis is always a serious condition. When just one bone is involved, the difficulty is, of course, much less than in the case of multiple osteomyelitis because cases are known in which the infection has attacked one bone after another, and in the past, cases have been seen in which twelve or thirteen different bone abscesses have developed in the same person.

Nowadays with the use of the X ray and modern methods of diagnosis, osteomyelitis is discovered and treated much sooner than used to be the practice thirty or forty years ago. Before the discovery of the sulfonamide drugs and of penicillin, there were few remedies which were able to get at a deep-seated infection in the bone. These newer remedies, however, which have a specific effect on the streptococcus, the staphylococcus, and the pneumococcus, are able to do much more in controlling osteomyelitis. Nevertheless, good medical practice still demands surgical treatment so that the bone is opened, the damaged and infected tissue removed, and the infected area treated directly with applications of penicillin as well as by injection of penicillin into the muscles or into the blood.

In a previous generation osteomyelitis affecting the jawbone was considered to be an almost invariably fatal disease. The astounding recovery of several such cases treated with penicillin was the most impressive observation early in the use of this amazing drug. Indeed the publication of the reports of these cases focused the attention of all the medical world on the great value of penicillin for the control of infections by the pus-forming germs.

OSTEOPATHY Osteopathy is a system of treatment of disease in which there is manipulation of the bones, joints, and other tissues of the body with a view to restoring what is conceived to be a deranged mechanism. The osteopaths themselves define osteopathy as "that system of the healing art which places the chief emphasis on the structural integrity of the body mechanism, as being the most important single factor to maintain the well-being of the organism in health and disease." In many states osteopaths are limited wholly to such manipulations. The osteopathic course of instruction now includes some college education and four years of osteopathic education in which osteopaths are taught something about germs and drugs. Thus in some states osteopaths are also permitted to prescribe certain drugs and to undertake surgical procedures.

OTOSCLEROSIS (See also *Deafness*) One of the most common causes of progressive deafness is a change in the internal ear in which spongy bone appears and in which the small bones of the internal ear fail to function. The experts in ear disease prefer to call the condition otospongiosis because of the changes that take place.

The exact cause of otosclerosis is not known. Innumerable studies have been made to determine whether or not it was hereditary or due to some vitamin deficiency or some failure of the glands to function, but unfortunately it has not been shown that any one of these factors is primarily responsible. Most authorities consider this to be a chronic inflammatory disease with the destruction of formation of new bone in the internal ear.

The condition seems to occur more often in women than in men and often the first complaint is an annoying and distracting ringing in the ears. Associated with this there is a gradual loss of hearing which goes on progressively. Although the condition may begin on only one side, eventually both ears become affected.

Sufficient hearing will remain in some cases to permit the person to follow ordinary conversation but in other cases the progress is so great that it becomes necessary for the affected person to learn lip reading or to avail himself of other technics in order to be able to hear the spoken voice. It has been found that the pitch of the raised voice is heard more easily in otosclerosis, so that some of these people hear better in noisy surroundings because the people who speak to them raise the pitch of the voice.

Whenever there is a gradual loss of hearing going on for months or even years, the suspicion is warranted that otosclerosis may be present. Indeed doctors have a saying to the effect that "otosclerosis is a disease in which the doctor sees nothing and the patient hears nothing."

Specialists in diseases of the ear have a good many different tests which they apply to such cases in order to make certain that the condition is actually otosclerosis and not any other disturbance of the mechanism of the internal ear which might develop similar symptoms.

As has already been said, all sorts of treatments have been applied to these cases but unfortunately the methods thus far developed, outside of certain surgical procedures, the use of lip reading and of hearing aids, have not been of special benefit. The doctor will, of course, make certain that all of the accessory factors involved in hearing are properly functioning. This includes cleansing of the Eustachian tubes by the technic which the doctor uses for blowing through the tubes. It includes also the administration of a suitable diet, the control of the dosage of vitamins, and the application of proper glandular materials when any glandular failure of function is found. Sometimes the ringing in the ears needs to be controlled by various sedative drugs. The operation for the making of a window from the outside into the internal ear, known as the Lempert operation, is still the subject of investigation but a good many cases have already been reported in which this operative procedure has been of definite benefit.

OVARY The ovary is the name given to the sex gland of women. There are two of these in a normal woman—one on each side in the lower portion of the abdomen.

It is the function of the ovary to provide the female egg cell which passes once each month down the fallopian tubes to the uterus. The ovary also develops various glandular secretions which are important in maintaining the female body structure and the functions which are peculiar to women.

In case the ovary becomes infected and it becomes necessary to remove it by surgery, the lack of these secretions brings about changes in the body. Hence one of the greatest discoveries in modern medicine is the determination of the nature of these secretions and the development of extracts or artificial substances which can be injected into the body and which serve to take the place of the secretions that are missing.

Since the ovary is supported in the abdomen by a tissue which holds it to the abdominal wall, it becomes possible for various symptoms to be associated with a stretching or twisting of these tissues, which are called ovarian ligaments. Twisting or stretching of these tissues may also affect the blood supply of the gland. Therefore symptoms of pain, swelling, or failure of functions in the ovaries which are associated with abnormal twisting or stretching of the ligaments may also require a surgical operation.

Occasionally also the ovary is subject to the formation of cysts, which are large collections of fluid in the form of glandular material or degenerated material of the gland itself. Cysts also occur when there is a hemorrhage into the gland. A cyst may remain small and not cause much disturbance. In other instances, however, the amount of fluid material develops tremendously, so that cysts may become exceedingly large and thus require surgical removal.

The ovary also becomes infected occasionally by the passing of infection along the tubes which carry the cells to the uterus. Infections like gonorrhea, tuberculosis, or streptococcic infections are accountable for more than 90 per cent of all infections of the ovary. When there is pus or infected material in the fallopian tubes—so-called pus tubes—it passes along by pressure to the ovary and thus carries the infection. In the presence of the pain, the swelling, and the fever which occur under such circumstances, the immediate treatment is the application of heat or of an ice bag. It is quite possible under modern circumstances to treat such infections with the sulfonamide drugs or with penicillin, and the physician must make the decision as to how long such treatment is to be carried on before surgical operation becomes necessary for the removal of the tube or the ovary.

Finally, tumors of all sorts may affect the ovary, including cancer. The doctor cannot determine from any examination that he can carry on from the outside of the body the exact nature of such a tumor. It is, therefore, generally believed that the treatment of all tumors of the ovary is the performing of an immediate operation, at which time the doctor decides the nature of the tumor and exactly what is to be done.

OXYGEN Oxygen once was just an emergency remedy rushed in when patients were at the point of death.

Today it is well established as a useful remedy in many forms of disease, and it is recognized that early use of oxygen may be far more beneficial than any attempt to delay its application, in certain types of cases, until an emergency exists.

New oxygen devices include incubators which keep premature infants in a high oxygen atmosphere. For grownups there are oxygen tents, oxygen rooms, and special devices for breathing oxygen on a more limited scale.

In use of the oxygen tent, the oxygen in the air is kept down at about a 50 per cent level in contrast with the normal level. About one standard tank of oxygen a day is required.

If an oxygen tent is not available, a temporary emergency type of apparatus can be made, consisting of an anesthetic mask with a rebreathing bag. It is also possible to introduce the oxygen through a tube in the nose. In setting up such a system, the oxygen must be passed through water to prevent too much drying of membranes of nose and throat.

Oxygen should be used in all cases in which breathing is difficult and in which the patient suffers from an actual shortage of air. This occurs in all types of asphyxia, such as carbon monoxide poisoning or pneumonia.

The shortage of air which occurs with diseases of the heart is seldom greatly benefited by treatment with oxygen, since this type of shortage is largely due to a slowing of circulation of the blood.

On the other hand, oxygen may help cases of angina pectoris, because in these cases there may be a deficient amount of oxygen in the heart muscle.

Persons whose attacks of angina pectoris are readily controlled by rest or by treatment with the usual drugs do not need oxygen, but those who have frequent and severe attacks of angina, which come on with the slightest amount of physical effort, may find themselves greatly benefited by this treatment.

All that is to be known about the value of oxygen in various forms of disease has not yet begun to be established, but investigations are being carried out in many hospitals and laboratories and increasing use is found for this substance.

Since there is danger of fire and of violent explosion of oxygen under wrong conditions, it is never to be used except under direction of an experienced attendant.

OZENA An extraordinary and unfortunate disease which affects the mucous membranes of the nose is called ozena, a word which comes from a Greek word meaning stench. The doctors have apparently never been very sensitive about describing the disease because the French word for this disease is *pue-nez,* which means stinking nose, and the Germans with their characteristic bluntness simply call it *Stinknase.*

In this disease there is a gradual degeneration of the membrane that lines the nose. Then a mucous or mucopurulent discharge collects and dries, so that there are large foul-smelling crusts. All sorts of investigations have been made to find out the cause of ozena and whether or not any special germs are present to produce the characteristic bad odor. The most recent point of view is that continued infection of the nose in infancy gradually produces atrophy and death of the nasal mucous membrane, so that the nasal opening becomes too wide and thus permits the collection of crusts and the secondary infection. Certainly this should be a warning to parents never to neglect infection of the nose in children but to see to it that infection is controlled as soon as possible.

Strangely also, from Great Britain comes the report that this disease occurs chiefly among young girls, mostly of the servant class, and that it is seen most often in public dispensaries and rarely in private practice.

Incidentally this disease, which was quite frequent in a previous generation, has now almost disappeared, as is the case of another disease in young women called chlorosis. This gradual disappearance of ozena is believed to be due to the improved diet, the outdoor life and exercise, and the increasing medical attention to infections occurring in childhood.

Formerly it was the custom to treat ozena by copious washing of the nose with alkaline lotions and antiseptic lotions. It was customary to keep the nose filled with gauze containing antiseptic materials. Modern treatment includes particularly proper attention to the diet and a glandular study so as to bring the patient into the best state of health possible. Attempts are made to stimulate the mucous membrane of the nose to restore, if possible, its lost function. Attempts have even been made by surgical procedures to transplant mucous membrane but fortunately the gradual disappearance of the condition by prevention and by the changes that have taken place in the general hygiene of the body are more important than surgical cure.

Unfortunately the large majority of people do not apply for treatment to infections of the nose until the damage has become well advanced. The occurrence of even a few cases of ozena should be a warning to secure prompt treatment in all such cases.

PAIN   Pain is one of four elementary sensations, the others being touch, heat, and cold. Studies by the physiologists show that there are in the skin little points or nerve endings specialized to detect pain, touch, heat, and cold. The ability to feel pain is a protective mechanism for the human being, since it warns us of danger.

When for any reason an area has lost sensation, pain is the first sensation to be recovered. Moreover, there are more pain spots in the skin than heat or cold, although the touch spots are just about as frequent. In other words, you can feel that something is touching you at just about the same time you feel pain, if the sensation is painful.

As with other sensations, the detection of pain varies in different people. Some people are much more sensitive to pain than others.

The scientists have been making special studies of the pain sensation in recent years, particularly with a view to measuring the effects of various drugs that are used to diminish the sensation of pain. One technic includes the use of heat to the point of feeling of pain; another, the use of cold or freezing to the point at which it becomes painful. It has been found that morphine raises the threshold at which pain is felt to twice its normal level; codeine raises it only 50 per cent; alcohol, 45 per cent; and aspirin, 33 per cent. Beyond a certain

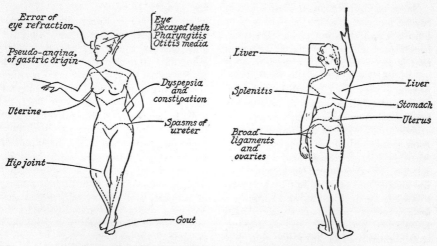

Areas where pains referred from other tissues are felt

dose extra quantities of any drug do not have any extra effect. Two drugs in combination do not raise the pain threshold any higher than one effective drug by itself. The only reason for using two drugs is that one has a more prompt effect and the other has a longer effect.

Studies also show that the speed at which a sensation moves along a nerve varies.

With our new knowledge of pain, it has become possible to diminish the pain during surgical operations by blocking the nerves, by cutting the nerves, and by the use of pain-relieving drugs.

The scientists also distinguish between pain on the surface, pain in the bones, in the blood vessels, or in the organs of the body. Pain is first felt in the little terminal points of the nerves which then carry the sensation, with a small change in electric potential, to the spinal column and up the spinal column to the area in the brain. From this point the feeling is reflected back to the point of origin, so that one feels the pain in the finger, the toe, or some specific spot. Because of the pathways by which the sensation is carried to the brain, there are instances in which pain is felt in a tissue that has been removed, as, for instance, pain that is felt in a leg that has been removed, because of irritation of the nerves along which that sensation would ordinarily pass.

Scientists also recognize what is called psychogenic pain, which is wholly mental. Such pain does not possess the qualities of pain that are associated with pain that is physical. The psychogenic pains are vague, they are irregular in their appearance, they are likely to be exaggerated in description, and they are usually accompanied by signs of excellent health otherwise. Pains that are more psychogenic than physical are likely to clear up when the mental reason for the pain disappears. Doctors refer, for instance, to the kind of pain that is felt by a person following an accident on a railroad or in a motorcar which promptly disappears when the person receives a check from the railroad or insurance company as compensation for his injury.

PALSY See *Paralysis Agitans*.

PANCREAS The pancreas is a large gland situated in the abdominal cavity near the stomach, liver, and gall bladder. Its functions include the development of secretions which are important in relation to the use of sugar by the body and to the digestion of proteins in the intestines.

The common association of inflammations of the gall bladder with inflammations of the pancreas has led doctors to believe that inflammations of the gall bladder are particularly dangerous because of the possibility of extension to the pancreas. Sometimes this glandular organ becomes infected directly with germs brought by the blood when people happen to have boils, mumps, influenza, pneumonia, or similar infections. Occasionally the pancreas is infected directly from an ulcer of the stomach. Men past middle age are much more frequently affected by inflammations of the pancreas than are women.

When this gland is infected, there are frequently attacks of dyspepsia and pains like those that occur with disease of the gall bladder. Often pains come on immediately after a heavy meal. There may be distention of the abdomen, vomiting, and localized pain and swelling. Usually also the doctor finds, when he examines the blood, that the white blood cells are greatly increased, which is usual when there is infection inside the abdomen. In a serious case of this kind the only definite life-saving measure is an immediate surgical operation to check the progress of the infection. In other instances the infection in the pancreas may not be sudden and severe but possibly in a milder manner over a long period of time. This is called chronic pancreatitis, or chronic inflammation of the pancreas. Associated with such infection, there are loss of appetite and weight, nausea and vomiting, a feeling of fullness, and occasionally much disturbance of digestion accompanied with diarrhea and the passing of a good deal of undigested material.

The pancreas may also be involved

by the formation of cysts, stones, and tumors. Under such circumstances there may be excessive secretion of the glandular materials, so that the symptoms are related to this fact. An excess amount of insulin in the blood, with an insufficient amount of sugar in the blood, gives the same symptoms as are associated with an overdose of insulin. This includes giddiness, unconsciousness—perhaps with convulsions—periodical attacks of intense fatigue, and shortness of breath. Indeed cases are known in which people who have been suffering with an excess amount of insulin in the blood have been diagnosed as intoxicated by alcohol. In one instance a man was arrested for murder with a motorcar due to driving while intoxicated, and it was shown later that he was suffering with an excess amount of insulin in his blood.

The pancreas is one of the vital organs of the human body, equal in its importance to the liver and the thyroid gland. Too few people really have any knowledge that there is such an organ.

PARALYSIS See also discussion of paralysis due to brain hemorrhage under *Apoplexy.*

PARALYSIS AGITANS In 1817 a London doctor named James Parkinson described a disease in which there was involuntary tremulous motion with lessened muscular power in parts of the body not in action and even when supported. He called attention also to a propensity to bend the trunk forward and to pass from a walking to a running pace. These are characteristic symptoms of what is now called Parkinson's disease or the shaking palsy, known scientifically as paralysis agitans.

The condition comes on most often in the sixth or seventh decade of life, but in rare instances a similar condition occurs in young people following epidemic infections of the brain.

Unfortunately nothing certain is known about the cause of paralysis agitans, although changes in the blood vessels of the brain and changes in the tissues of the nervous system and brain

have been found. The disease is not especially associated with high blood pressure or brain hemorrhage.

In the very early stages of paralysis agitans a cessation of the ordinary swing of one arm may be the first visible sign. Another sign is a gradual appearance of fixity in the facial expression and slowness with which the ordinary movements of expression come and go. The condition tends to appear first in one limb and then to spread to the other limb on the same side and finally to the opposite limbs. The usual order of involvement is arm, leg, opposite arm, and opposite leg. After rigidity invades the muscles of the trunk of the body, the person with paralysis agitans tends to take a stooping attitude and to take shorter steps when he walks. Then he tends to take increasingly rapid steps, so that he breaks into a shuffling trot when he walks. Gradually all movements become slower and more limited in range.

The rate of progress of paralysis agitans varies. In many instances the condition may be confined to one limb for months or even a year before any other portion of the body is affected, and similar periods may pass before the condition spreads to other parts of the body. The general health of such a patient may remain remarkably good for many years.

Palliative treatment tends to postpone the arrival of complete disability and to give the patient relief from some of the disturbing symptoms. The drugs that influence rigidity are drugs of the belladonna type, and several technics have been developed for giving these drugs so as to bring about ease and apparent improvement. A new surgical approach involves stopping the flow of blood in certain blood vessels of the brain.

A specialist has observed that some strong emotional stimulus may suddenly bring about temporary amelioration of the disability. Sudden fright or danger may do this, but soon after there is a relapse into the previous condition.

Everything possible should be done for these patients to improve their general health and strength. Massage and suitable baths tone the skin and muscles. Sedative drugs tend to reduce the restlessness and the tremors.

PARANOIA When human beings develop a mental disorder which is characterized by extraordinary ambitions and suspicions about persecution and grandeur expressed in logical form, the condition is called paranoia. There are many different types of paranoia.

PARATHYROID GLANDS The parathyroid glands are the smallest known organs of internal secretion. Usually there are four parathyroid glands —two on each side. They lie in the throat behind the thyroid gland. They are small, so that the entire four glands weigh only a tiny fraction of a pound.

Apparently the effect of the secretion put out by the parathyroid glands is to influence calcium and phosphorus as used in the human body, raising the total amount of calcium in the blood and lowering the total amount of phosphorus. When it is necessary to increase the amount of calcium in the blood, the material is obtained either from the bones or from extra calcium taken into the body. The great importance of calcium in the human body has often been emphasized, since it is the material which makes up the bones and teeth and since it is also involved in stabilizing nervous reactions. Thus in certain convulsive disorders, such as tetany, there may be too small an amount of calcium in the blood.

The condition called tetany, which is a sign of insufficient activity on the part of the parathyroid glands, is characterized by a tendency of the muscles to go into a condition of painful, prolonged spasm. This involves the muscles of the forearms and hands and the throat but may involve almost any muscles of the body. Associated with the spasms there may be tingling sensations, a feeling of weight on the chest, and general numbness. Occasionally twitchings occur in various muscles. People with tetany due to insufficiency of calcium may also be nervous, self-centered, emotional, or depressed.

Once it was exceedingly difficult for doctors to treat such patients successfully, but nowadays there are many ways in which calcium may be put into the body promptly. In many instances, however, the symptoms of tetany are produced by other conditions which are not related to a deficiency of action of the parathyroid glands. Thus the condition called rickets, or osteomalacia associated with characteristic changes in the bones may produce similar symptoms. In all such conditions the calcium in the blood is low due to defective absorption of calcium from the food. In many instances symptoms like those of tetany are due to excessive alkali in the body.

The first step for the doctor in all such cases is to find out exactly what is the state of the blood and the cause of the symptoms. Sometimes the condition is controllable by providing a diet with a low amount of phosphates, supplemented by the giving of large amounts of calcium salts. A diet low in phosphates would eliminate meat, yolk of egg, and also cut down the amount of milk.

The opposite condition is excessive action of the parathyroid glands, likely to be characterized by serious changes in the bones. This produces a condition called fibrous inflammation of the bones, or osteitis fibrosa. In this condition the bones are soft and can be cut with a knife due to the elimination of calcium from the bones. The bones actually become porous, producing a state that is also characterized by the name osteoporosis. Because of the excessive mobilization of calcium in the blood derived from the bones, stones are often found in the various organs of the body. Softness of the bones and the failure of the calcium to be used properly in their development may produce strange deformities in the body. To the twisting and disturbance of the bones the name "osteomalacia" is given. Sometimes the excessive action of the parathyroid glands is due to a tumor growth in these glands. In such cases surgical removal of the gland is the only help.

PARESIS   About 3 per cent of people who became infected with syphilis in the past developed late in life a condition called variously general paralysis, general paresis, general paralysis of the insane, or, by the doctors, dementia paralytica. In this condition the syphilis is found to have infected the brain and the coverings of the brain with damage to the tissues sufficient to result in paralysis and mental disturbance. Strangely, this form of syphilis occurs three to five times as often in men as in women.

Customarily the person who has had syphilis and who is developing paresis first shows the condition by slight changes in manner, including irritability, carelessness about the clothes and the body generally, lack of judgment, absent-mindedness, inability to concentrate, slowness of comprehension, and similar irregularities. Since all of these symptoms may occur as the result of a variety of other conditions, their appearance in a person should not necessarily be considered the sign of beginning paresis. It is the assemblage of the symptoms and their characteristic development and continuance that permit the expert to make the diagnosis.

Associated with the mental symptoms affecting the nervous system there are others of a motor character, such as disturbances of dexterity, tremors of the hands, inability to make co-ordinated movements, even changes in the facial expression and often speech defects, so that the patient cannot say such trick phrases as "she sells sea shells," "third riding artillery brigade," "Methodist Episcopal," and similar phrases.

One of the signs long known to be associated with paresis is the change in the pupil of the eye, so that when the doctor makes the test the pupil of the eye does not react to light but does react to accommodation; that is to say, the pupil will not grow smaller with light and larger without light but will adjust itself to looking at objects close up or at a distance.

As paresis develops, there comes one of the symptoms which is most dramatic, namely, a condition called euphoria, an extraordinary sense of well-being in which these people are grandiose, elated with delusions of wealth and great power, and in which they feel better than ever before. This appears in around 15 to 20 per cent of the cases. These delusions take strange actions. One man of ordinary income went into a department store and ordered a thousand dollars' worth of silk underwear. A baker doing an ordinary business ordered twenty-seven delivery trucks to take care of an increase in business which he thought was going to occur.

In other cases there are depression, anxiety, fear of danger, and self-accusation. In still others there are loss of memory, difficulty in calculation and writing, and difficulties in judgment.

Eventually the damage becomes so great that the patient with paresis has to be put to bed, and a general paralysis of all of the muscles of the body ensues.

Once paresis was considered to be an invariably fatal disease. If a man or woman developed this condition, which was often called softening of the brain around 1900, the outlook was bad. There was the possibility of death, the likelihood of years of confinement in an institution for the insane. Today the outlook for such a person is far from hopeless.

The improvement in outlook has resulted from the gradual development of a number of important discoveries in medical science related directly to an understanding of this disease. The famous Japanese investigator Noguchi was the first to prove that general paresis is caused by syphilis. Another investigator found that the injection of such patients with the germ that causes malaria resulted in a fever which tended to stop the progress of the paretic condition. Next came treatment by the use of heat, which is developed either through passing an electric current through the body or by putting the patient in a body-baking device. Then came various drugs of the arsenic type, such as salvarsan or 606, scientifically called arsphenamine, and another more specific arsenic drug called tryparsamide. All of these methods are difficult to administer and are used only in a hospital.

Most recent in the treatment of paresis and of other forms of syphilis of the nervous system is the use of penicillin. It is now rather well established that penicillin is effective in the treatment of early syphilis, often bringing about recovery, as nearly as can be determined by modern methods, within weeks or months. In many instances excellent results are secured by combining the treatment of syphilis with penicillin and one of the arsenic preparations.

A joint investigation conducted by experts in various parts of the country under the direction of the National Research Council has shown that 80 per cent of 30 cases treated with penicillin improved to some degree, nearly half improved 50 per cent or more, 8 improved 75 per cent and 1 was restored to normal. Even in long-continued paresis in which deterioration had occurred, 2 out of 10 improved 75 per cent, 1 out of 10 improved 50 per cent, but in 7 the deterioration had been so great that improvement was not possible.

Apparently there is new hope for the person with paresis.

PARKINSON'S DISEASE See *Paralysis Agitans.*

PARTURITION (See discussions under *Pregnancy* and *Prenatal Care*) Parturition is the process of giving birth to a child.

PATCH TEST The patch test is a technic in which a small patch of adhesive, containing a substance to which a person may be sensitive, is applied to the skin. The appearance of redness and inflammation is considered to be a positive test.

PEDIATRICIAN A pediatrician is a specialist in the treatment of children's diseases. This specialty is called pediatrics.

PELLAGRA Certain diseases are called deficiency diseases, which means they result from failure of the body to receive something that it needs for growth, repair, and development. One of the most serious of the deficiency diseases is called pellagra, which for many years has caused great harm and suffering to mankind. At one time many thousands of cases of this disease occurred throughout the United States. Today it is seen only in certain areas where the diets of people are greatly limited because of economic, social, or agricultural conditions. In 1917–18 at least 200,000 people in the United States suffered from this disease. In 1915 it was reported that 10,000 people had died of pellagra.

Today we know that the condition occurs largely because of the absence of certain necessary vitamins and proteins from the diet. Most important is nicotinic acid, also known as niacin. This substance, which is a part of the vitamin B complex, is absolutely necessary for the health and growth of the human body. When it is absent from the diet, there occur changes in the skin with redness and irritation and secondary cracking and ulceration. Soreness of the mouth and a violent red appearance of the tongue are other serious manifestations. We know from postmortem examinations that this redness and irritation may extend along the entire intestinal tract. Superimposed on these conditions there may be irritability, anxiety, delirium, and burning sensations in the nerves. The soreness of the mouth and of the intestinal tract prevent people with pellagra from eating as they should. Hence the condition develops into what is called a vicious circle.

Experiments have shown that feeding of people who have pellagra with yeast, liver extract, fresh milk, eggs, and lean meat brings about prompt recovery. Also the necessary vitamins may be either injected into the body or provided in other ways. Whenever a single vitamin is absent, it is likely that other vitamins also will be missing from the diet. This means that the diets of all of those with pellagra have to be investigated. Often it is found that these people have been living on pork fat, corn bread, soda biscuits, and corn syrup. Their diets need to be supplemented not only with the foods that have been mentioned but also with tomatoes, green peas, other green and yellow vegetables, and similar foods.

An interesting sidelight on pellagra is the suggestion that Job, when he complained about his boils and when he was stricken with a terrible skin disease that involved his entire body from the soles of his feet to the crown of his head, was actually suffering from pellagra. The condition appears wherever poverty exists. It will be remembered that Job had lost his money and had become a pauper.

PELVIMETRY The obstetrician before childbirth measures the dimensions and capacity of the pelvis of the woman who is going to have a child. The pelvis is the basin-shaped ring of bones at the bottom of the trunk. It joins the legs below and the spine above.

PEMPHIGUS A disease of the skin in which there are large blisters which break and leave pigmented spots is called pemphigus. Frequently itching and burning appear in connection with the development of the blisters. There are many different forms of skin disease in which such blisters appear and there are many different varieties of pemphigus.

PENICILLIN A mold known as *Penicillium notatum,* when grown in a suitable mixture, gives off a secretion that can be dried and extracted as a powder. This material is called penicillin. It has been found to be immensely effective in the treatment of all sorts of infections by germs of many different varieties.

PENIS The penis is the male sex organ used in sexual intercourse. Various disorders as well as infections may affect the organ. Surgical procedures have been developed for correcting structural disorders, particularly when there is an abnormal opening of the tube called the urethra which carries the urine from the bladder to the outside. One of these disorders is called hypospadia, in which there is a splitting of portions of the penis so that the opening comes on the inner side instead of at the front.

PERICARDITIS The heart lies in a sac which is called the pericardium. This sac may become infected and inflamed, in which case there is pain over the heart, a rapid pulse, and often severe coughing. Since the infection tends to roughen the lining and to produce fibrinous material, the doctor can hear a sound of the rubbing of the roughened portions when he uses the stethoscope in cases of pericarditis. There are many different varieties of pericarditis, depending on the nature of the germ that produces the infection and on the extent of the symptoms.

PERINEUM The space between the genital organs and the anus or lower opening of the bowel is called the perineum. Women frequently have disturbances in this area associated with tearing and pressure because of childbirth. The area may also become infected by the ringworm that attacks the groins, in which case there is severe itching and sometimes blistering in this area.

PERITONITIS The peritoneum is the name given to the membrane that lines the abdominal cavity just as the lining of the chest cavity is called the pleura. This tissue is subject to such conditions as affect linings elsewhere in the body. Thus it may rupture through the wall of the abdomen in the case of a hernia, or rupture. There may be cysts of the folds of the peritoneum that go down to the organs. This part of the peritoneum is called mesentery and the cysts are called mesenteric cysts.

The most serious condition that affects the peritoneum is peritonitis, which means inflammation of the peritoneum. When this tissue becomes inflamed, the results are always serious. Sometimes inflammation of the peritoneum develops after injury to the abdomen but in most instances the peritoneum is infected by germs which come by way of the blood or by secondary infections by the organs that lie within the abdomen, like the appendix. If, for instance, the appendix becomes infected and ruptures, the most dangerous complication is secondary peritonitis. Sometimes the peritoneum becomes infected by the rupture of an ulcer of the abdomen or the stomach. Pain begins almost immediately with infection and is felt at the point where the infection originated. As the inflammation progresses, the patient becomes seriously ill because of the absorption of the poisonous materials. There is fever, rigidity of the abdominal wall, and tenderness when the wall is touched. Thus whenever there is severe abdominal pain accompanied by tenderness of the abdominal wall, by vomiting and fever, the doctor suspects peritonitis. Unless acute peritonitis is promptly treated, it may be fatal. The time between the occurrence of the peritonitis and death may be only a matter of a few hours to a few days, depending on the severity of the infection. Obviously, therefore, the prompt diagnosis of peritonitis is of the utmost importance in saving life.

In most instances treatment of this condition is surgical. The doctor opens the abdomen and removes the infectious material, sometimes applying drug treatments directly to the peritoneal cavity.

Since the germs which affect the peritoneum are in most instances of the types that yield to sulfa drugs and to penicillin, physicians anticipate great improvement in the records of deaths from peritonitis in the forthcoming years. It is doubted that the condition will be considered as seriously fatal in the future as it has been in the past. However, even the sulfa drugs and penicillin cannot be considered helpful in cases of this type unless the diagnosis is made promptly and treatment given at once.

PERSPIRATION In hot weather human beings get especially interested in perspiration, the chief use of which is to regulate the heat of the body and keep it normal. The sweat glands are the chief paths by which water reaches the surface of the skin; a good deal of water passes through the skin by what is known as insensible perspiration. Perspiration is about 98 to 99 per cent water.

Tests have been made in the hot desert to determine how much fluid may be lost from the body by way of sweat. People vary as to the speed with which they begin to perspire and as to the amount of salts and water that they lose from the body during perspiration. People vary also as to the amount of perspiration from various portions of the body. One investigator found that the perspiration from the palms and soles is five to ten times as much as from other parts of the body. Incidentally, people who do not perspire fairly easily should not live in tropical countries.

The odor of the sweat varies according to the part of the body from which it is secreted. Ordinarily it is acid, but after profuse perspiration it tends to be neutral or alkaline.

There is a division of work between the skin and the kidneys in excreting water. For that reason the urine is light-colored in winter when perspiration is slight and darker in summer when the skin is secreting a great deal of water.

Perspiration is increased by heat, by the drinking of warm drinks, by psychic causes such as fright and anxiety, and by a number of the drugs which are known to increase the flow of water from the skin. Perspiration is decreased by external cold and by various drugs which have been proved capable of decreasing perspiration.

A number of special diseases affect the sweat glands. One of them, which describes excessive sweating, is called hyperhidrosis, in which the hands are continually moist, clammy, or dripping with fluid. This perspiration is usually cold. Serious states of this kind should be treated by specialists in diseases of the skin who have special remedies that can be prescribed.

Excessive perspiration may be the

symptom of a serious general condition. Often perspiration is affected by the emotional state. People who perspire freely should wear underwear that does not retain moisture—a mixture of silk and wool, light in weight, for winter, and cotton and silk in summer. More important, however, than the type of underwear is the amount of clothing. Care should be taken not to wear too much clothing, particularly by those who perspire excessively. Many people now find it advantageous to wear the same weight of underwear all year round. Medicine has developed several different substances which are useful in limiting the amount of perspiration. These drugs, however, are in most instances sufficiently potent so that they should be used over large sections of the body only when specifically prescribed by the doctor. Many different dusting powders useful in excessive perspiration are also available.

There is another condition in which sweat fails to be secreted by the body. This is exceedingly rare.

In a third type of case there is an offensive odor to the sweat. This is known as bromidrosis.

In another condition the sweat is colored, and this condition is called chromidrosis. The appearance of colored perspiration is believed to be due to infections with various kinds of germs.

PERTUSSIS See *Whooping Cough.*

PHARYNX In the throat, between the mouth and the opening of the esophagus which leads into the stomach, is an area that is commonly called the pharynx. In the pharynx are found the tonsils and a good deal of lymphoid tissue. It is customary to divide the pharynx into parts, including the nasal pharynx, which is the part that goes up toward the nose, and the laryngeal part, which goes down toward the larynx and trachea.

Whenever anyone catches a severe cold or gets a sore throat or acute tonsillitis, the pharynx is likely to be inflamed at the same time. When the infection is caused by a streptococcus, usually known as the hemolytic streptococcus, the condition known as septic sore throat develops. In this condition the mucous membrane becomes swollen, purple, and glazed. The uvula, which is the little piece of tissue which hangs down into the throat from above, may become swollen and the tonsils may become seriously infected. Sometimes this swelling is so severe that the patient finds it difficult to breathe.

With a septic sore throat the patient is gravely ill, the breath develops a foul odor; it is difficult for the patient to eat. Moreover, the infection is rapidly absorbed from the throat, so that the patient may become generally ill and secondary infections may be set up in other parts of the body.

Fortunately the streptococcus of septic sore throat is susceptible to treatment with the sulfa drugs and penicillin, so that this condition has been largely brought under control by modern technics.

Most important when an epidemic of septic sore throat strikes a community is to find out exactly where the epidemic originated and how it spreads. In the past, before strict control of milk supplies was the rule, epidemics were usually due to infection from the udder of the cow, often from a milker who was himself infected with septic sore throat, and often from a milker with severe infections of the fingers. Septic mastitis in the cow, which merely means streptococcus infection of the udder, is associated with epidemics of septic sore throat in the communities that use the milk.

Another condition that affects the pharynx is Vincent's angina, a form of infection of the throat caused by germs. This condition also requires special treatment since the organisms of Vincent's angina are known to be susceptible to treatment with several specific remedies. Most important, however, in such cases is for the doctor to make certain of the diagnosis of the condition so that specific remedies may be applied.

PHENOLPHTHALEIN Phenolphthalein is a neutral drug that acts on the large bowel as a purgative. Some people are allergic to it and break out with skin eruptions. In general, however, it is among the least toxic of the usual laxatives. It is a constituent of a good many patent laxative drugs.

PHLEBITIS The human being walks upright so that the veins in his legs have to carry the burden of a column of blood returning to the heart. These veins have valves which may remain capable of holding up the column of blood throughout life. In many instances, however, the valves break down, and the result is the appearance of varicose veins.

If infections occur, the linings of the blood vessels become inflamed. Clots may be formed which are then carried off from the veins to appear elsewhere in the body. The blood may accumulate in the tissues of the legs, causing swelling and pain. Any illness which slows the circulation of the blood and during which there is a long period of lying in bed may induce the formation of clots in the blood vessels. If you happen to be walking when a clot forms, there is lameness in the leg, and the foot may swell and become blue.

In such cases relief is had by elevating the foot of the bed moderately or sleeping with the legs elevated. After about ten days of cautious exercise and the wearing of a semielastic bandage recovery will usually occur.

Inflammation of the blood vessels with the formation of such clots is known as thrombophlebitis, which comes from the words "thrombo," meaning clots, and "phlebitis," meaning inflammation of the veins.

After about 1 per cent of cases of childbirth and after about 2 per cent of severe operations in the abdominal cavity, thrombophlebitis occurs as a secondary complication. Sometimes if the infection is severe, there will be fever with chills. The chief danger from thrombophlebitis is the possibility that a portion of a clot may break away and get into the blood stream, eventually blocking an important blood vessel in the lungs, heart, or brain. Fortunately this complication is not exceedingly frequent. More frequent is the possibility that a clot may get into some other part of the body and set up a secondary infection or abscess.

A vein with thrombophlebitis is frequently painful. The doctor may prescribe many soothing remedies to overcome the pain and also to bring about relief. Since the pain may be due to a spasm of the blood vessels or of the muscles, remedies used to overcome spasm are helpful. Carefulness in keeping the legs elevated and taking pressure off the veins whenever possible often brings about complete relief in these cases.

PHTHISIS (See *Tuberculosis*) Pulmonary consumption, or tuberculosis, used to be called phthisis because this condition produced progressive wasting and emaciation of the body.

PICA Children frequently crave unnatural articles of food, eating dirt, sticks, plaster, or all sorts of similar materials. The condition is known as pica.

PILES See *Hemorrhoids*.

PILONIDAL CYSTS At the very bottom of the human spine there is occasionally a glandular organ that does not close completely at the time of birth or that perhaps continues to secrete material which does not find an easy outlet, so that the end result is a cyst, a collection of fluid in a gland without any outlet. The point where the cyst appears is at the very end of the spine, where the tail would be if human beings had tails.

These cysts apparently cause greatest disturbance in men between the ages of twenty and forty-five, and they were a real problem for the surgeons of the United States Army and Navy during the war.

Ancient people gave the pilonidal cyst

its name, since the words "pilus" and "nidus" simply mean a place where there is hair or a nest of hair. If the little opening becomes infected, there is inflammation with pain on sitting or motion. Sometimes attempts are made to treat this by the use of hot sitz baths, the application of hot-water bottles, minor incisions merely to let out the fluid that is under pressure, and similar temporary procedures. When, however, the openings get blocked with hair, with dirt or with body secretions, competent surgical action is needed.

With soldiers in jeeps, fliers who sit for long periods of time and come down with a bump, or truck drivers, the cyst frequently becomes inflamed. If the blocking is sufficient to cause large accumulations of material, the cyst may grow to the size of an egg.

A proper surgical operation for pilonidal cyst includes the cutting out of the abnormal tissue and sufficient time in the hospital to permit complete healing. Since this may involve the removal of a large amount of tissue, some reparative or plastic surgery procedures may ultimately be necessary to bring about completely satisfactory results.

Attempts have been made by experimentation to find ways to inject the area with caustic substances and to obliterate it as one obliterates varicose veins. However, these methods are still considered in the experimental stage.

PINEAL GLAND The pineal gland is another gland whose activities seem to cease at the time of maturity. This gland lies within the skull at the lower portion of the brain. As yet we do not know with certainty what its functions in the human body actually are. The gland is tiny—about the size of a pea when it is flattened out. When, however, it becomes enlarged from any cause, it tends to close up the canal by which the cerebrospinal fluid circulates from the brain into the spinal cord. If this canal is closed, the fluid in the brain develops a high pressure with symptoms so serious that they may lead to death. We learn about the functions of the

glands in various ways. One of the methods is to destroy the gland completely in an animal or to remove it from the animal's body and then observe the animal to see what happens. Another method is to make an extract of the gland and feed it to animals in excess to see what an excess of this glandular material will do to the animal.

Various effects have been observed following the injection of extracts of the pineal into animals. It is supposed to have some effect in stopping overaction by the sex glands and also to inhibit too rapid growth. These effects are doubtful. No method has yet been found for making an extract of the pineal gland which with certainty has definite activity. Generally animals fed with this material grow larger and stronger muscularly, although there may be trouble with the development of the genital organs. In guinea pigs, if the gland is destroyed, the sex organs grow more rapidly and become larger than those of animals which do not have their pineal gland destroyed.

Here is a gland in the internal system which is obviously of some importance in the life of the human being but which needs to be studied far more extensively before we can say exactly what its functions are.

PITUITARY GLAND The pituitary gland is a veritable storehouse of hormones or important glandular principles. At least five of these are already well recognized. One is known as the growth hormone, another as the sex hormone, the third as the thyroid-stimulating hormone, the fourth as the milk-stimulating hormone, and the fifth as the adrenal-gland-stimulating hormone.

Any trouble with the growth hormone is promptly reflected in the size of the animal or child concerned. If the hypophysis, as this gland is sometimes called, is removed from a young animal, its growth is stopped. In a few weeks its long bones will discontinue increasing in length. Moreover, the body weight as a whole remains low.

The pituitary gland secretes a substance which is definitely related to the activities of the sex glands. Unless this portion of the gland is functioning adequately, the sex organs and the glands do not grow satisfactorily, and the person does not mature.

When a woman becomes pregnant, the substance secreted by the gland which maintains her periodic functions is no longer needed by the body and is found in the urine. This fact is the basis of the tests which have been developed for determining whether or not a woman is pregnant. In these tests, known as the Aschheim-Zondek test, the urine of the patient is injected into immature mice or rabbits. Within a few days, if the hormone is present in the urine, these animals become mature. Urine from a woman who is not pregnant will not produce maturity in the animals. This test is known to be effective in from 98 to 99 per cent of cases and constitutes one of the greatest advances of medical science in recent years.

Since the hormone is known to exist in the urine of pregnant animals, it has become possible to isolate it and to use it as a medicine in the treatment of various conditions. These conditions are practically all of the type involved in action of the sex glands. The determination as to whether or not the pituitary principle is to be used must rest with the physician after a most thorough study of the condition in the individual patient.

In the same way it is recognized that there lies in the pituitary gland a substance which is important in relation to the secretion of milk and other substances which are definitely related to the flow of the urine. There is, moreover, a portion of the gland which seems to be primarily concerned with the action of the thyroid gland.

These glandular substances are used in the treatment of a variety of conditions. Some are still in an exceedingly early experimental stage. But more and more is being learned as to how the human body may be influenced through this interlocking directorate of glands.

The posterior portion of the pituitary gland has a definite effect on the un-

striped muscle mechanism in the human body, serving to stimulate it when it is not active. It is, therefore, used to aid the action of the organs in childbirth, to stimulate motion of the bowels when they seem to be paralyzed under various circumstances, and, finally, to have some effect in stimulating the development of the blood sugar.

In general, when the pituitary gland is inactive, the patient is slow and sluggish, both mentally and physically. Fat increases in various portions of the body, and the patient falls asleep readily. If the condition occurs before the child i; grown, mental development is retarded, the sex glands remain small, and maturity is delayed.

When there is overactivity of the gland as a whole, there may be all sorts of symptoms due to the enlargement of the gland in addition to the overgrowth and overdevelopment already mentioned.

In addition to the functions of the pituitary gland that have already been mentioned, it has a definitely established place as a controlling gland over some of the other glands in the system. For instance there is one substance from the pituitary which is called the diabetogenic substance, because it is known that the pituitary can definitely influence the use of both carbohydrates and fats in the body.

The investigators are convinced that the pituitary has some definite relationship with the islands of Langerhans of the pancreas, important in the control of sugar. When these islands are deficient, diabetes develops. For instance it is known that removal of the pancreas will result in the appearance of sugar in the blood and the urine of the animal, after which removal of the pituitary will considerably ameliorate these symptoms. The death of an animal with the pancreas removed is considerably postponed if the pituitary gland is removed at the same time.

Moreover, the removal of the pituitary gland from an animal in which the pancreas is intact will result in a lessened amount of sugar in the blood and in the urine. At the same time the amount of sugar stored in the muscles and in the liver as glycogen is lessened.

Next the pituitary gland secretes a substance which helps to control the thyroid gland. Whenever there is a deficient action of the thyroid gland, the pituitary increases in size. Patients who have a deficient action of the pituitary gland tend to have a basal metabolism that is lower than normal. Administration of the substance from the pituitary which is known to control the thyroid will result in enlargement of the thyroid.

Another principle of the pituitary controls the adrenal glands. Removal of the pituitary is followed promptly by a breakdown of the adrenal glands. Thus it is thought to be possible that the substance in the pituitary gland may set up the first steps of the disease which follows complete destruction of the adrenal glands. This disease, which is called Addison's disease, may be treated by the administration of the cortex of the adrenal glands. Formerly patients who had a breakdown of the adrenals invariably died. Now by the use of this extract, which is called cortin, their lives may be lengthened. It is conceivable that the giving of the pituitary adrenal principle would also help in such cases.

Finally, there is a definite effect of the pituitary on the parathyroid glands, which are largely concerned with the handling of calcium by the body and with the growth of bones.

The substance in the pituitary that controls the adrenal cortex is ACTH or corticotropin. Investigators also believe a substance in the pituitary that controls growth may have some relation to various forms of cancer. Experimental removal of the pituitary in one case stopped a cancer of the prostate gland.

PLAGUE In the Middle Ages plagues of various kinds used to devastate mankind. Now we have learned that these plagues were due to the spread of certain germs which are known as the germs of plague or pestilence. The two most common forms of plague are bubonic and pneumonic plague, depending on whether the germs infect the lungs or are associated with the appearance of a swollen abscess in the groin, commonly called a bubo. Modern medicine has developed methods of vaccination against plague and technics of control which prevent the spread of the disease so that it is exceedingly rare in civilized countries. There have been only a few cases of pneumonic or bubonic plague in the past fifty years.

PLEURISY The lining of the cavity of the chest is called the pleura. Any inflammation or infection of this lining leads to symptoms which are grouped together under the name "pleurisy."

The pleura covers the inside of the chest wall, the top of the diaphragm, and the outer side of the lungs. When the pleura becomes inflamed, it tends to give off a good deal of fluid. The accumulation of this fluid in the chest cavity develops a condition that is called pleurisy with effusion. If the fluid given off becomes secondarily infected with pus-forming germs, there is a purulent pleurisy or an empyema. If the condition heals, there may be thickening of the wall. Inflammation and the accumulation of fluid also limit the breathing, displace the heart and other organs, and cause a good deal of pain.

Usually pleurisy is secondary to disease in some other part of the body, so that the infection of the pleura follows a disease of the lung or the carrying of germs from an abscess elsewhere in the body to the pleura. Occasionally pleurisy follows damage to the chest wall.

Pleurisy may begin with a sudden, severe stitch or pain in the side. Difficulty in breathing brings on a cough. There is expectoration. If there is a severe infection, there may also be chills and fever.

Pleurisy is a painful condition, and the patient who has it will show evidence of his distress. He will try to lie so that the pain is relieved. When the doctor listens to the chest, he can hear a rubbing that is characteristic of the roughened lining membranes when they touch each other.

The control of pleurisy, when there is not any outpouring of fluid into the chest cavity, involves rest in bed and treatment of the disease so as to eliminate the infection. The pain is relieved with heat. Often it becomes necessary, however, to strap the chest tightly with adhesive tape so as to reduce its motion.

Once fluid has developed in the chest cavity, it is necessary to determine its presence by the usual methods which the doctor follows and also by use of the X ray. The doctor can put a needle into the chest wall and remove the fluid, which brings about prompt relief. In case of serious infection with the production of empyema, surgical operation may be necessary. However, the development of the sulfonamide drugs and of penicillin now makes it possible in many instances to produce cures by draining the cavity and by putting in solutions of these remedies which act directly on the infecting germs.

PNEUMONIA In the vast majority of cases of pneumonia the cause is a germ known as the pneumococcus. There are at least thirty-four different types of this germ, and they may be identified by the physician through laboratory tests of the sputum. Many cases of pneumonia are caused by germs other than the pneumococcus. In some instances the streptococcus produces pneumonia that is even more serious than that caused by the pneumococcus. Recently there have been many cases of pneumonia associated with infection with specific viruses. In most instances pneumonia comes on after a severe cold or in association with some other infectious disease.

Until recent discoveries, such as the sulfonamides and penicillin, pneumonia was among the most feared of all diseases. That fear has not entirely disap-

peared. Any condition that attacks a vital organ of the body is serious. Diseases that strike the heart, lungs, and brain are more feared than those that affect the digestion or the muscles of the body. Some diseases cause death in a short time; human beings fear most those diseases that produce death rapidly.

Doctors combated pneumonia twenty-five years ago chiefly by good nursing, by the use of drugs to support the heart and the circulation, and by controlling excessive fever and intoxication of the body. Nowadays the mainstays in the treatment of pneumonia are the sulfonamide drugs, penicillin, and the use of oxygen. With these new methods of treatment the number of deaths from pneumonia has been cut more than two thirds. The death rates for pneumonia in the Army are the lowest that have ever been recorded. Whereas 17 per cent of the men in our Army who were infected with pneumonia died of the disease in World War I, less than 1 per cent of those infected with pneumonia died in World War II.

In a typical case of pneumonia the person who has had a light cold or some infectious disease is taken suddenly with a shaking chill and a sharp, stabbing pain in the side. This pain is made worse by breathing. Then comes a cough with bloody or brownish expectoration and fever. Frequently headache and nausea disturb the patient, and occasionally there is vomiting. Sleep is difficult because of the general misery and the pain. Among the worst of the symptoms are prostration and weakness. However, in some instances, weak as the patient may be, he has delirium and sudden urges which may cause him to attempt to leave the bed.

As the infection develops, the outpouring of blood and serum into the lung causes it to solidify, so there is insufficient breathing space and great difficulty in causing the blood, which comes back to the heart through the veins, to go through the lungs in order to receive new oxygen. As a result, the fingernails and the skin turn blue, and there is great shortness of breath. The breathing is shallow and grunting.

As the disease continues to become worse, the abdomen becomes distended, there is delirium and occasionally even jaundice. The fever becomes higher and the illness profound.

As the patient recovers, the temperature and the pulse return to normal, but the patient will remain weak for weeks or months and only gradually regains strength. Sometimes the recovery is delayed by complications, such as secondary infection in the chest, producing the condition called empyema. Such collections of pus cause the temperature to be high in the evening and low in the morning, and surgery may be necessary to let the pus out of the chest. However, the use of the sulfonamide drugs and penicillin has greatly lessened this complication.

The care of a patient with pneumonia taxes to the utmost the skill of the doctor and the nurses. Pneumonia patients must be kept at rest and should remain in bed for at least a week after the temperature, the pulse, and the breathing rates have returned to normal. The diet of the patient with pneumonia is usually ample, with plenty of salt and enough fluids to maintain the fluid content of the body. If there has been purging or elimination of great amounts of fluid by vomiting or by the bowel, this fluid must be restored.

Relief from pain and discomfort can be had by the prescription of suitable drugs. Especially valuable also for the relief of the pain in pneumonia is strapping of the chest to prevent excessive stretching of the ribs. The application of poultices, jackets of various kinds, and electric applications may afford comfort but certainly do not have any direct action on the pneumonia, and they sometimes interfere with the breathing of exhausted patients.

The greatest danger to life in pneumonia is in the extremes—that is, in the very young and in the very old. The disease is usually more dangerous to women than to men. It occurs more frequently to those who suffer from exposure to bad weather by their occupations, who are weakened through undernourishment, or who have indulged excessively in alcohol.

For a long time physicians depended in the treatment of pneumonia on a variety of serums which had been developed and which were specific to a certain extent against the individual types of infection. Today the sulfonamides and penicillin have been found so efficient in this condition that the use of serums is likely to disappear except in occasional cases when the physician may consider it necessary.

Particularly valuable against pneumonia is that form of the sulfonamides known as sulfadiazine. Combinations of sulfadiazine with other sulfonamide drugs are also useful in pneumococcus infections.

The shortness of breath in pneumonia is one of the most serious of the symptoms and used to be treated by making sure that the windows were kept wide open and that there was plenty of fresh air in the room. More recently the value of oxygen has been established, so that the shortness of breath and the blueness associated with insufficient oxygen are overcome by the use of oxygen chambers or oxygen tents for those seriously ill with pneumonia. Sometimes also the patient who is short of breath is helped by a semisitting position rather than being permitted to lie flat on the back.

It used to be said that recovery from pneumonia depended on the heart, and drugs to stimulate and aid the heart were frequently given. Nowadays so much benefit is derived from overcoming the infection itself and the intoxication caused by the infection and by the use of oxygen that remedies directed to enforcing the action of the heart are less often used. However, the constant attention of the physician in a case of pneumonia is exceedingly important, since he can detect difficulties related to the heart at the earliest possible moment and give the relief that is indicated when symptoms affecting the heart appear.

Especially important in all cases of

pneumonia is the period of recovery. The greatest danger lies in the endeavor to get the patient up and back to work too soon.

In most cases the fever persists from five to ten days, although occasionally even longer. Then the condition improves by a crisis, which is one of the most striking features of the disease, or by a gradual improvement. When a crisis occurs in pneumonia, the patient seems to be on the verge of collapse; suddenly he begins to perspire freely, there is a rapid drop in the temperature to normal or subnormal, a slowing of the breathing and pulse rates, and in a few hours the person looks and feels better and drops off into a quiet sleep. There is no truth to the statement that the crisis always occurs on an odd day, like the fifth, seventh, or ninth.

Unlike other acute infectious diseases, pneumonia may occur more than once in the same person. Indeed there is a belief that recurrence of pneumonia appears more often than that of any other infectious disease. There does not seem to be any truth in the belief that a person who has had one attack of pneumonia is likely to have others of the same type; rather we now know that there are several different kinds of pneumonia and the person who has had one kind of pneumonia may get one of the other types.

PNEUMONIC PLAGUE See discussion under *Plague*.

POISONING Hardly a substance exists in nature but is capable of producing unsalutary effects on the human body if taken in sufficient amounts or under the wrong circumstances or in relationship to certain tissues. Any substance capable of producing such deleterious effects is known as a poison. For every substance there is a safe dose and a poisonous dose.

When a physician is confronted with a case of suspected poisoning, he must provide first aid, which is designed to remove the dangerous substance from the body and overcome the dangerous

symptoms. First try to ascertain the nature of the poison taken. An empty bottle in the vicinity, the presence of some of the substance in a cup or utensil, or the presence of some of the substance on the tablecloth, the floor, or the clothing may be a valuable sign. By examining the breath or the mouth of the patient one may sometimes determine the possibility of poisoning. If the person has taken the poison accidentally, he may be willing to tell the doctor, provided, of course, that the patient is still conscious.

If poisoning is suspected, the doctor should be called immediately. Before the doctor arrives, it is well to give whites of eggs, milk, or strong tea, which are antagonistic to many poisons.

In order to get the poison out of the body as rapidly as possible, one may provoke vomiting. This may be done by tickling the back of the throat or by giving a cup of warm water with salt or by using a stomach tube, provided a stomach tube is handy and one knows how to use it. Perhaps the simplest procedure is to put a heaping teaspoonful of salt in a cup of lukewarm water, stir until the salt is dissolved, and have the patient drink the mixture, repeating every three or four minutes until vomiting is provoked. Usually vomiting will occur promptly and will serve to wash out the stomach. Thereafter the case must be treated as any other case of dizziness, faintness, or shock.

The symptoms must be treated according to the severity of the poisoning. If the patient is greatly weakened or prostrated, he must be kept reasonably warm, recumbent, and his general strength must be sustained.

In poisoning with narcotic drugs it is customary to provoke vomiting and then to give strong black coffee, at the same time doing everything possible to keep the patient awake. Sometimes it is necessary to walk the patient about forcefully. As long as the person is awake, he will continue to breathe; if he is permitted to sleep, breathing may stop.

For many common poisons there are

special antidotes. Few people have time to consult tables of antidotes; few people remember where an antidote is to be found.

In considering the care of cases of poisoning for purposes of first aid, it is preferable to consider them in groups according to the nature of the poison. More deaths are due to carbon monoxide gas than to any other poison. Many of these deaths are suicidal; others are accidental; and in a few instances carbon monoxide gas has been used for homicide. The person who has been poisoned with carbon monoxide gas has a purple appearance, the blood is fluid and cherry-red in color. All of the organs are congested and cherry-red in color. The most important sources of carbon monoxide gas are coal and coke in charcoal stoves, various industrial and chemical industries, the exhaust gas from motorcars, the exhaust gas from internal-combustion engines, mine explosions, blasting operations, factory furnaces, blast furnaces, and tunnels in which carbon monoxide gas accumulates.

As soon as a person has been removed from the gas, the cherry-red coloration may be considerably reduced. After recovery from carbon monoxide poisoning, depending on the severity of the poisoning, there may be headaches, inflammations of the nerves, and in some instances mental disturbances.

In warfare many gases capable of poisoning the human body were once used. These include blister gases, mustard gases, and lewisite, which gives burns like those of mustard gas. The blister fluid from lewisite contains arsenic.

There are also lung-irritant gases which are sometimes found in industry. These include chlorine, phosgene, and chloropicrin. Their effects are primarily on the lungs.

Other gases are tear gases which cause the eyes to fill with tears and make vision difficult if not impossible. Such gases as methylchloride, sulfur dioxide, and ammonia, used in various types of refrigeration apparatus, have also the possibility of poisoning the human body when the person is exposed to a considerable dose.

In connection with war defense, technics of detection and protection against all these gases have been developed.

The corrosive acids include hydrochloric acid, nitric acid, and sulfuric acid; the alkalis include potassium, sodium compounds, and ammonia. The taking of these substances in fairly large amounts will so damage the tissues that death ensues, often in a few minutes.

Following the taking of such substances, there is immediate burning, pain from the mouth to the stomach, with destruction of the mucous membranes of the mouth. Then come shock and collapse, with a rapid feeble pulse, coldness of the extremities, clammy sweating, thirst, and depression.

The treatment of acid poisoning involves the giving of alkalis, but the carbonates and bicarbonates are usually avoided because they create carbon dioxide gas. The substances best given are solutions of lime water and, in an emergency, soap solutions may be used. Substances like milk, oil, or barley water also help to control the damage.

In acid poisoning or alkali poisoning the damage is usually so severe that hospitalization and the constant care of a physician may be required.

When a person is poisoned with an alkaline substance, it is customary to give him a dilute acid like vinegar or lemon juice. If a carbonate has been taken, it is customary to give potassium salts, which means magnesium sulfate. The whites of egg, barley water, or oily solutions may help to overcome the damage. The great danger of poisoning with such substances is the scarring that occurs with complete closure of the throat or the esophagus, so that long-continued treatment, or even surgery, may be necessary to make it possible for the patient to live.

There are innumerable drugs which can poison the human being. (Each of these is discussed under the appropriate alphabetical designation.) Reports have been made of unnecessary deaths due to bichloride of mercury, kerosene, and gasoline. Commonly used in households for cleaning purposes are substances like benzene and carbon disulfide, which also have poisoning possibilities.

More rare are cases of poisoning by substances like arsenic, zinc, and thallium. In connection with poisoning by substances of this kind, it is well to remember that we are confronted with the possibility of chronic poisoning through the taking of small amounts over a long period of time as well as with the acute cases which follow the taking of a large dose.

Children have died from strychnine poisoning because they ate large amounts of sugar-coated cathartic pills which contained strychnine. There are numerous reports of people who have taken overdoses of medicines for sleeping or for relieving pain. These substances are not poisonous in ordinary amounts but become poisonous when too much is taken.

People have been poisoned by nicotine sprays used on plants.

Once great numbers of people suffered from lead poisoning. Babies have suffered from such poisoning due to chewing paint on cribs, baby carriages, play pens, or toys. Lead pipes occasionally are used in plumbing and enough lead has been known to get into water or beer or wines conveyed in pipes to produce cases of poisoning. An unusual instance of lead poisoning was brought about by the burning of discarded storage-battery casings as fuel. Altogether, however, the danger of lead poisoning is much less than it used to be because scientific controls have been developed in industry following the detection of this hazard. For years people have joked about the possibility of dying from lead poisoning due to bullets. Finally, however, a scientific report has appeared which proves definitely that lead could be discharged from bullets in the body and produce damage.

ACETANILID POISONING — Acetanilid and phenacetin, as well as pyramidon, are frequent constituents of headache remedies which in sufficiently large doses will bring about death. In addition to the measures usually tried in poisoning, it may be necessary in severe cases to use artificial respiration in order to force the breathing to continue.

ARSENIC POISONING—No matter how arsenic gets into the body, it is eventually passed into the intestines from the blood, although small amounts are eliminated in the hair and considerable of it may be carried to the skin to produce pigmentation.

If small doses of arsenic are taken into the body over long periods of time, irritation of the nerve endings is produced.

Years ago arsenic was found to contaminate beer made under bad conditions in England, and there was an epidemic of such irritation of the nerves among persistent beer drinkers.

Workers in arsenic may have the skin of the hands so severely affected that there will be ulceration down to the bone.

BARBITURATE POISONING—Stories continue to appear about people who die either purposely or by accident from large doses of "sleeping pills." The most common ingredient of sleeping pills is barbituric acid in the form of salts called barbiturates. Among the most commonly known of those are luminal, seconal, phenobarbital, pentobarbital, amytal, dial, ipral, nconal, and ovipal. Every drug manufacturer deals in products of this kind.

Most states have laws that require prescription of the tablets by a physician; some states require a new prescription before an old prescription can be filled. All these drugs can put people to sleep. They differ in the speed of their action, the duration of their effect, and the extent to which the body can get rid of the drugs. With excessive doses people find themselves unsteady in their walking. At the same time the drug slows the breathing, increases the heart rate, causes a fall in the blood pressure and the temperature. Some people become used to the drugs and think they are able to take larger and larger doses without hazard. Eventually many pass the margin of safety and are found unconscious or dead.

The doctor when called to see such patients must find first the cause of the unconsciousness. Cases are known in which people have taken from five to ten times enough to produce sleep and have still recovered. Once the average dose is exceeded the risk begins. The doctor must make sure that the throat is clear of mucus and that the patient will get enough air. If there is blueness, oxygen is given at once. The oxygen will cause the blueness to disappear if the patient is able to use the lungs. If, however, the breathing is feeble it may be necessary to supply artificial respiration with one of the machines available for this purpose. A suggestion has been made to put a small amount of a drug that can cause vomiting in each pill. If too many pills are taken the patient vomits and thus gets rid of the poisonous sedative.

Several drugs are antidotes for this condition, the most important of these being picrotoxin. This is given promptly, particularly when the blood pressure is falling or when the respiration is seriously depressed despite the giving of oxygen.

BENZENE POISONING—Benzene, also called benzol, has many uses in trade and commerce. It is used as a motor fuel; as a solvent in the manufacture of rubber goods of one type or another; sometimes also in the manufacture of spray paints, floor cleansers, floor waxes, varnish removers, and indeed as a solvent for all sorts of materials. Benzene is a clear fluid known as a coal tar product.

Ordinarily the vapors are heavier than air, which is important in relationship to poisoning, as is also the fact that the heating of benzene will cause it to become lighter, to rise, and to spread throughout the air.

A person who has been poisoned by benzene acts much like a man who has become intoxicated by too much alcohol; either he will become unconscious or appear to be dazed. He will stagger when walking or, if sufficiently affected, become drowsy and gradually unconscious, so that finally he dies.

In milder cases there is depression, nausea, vomiting, and a tendency to sleep. Moreover, there are likely to be changes in the blood which are revealed by other symptoms, such as bloody spots appearing suddenly over the body.

A person subjected to repeated inhalations of benzene shows loss of vigor and fatigue. Of course the most important point in making a diagnosis of this condition is to determine that the person concerned has been in contact with benzene.

If a man who has been cleaning a still or a tank, or one who has been painting the inside of a tank with a paint containing benzene, suddenly develops these symptoms, it may be taken for granted that he probably has benzene poisoning. If anyone engaged in spray painting or removal of various paints or varnishes develops such symptoms, the paint or material used should be investigated at once as to its benzene content.

It is, of course, of first importance for the person concerned to be removed as soon as possible from the situation in which he is exposed to the benzene.

The physician sees to it that he is put immediately at rest, that he gets sufficient sleep, that his heart is properly supported by the right kind of remedies, that there is plenty of fresh air, and that his nutrition is adequate. If the blood damage has been great, it is, of course, important to pay special attention to building it up.

BORIC ACID POISONING—Boric acid in ordinary quantities is not a dangerous poison but infants have been seriously poisoned by drinking boric acid solutions instead of water. Thirty grams of borax also have been reported as being fatal to adults. For this type of poisoning it is necessary to clean out the stomach and bowels as soon as possible, to give coffee for stimulating, and to protect the kidneys by giving fairly large doses of alkaline drinks.

COAL OIL POISONING—Occasionally children drink kerosene or coal oil by mistake and as a result may develop poisoning.

Dr. Julian P. Price has reported four cases of children who drank kerosene, one without any serious effects; one with immediate collapse from which he recovered; one who developed fever, difficulty in breathing, and later recovered; and one who died. The patient who died was a white boy, eleven months old, who while crawling around the floor picked up a container holding coal oil and started to drink.

Immediately he began to cough and attracted the attention of the nurse, who rushed him to the office of the family doctor. The family doctor gave him some sweet cream, followed by a drug, which caused the child to throw up the mixture in the stomach. Everything possible was done to keep the child stimulated and to restore his circulation and breathing, but the next day he died from terminal pneumonia.

When coal oil is first taken into the stomach, there is a burning feeling in the mouth, throat, and stomach, colic in the abdomen, vomiting, and thirst. If the poisons of the coal oil are absorbed, the patient develops drowsiness, shallow breathing, feeble pulse, and turns blue, then becomes unconscious and not infrequently dies.

In grown-up persons who take a small amount of coal oil or who work for a long time in an atmosphere where they inhale a great deal of coal oil, symptoms develop like those of a mild jag which is called a "naphtha jag."

The first symptoms are a sense of excitement and lack of self-control; later, however, there is depression, headache, nausea, roaring in the ears, irritation in the throat, and a trembling in the hands and arms.

If a sufficient amount of the fluid is absorbed, signs of shallow breathing, weak heart, convulsions, and death follow.

Thus far medicine knows no specific antidote for coal oil poisoning. Therefore under such circumstances the first thing to do is to wash out the stomach and give a mild laxative.

Then stimulants are used in order to sustain life and the patient is watched constantly so as to lend him such support as can be given by medicine for the organs that need it.

CYANIDE POISONING—For years the writers of detective stories have depended on cyanide poisoning as a technic for quickly getting rid of someone in a novel. Cyanide poison is commonly believed to be invariably fatal. Since the product is used in the silver industry and also for the destruction of insect pests, it is fairly well known. Of course every pharmacist is exceedingly careful to make certain that purchasers of cyanide are properly registered. Every year in the United States anywhere from 80 to 245 people die as a result of cyanide poisoning. The medical records show that 22 people who had taken such poison have recovered.

Usually it is difficult to find out how much cyanide the person took and this makes difficult the determination of its exact poisonous character. Treatment of cases of cyanide poisoning has usually been unsatisfactory because the drug is actually rapidly fatal. Many studies have been made on the use of a variety of substances which might act as antidotes to cyanide poison. One of these was methylene blue. Another substance frequently used is glucose, which is given by injection. More recently pharmacologists have tried the effects of amyl nitrite, sodium nitrite, and sodium thiosulfate, which have been found more effective than methylene blue alone in protecting animals from the effects of such intoxication.

LYE POISONING—Household lye is a menace to little children. The substance is commonly used as a cleansing agent. Lye is a caustic alkali. Such substances are found also in washing powder, drainpipe cleaner, and paint removers.

When lye gets into the throat of a child, burns of the throat, the larynx, or voice box and of the esophagus or swallowing tube occur. These result in secondary scarring which may block the passages and even lead to death. Immediately following the swallowing of lye the lips and the tongue and the throat become swollen and ulcerated.

First try to neutralize the alkali with a weak acid such as diluted vinegar, lemon juice, or orange juice. Nothing is gained by trying to pump the stomach to get the substance out because it has already produced its maximum damage. The substance is never taken in sufficiently large amounts to offer any possibility of recovery of any of it.

The visible burns have to be treated by application of oils like olive oil. Usually sedatives have to be given to control the pain.

Once the first wounds have healed, doctors have a technic for reopening the passages so that the child may breathe and swallow. This is accomplished by causing the child to swallow a piece of string. Then bulbs which are gradually increased in size are forced down the string to dilate the passage.

Caustic substances should always be labeled "poison." Following the passage of laws regulating labeling, there has been a decrease in the number of such accidents. Nevertheless, enough cases still occur to indicate that carelessness in leaving caustic substances such as lye around the house continues to result in serious damage to great numbers of children.

MERCURY POISONING—Bichloride of mercury is one of the most dangerous poisons. A doctor should be called at the earliest possible moment because this drug acts on the tissues of the body and, if not removed soon enough from the tissues, the effects of bichloride of mercury are usually fatal. In severe cases a person who has been poisoned with bichloride of mercury suffers from pains in the abdomen, vomiting, and a good deal of purging. In bichloride of mercury poisoning it is customary to give egg white as soon as possible and also some milk. Every case of bichloride of mercury poisoning is so serious that the attention of a most competent physician should be secured immediately.

MUSHROOM POISONING—Two couples went out into a near-by woods and picked a large quantity of mushrooms. Into the pan in which these fungi were cooked a quarter was dropped, in the belief that any poisonous mushrooms would be revealed if the silver coin became tarnished.

The quarter did not tarnish, so that night the four sat down and had a hearty meal of the delicacies.

At two in the morning one of the women awoke with a severe abdominal pain, associated with nausea, vomiting, dizziness, and prostration. At four, her husband suspected that the mushrooms might have been poisonous, so he took a large dose of salts.

A doctor was called at six to treat the woman. Later the other couple felt the same symptoms. For thirty-six hours all four were exceedingly sick, developing severe jaundice. Finally two died.

When their bodies were examined, the livers and the kidneys were found to be badly damaged. Even the nervous systems and the brains showed signs of severe damage.

This incident should bring home to you two important lessons:

1. To be sure that mushrooms are not poisonous, buy them from an experienced dealer who can take the responsibility.

2. If you do happen to feel any symptoms of mushroom poisoning, as I have described above, call a doctor immediately, because prompt action means the difference between life and death.

Mushrooms have been eaten by human beings as far back as history can record. The ancient Babylonians used to enjoy them and the early Romans sold them as delicacies.

There are more than eighty species of poisonous mushrooms in this country, the most deadly type being the *Amanita phalloides*. It is responsible for more than 90 per cent of the deaths from mushroom poisoning.

MUSSEL POISONING—At certain times of the year the form of shellfish known as mussel is poisonous. Outbreaks of poisoning have been seen on the Pacific coast, Nova Scotia, Canada, and in Belgium. Now studies of such poisoning have been made by Drs. Hermann Sommer and K. F. Meyer of the University of California, who find that the original source of the poisoning is a microscopic organism that grows in the ocean. Like all plankton organisms, it is most abundant in the summer, and at times may multiply so largely that there will be 40,000,000 of these germs in a quart of water.

When the germs are present, the water develops a deep rust-red color, so that it is red in the daytime and beautifully luminescent at night. Apparently the organism develops largely in the summer because of the strong radiation of the sun, which offers ideal conditions for the growth of these germs.

The poison developed by these germs has been analyzed and found to be one of the strongest poisons known. It is an alkaloid like strychnine, muscarine, and aconitine. So powerful is this poison that one millionth of a gram is sufficient to kill a mouse if it is injected into its body. A fatal dose by mouth for human beings is just a few milligrams, or a thousandth of a gram. It represents about one two hundred thousandth of a pound.

Plankton, which is found in the ocean, serves as a food for animals on the seashore. When the mussels take in the plankton, they store the poison in their digestive glands. This poison is not harmful to the mussels but is harmful to the person who eats them. The mussels gradually get rid of the poison in a few weeks, provided they do not absorb any additional organisms.

The muscular tissue, or white meat, of the shellfish does not contain much of this poisonous material because practically all of it is concentrated in the digestive gland—the dark central portion of the mussel.

The condition is not confined exclusively to the mussels, but may also be found in certain clams. The only shellfish which are entirely free from the poison are those which live far from the open ocean, such as the softshell clams, native oysters, and scallops. Abalones and crabs do not eat the plankton.

While death from this poisoning is not frequent, it occurs with sufficient regularity to warrant a warning. In July 1936 there were two deaths caused from this source. During 1939 there were several outbreaks on the Pacific coast.

Anyone who gets enough of the poison feels first a prickly sensation in the lips, the tongue, and the finger tips, followed by numbness, then failure to co-ordinate properly in walking, and, finally, ascending paralysis, so that death may result from respiratory failure in from two to twelve hours after eating the poisonous shellfish.

Unfortunately we do not know of any antidote that will stop the action of the poison once it is absorbed. This means that prevention is most important. Drs. Sommer and Meyer suggest the following rules:

Do not eat the viscera (dark meat) or drink the juice from mussels, clams, or similar shellfish from the open Pacific coast between the first of May and the first of November. The white meat must be thoroughly washed before cooking. The addition of baking soda in cooking shellfish, which has been advocated, helps to reduce the toxicity but is no safeguard against poisoning if highly toxic whole shellfish are prepared.

NARCOTIC DRUG POISONING—Narcotic drugs are poisonous when taken in sufficiently large doses. When people are poisoned by these drugs, they incline to fall asleep and to sleep into death. It is customary to treat the patient by bringing about vomiting so as to get as much of the poison out of the body as possible. Strong black coffee is given to stimulate the higher centers of the brain. Frequently it may be necessary to pick the patient up, walk him about, and stimulate him in other ways in order to keep him awake. As long as he is awake, he will continue to breathe, but when he is asleep, breathing may stop.

THALLIUM POISONING—Thallium is related in its action to that of lead and arsenic. Among the first uses to which the product was put was to mix it with various grains and other substances in the form of a paste which permitted its sale as a rat poison. Its special value as a poison was due to the fact that it would not warn a rat away by any special odor or taste. It would severely depress the heart and injure the nervous system and thus produce death.

The very factors which made it especially useful as a rat poison made it dangerous to human beings and particularly to children.

Occasionally reports appear of thallium poisoning in children who have received overdoses.

There is unfortunately no certain antidote for thallium poisoning. The physician may administer sodium thiosulfate, which is found to be effective to some extent in poisoning by arsenic, and he may use all of the usual measures for supporting life while the body tries to overcome disease.

ZINC NOT POISONOUS—The feeding of animals with zinc has been the chief method used for determining the possible deleterious effects. No noticeable harmful changes were found, however, on the feeding of zinc. Through three generations of animals their chemical tests did not reveal any accumulation of this matter in the organs when the animals were examined after death.

Buttermilk normally contains a small amount of zinc, which increases after contact with zinc containers.

Zinc is regularly present in the internal organs of animals fed with ordinary foods. The amount present does not increase appreciably when the animals are fed with foods containing additional amounts of zinc. Apparently the zinc taken into the body is promptly excreted by the usual routes.

POLIOMYELITIS See *Infantile Paralysis*.

POLYCYTHEMIA When the red blood cells are increased far above the normal amount, the condition is called polycythemia. The average number of red blood cells is about 5,000,000 to 6,000,000 in each cubic millimeter of blood. In polycythemia the number may increase to reach as high as 15,000,000 in each cubic millimeter of blood. Too many red blood cells make it difficult for the blood to flow.

A slight increase in red blood cells is found in certain chronic diseases and is also associated with slight degrees of poisoning of various types. Usually such slight increases indicate that the body is trying to make up for lack of oxygen brought about by the interfering factor.

Sometimes the total number of red blood cells is not actually increased but they are concentrated in the blood to give a much higher red blood cell count. For example the blood may lose great amounts of water because of diarrhea as in cholera, or there may be failure to get sufficient water into the body.

It is said that hard exercise will increase the number of red blood cells in the circulation and also that massage may bring about this result.

In certain unusual tropical diseases the spleen becomes much enlarged and there is also a tremendous increase in the number of red blood cells. In such cases the person appears constantly flushed but with a blue rather than a red appearance, the small veins are prominent, and all of the blood vessels seem full because of the extra amount of red blood cells.

The symptoms associated with an excessive number of red blood cells are dizziness, fainting, a feeling of fullness in the head, nosebleed, and sometimes disturbances of vision and constant ringing in the ears. The condition usually affects older people rather than young ones, coming on rather gradually and increasing steadily. Headache is not an infrequent symptom because of the congested blood vessels. Frequently people with these conditions are told by their friends that they are getting dark-colored, and there may be some associated disturbances of the nervous system.

When these conditions occur, a careful examination of the blood will show the greatly increased number of red blood cells and lead to a prompt diagnosis. This is the type of condition in which a simple laboratory procedure gives a definite clue to the nature of the disorder.

Recently new methods of treatment have been developed. It has become possible to apply radium and the X ray to the spleen and to the long bones which are concerned with the manufacture of red blood cells, and certain drugs have been developed, like benzol, which seem definitely to reduce the large amount of red blood cells. In many instances the combination of the three methods of treatment seems to bring about cure.

It is, of course, important to know whether or not the condition is actual or is simply a temporary apparent increase in the red blood cells due to living at high altitudes, inhaling carbon monoxide over long periods of time, or some similar temporary factor.

POSTURE   The human body is in many ways a machine—probably the most efficient, complex, and intricate machine that was ever put together—but with all its efficiency it suffers with certain weaknesses and defects that result from the way in which the machine was evolved.

Fundamentalists are convinced that man sprang in his present form into life. Evolutionists are equally if not more convinced that the human being evolved from a species that once walked on all fours. After the human being began to straighten up so as to use two of the feet as hands, he put stresses and strains on parts of the body that were not constructed to bear that burden. The experts in orthopedic surgery say that the mechanics of the body resulting from this evolution make a good many people round-shouldered, stoop-shouldered, with sunken chests, twisted

backs, protruding abdomens, and lame hips. Much of the difficulty arises because insufficient attention is given to strengthening the weak points during the years of growth.

When the little baby first reaches up a tiny hand to pull himself up to his feet, the stresses on certain portions of the body begin.

Good posture means that the body is held in the correct position when standing, sitting, or lying down, and also in motion. In standing, the human being must stand tall, the abdomen drawn in, the shoulders square and high, the chin straight back, the weight properly distributed on the feet, the curve of the back well within normal limitations.

In the correct sitting position the body is erect, the head poised to bring the center of gravity in the line joining the bones of the hips. It does good to practice this position while sitting. Constant assumption of a bent posture or a droopy position while at work or at rest results in stretching and relaxing of ligaments with a tendency toward permanent sagging. As a result, the back becomes rounded and the chin is shoved forward.

Here are some simple exercises which help to strengthen the muscles of the back and abdomen and thus improve posture:

1. Lie on the back, hands back of the neck. Take a deep breath and raise chest high; keep chest up and exhale by pulling abdomen in.

2. Same position; knees bent, feet pulled up. Pull abdomen in hard and then relax part way.

3. Sit in a chair, trunk bending forward. Incline trunk forward from the hips, keeping spine straight. This exercise may be done standing.

4. Standing; abdominal retraction. Stand with the heels four inches away from the wall but with the hips, shoulders, and head touching the wall; flatten the lower part of the back against the wall by pulling in the abdominal muscles. Holding this position, come away

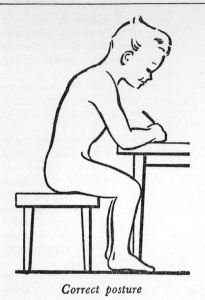

Correct posture

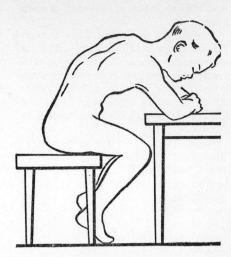

Incorrect posture

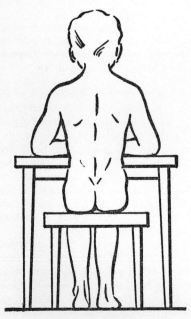

Correct posture

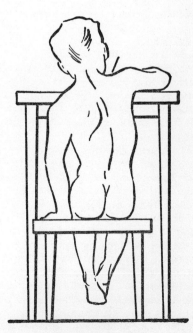

Incorrect posture

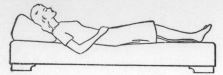

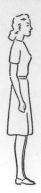

Lying down requires the least energy

Standing requires 12 per cent more
energy than lying down

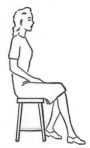

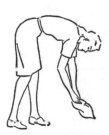

Sitting requires 4 per cent more energy
than lying down

Bending requires 55 per cent more energy than lying down

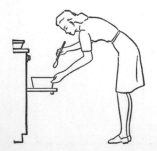

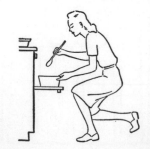

Incorrect posture for low oven

Correct posture for low oven

Handle too short

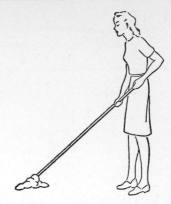
Longer handle eliminates stooping

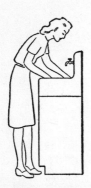
Sink too low

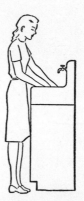
Correct height

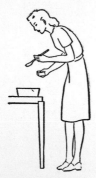
Table too low

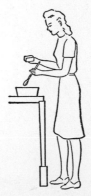
Table correct height

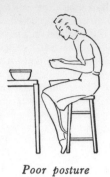

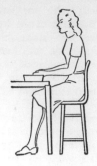

Poor posture   *Good posture*

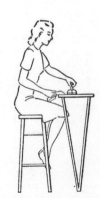

Standing is fatiguing   *Sitting is more comfortable*

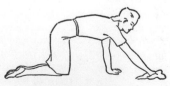

Kneeling is fatiguing

from the wall with the weight well forward on the balls of the feet.

5. Standing; leg raising. Stand with hands on hips, back flat, and chin in; raise leg forward without bending the knee; lower it; repeat with other leg. This exercise teaches how to hold the back flat.

6. Carrying the head forward, clasp hands behind the head. Force the head back against their pressure, keeping chin in. This strengthens the muscles of the back of the neck.

7. Spinal curvatures. "Stand tall," holding the back straight. Rise on the toes with the arms extended forward and up, stretching the arms and the body.

8. Distended abdomen. This condition may be successfully prevented and largely overcome by doing exercises 2 and 4.

PREGNANCY During 1943 there was an excess of several hundred thousand births in the United States over the number that would ordinarily have been expected. This situation was definitely related to the war and to the fact that some 10,000,000 men were removed from civilian life into a military career.

During the period of 280 days from the time when a child is conceived until his birth, many changes take place in the body of the prospective mother. While the greatest changes take place in the organs immediately concerned with childbirth, every organ of the body of the mother is influenced by the pregnancy. At the time the child is conceived, the egg cell which has come from the ovary of the mother is fertilized by the male cell. About the middle of the menstrual cycle an egg cell, or ovum, passes from the ovary of the woman down the fallopian tube to the uterus, or womb.

The time when the woman is most likely to become pregnant is the period between the tenth and seventeenth days after the first day of menstruation. This is now considered to be the period of greatest fertility.

When pregnancy occurs, the uterus becomes thickened and enlarges with the growth of the prospective child. The breasts of the mother begin to enlarge as early as the second month and in very young mothers who are having their first baby as early as the second or third week. These changes also increase during the course of pregnancy. The various glands of the body are affected by the pregnancy, since most of them have to increase their work by producing greater amounts of secretion. The whole rate of chemical changes going on in the body, measured by the basal metabolism, is also likely to be increased during pregnancy.

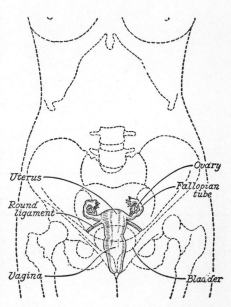

Diagram of the female organs involved in reproduction

The mother needs extra calcium at this time because of the demands of the growing baby for this substance used in the building of bones and teeth.

In a healthy pregnant woman the number of red blood cells and the amount of red coloring matter also increase to the upper boundaries of normal. This is associated with increased nutrition and the demands of the growing baby.

Diagnosis—There are certain definite signs by which the doctor can determine whether or not a woman is pregnant.

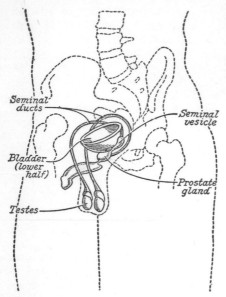

Diagram of the male organs involved in reproduction

In the majority of cases the regular menstruation disappears after the woman has conceived and does not appear again during the course of pregnancy. Physicians, therefore, are likely to say that the first cause of the disappearance of menstruation is prospective childbirth. A discontinuance of menstruation in a woman who has always been regular before means in the vast majority of cases that she has become pregnant. In some instances, however, the woman may have a discharge of blood from the uterus once and occasionally twice after conception has occurred. The duration and the quantity are usually much less than normal.

A common sign of prospective motherhood is some nausea and vomiting in the morning. This usually develops during the second month and rarely lasts beyond the end of the fourth month. It may, however, appear during the first month and may extend beyond the fourth month in occasional cases. There are many variations in the appearance, intensity, and duration of this disorder. Some women are troubled several times a day. In rare instances the disturbance occurs only at night when the woman goes to bed.

Many women during this time become increasingly emotional. Peevishness, fretfulness, irritability, and unreasonableness are not uncommon. Some women are more or less depressed, but many are increasingly buoyant and joyful.

The craving for strange foods which appears is a manifestation of the mental changes that may occur. Indeed this mental state may be reflected not only in unusual appetites but by a complete change of habits, so that a woman who has been exceedingly cleanly and meticulous in her habits may suddenly become careless and slovenly.

Between the sixteenth and eighteenth week the prospective mother is likely to feel a feeble fluttering, which is called quickening. The symptom is not a certain one because there are many things that go on inside the abdomen related to digestion that might simulate movements of the prospective child. Women who are greatly worried as to whether or not they are actually pregnant frequently imagine they feel movements that are actually not there.

The usual changes in shape and size of the body are well known to most people as signs of pregnancy. There are, however, certain signs which are so positive that they do not permit any contradiction. One of these is an X-ray picture, which will show the presence of the child. Another is the hearing of the heartbeat of the child, which, incidentally, appears between the eighteenth and twentieth weeks and occasionally earlier. Finally, there are the laboratory tests like the Aschheim-Zondek test which have a very high degree of positiveness in making a diagnosis.

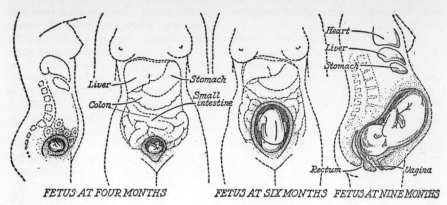

FETUS AT FOUR MONTHS   FETUS AT SIX MONTHS   FETUS AT NINE MONTHS

The relative size of the baby at various periods before birth

SUPERSTITIONS—There are many strange notions about pregnancy which persist and which are hard to destroy.

Of all the persistent notions not founded on fact, the one that prevails among people to the greatest extent is the idea that the mother can in some way mark the baby while carrying it. We know with certainty that there is no nervous connection between the mother and the unborn child. The mothers of Sparta in ancient Greece were commanded to look only on pictures and statues which showed the strong and beautiful so that their children would be strong and beautiful. We know today that it is not possible to affect the child, who is actually the sum of his parents, by any such activity.

The idea most widely prevalent is the belief that a shock to the mother will mark the child. Yet during all great wars, when mothers all over the world are exposed to unusual horrors, the number of babies born with markings is no greater than in normal times. Thousands of babies with birthmarks or defects have been born to mothers whose mentalities have not shown the slightest sign of any disturbance.

Many strange beliefs are associated with determining whether the baby will be a boy or a girl. Some people think that a girl's heart beats more rapidly than 140 times a minute and that a boy's heartbeat is likely to be slower.

True, large babies usually have slower rates than small babies, and boys are generally slightly larger than girls; there is not enough difference, however, to make it possible for anyone to determine with certainty before birth which babies will be boys and which will be girls.

Some people think that the sex of the baby is indicated by the shape of the mother. There is no basis for this belief. Some people think that a baby will always be lucky or will have second sight if he is born with a caul or a veil. That is just a condition of birth and has not the slightest significance. Anybody who believes in second sight will believe anything.

Not long ago a man listed the superstitions in Adams County, Illinois, relative to pregnancy. Here are some samples:

1. A woman who lays her coat and hat on a strange baby's bed will get a baby.

2. If outgrown baby clothes are given away, the mother will soon need them again.

3. If a couple get married and go to a picture show within the first three days, they will have twins.

4. A poor man is certain to have many children.

5. When a boy is born, it means that the husband has more strength than his wife.

6. Boys are born more frequently to youthful than to elderly parents.

7. A baby born on a stormy night will be cross and nervous.

8. A child born at four o'clock in the afternoon will be moderately rich.

9. A baby born with an open hand will be openhanded and of a generous disposition.

10. There are still people in Adams County who think that the stork brings babies, that the doctor brings the children in his satchel, and there are some who say that babies are found in hollow tree stumps. This is not peculiar to Adams County. There are still people all over the world who do not know even a fraction of the simplest facts about life and living.

DIET OF THE PROSPECTIVE MOTHER —A woman who is going to have a child must remember that her food supplies the child with the essential materials for his growth. The food supply of the child comes to the baby through the blood vessels which connect him to the mother. If the food of the mother lacks these necessary substances, they are likely to be extracted from her tissues and organs for the growth of the child.

There used to be an idea that a mother had to lose a tooth for every baby. Now we know that proper attention to the teeth of the mother and to her diet makes unnecessary any loss of teeth during pregnancy. This does not mean that the prospective mother ought to overeat. Overeating will throw an excess burden on her digestive organs and make her carry around extra weight, which will mean increased fatigue and disability. A slight increase of weight in the prospective mother is normal. Any abnormal increase in weight will have a bad effect.

The prospective mother should not think that she can keep down the weight of the baby by starving herself. The baby's weight is not dependent entirely on the amount of food that his mother eats. A good general rule for the prospective mother is to eat the foods that she usually eats but to make certain that she gets plenty of milk and more fresh fruits and vegetables than she would take ordinarily. She should watch particularly her supply of vitamins and such mineral salts as calcium, phosphorus, iron, and iodine. She ought to have eight to ten glasses of water each day unless her doctor tells her that she should restrict her fluid for some reason. The necessary proteins are supplied by meat, eggs, milk, and such vegetables as peas and beans. Fats are important—particularly butter, cream, and cheese because they provide vitamin A. The sugars and starches, including bread, potatoes, and cereals, are needed to provide the materials for energy.

Besides getting a rich supply of vitamins A, B, and C from fresh fruits and vegetables, particularly citrus fruits and tomatoes, the prospective mother may require extra cod-liver oil or halibut-liver oil, as prescribed by her doctor, so that she will get adequate amounts of vitamins A and D.

Alcohol should be avoided altogether, and cigarettes should be smoked in moderation. Moderation means around five or six cigarettes daily as a maximum for the prospective mother.

The nausea and vomiting that occur during the early months of pregnancy are sometimes helped by replacing the regular three meals daily with small amounts of food taken every two and one half hours.

HYGIENE—The amount and kind of exercise that the expectant mother takes depends largely on her previous habits. She should never exercise to the point of fatigue but should stop as soon as she begins to feel tired.

Walking is the best exercise. It may be taken outdoors except during extremely bad weather. When walking, the pregnant woman should wear shoes with low heels and wide toes because high-heeled shoes may cause her to slip more easily, with the possibility of accident.

Women who are accustomed to strenuous sports, such as tennis, can stand more exercise than those who have usually led an indoor life.

In summer the expectant mother

should be cautious about walking in the hot sun. She should walk slowly and avoid crowds. Two miles daily is an average distance.

Among the strenuous sports particularly to be avoided are running, tennis, swimming, skating, and horseback riding. A little dancing may be enjoyed in the early months. The prospective mother should never dance in a crowd where she is likely to be bumped or pushed about.

If the woman is used to driving her own car, she may continue to do so during the early months but should certainly give up driving later. Rough roads and bouncing should always be avoided.

The prospective mother must remember to rest frequently. If she has not been taking a nap in the afternoon, she should develop the habit and lie down for half an hour daily if circumstances permit. If she is not able to sleep, the reclining position will rest the heart and relax the body generally.

A pernicious notion is the belief that bathing during pregnancy is harmful. Cleanliness at all times is necessary for the health of the human body. There are many kinds of baths, including shower, sponge, or tub. Hot baths cause fatigue but produce some relaxation. The best temperature of water for ordinary baths is between 85 and 90 degrees Fahrenheit. Even those who are accustomed to cold baths in the morning will find it best to increase the temperature of the bath while carrying a prospective child. Extraordinary kinds of baths like cold showers, ocean baths, Turkish and Russian sweat baths should never be taken during pregnancy except with the advice of the doctor.

BIRTH OF THE BABY—Before the baby comes, the mother should assemble the materials that will be required at childbirth. If she is going to a hospital, and the vast majority of women now have their babies in the hospital, she will need at least two nightgowns, a bathrobe, two pairs of stockings, a pair of slippers, a few handkerchiefs, a toothbrush, some toothpaste or tooth powder, and a comb and brush.

In most hospitals the baby's clothes are provided until the baby is ready to leave. The day before the mother expects to leave the hospital with the baby she should be provided with a shirt, a band, a petticoat, a pair of stockings, some safety pins, a few diapers, a sweater, a cap, and two blankets, all of which may be necessary for the baby en route to his home. The more experienced mother will have available a good many other clothes for the baby because babies grow fast and need many changes before they become one year old.

In most cases the time required for childbirth for a first baby will be between sixteen and eighteen hours and for later babies between eight and ten hours. There is no reason to be panicky when the first symptoms appear. A wise mother will have consulted her physician about having a baby even before pregnancy begins and will be in touch with her doctor throughout the pregnancy and after the baby is born.

There is a common belief that more babies are born at night than in the daytime. Actual investigations show, however, that births vary little from hour to hour in the course of a day. A slightly larger number occur between three and four o'clock in the morning than between nine and ten o'clock at night, but the number from hour to hour varies little indeed.

The body of the woman returns in most instances to normal six to eight weeks after childbirth. During this period rest and quiet are important. About the fourth day after childbirth the mother may begin light exercise, sitting up in bed and increasing her activity. The tendency nowadays is to get the mother up much earlier than used to be the case. Nevertheless, it is still not advisable for the mother who leaves the hospital on the tenth or twelfth day following childbirth to go up three flights of steps to an apartment, if she lives in an apartment building. If possible, someone should carry her. If she must walk, she should walk slowly and rest frequently.

It is usually best for the mother to leave the hospital in the afternoon so that she can go home and get right to bed.

Women of different races and different spheres of life have different habits in regard to how much they undertake after childbirth. Many women incline to overdo the social side of pregnancy. Too many visits and visits that last too long cannot do any good. Long telephone calls are frequently more boring and weakening than actual conversation with visitors. People with colds or infections should never visit a woman who has just had a baby and certainly should be kept out of any contact with the baby or baby's room.

PRENATAL CARE

In accordance with the dictates of modern medical science, a woman should consult her physician even before she becomes a prospective mother. He is able from a study of the heredity of the husband and wife, from a study of the incidence of disease in the family, and from an examination of the physical condition of the woman, to give advice as to whether or not it is desirable for the parents concerned to have a child.

Certainly just as soon as a woman believes she is to become a mother she should consult her physician. He will then make the necessary scientific examinations to determine with certainty that she is in the expectant state. These examinations include laboratory studies which are now well-nigh positive as to whether the answer is yes or no. They include also physical examinations, tests of the excretions of the body, and a record of symptoms.

Then the physician makes a complete physical examination, which includes a study of the blood, the blood pressure, and the kidneys, to determine the presence or absence of inflammations and of diabetes. He makes accurate measurements of the organs concerned in childbirth and thus is able to anticipate any difficulties which are likely to arise.

Examinations continue at first at intervals of one month, unless extraordinary symptoms arise, later at more frequent intervals of perhaps two weeks, or indeed every week if that seems necessary. On each occasion the doctor will question the prospective mother carefully as to fatigue, vision, and the presence of any unusual swellings or headaches. Should the answers be suggestive, he will then make the necessary examinations to determine the exact significance of any such symptoms. By those examinations he is able again to anticipate difficulties and in most instances to prevent serious complications.

DIET—A prospective mother usually gains about 14 per cent in weight during the nine months previous to the birth of the child. Most experts are convinced that a gain of anything more than twenty pounds is far too much.

The authorities are agreed, however, that the prospective mother requires in addition to her normal well-balanced diet, more protein, calcium, phosphorus, iron, and the established vitamins. We know that some proteins have higher biologic values—that is, more value for the building and conserving of human tissues—than others. The proteins especially important are the so-called animal proteins, including milk and meat. The proteins of cereals and vegetables and fruits are less important.

The prospective mother must have enough vitamins A and D, calcium, and phosphorus, to provide for the calcium needs of her baby and also those of the growing baby. Milk and milk products provide most of the necessary calcium, but the doctor may choose to recommend additional calcium in the diet if he thinks it necessary.

Our diets are ordinarily low in iron, and iron is absolutely necessary for the building of red blood cells. Obviously the prospective mother needs extra iron. The fact that many a baby is born slightly anemic is now demonstrated by careful scientific studies. Therefore the mother should be sure to eat plenty of the iron-containing foods and, if necessary, should have extra iron prescribed by the physician.

Finally, among the mineral salts iodine is of great importance. Much of our modern salt is enriched by the addition of extra iodine or indeed by the restoration of iodine that has been removed in the refining process. We know that a lack of sufficient iodine in the diet of the mother may influence not only her own thyroid gland but that of the prospective child.

HEALTH OF THE PROSPECTIVE MOTHER —When a prospective mother finds that her wedding ring is getting too tight or that her shoes feel too tight or that her vision is becoming blurred, she must realize that these are danger signals. She should never disregard persistent vomiting, bleeding, nausea, or any difficulty with her vision.

During the months before the child is born the prospective mother should wear comfortable clothing. She should avoid any constrictions around the waist. She should be careful about wearing elastic garters that constrict the blood vessels because this helps to cause varicose veins.

The prospective mother should try to be contented and avoid undue emotional reactions or excitement. She need not fear that her mental condition will affect the physical body of the prospective child. However, nervous irritation, undue fatigue, or exhaustion associated with excess emotional reactions may harm both her and the developing child.

EQUIPMENT FOR BABY—After the end of the third month the prospective mother can begin to prepare for the baby by providing some necessary equipment. This includes as a minimum the following:

Three abdominal bands, about 6 inches by 20 inches, torn from fine, firm flannel and not hemmed. A half yard of 22-inch flannel may have the selvage torn off, then may be torn in three equal strips. Bands are not necessary after the navel heals, unless the physician particularly orders them.

Three shirts, size 2, silk and wool, or cotton and wool mixed, for the winter baby; cotton for the summer baby. These shirts should be large enough to slip on easily and not be outgrown too rapidly.

Those that open down the front and are tied in place are most convenient.

Three dozen or more diapers, size 20 by 40 inches, preferably of bird's-eye or good quality outing flannel; the new gauze type is quite popular with some mothers. A more expensive type is the paper or cotton-filled diaper that may be used once and destroyed. These are especially nice for traveling or for people who can afford such luxuries. Knitted soakers are also used and are preferred to rubber diapers or pants, but neither is advisable for constant wear because they cause irritation of the skin.

Three nightgowns, made of soft outing flannel, 27 inches long, with drawstring in hem and wrists. These should open down the back.

Three or four kimonos of medium weight, flannelette, with little or no trimming, opening down the back and fastening with ties. Simple dresses with "gertrudes" are preferred by some mothers but kimonos are more practical.

Sleeping bag or baby bunting, a sleeveless square slip with hood attached, with zipper or tie front, will be useful for out of doors for a cold-weather baby.

Three pairs of soft stockings, socks, or booties. For small infants many prefer to wrap feet and legs in extra diaper.

Blankets, three cotton and two wool, 1 yard square.

Two flannel or cashmere sacks or crocheted jackets are useful.

Two quilted pads for lap protectors or square of rubber sheeting.

It is also desirable to have suitable preparation in the home, including a bed or a bassinette. A new clothesbasket will make an ideal bed for the first six months. If the husband can do a little plain carpentering, he can make a platform with legs which will hold the basket securely and which will raise it above the floor level. In this basket is put a plain mattress which is also made of quilting or padding material. A rubber sheet is placed over the mattress.

The mother will need a tub in which to bathe the baby and a tray to hold sterile water, a jar of sterile cotton, nipples and bottle caps, nursing bottles for holding water and artificial feedings if they are to be used.

PRESBYOPIA When people get old, their eyes change. The word "presbyopia" merely means "sight of an old man." The ability to see normally slightly changes after the age of forty, increasingly toward the age of 70. There is a gradual decline of the power of the eye to accommodate due to a loss of elasticity of the lens of the eye, which becomes more rigid and flatter. As a result the near point of distinct vision moves and reading becomes increasingly difficult at the usual distance. At this time it is difficult for anyone who has the condition to read fine print or to do any kind of near work without the aid of convex glasses.

This change in the eye is not a disease but a natural change which occurs in the human being with age. The lens of the eye in youth is an elastic tissue. By action of one of the muscles of the eye the elastic capsule of the lens becomes relaxed, which allows it to become more globular. However, as age goes on, the lens becomes hardened and cannot easily become more globular.

People with presbyopia see well at a distance. This is likely to give them a great deal of encouragement, particularly on a golf course when they can see the flight of a golf ball for hundreds of yards. When, however, they try to read the telephone book, they find that that is an entirely different matter. As the condition becomes worse, the person with farsightedness pushes the book away and holds the head back. However, even with this help it is still difficult to see the book well. Reading at night becomes especially troublesome because the pupil of the eye dilates, owing to poor illumination.

One of the chief symptoms of presbyopia is a feeling of tiredness on reading, culminating in many people with headaches toward the end of the day. Women find it especially difficult to thread needles or to work on fine patterns because the patterns fade away and become almost obliterated and the eyes become tired if they persist in the work.

There is just one thing for a person with such a change in the eyes to do and that is to consult a specialist in conditions affecting the eyes, who will measure the amount of change that has taken place and will prescribe suitable convex lenses to meet the situation. The specialist in conditions affecting the eye is likely to take into account the occupation of the person concerned because the distance at which the work is usually done is important. In reading, writing, and sewing, 13 inches is usually a comfortable working distance but a piano player may require 20 to 25 inches, so that the glasses that he will need would be weaker than those required by a printer. Some people require two sets of glasses, one for reading and the other for their work.

Every few years it is desirable to consult a specialist again because the eyes continue to change up to a certain point.

PRESCRIPTIONS Many a patient has puzzled inordinately over the prescription handed to him by the doctor. Once prescriptions were written almost altogether in Latin. This was not done to mystify the patient. Latin was the classical language used by all learned men in the Middle Ages; at that time medicine was studied in Latin. True, there is some advantage in having the confidence of the patient in the prescription. He is more likely to respect a long technical term that he does not understand. However, modern times tend to remove the mystery and secrecy from science. People are being educated in medical matters. Furthermore, the writing of prescriptions in English tends to oppose charlatanism and quackery.

The official books used by doctors and druggists as guides to the drugs that are prescribed by the doctor and put into prescriptions in the drugstore will, during the coming years, use the English titles as the main titles, with the Latin supplementary.

Many people wonder why there is

an R with a cross on the top of the doctor's prescription. Some have suggested that this sign represents an invocation to Jupiter and that it is a carry-over from the days when people believed in mythical gods and goddesses. More recent studies indicate that the cross at the end of the R is not a symbol but a substitute for a period to indicate that this R is an abbreviation. The letter R is the first letter of the Latin word *recipe,* which means take. Thus the doctor instructs the druggist to take the amount specified of each of the substances mentioned in the prescription and to mix them according to the directions, which are usually given in Latin at the bottom of the prescription. The most common direction in any prescription is the word *misce,* which is another Latin word, meaning mix. Quite often the doctor abbreviates this with a capital letter M.

Once prescriptions were noted for the large number of ingredients that they contained. A doctor of an earlier day would inquire as to the various symptoms about which the patient complained and would put something in the prescription to cover every symptom. Nowadays, however, scientific medicine limits itself to a smaller number of drugs of higher power and of more specific effect on the human body. The modern doctor is likely to include only a few ingredients in any prescription. He is more concerned with controlling the cause of the disease and healing and somewhat less with relieving all of the individual symptoms. Control of the cause and healing of the disease remove the symptoms.

PROSTATE In the male human being just at the neck of the urinary bladder is an organ known as the prostate. The prostate surrounds the urethra, the tube which carries the urine from the bladder, like the insulation around a pipe. The muscle fibers of the prostate act as a sort of valve mechanism which shut off the urinary bladder so that urine does not come into contact with the male sperm cells.

When the prostate becomes infected, as it usually does in severe cases of gonorrhea, there are all the usual signs of infection including a rise in temperature, pain at the area of infection, and frequently a discharge. Sometimes an infection in the prostate persists to the point of abscess, which either breaks into the urethra or the surrounding tissues or else is evacuated by a surgical procedure.

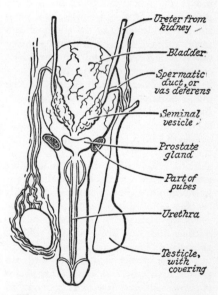

The anatomy of the genito-urinary system in the male

The most common condition affecting the prostate gland is the simple enlargement that comes on with advancing years. The exact cause of this enlargement of the prostate is not known. Sometimes it enlarges slowly for many years without symptoms, the chief sign being a falling off of the power to urinate.

Another sign, however, is a more frequent desire to urinate, so that the man who is affected gets up frequently at night. Associated with this there may be some retention of fluid in the bladder, so that it is not completely emptied at the time of urination.

Among the greatest advances made by medicine in recent years is the improvement of treatment in this condition. Modern treatments include the use of glandular substances which help to bring about control of the hypertrophy of the gland. In an earlier day the operative procedure for enlargement of the prostate included a two-stage operation which was a major operation in every sense of the word. Nowadays a new technic permits removal of the enlarged material through a tube which is passed up from the outside and through which the gland is removed by electrical dissection. Formerly the death rate in surgical operations on the prostate was very high; nowadays it is minimal.

PRURITUS See *Itching*.

PSITTACOSIS The popular name for psittacosis is parrot's disease. However, the disease is transmitted not only by parrots but also by all kinds of birds, including parakeets, lovebirds, and canaries, and also by infected human beings.

Just as human beings who are apparently well can transmit infectious disease, so also may a bird that is apparently well transmit psittacosis. In most cases, however, the parrot will seem to be ill. Because of the illness of the bird the owner is likely to fondle it and give it much more personal attention, with the result that the owner gets the psittacosis. As might be expected, a disease that can pass from a parrot to a man may also infect chickens, rabbits, mice, and guinea pigs. Strangely the disease affects chiefly the intestinal tract of birds but in almost every instance specifically the lungs of human beings. Cases are recorded in which the infection has reached a human being because he fed the parrot by the mouth-to-mouth

method. Most often it occurs merely from handling the sick birds. Not infrequently a person who becomes sick will pass the disease on his infected hands to other members of the same family.

In the United States during the past few years there have been several serious outbreaks of psittacosis in California, Pennsylvania, and in Boston, Massachusetts. The United States has forbidden the importation of birds, particularly during the war period, because of the danger of bringing psittacosis into the country.

The cause of psittacosis is another one of those filtrable viruses—the toxic agents which are so small that they can pass through the pores of a clay filter.

Usually from eight to fourteen days after a person has been exposed to the infection he will feel sick, have a headache, backache, pains in the eyes, and chills. Soon he begins to cough, and in at least one fourth of the cases serious nosebleeds occur. There is an inflammation of the lungs which has the symptoms of pneumonia but does not have the congestion of the lungs and other signs that are typical of pneumonia. The disease is likely to be confused with all forms of pneumonia caused by other germs and viruses. The disease may be exceedingly serious, causing death, but many cases probably recover and, because they are exceedingly mild, are never diagnosed as psittacosis.

Regardless of the love or attachment of the owner to the bird, any bird that is shown to be infected with psittacosis should be sacrificed. Not only the bird but the cage and any other materials which have come in contact with the bird should be destroyed by fire.

PSORIASIS Psoriasis is one of the ten most frequent of all skin diseases, actually making up about 6 per cent of all of the cases of skin diseases for which people consult specialists.

Cases have been reported in babies six days old, but usually psoriasis does not appear until after fifteen years of age. This skin eruption affects women and men alike. It is non-infectious, but there seems to be a tendency to psoriasis in certain families.

Psoriasis is the most puzzling of all skin diseases because exact information as to its source is not available. Many dermatologists believe that psoriasis is related to difficulty in digesting fat. Some believe that it is related to a disturbance of the nervous system. There are from time to time papers published which seem to indicate that certain germs or viruses may be responsible, but thus far the evidence in behalf of any of these causes is not considered well established by the medical profession.

Usually psoriasis begins by a little pinhead-size, bright red eruption. These little spots group to form larger ones, finally resulting in great patches of reddened skin. The healing occurs from the center, leaving a red or reddish-brown stain. Characteristic of psoriasis also are the scales, which are thick and silvery white. When the scales are pulled off, small bleeding points remain.

Eruption is seen most frequently on the elbows, knees, and backs of the arms and legs; less frequently the chest and abdomen are involved. Occasionally the lesions become infected, and this results in the usual formation of pus. Also in chronic psoriasis the fingernails and toenails may be affected.

When the cause of the disease is unknown, treatment is likely to be widely varied. Psoriasis has been treated by diets, most of which seem to have been ineffective, except low fat diets. Vitamins are usually prescribed because people who are on special diets may miss important vitamins. Arsenic is frequently prescribed by specialists. Because it is a poisonous drug, it should never be taken except in doses prescribed by the dermatologist. As might have been expected, all of the sulfonamide drugs and the antibiotic drugs have been tried in psoriasis but without any special effect.

Many patients with psoriasis improve with sunlight or with artificial sunlight such as comes from ultraviolet rays. Here again the dosage must be carefully selected by a specialist in diseases of the skin, since overexposure may make the condition worse.

Several special drugs have been developed for the treatment of psoriasis, including particularly one called chrysarobin, which has been found by dermatologists to bring about improvement in many cases.

With the point of view that psoriasis might be due to glandular deficiencies, some cases have been treated recently with male and female sex hormones. In a few instances, but certainly not in all, these hormones occasionally bring about improvement.

A few cases have made great improvement when treated with Cortisone and later relapsed.

PSYCHOSIS This term is used to describe any disturbance of the mind, varying from exaggerated emotional outbreaks to serious disturbances such as used to be called insanity.

PTOMAINE POISONING See *Food Poisoning.*

PULSE When blood passes through an artery, the impulse of the pumping by the heart is carried down so that a finger applied to the artery anywhere near the surface permits a counting of the pulse rate. The number of pulsations in a minute varies with adults from 67 to 72. Infants may have a normal pulse rate anywhere between 100 and 120. The most rapid pulse rate ever recorded was something over 300 beats per minute. This condition is called tachycardia. A slow pulse is known as bradycardia. Many long-distance runners have exceedingly slow pulses—indeed as low as 40 to 65.

PURPURA HEMORRHAGICA Whenever there is a shortage of platelets—certain formed elements—in the blood, bleeding will occur almost spontaneously, particularly from the mucous membranes in the nose and in the mouth. Bleeding underneath the skin is frequent, giving the appearance of bruising. Sometimes this condition is associated with poisoning by drugs of the benzol type or with the poisoning that occurs from the action of certain types of germs, such as those of diphtheria, tuberculosis, and the streptococcus. Cases occasionally follow poisoning with the drugs that are used in the treatment of syphilis. The number of platelets may be lessened as a result of some action on the bone marrow, in which the cells giving rise to the platelets are formed. A lessened number of platelets may result from a lessened formation of the cells or from a toxic action which destroys these cells more rapidly than they are formed. In many women a lessening of the platelets occurs with each menstruation.

By a safety mechanism of the body the number of platelets tends to increase whenever a slight hemorrhage starts in the body of a normal person. Also the platelets that are left develop increased ability to form clots. If there has been an extensive attack on the blood-forming organs, the lessening of the number of platelets is associated with the lessening of the number of red blood cells and of the white blood cells as well. In some instances the lessening of the number of platelets occurs only at irregular intervals, between which the bleeding does not occur.

Purpura hemorrhagica occurs most commonly in people between the ages of twelve to twenty-five years, although it may occur at any age. The condition may come on gradually so that it is not possible for the person concerned to say just when the condition started. Some cases are so severe that the person bleeds to death in a few days or weeks. In others the condition goes on with varying severity throughout a long life.

Many different methods have been discovered for treating patients with this condition with a view to bringing about benefit, if not cure. One of the simplest methods is the injection of blood directly into the body, sometimes into the veins, sometimes into the muscles or under the skin. Transfusion of blood is today one of the most useful methods in the treatment of disease. The use of the venom of the moccasin snake has been found to be of value, and tests have been discovered for determining whether or not the case is of the type which will be benefited by the use of the venom.

In severe cases the removal of the spleen by surgical operation has been shown to be of value. This operation has been used now in many hundreds of cases, apparently with advantage in most instances. Still other treatments involve the taking of large amounts of vitamin C, the feeding of a high vitamin diet, and the use of a new chemical called vitamin P.

Most of the methods of treatment are considered to be experimental for the individual case. In every case a study should be made to see if the person is sensitive to some protein and if the platelet disturbance is associated with such sensitivity.

PYELITIS (See also *Kidneys*) Inflammation of the kidney is called pyelitis. Infection is usually associated with pain and tenderness, irritability of the bladder, fever, sometimes blood or pus in the urine. Pyelitis is described as hemorrhagic or suppurative, depending on whether or not the blood or the pus is the most prominent feature. A pyelogram is an X-ray picture of the kidney. Pyelonephritis is another term for infection of the kidney and its pelvis. The treatment of pyelitis nowadays involves, first, a scientific diagnosis as to the nature of the condition and, second, the use of such drugs as the sulfonamides, penicillin, streptomycin, and mandelic acid, which are known to be efficient in removing the infection. When, however, control by drugs becomes impossible, surgical procedures are used.

PYEMIA Any infection with germs that produces pus which gets into the blood is known as pyemia.

PYLORUS The pylorus is the valve which releases food from the stomach into the intestines. Ulcers may occur in this area with subsequent scarring and constriction. Sometimes a spasm of the pylorus occurs, particularly in babies. Serious conditions affecting the pylorus are usually treated by surgery.

PYORRHEA Pyorrhea alveolaris refers to a purulent inflammation of the gums and the outer covering of the roots of the teeth. As a result the teeth become loose and there is a flow of pus from the roots of the teeth. Pyorrhea can be prevented by suitable dental attention to the teeth at regular intervals. Treatment involves not only a high quality of dental care, including the use of specific remedies against infection, but also a study of the general health of the person concerned.

Q FEVER Q fever is a disease something like influenza or atypical pneumonia. It is caused by a rickettsial organism similar to the type of organism that causes typhus. The condition was first definitely established in Australia but now cases have been reported in Texas, Illinois, Montana, Arizona, and California. In Los Angeles doctors have seen more than 300 cases and three deaths have been reported. Apparently the condition can be carried by raw milk that has not been properly pasteurized. Cases of Q fever have been found also in Italy, in the Balkans, in Panama, and in Switzerland.

Q fever usually begins suddenly with symptoms like those of any common infectious disease, including fever with slowness of the heartbeat, headache, occasionally chills and drenching sweat. When the doctor examines the patient he finds that there is some inflammation of the lungs accompanied by a mild cough but with little expectoration and accompanied also by pains in the chest but examination by stethoscope or X ray does not reveal changes such as those typical of pneumonia or tuberculosis. In many ways the appearance of Q fever under the X ray is more like atypical virus pneumonia. Q fever has been treated with the sulfonamide drugs and with penicillin but without definitely affecting the course of the disease. Streptomycin has been more beneficial than

either of these drugs, and aureomycin is even more beneficial than streptomycin. All of these drugs must be prescribed by the physician in the amounts suited to the individual case. In exceedingly severe cases transfusions of blood and inhalation of oxygen have been helpful. Such diseases as Q fever indicate how important is proper pasteurization and control of milk as a means of preventing the spread of infectious disease.

QUACKS In times of great stress, in pain or in sorrow, human beings frequently forget everything they have learned about science and truth and resort to incantation, prayer, and magic. The human being in fear of an incurable disease will grasp at any suggestion that may be offered to him, never stopping to inquire as to the motives of those who sell the cures and never inquiring as to the basis on which the claims of cures may rest.

All over the world there are still people who explain all disease as a seizure of the body by some evil influence. To them the cure of disease rests on conjuring that evil influence out of the body. Out of that belief have come all of the magical cures, which include charms, amulets, suggestion, and a good many medicines that are without any virtue except such as resides in the faith that the patient has in the medicine and in the doctor.

Human beings crave miracles. Modern science gives them miracles like penicillin and the sulfa drugs, like modern surgery and blood plasma. But familiarity with these miracles soon takes away their magic.

The quack in medicine today does not have the opportunity he had in a previous generation to victimize millions of people. Once quacks had unlimited use of the radio, the mails, and newspaper advertising. Today the new Food, Drug and Cosmetic Act, the regulations of the Federal Trade Commission, the ethical standards adopted by newspapers, radio stations, and similar mediums of public education limit the most gross varieties of quacks from any use of their mediums for securing public attention. A few quacks still prevail, but they are largely limited to local areas and to small groups of susceptible people who are always willing to try something weird or mystical before they try science in the healing of disease.

The quacks are marked by certain definite characteristics. They claim knowledge that they do not possess. They put after their names long appendages of degrees, most of which were never conferred on them by any university. They make exaggerated claims as to their ability to cure disease. They do not even hesitate to guarantee a cure if that seems necessary to secure a patient. They are likely to charge far more than the traffic will bear or else to build up a tremendous group of followers by charging just a trifle to thousands of people. Finally, they always claim to be able to perform functions in the field of healing which are far beyond the ability claimed by others in the community.

The public can tell a good doctor by the fact that he is just the opposite of the list of attributes that has just been mentioned. A good doctor will have graduated from a good medical school, he will have had an internship in an approved hospital, he will be a member of leading medical organizations, and he will be a member of the staff of a reputable hospital. If he is a specialist, he will have the certificate of one of the certifying boards in the various specialties. He will not be an advertiser. He will not pass out handbills. He will not have a big electric sign in front of his office. He will never guarantee a cure or promise to cure a serious disease in one or two treatments. He will be a reputable citizen of his community.

QUARANTINE The word "quarantine" comes from an Italian word meaning forty. The Italians of the Middle Ages would prevent people who arrived on ships from entering port until forty days had passed if there was a case of plague aboard the ship. Nowadays the word "quarantine" is applied to any instance in which a human being or an animal is detained for the purpose of preventing infection. For instance it is impossible to take a dog into England or Hawaii without a quarantine period, which is used to make certain that the animal does not have rabies, or hydrophobia.

A sick person who is kept to himself is not quarantined but isolated. It is customary to isolate sick people with infectious conditions until they are well and free from germs of contagious disease. For every infectious disease there is a period of quarantine and a period of isolation. For example, if a child has scarlet fever, other members of the family are likely to be quarantined for a certain period of time to make sure that they will not spread the disease. The patient himself is isolated until he is free from the infection, including discharges from the nose and throat.

The isolation and quarantine periods vary for different diseases. For meningitis the period of quarantine is two weeks. For measles and for German measles the minimum time is one week from the appearance of the rash or the first symptoms of the disease.

A child who has had diphtheria is not released to play with other children while there are still germs of diphtheria in his throat. In most cases of diphtheria germs can still be found in the throat a week or two after all other signs of the disease have disappeared. It is customary, therefore, not to release the child until at least two cultures from the throat have been negative—that is, free from germs of diphtheria.

Whooping cough is one of the diseases in which the practice of quarantine and isolation is most difficult. Cases are known in which the germs that are associated with whooping cough may still be found in the throat for months after all the other symptoms have disappeared. Therefore, if the weather is pleasant, children who have had whooping cough are permitted to be outdoors in the sunshine, but they are not permitted to make close contacts with other children as long as the whoop and the germs persist.

Mumps is most contagious during the early days. Once the patient begins to convalesce, the danger of catching mumps is not so great.

It is a safe rule, whenever a child has an infectious disease, to make certain that he is entirely free from secondary complications like running nose, cough, infection in the ear, and similar disturbances before the child is permitted to go back to school or to mingle otherwise with other children.

QUICKENING When a pregnant woman feels motion inside the uterus, commonly called "feeling life," this is called quickening. The first recognizable movements appear usually from the sixteenth to the twentieth week of pregnancy.

QUININE Quinine is a drug used specifically in the treatment of malaria. Because of the shortage which occurred during World War II, a substitute called atabrine was developed which is also used as a specific against malaria. This product is called quinacrine hydrochloride in the United States Pharmacopoeia. Quinine was long used as a tonic and as bitters. It has also been used for certain forms of muscle weakness. The great shortage of quinine during World War II has limited its use almost exclusively to the treatment of malaria. One of the substances derived from quinine called quinidine is used in the treatment of fibrillation of the heart muscle. It acts to slow the heart and lengthen the time of conduction of the heartbeat.

All of these drugs are toxic when taken in wrong dosage and should never be used except when prescribed by the physician.

QUINSY (See also discussion under *Tonsils*) Quinsy is a term applied to abscess in the area around the tonsils. Such abscesses must be treated by a specialist in conditions affecting the throat; he will open the abscess and

supply treatment against the infection, such as the use of the sulfa drugs.

RABBIT FEVER See *Tularemia*.

RABIES Summer is the time of the year when pet and domestic animals run free and, therefore, the time when rabies is most frequent.

The dog is the animal most frequently attacked by rabies, although any animal may be infected. Most people think that a dog with rabies, or hydrophobia, will run wildly through the street, snapping at every human being who crosses its path. Not every animal with rabies has reached this stage of the disease when it bites a human being. In many animals the first signs of rabies are merely irritableness and restlessness. Ultimately, however, the animal develops difficulty in swallowing, paralysis which makes the mouth hang open, and the drooling of saliva, which are the marks of the animal with hydrophobia.

In the final stages of rabies an infected dog will howl, snap at people and other animals, will run and bite. Eventually the infected animal becomes paralyzed, has convulsions, and dies. Under modern conditions, however, such an animal will probably be picked up if it is in the city or killed if it happens to be in the country before it reaches the final stages of rabies.

Human beings get rabies from the bite of an animal infected with the disease. Rabies is caused by a virus which appears in the saliva of the animal several days before it has serious symptoms. When this virus gets into the body of a human being, either by the bite of an animal or in any other way, the virus affects the nervous system and eventually reaches the central nervous system, including the spinal cord and brain. The closer the entrance of the virus to the brain, the quicker come the serious symptoms. Bites on the face, lips, and hands are more serious than on the feet and legs because the point of inoculation of the virus is nearer to the brain.

Considerable epidemics of rabies have appeared in the United States in recent years. During 1944 the disease was especially prevalent in Maryland, Indiana, and in the Bronx in New York.

People can do a great deal to prevent the spread of rabies by taking proper care of dogs. Dogs should wear muzzles when out of doors. The dog that is kept in a good home is usually watched carefully, kept from contact with savage dogs, and therefore is not likely to be involved as is the dog that runs free. Homeless animals should be picked up and disposed of by the methods that prevail in the particular area.

Because of the terrible possibilities of rabies, just one course should be followed after every dog bite. The animal should be captured alive, if possible, and kept secured for at least ten days, during which time it will either die or develop the symptoms of hydrophobia if it has that disease. If the dog dies (or, in fact, if the dog does not die, it may be desirable to destroy the animal), the brain should be examined in order to make certain whether or not it has the signs in the brain that are characteristic of rabies.

If a person is bitten on the face or on the hands, the Pasteur treatment should be begun immediately because of the short time that may elapse between the time the bite occurs and the time the virus reaches the brain and nervous system.

The onset of rabies usually follows the bite of an infected animal in from twenty to ninety days. During this period the symptoms may include restlessness, apprehension, with irritation and tingling at the site of the bite. When the disease begins, the horrible symptoms which give hydrophobia its name appear. A slight huskiness of the voice is followed by a sense of choking because the muscles of swallowing and breathing go into spasms. The infected person may refuse to take water because of the pain associated with swallowing. The physician who is called to see such a patient will wish to treat the bite by cauterizing it with a strong acid, sometimes by laying the wound open with a knife in order that the treatment may reach all parts of the wound. Then the Pasteur treatment is given, during which the patient may usually go about his business.

The old term "dog days" refers to the period when dogs were thought to be most likely to run about mad. It is a misnomer. Dogs may run loose and bite people in any season of the year.

RADIATION   Radiation is used in medicine to describe the action of rays of various types and also the divergence from a common center of sensations and stimuli. The term "radiography" is used to describe the use of the X ray as well as roentgenography, which comes from Roentgen, the inventor of the X ray.

RADIUM   Radium is a rare metal discovered by Pierre and Marie Curie in 1899 and is known particularly because it emits rays which have the power to control the growth of human tissue. Radium rays have been used in the treatment of all sorts of skin diseases, cancers and other new growths of the skin, hemorrhage, and infections.

RÂLE   The word "râle" comes from a French word meaning rattle and refers to the various sounds that are heard in the lungs when the doctor listens with his stethoscope. He describes all kinds of râles, such as dry, moist, bubbling, clicking, gurgling, and sibilant, as well as râles related to certain areas of the respiratory tract.

RATBITE FEVER   The bite of a rat, or less commonly of other animals like the ferret, the cat, the dog, the weasel, the squirrel, and the pig, sometimes injects into the body of human beings organisms which are capable of setting up infection with fever, nervous symptoms, and serious disability. The infection is called ratbite fever.

Another condition like ratbite fever is called Haverhill fever. It also is caused by the bite of a rat, and sometimes by taking food and drink which have been contaminated with an organism similar to that conveyed by ratbite.

Japanese investigators were first to discover that the bite of the rat injects into the body of the person bitten a spiral organism which is responsible for the symptoms.

Haverhill fever is so named because the first epidemic which was studied occurred in Haverhill, Massachusetts. Since that time other cases have been found in other portions of the United States.

It is apparent that the germs responsible live in the noses and throats of rats without disturbing them, but cause a variety of diseases with fever when conveyed to human beings.

Ratbite fever has been found in practically every part of the world. It is seen most often in infants and children, the youngest child on record being an infant who was bitten on the eleventh day of his life and died from the infection.

Not every rat has the infection. In the United States the largest and most vicious species are the Norway or sewer rats which are found mostly in underground places and the sleeping quarters of poorly constructed houses. This is the type of rat responsible in most cases of ratbite fever.

There is an incubation period for infection from ratbite fever ranging from one to four weeks. Then when the disease begins, there is fever which goes up and down and which disappears briefly from time to time. Occasionally there is a skin rash.

Haverhill fever is distinguished from ratbite fever by the fact that its incubation period is much shorter and the fever does not come and go as in ratbite fever. If there is any skin eruption, it is small. Usually in Haverhill fever the joints are involved as part of the condition.

Most patients recover, particularly if the condition is diagnosed early and if treatment is given promptly. Anyone bitten by a rat should, of course, have the wound cauterized at once by a physician, who will use a solution of carbolic acid; then strong antiseptic solutions are applied to destroy such germs as may remain in the wound.

The spiral germs of ratbite fever are controlled by the giving of preparations of arsphenamine. The treatment of Haverhill fever is still under investigation. It has been found, however, that the sulfonamide drugs and salicylic acid do not control this infection.

RAT CONTROL Scientists estimate that rats cause an annual loss of property in the United States of almost a billion dollars.

A new rat killer called ANTU can destroy rats as DDT destroys insects. The letters ANTU stand for a chemical substance known as alpha-naphthyl-thiourea.

A similar product was first used to test taste because of a special bitter quality. Tests were carried out first on rats because rodents have the special ability of being able to select nourishing foods and to avoid poisonous substances.

The day after the first test made with this chemical on the rats all of them were dead. Human beings had tasted the substance without harm. The investigators found that laboratory rats would eat enough of this chemical, which was called phenylthiourea, to poison them; but that wild rats, which had been trapped in city dumps, objected to the bitter taste and would not eat bait that had been treated with it. The chemists then selected twenty-four different substances like phenylthiourea for tests and finally chose ANTU.

ANTU affects dogs, cats, and other pets but it is so much less poisonous for them that it will not injure them. A single dose will kill a half-pound rat quickly but will have little effect on a ten-pound dog.

ANTU kills rats in a peculiar manner. After the rat has taken a small quantity the lungs fill up with body fluid, which suffocates the rat exactly as if it had been drowned. Strangely, ANTU is less effective against the common house mouse than against the brown Norway rat.

As an indication of the effectiveness of ANTU, one pound of the substance is sufficient to kill 200,000 rats. The product is mixed with finely ground corn or wheat or as a spray or dust on cut-up vegetables, tomatoes, or potatoes that are readily eaten by rats.

REFLEX The word "reflex" is used to describe a reaction or movement which is reflected from some stimulus far away. Essentially a reflex is an involuntary action. Among the reflexes most commonly known are the knee jerk, which is absent in many diseases of the brain and spinal cord, and other similar responses related to tests on other parts of the body. The oculocardiac reflex is a slowing of the rhythm of the heart that follows compression of the eyeball. A slowing of 5 to 13 beats per minute is normal. Anything more or less than that is not normal. Laughter brought on by tickling is also a reflex action, also vomiting when the throat is tickled with a feather. The swallowing reflex takes place when some substance is put on the back of the tongue. If a baby jumps when he hears a loud sound, that is called a startle reflex.

RESPIRATORY TRACT See *Colds, Rhinitis,* et cetera.

RESUSCITATION The human being can do without food for about forty days, without water for about four days, and without air for about four minutes. Whenever people become unconscious due to inhaling carbon monoxide, because of electric shock or drowning, the first essential is to restore the breathing. This fact was recognized as long ago as 1633, when an English doctor named Stephen Bradwell described a method for taking care of people who were apparently drowned. He wrote, "Turn the feete upward, head and mouth downward and so hold by the heels that the water may come out. Let others help forth the water by stroaking, crushing, and driving his belly and stomach reasonably hard, from the bottom of his belly toward his throat. If it be cold weather let all this be done in a warme roome before a good fire."

The average person breathes from six-

teen to twenty times a minute. Most experts believe that the movements for artificial respiration should be given more rapidly than this, since sufficient air will not be taken in at that rate to comfort the patient. Some recommend that the rate be between twenty-four and forty movements per minute.

Among the most serious of emergencies which may occur, demanding first aid, is resuscitation after asphyxiation, which may result from drowning, from electric shock, and from exhaust-gas poison. Occasionally also there may be asphyxiation from other sources, such as gas escaping from electric refrigerators.

It has been estimated that 25 per cent of men and boys past twelve years of age do not know how to swim, and there are few women who would be capable of swimming long enough or far enough to save themselves in an emergency. When a person has been under water long enough to become unconscious—about four or five minutes—first aid measures are of greatest importance to save life. The practice of resuscitation by the manual method is important because it is the quickest and most readily available. There are numerous devices for artificial resuscitation, but it is usually not well to wait until these come. Until 1952 the most commonly practiced method was the Schaefer technic. Then the American Red Cross, the American Medical Association and other agencies after extended research adopted a new method called the Holger. The Holger method and a few of its variations are described below.*

The Holger: The unconscious person is placed face down with the hands on top of each other, the forehead resting on the hands with the face turned slightly to one side. His elbows are extended toward the side. The operator

*The description of the Holger method and its variations is reprinted by permission of the *Journal of the American Medical Association,* from the article "Critical Survey of Manual Artificial Respiration," by Dr. Archer S. Gordon, et al., 1951, 147–15: 1445–47.

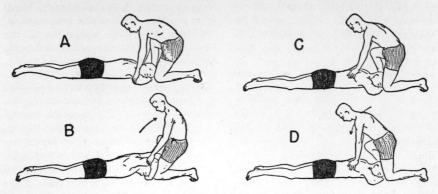

*Arm lift-back pressure method of manual artificial respiration (after Holger Nielsen).
A, placing hands for arm lift. B, arm lift. C, placing hands for back pressure. D, back
pressure.*

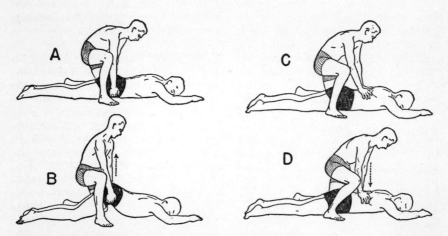

*Hip lift-back pressure method of manual artificial respiration. A, placing hands for
hip lift. B, hip lift. C, placing hands for back pressure. D, back pressure.*

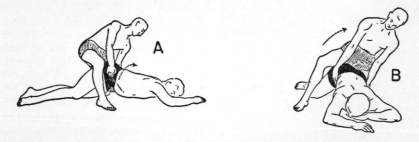

*Hip roll-back pressure method of manual artificial respiration. A, side view of hip roll.
B, front view of hip roll.*
(*Courtesy of the* Journal of the American Medical Association)

kneels on one or both knees in front of the head of the unconscious person. The operator places his hands under the victim's arms above the elbow and rocks backward drawing the arms upward and toward himself. The arms are elevated until firm resistance is met, then replaced on the floor. The operator then moves his hands to the back just below the shoulder blades and rocks forward exerting pressure on the back. The operator's thumbs lie close to the spine and the fingers are separated extending backward and toward the side. The operator's arms are kept straight during both the lift and the pressure phases and the complete cycle is repeated about ten to twelve times a minute.

Hip Lift: The victim is placed in the prone position, face down, as for the Schaefer method. The operator kneels on one knee at the level of the hip, straddling the victim and placing the other foot near the opposite hip. He places his hands under the hips (at the anterior superior iliac spines) and raises the pelvis vertically upward 4 to 6 inches. The hips are then replaced on the ground, and the cycle is repeated. The hip lift is performed at 12 times per minute. Lifting of the hips produces active inspiration as a result of several mechanisms: (*a*) When the hips are elevated, the abdominal contents sag downward toward the floor; this results in an intra-abdominal negativity that tends to draw the diaphragm downward. (*b*) Because of the ligamentous attachments between the viscera and diaphragm, the downward movement of the abdominal organs is followed by a similar action of the diaphragm. (*c*) Elevating the hips hyperextends the spine and increases the intercostal spaces of the lower ribs.

Hip Lift-Back Pressure: The hip lift-back pressure method combines alternate lifting of the hips, as described, with pressure on the midback (just below the scapulas) with the fingers spread and the thumbs about an inch from the spine. As the operator lifts the hips he rocks backward, and as he exerts back pressure he rocks forward. In each phase he keeps the arms straight, so that the work of lifting and pressing is distributed over the shoulders and back, rather than being imposed primarily on the arms.

Hip Roll-Back Pressure: This is a modification of the hip lift-back pressure method in which a roll is substituted for the lift in order to increase the ease of performance. The operator kneels astride the prone subject as described for the hip lift method; instead of lifting both hips, he uses the knee on which he is kneeling as a fulcrum on which to roll the victim. The operator keeps his arms straight and rolls himself in the same direction in which he rolls the victim. Great care must be exercised to insure that the victim is rolled up onto the operator's knee or thigh so that both hips are raised from the ground.

RETINA Vision in the human being is brought about through the passing of light rays through the eye to the nervous tissue at the back of the eye called retina. A serious condition is detachment of the retina. An operative procedure has been developed which is helpful in such cases. The doctor can see the retina at the back of the eye by the use of the device called the ophthalmoscope. An inflammation of the retina is called retinitis. This may be due to either infection, hemorrhage, or other types of injury. Sometimes it is associated with inflammation of the kidneys or hardening of the blood vessels.

RHEUMATIC FEVER (See also discussion under *Heart*) Rheumatic fever has come to be recognized as one of the most important public health problems of the country. It is important not only as a cause of death but as the chief disabling heart disease.

Fortunately, research has established a method of controlling rheumatic fever and relapses by treating sore throats promptly with sulphadiazine and penicillin. This eliminates the hemolytic streptococcus and its toxins.

Apparently infections coming into

the body by way of the nose and throat and lungs are followed not infrequently by attacks of rheumatic fever. Nevertheless, great numbers of children with infected tonsils and adenoids do not get rheumatic fever, so that some additional factors must be concerned.

Studies have been made to find the part played by crowded, unhygienic living conditions and poor nutrition, but the occurrence of cases not infrequently in families that are well to do and in which the children are well nourished causes skeptics to doubt that the social-economic factors are primarily responsible. For a long time it has been thought that climate was one of the most important factors. Yet we now know that the disease may occur in warm as well as in cold, damp climates.

When rheumatic fever gets in the heart, it produces changes in the muscles of an inflammatory character, damaging the strength of the heart and permitting it to dilate, making it impossible for the heart to do its work. Often rheumatic fever comes on insidiously. Occasionally the so-called rheumatic lesions affect the joints, giving symptoms like those of growing pains, and these seem to be of great importance. Sometimes there are severe attacks of pain in the abdomen related to infections of lymph glands. Sometimes there are mild, fleeting pains in the tendons or muscles. Pains in the heels are not infrequent. Also associated with this condition are symptoms like those of St. Vitus' dance, which may be the first sign of rheumatic fever. The attack on the heart, however, is the fundamental problem and the one that deserves greatest consideration.

Any infectious disease is a grave risk for children who have had rheumatic fever. The secondary infection brings on a recurrence of the attack on the heart. Yet this seriousness need not cause despair, for more attention is now being given to the disease. Hospitals and sanatoriums are being developed in which everything possible is done that can be done. The outlook seems brighter every day for the appearance of new knowledge which will permit proper control of rheumatic fever.

The doctor who studies the patient with rheumatic fever will find signs and symptoms which are not easily apparent to the non-medically trained person.

Over half of the patients with rheumatic fever have tonsillitis or sore throat from one to four weeks before the rheumatic symptoms appear. The rheumatic symptoms may come on gradually or suddenly, usually associated with overexertion or chilling. Then the fever rises to 102 or 104 degrees, the pulse becomes rapid, there is profuse sweating, pains in the joints, and prostration. Seldom do the pains begin in all of the joints at once. Those most subjected to stress and strain are first affected. Sometimes the joints swell because of the accumulation of fluid in the joints. It is quite possible for the doctor to control the pains in the joints and the symptoms of the rheumatic type with drug preparations that are now available and with other methods of treatment.

The detection of the first signs of the disease in the heart is somewhat more difficult. In cases in which these patients come early to the hospital, the electrocardiogram shows transient abnormalities in the heart early in the condition. The obvious signs of damage to the heart, like irregularity, rapidity, pain, changes in the size of the heart, and the accumulation of fluid in the heart sac, come on somewhat later and are easily detectable by the physician. Just as soon as the heart enlarges and becomes incompetent, there are changes in the sounds of the heart as they are heard by the doctor with the stethoscope. The pulse generally reflects the condition of the heart, and the physician trained to detect changes in the pulse will find these early. In rheumatic fever there are also changes in the skin, with the appearance of eruptions. There are also nodes which appear under the skin and which are typical of rheumatic conditions.

When the blood is examined, it is found that the white blood cells increase with the infection. Especially important, however, from the point of view of laboratory study, is the sedimentation rate of the red blood cells. This is considered, in general, to be a good index of the activity of rheumatic disease. The sedimentation is high when the disease is active and low as improvement occurs.

Sometimes infections of the kidney and of the intestinal tract will accompany the rheumatic condition. Such conditions may also give severe pain in the abdomen like an attack of appendicitis. In some instances these attacks have been so severe that operations have been done when the condition was actually due to involvement of the heart with rheumatic fever.

When a child has been attacked by rheumatic fever, there comes a time in many cases when the acute disease becomes chronic or, in other words, when the activity lessens and the infection becomes relatively inactive. For that reason any improvement is welcomed by the doctor because it means that the condition may be tending toward the quiescent stage.

When the condition finally becomes stabilized, the doctor will usually want to make another complete examination, testing the blood for the white blood cell count and the red blood sedimentation rate, determining the function of the heart with the electrocardiograph, measuring the vital capacity of the patient to see if his lungs are working efficiently, perhaps getting a measure of the ability to respond to mild work. If the rate of the pulse of the patient continues high while he is asleep or if the pulse does not come back fairly promptly to its normal rate following slight activity, the doctor knows that it is too soon for the infected child to begin work and exercise. On the basis of these tests the doctor can tell what the likelihood is of partial or complete recovery.

The chance of complete recovery is less if the condition comes on very early in childhood. Obviously also the condition is not good if there are repeated attacks of fever with inflammation of the heart. In general doctors are inclined to believe that the worst side of this disease has received too much emphasis. There are now great numbers of people alive and active in this country who had rheumatic fever when they were children and who in adult life carry on vigorous activity, although perhaps they are unable to submit themselves to excessive exposure or stress.

As I have already said, the child with rheumatic heart disease or with any congenital heart disease is especially susceptible to secondary infection and must be guarded against dangers of this kind. Nevertheless, a significant proportion of children with rheumatic fever escape fatal damage to the heart. The life insurance studies show that young adults who have had a single attack of rheumatic fever without too much damage to the heart have an almost usual life expectancy. All this means, therefore, that the child with rheumatic fever must be given special care for a long time not only when the disease is active but also when it has become inactive.

At present children with rheumatic fever and adults as well are treated during the active stage of the disease with a variety of treatments, few of which are known, however, to be absolutely specific against rheumatic fever.

All sorts of treatments have been tried, including the sulfa drugs, penicillin, heat, vitamins, and blood transfusion, but it cannot be said that any of these methods has shown ability to conquer rheumatic fever. The failure to have as yet a specific treatment for rheumatic fever means that the general care of the patient, the kind of nursing he receives, and the regular watchfulness of the doctor to meet every change as it develops are of the utmost importance in controlling the progress of rheumatic fever.

For many years it has been shown that drugs of the salicylic acid type are especially useful in controlling the fever, the pains, the swelling in the joints, and such symptoms. These are called symptomatic drugs, however, because they do not cure the disease. They do relieve the painful symptoms.

When the heart is especially involved, extra attention must be given to supporting its work so that every possible strain can be kept from the heart. Continuous rest in bed for the duration of the active stage of rheumatic fever is the one technic of which we are certain. The rest may involve weeks, months, or even more than a year in bed. As the condition improves, the doctor begins to permit a certain amount of physical activity, first from the bed to a chair, then walking, and finally return of the child to school. Nevertheless, I have just heard of a case of a child fourteen years old who had recovered from the acute stage of rheumatic fever. On the second day that the child was home from the hospital the father called the doctor and asked if the child could go swimming in the lake. Parents must simply learn that the child with rheumatic fever must be carefully guarded by those responsible for him until he reaches the age when he is able to make wise decisions for himself. The gradual resumption of physical activity must be most carefully controlled. For instance the child is allowed to sit in a chair half an hour twice a day for one week. Then the next week this allowance may be increased by fifteen minutes a day if there have been no untoward symptoms. At the end of two weeks the child may perhaps be permitted to go to the bathroom himself. Then moderate exercise may be allowed for fifteen minutes a day for two or three weeks. Perhaps after five or six months the child is able to have physical activity.

The most disappointing part of the treatment of rheumatic fever is the fact that it tends to come back again after it has apparently gone. This means that the doctor must determine, after the active stage has passed, that the heart has either been permanently damaged or not damaged. It means also that the child must come back for examination at regular intervals for a fairly long period of time to make certain that new activity has not begun and to make certain also that everything possible is being done for improvement of personal hygiene.

There is no doubt that children with rheumatic fever are best cared for in special institutions like Irvington House, Irvington-on-Hudson, New York, or La Rabida Sanitarium, Chicago, where the child may remain for weeks or months under the best possible conditions of ventilation, rest, sunshine, and nutrition. If it is found while the child is in the sanitarium that the conditions at home are not suitable, everything possible must be done to improve those conditions so that the child will return to a better place.

If the child with rheumatic fever has blood that is not up to normal, the anemia must be improved with suitable foods and drugs. Infected tonsils and adenoids are removed during the quiet periods. Nowadays we know that secondary infections with the streptococcus are fatal to such children. It becomes possible by the use of the sulfa drugs or penicillin to prevent any secondary streptococcus infection at the time when the tonsils and adenoids are removed.

The vast majority of children with rheumatic heart disease can and should attend regular schools and engage in a normal school life. In many of our large cities there are special schools for children with handicaps related to the heart or other parts of the body. The program for these children should be planned, however, not to make them invalids with rheumatic heart disease but rather toward teaching them that they can lead a reasonable and well-regulated life and be useful members of society.

In climates that are warm and dry there is less chance of secondary infections of the nose, throat, and lungs, which are so fatal in rheumatic fever. Probably for that reason the warm, dry climate is better for children with rheumatic fever than the chilliness and dampness that sometimes prevail in more northerly climates.

In a recent report by experts in the care of rheumatic fever there were six definite directions given to be followed while the disease is inactive:

1. Take measures to improve the general health and resistance of the child.

2. Observe the patient regularly for signs of recurrence and alterations in cardiac status.

3. Encourage physical activity, to the limit of the child's capacity. Only a small percentage of children at adolescence are found to have sufficient permanent heart disease to preclude normal activity.

4. Provide vocational guidance and occupational training for the relatively small group who cannot engage in normal physical activity.

5. Discourage parents and teachers from making a chronic invalid of the child. Educational authorities need to know that the vast majority who attend regular schools when the disease is inactive can and should engage in normal school life.

6. Minimize exposure to upper respiratory infections, if possible, by improving unfavorable living conditions—for example, overcrowding in the home, particularly in bedrooms—and by controlling the spread of infection through school and family contacts.

Newest in the treatment of rheumatic fever as in rheumatism is the use of Cortisone (compound E) or the adrenocorticotropic hormone (ACTH). These new substances seem to be able to control the inflammation in this condition.

RHINITIS Any inflammation of the mucous membranes that line the nose is called rhinitis. This is of various forms, chief of which are those that are due to infection and those due to sensitivity to various substances. The infections are described according to the name of the infecting germ. A condition called ozena (see discussion under *Ozena*) is also known as atrophic rhinitis.

RHINOPHYMA Occasionally, due to changes in the blood vessels, the nose becomes swollen with great nodules. This change in the nose is called rhinophyma, which merely means a nose that grew. There is not much that can be done for this condition except by what is called rhinoplasty, or plastic surgery of the nose.

RHUBARB Rhubarb used to be much used in medicine as a laxative and particularly in that form of constipation which was related to the intestine. The product is still included by many physicians in prescriptions for purgatives.

RIBS There are twenty-four ribs in the human being, each of which extends from the bones of the back around toward the front. Because they act as a protective case for the organs of the chest, they are subjected to injuries so that they become bruised or broken. Frequently a broken rib heals simply by having it properly strapped in place. Whenever there is a suspicion that a rib has been broken, an X-ray picture should be taken. Sometimes there is an extra rib high up in the chest which may cause disturbances by pressure on tissues. This is called a cervical rib. Sometimes the lower pairs of ribs do not make connections except at the back. They are called floating ribs.

RICKETS When lime salts fail to be deposited in sufficient amounts in growing cartilage and in newly formed bone in the body, deformities result which, taken together with the other symptoms that occur, make the disease called rickets.

Once rickets was a disease little understood, but today the condition is recognized to be a deficiency disease caused by insufficient amounts of vitamin D, calcium, and phosphorus during the age when growth is rapid. Incidentally, with rickets, as with every other deficiency disease, the failure to receive sufficient amounts of one vitamin is likely to be associated with the failure to receive sufficient amounts of other vitamins and minerals.

Human beings once spent much of their time in the sunlight and developed vitamin D in their own bodies by the action of the sun on a chemical substance in the skin. Then mankind moved into tenements and apartment houses; playgrounds disappeared; smoke poured over the sky, and sunlight became absent from the human environment. As a result it became necessary to supply children with their vitamin D from artificial sources or otherwise provide them with artificial sunlight.

As far back as 1905 there were from 94 to 98 per cent of children in cities who had rickets. As recently as 1920 from 44 to 60 per cent of children in Baltimore were found with symptoms of rickets. Today the percentage is much less because of the provision of cod-liver oil, cod-liver oil substitutes, vitamin D milk, artificial sunlight, or similar dietary accessories.

Rickets is diagnosed with certainty by the use of the X ray, which shows the failure of the skeleton of the body to develop as it should. There are, however, other symptoms which result from the failure of the bones to develop properly, including beading of the ribs, the development of potbelly, bending deformities due to the fact that the bones are soft. Commonly the child with rickets sits with his thighs slightly spread apart and with one leg crossed over the other; the hands are placed on the floor or on the thighs to assist the backbone in holding the body erect. The pull on the tissues by the muscles and ligaments and the softness of the bones cause bending, so that the bowlegs and knock-knees of rickets are characteristic. Rickets also leads to delayed eruption of the temporary teeth and to deformities of the unerupted permanent teeth.

It is much better to prevent rickets than to try to cure it. Parents should make certain that children, even in the nursing period, receive sufficient amounts of vitamins A and D and vitamin C as well, also adequate amounts of calcium in the diet, best taken perhaps as milk, to insure proper and healthful growth. The dosage of the vitamins and of calcium received through the diet and in other ways will be determined by the doctor.

RINGWORM In addition to the infection of the feet called athlete's foot, ringworm may affect any portion of the body. One form of ringworm produces coffee-colored scales on the inner side of the thigh. Associated with this infection there is irritation of the skin and itching. Ringworm of the groin is apparently more easily controllable than ringworm of the foot.

In the treatment of ringworm of the groin physicians usually recommend that underwear be boiled so as to prevent reinfection of the area by the clothing. The specialist prescribes a variety of treatments depending on the nature of the infection. Often weak ointments of sulfur or salicylic acid and lotions containing such substances are prescribed for the condition and bring about healing. The dryness of the area is also important for the prevention of reinfection.

Another form of ringworm attacks the skin of the body away from the hair and produces spots of infestation like circles. Ordinarily this form of infection is treated with ointments of salicylic acid. If this ointment is rubbed well into skin in the infested area, the skin will peel and the infection will be eliminated.

In addition to treatment with salicylic acid, several different dye substances like gentian violet, crystal violet, and brilliant green have been used against ringworm.

Ringworm which attacks the scalp may be still a different variety and may be much more difficult to control because of the necessity of removing the hair. There is no single salve or ointment that can be placed on every case of ringworm with a useful result. Because the ringworm gets into the hair follicles, repeated infection may occur. In such cases it is necessary to cut the hair, to shampoo it daily with tincture of green soap, and to apply an ointment capable of destroying the ringworm. Sometimes it is necessary to cause the hair to fall out by other technics.

ROCKY MOUNTAIN SPOTTED FEVER

Since the first settlement by white men the disease known as Rocky Mountain spotted fever has been prevalent in Idaho and Montana. Now we recognize that this condition prevails throughout the world, and cases have been found in many of the states of the United States; the only ones escaping have been Maine, Michigan, Mississippi, New Hampshire. Vermont, and Wisconsin.

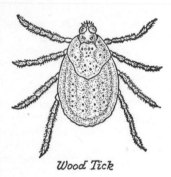

Wood Tick

The wood tick, which may carry a variety of virus diseases including Rocky Mountain spotted fever

Rocky Mountain spotted fever is an infectious condition which is transmitted by wood ticks in the Rocky Mountain Pacific coast states and by dog ticks in the Southern and Eastern states. The time when spotted fever appears is usually the time when the ticks are prevalent. Not only the ticks that have been mentioned carry the disease but almost any kind of tick. In the mountain states where the rabbits may be infected by the virus of Rocky Mountain spotted fever, the rabbit tick can carry the disease. In the United States for a period of four years, 1933–37, 2190 cases were reported with 420 deaths.

After a person has been bitten by an infected tick, there are a few days of moderate illness accompanied by chilly sensations and loss of appetite. Then come the chill, with pains in the bones, muscles, back, and joints, headache, and general illness with not infrequently a short dry cough. A fever develops, which may go as high as 105. About the third, fourth, or fifth day of the fever there is a rash which appears first on the wrists, ankles, and back and then spreads over the body. This takes about twenty-four to thirty-six hours. People with this condition sometimes also develop restlessness and insomnia, occasionally delirium and convulsions.

In general one attack of this disease will protect the person against future attacks of the same disease, although second attacks have been reported in some cases eight or more years after the first attack.

A vaccine has been developed which protects people against the disease. Of course the best way to control Rocky Mountain spotted fever is to reduce the number and limit the distribution of ticks. In the Bitter Root Valley this is done by destroying the small animals and dipping the cattle. Clearing and cultivation of land also make it impossible for the ticks to thrive. People themselves can avoid tick bites by wearing a specially designed working costume with the trousers worn inside of heavy woolen socks and high laced boots. It is also customary to interpose strips of felt or other absorbent material in the neckband and wrists to prevent the ticks from getting under the clothing.

Arrangements should also be made to be certain that dogs, cats, and other pets are free from ticks.

Children are examined twice a day to make certain that the ticks are not on their bodies.

When a tick is found on the body, it should be removed by gently pulling it off with the fingers. Crushing of the tick should be avoided.

Because of the severity of this infection, every necessary supportive treatment is used by the doctor to bring the patient safely through to recovery.

A new antibiotic drug especially valuable in this condition is chloromycetin or choramphenicol.

RUBELLA Another name for *Measles, German,* which see.

RUPTURE See *Hernia.*

SACROILIAC See *Backache.*

SACRUM At the lower end of the spine there is a triangular bone which is formed of five united bones of the spine. This is called the sacrum. Many a case of backache is ascribed to a disturbance of the joint between the sacrum at the back and the bones of the pelvis in front.

SADISM Some people derive pleasure of a sexual character from inflicting cruelty on others. The scientific term for this is sadism. It derives from a man named Marquis de Sade who lived around 1800 and who wrote a book on the subject, describing his own experiences.

SALIVA The saliva is a fluid put out by the salivary glands, of which there are some under the jaw in front of the ear and under the tongue. It contains a starch-digesting ferment. It serves also to moisten and soften food and to keep the mouth moist.

SALPINGITIS (See discussion under *Fallopian Tubes*) Infection of the fallopian tubes is called salpingitis.

SALT Pure sodium, which is one of the two elements in sodium chloride or common salt, is seldom found except in chemical laboratories. Many combinations of sodium with other elements are used in diet and in industry. Table salt is sodium chloride. Baking soda is sodium bicarbonate.

The average man takes in his diet about half an ounce of sodium chloride every day. It is easy, on a low salt diet, to reduce this to about one fifth as much. This is done particularly when excess of fluid accumulates in the tissues as in dropsy. No one knows exactly the minimum or maximum of sodium chloride that any one person ought to have, but fortunately the human body is equipped with factors of safety so that it can get rid of excesses of various substances. The average human body contains at all times about three ounces of sodium chloride. The use of salt by the body and its elimination by the kidney are apparently controlled by the cortex or outer layer of the adrenal gland.

Many vegetables contain another salt with an element similar to sodium, namely, potassium. A person who subsists on a vegetable diet craves salt because vegetables contain less sodium than meat. The moment the salt in the human body falls below the amount necessary, a craving is set up.

Salt is also important for supplying the chlorine element since hydrochloric acid is secreted by the stomach regularly as an aid to digestion. Pepsin works as a digestive substance only in the presence of hydrochloric acid. However, hydrochloric acid should not be taken by the average person in that form except on the advice of a physician.

Various diets free from large amounts of sodium chloride have been developed. Most physicians are convinced that there is a definite relationship between salt in the diet and the occurrence of various conditions affecting the blood pressure and the kidneys. However, in the presence of unusual craving for salt, or, in fact, in any disease condition, it is well to be guided in such matters by competent advice.

SARCOMA Tumors which are malignant but not made of epithelial tissue (like cancer) are usually of the sarcoma type. They may involve cartilage or bone or fibrous tissues. The diagnosis is made by the doctor, who takes a piece of the tumor and examines it under the microscope.

SCABIES See discussion under *Insect Pests.*

SCARLET FEVER The story of an attack of scarlet fever is rather typical. From two to four days after a person has been in contact with someone who has scarlet fever, a chill occurs. Then there is sore throat with some nausea and vomiting. Promptly the pulse becomes rapid. The fever rises as high as 102 to 104 degrees. Bright red spots about the size of a pin point begin to appear, usually first on the neck and chest. This eruption spreads rapidly over the rest of the body. The face appears red, usually because of the fever and not because of the eruption. After a few days the rash begins to fade, and in about a week the skin is normal in color.

There is usually a severe sore throat and an intense redness of the inside of the mouth. The tonsils are swollen. The tongue develops a peculiar appearance which has given it the name of strawberry tongue. Sometimes the glands in the neck enlarge because of the infection.

Infection with scarlet fever varies in severity. There have been times when exceedingly severe forms of scarlet fever have attacked whole communities. More recently scarlet fever seems to have become a relatively mild disease, and the number of deaths has greatly decreased. Each winter brings an increase in scarlet fever, as does also late spring.

Many people believe that scarlatina and scarlet fever are different conditions—one milder than the other. Actually there is just one disease of this type, although from time to time cases of German measles and eruption due to sensitivities of various kinds are mistaken for scarlet fever.

Scarlet fever seldom occurs during the first year of life, probably because babies inherit from their mothers some resistance to the disease. Most cases occur in children between six and ten years of age. Incidentally these are the ages when children first begin to have contacts with other children in schools and on playgrounds. Scarlet fever is not, however, exclusively a disease of childhood. More than 15 per cent of those who have scarlet fever are more than sixteen years old.

The height of infectivity in scarlet fever occurs when the nose and throat are filled with discharges contaminated with the germs that are now recognized as being responsible for scarlet fever. Most people are now convinced that the cause of scarlet fever is a special type of streptococcus. In most cases the infected person has the germs in the discharges of the nose and throat for from ten to fourteen days.

Since 1924 great advances have been made in our knowledge of scarlet fever. Among these has been the development of a test of the skin called the Dick test (like the Schick test in diphtheria), which shows whether or not a child is likely to have scarlet fever if exposed to the disease. This is known as susceptibility.

In the skin test for susceptibility to scarlet fever the toxin is injected under the skin, and a simple salt solution is injected as a control. Reddening in the area in which the toxin was injected is taken as a positive test. There is also available an immunizing toxin which, when injected into the body, causes the child to develop resistance against scarlet fever. In times of epidemic immunization with the scarlet fever streptococcus toxin is recommended for any person who shows a positive reaction to the Dick test.

Sometimes there is a local reaction to the injection of the toxin, but this usually disappears within forty-eight hours. In other instances there may be a general reaction, with pain, some fever and nausea, sometimes even a slight rash. However, immunization against scarlet fever avoids long isolation, serious complications, and makes the disease much milder.

Various communities in the United States differ as to the length of time children with scarlet fever should be kept at home. The recommendations vary from a minimum period of twenty-one days to a maximum of six weeks. The decision as to whether or not schools shall be closed during an epidemic of scarlet fever depends on the extent to which the closing of the school helps or interferes with the spread of the disease. In country districts, where children go to widely separated homes, closing of the school may be of value. In cities, where children mingle much more closely at home and in the neighborhood than they would in the school, it is customary to keep the schools open.

Children in families where there are cases of scarlet fever will stay home during the time of the infection. Every person who has scarlet fever should be isolated and remain isolated until the doctor declares that it is safe for that person to mingle with other people.

If every case of scarlet fever is diagnosed promptly, if the patient is put to bed, and if proper measures of disinfection are carried out in relation to discharges from the nose and throat and in regard to contaminated materials, and if, in addition, we apply all that we now know about the specific prevention of scarlet fever, this disease may someday soon be eliminated as an infection threat to human beings.

From ten days to two weeks after scarlet fever first appears the skin begins to peel or scale. Great patches of skin may come off the hands and feet. Over the rest of the body the skin usually comes off in small scales. The scales of the skin and the skin that peel off are not important in spreading the disease except when they are contaminated with secretions of the nose and throat. These secretions do contain the germs and will themselves spread the disease or do so by contaminating the skin, the patient's dishes, or anything else which he soils.

Since infection with scarlet fever is a menace not only because of itself but particularly because of the secondary complications, special attention is given in scarlet fever to protecting the kidneys and the heart during the time when the person is sick. Every patient with scarlet fever should remain in bed for three weeks.

The severe inflammation and swelling in the throat may extend into the Eustachian tubes, which pass from the back of the nose to the ears. Thus the scarlet fever infection may spread into the ear and bring about a serious complication, even mastoiditis, with permanent damage to hearing.

The antitoxin for scarlet fever is successful in controlling the disease and in greatly decreasing its severity. The decision as to whether or not the antitoxin is to be given in scarlet fever must, of course, rest with the physician. New methods of treatment, including the sulfonamides and antibiotics like penicillin and tetracyn make scarlet fever a much milder disease than it used to be. The antitoxin for scarlet fever is given particularly in those cases in which the disease is severe. The antitoxin of scarlet fever does not affect the germs themselves but does affect the toxin, which is responsible for the symptoms of scarlet fever. The drugs of the sulfonamide type act directly on the germs, preventing their growth and thus decreasing the menace of the infection and the amount of toxin that develops. Deaths from scarlet fever are now exceedingly rare.

The doctor who takes care of the patient with scarlet fever will prescribe remedies which prevent headache and other pains, also lotions to take care of itching and irritation of the skin. He advises the family as to the cleaning of linens, utensils, and other materials used by the patient, in order to prevent the spread of the disease. After the patient has recovered, the bed and body linens and any other material that may have come in contact with discharges from the patient and all objects, such as thermometers, spoons, cups, and toys that have been used by the patient, should be boiled, steamed, or soaked in a suitable germicidal solution. The permanent furniture should be thoroughly washed and cleaned, and the room aired and sunned for at least one day as a means of eliminating infection.

SCIATIC NEURITIS A long, large nerve known as the sciatic nerve passes from the lower part of the spinal column out of the spinal canal through some openings between the bones, then down to the back of the thigh and onward to the leg. Whenever this nerve becomes irritated or inflamed, there is pain in back of the thigh and in other portions of the body through which this nerve passes. The sciatic nerve is the longest nerve in the body. Frequently the pains that result from inflammation of the sciatic nerve are confused with rheumatic pains. Pain develops in this nerve as a result of pressure on it due to changes in the blood vessels, by disturbances of the spinal cord in the area in which the nerve arises, as a result of falls or strains, by exposure to rain, wading in cold streams, working in damp places, or similar experiences. Sometimes pain in the sciatic nerve is associated with severe constipation either from pressure of material in the loaded bowels or from absorption of toxic materials from the body which affect the nerves.

When the doctor studies the patient for the presence of sciatic neuritis, he will make a number of tests to determine whether the pain is due to the sciatic nerve or to some other cause. He will examine the back for any unusual curvature of the spine or any pressure that might result from bones in the wrong position. He will study the legs for signs of spasms of the muscles or for wasting. He may test the effects of raising the leg in a straight position while the patient lies flat on the back. This puts a strain on the large hamstring muscles which, in turn, refer the strain to the nerve. It is also important to determine whether the pain is the result of difficulty with the nerve or with the sacroiliac joint.

In treating a sciatic neuritis the doctor must overcome any unfavorable conditions of work or climate which may be contributing factors. He studies the diet to make certain that there are adequate amounts of such nutritional substances as thiamine. He prescribes rest and arranges the bed so that there is relief from tension and support to the inflamed tissues. Heat is helpful in relieving the pain.

After the pain has subsided, the patient must continue to avoid strenuous exercise, which is often followed by twinges in the nerves.

There are a variety of methods of special treatment, including injections of various substances in and around the nerve.

Finally, there are surgical processes involving work on the bones and muscles or on the nerve. In a severe case of sciatic neuritis determination of the causative factors and treatment applied specifically to control these conditions involves the highest art of the physician.

SCLERODERMA Sometimes the skin of a human being becomes altered in its consistency and color, so that there are large or small areas of the skin that become hard and yellow, occasionally hard and white. No one knows the cause of this condition. Women are far more commonly affected than men, and most often between twenty and forty years of age. It has been thought from time to time that glandular changes have been responsible. Many physicians are convinced that the disturbance is definitely related to some condition in the nervous system because changes in certain areas of the spinal cord have been found on post-mortem examination. There are many methods of treatment, including the use of the electric needle for removing the area or various ointments for softening the tissue. In general, however, treatment is unsatisfactory in stopping the progress of the disease or in curing it.

SCLEROSIS This is a scientific term derived from a Greek word meaning hard. It is used to describe a hardening of any tissue of the human body. There are many different forms of sclerosis, involving tissues of the eye, tissues of the spine, tumors of the breast, and other tissues.

SCOLIOSIS See *Spinal Curvature*.

SCURVY See discussion under *Vitamins*.

SEASICKNESS The immense amount of ocean transportation during the war has kept attention focused constantly on seasickness, a condition which, of course, must be considered in relation to carsickness and airsickness.

The investigators are convinced that there is some relation between the eye, the ear, and the sensation of air-, car-, or seasickness. The exact cause of seasickness has not yet, however, been determined—at least not to the extent that there is a specific remedy related to the cause.

People in trains, ships, and airplanes who are confined in stuffy rooms and who are unable to move around are more likely to become sick than those who are comfortably located. People who travel on trains and who get carsick in a compartment or room may not be carsick if they sit in the open car. Overloading the stomach increases the tendency to seasickness or airsickness. Small amounts of food taken frequently are sometimes helpful.

People who become nauseated easily have their symptoms of seasickness intensified when there is an oily smell from the engines. Sometimes people become nauseated when the odor of food spreads through a plane as the stewardess begins serving dinner.

The semicircular canals in the internal ear, which are associated with balance, seem to have a definite part to play in the symptoms of seasickness. It has been found, for instance, that quick vertical movements of an airplane are a factor in producing airsickness. Many people become airsick or seasick when noises and vibration are excessive. Some people become sick in trains while riding backward but not while riding forward. People who have chronic infections of the sinuses and of the ears are more likely to be airsick than those who are without such infections.

Among the various remedies that have been offered for seasickness are the following:

1. A tight belt.
2. Champagne before sailing.
3. Hold a bag over the nose and breathe into the bag.
4. Stuff cotton wool in the ears.
5. Keep a bandage over the eyes.
6. If you are smoking, don't stop smoking.
7. If you are smoking, stop smoking.
8. Lie flat on the back.
9. Dance in rhythm with the ship's movements.
10. Eat heavily of fruits and alkaline foods.
11. Take baking soda.

In general, however, it is well to be advised by a doctor such as the one who for years traveled on the *Aquitania* and who made a record of some of his experiences with seasick passengers. He says that seasickness, when not complicated by a hangover from too much celebration before going on board, is due to unusual reactions that occur in the nervous system because of excessive stimulation reaching the parts of the body that are concerned with balance. This means particularly the semicircular canals in the internal ear. For the prevention of seasickness he has recommended fresh air with bodily warmth. Have plenty of sleep before going on the boat. Because of uneasiness around the center of the abdomen, many people find the wearing of a firm abdominal binder comfortable and helpful. Be moderate in drinking and eating before going on the boat and make sure that the bowel is working satisfactorily. Alcohol tends to take the edge off the apprehension but will not itself prevent seasickness. Take such sedative drugs as the doctor may prescribe.

Up to recent times medicine has not had information concerning any drug or method of treatment that has been quite satisfactory in preventing, relieving, or curing motion sickness. The United States Navy during World War II made extensive studies and proved that psychosomatic factors are unimportant in seasickness. Studies were made of keeping sailors in different positions from lying down to crouching and standing. Almost by accident a discovery was made in

1947 that seems to be the answer to the problem of motion sickness. It is a drug called dramamine, one of the antihistaminic products similar to those that are used against hay fever and food sensitivities. It was sent to the clinics for experiments in these conditions. In the course of the trials the drug was given to a pregnant woman who was sensitive to foods and who all her life had been sensitive to carsickness. When she took this drug for food sensitivity, she was completely relieved of carsickness. Repeated tests using the new drug and using a simple capsule of milk sugar proved that only the new drug gave her relief. Later the drug was used on other people who suffered from airsickness and they too obtained relief.

Extensive studies were then made on sailors on one of the large ships and proved again that the drug was excellent. Dramamine is now recognized as being effective for both preventing and treating motion sickness. The drug may be taken by mouth or given in other ways. It is supplied on prescription of doctors and is worthy of trial by people who look on ocean voyages with dread because of invariable seasickness. The drug is also successful in airsickness and carsickness and possibly in some cases of Menière's disease and migraine.

SEBACEOUS CYST   See *Wen.*

SEBORRHEA   (See also discussions under *Dandruff* and *Hair*) Some people perspire more than others. Some people have more dandruff and peeling of the skin than others. Many specialists in diseases of the skin are convinced that seborrhea or dandruff is an infectious condition which arises from germs which are normally on the skin but which are especially prevalent on a greasy skin.

Some physicians are convinced that seborrhea represents a special type of constitution in which there is an increase of the secretion from the glands in the skin, an overgrowth of such glands, and an enlargement of the pores. Associated with this there is usually a thickening of the skin and also an increased activity of the sweat glands.

One British physician is convinced that seborrhea is associated with similar activities which affect the mucous membranes of the mouth and the other orifices of the body, and that sometimes there is also change of the mucous membrane of the nose in conditions like hay fever and asthma.

For this reason it has been suggested that the person who has an unusually greasy skin with excess secretion might well take a diet which is rich in proteins but restricted as to sugars, fluids, and salt. It should also be a diet that is high in vitamins, particularly leafy green vegetables and fresh fruits. Irritating foods and highly seasoned foods like fried foods and pork are also to be avoided.

In the worst types of seborrhea it is obviously necessary for the physician to treat the entire body from the point of view of rest, exercise, and hygiene generally. In certain cases, however, where the condition is largely confined to scurf on the scalp, treatment applied directly to the dandruff is itself sufficient to bring about a successful result.

Certainly anyone with dandruff ought to wash the hair at least once a week, bathe the body regularly at least once a day, and avoid the wearing of clothing that produces heat next to the skin with maceration and softening caused by the fluid.

Dandruff of the scalp is, however, only one manifestation of the seborrheic constitution. The regular washing of the hair and the application of suitable scalp treatments can keep dandruff under control week by week. When, however, there is an eruption of pimples on the face with a greasy complexion and enlarged pores, when there is scaling and inflammation of the skin behind the ears and in the groins, the condition demands much more serious attention.

Patients of this type must be kept in a good mental frame of mind, must get plenty of sleep, must be given proper treatments to avoid itching and irritation. They must have their blood brought up to par by the suitable administration of the necessary vitamins, iron, and similar substances.

A new drug specifically against seborrhea is called Selsun. This is used as a shampoo, left on for ten minutes, and then rinsed away.

SENESCENCE Old age can be divided into two periods—senescence, which is the gradual aging of the body, and senility, in which the aging process is complicated by a variety of conditions.

Unfortunately uncomplicated old age is exceedingly rare. As people get old, the cells of the body lose their power of repair. When this happens, tissues become fibrous, occasionally even calcified. The rareness of uncomplicated old age is shown by the fact that one famous pathologist reported that he had never seen a case of a completely natural death in an experience of thirty-eight years, during which he had examined by post-mortem examination many thousands of bodies; another pathologist, who had examined post mortem more than 20,000 bodies, said that he had seen only twenty-five which could be called examples of healthy old age. In these twenty-five death occurred simply through a gradual wearing out of the heart.

Normal old age comes on gradually and is usually well established by the age of sixty-five, although there are exceptions. For that reason the age of sixty-five is usually set up as the age for retirement from public office or positions of administration. Longevity and the postponement of senility depend on several factors, the first of which is the influence of heredity. In many families youthfulness persists much longer than in others. Much can be done to prevent the development of the changes associated with old age by practicing temperance in food and drink, by relaxation of the mind through hobbies and vacation periods, by healthful but moderate exercise and other practices in the field of good hygiene.

Unquestionably the condition of the blood vessels is the most important single factor in the aging of the human body. Hardening of the arteries is likely to be associated with more rapid degenerative changes, since the tissues depend on the blood vessels for their supply of nutriment, especially oxygen. Associated with rapid old age also is the wearing out of muscular tissues in the bowels and in the walls of blood vessels.

The diseases most likely to occur in old age are enlargement of the prostate gland, which is said to occur in at least half of all men over the age of seventy; cancer, which is especially a disease of old age, although cases do occur in the young; and arthritic changes in the bones and joints.

Pediatricians say that the first year of life is the most critical. Others insist that the first ten years are the hardest. Some call adolescence, with the transition from childhood to adult life, the most critical period.

The great control that is now asserted over infant mortality and the elimination of many of the diseases that used to affect youth make the majority of doctors today think that the most serious age is the period of transition from maturity to old age. Men enter the most critical period of their lives at fifty. This is the time when they begin to need glasses to read the print in the telephone book. Now they begin to get tired a little earlier in the afternoon.

Occasionally the onset of these conditions induces resentment. Many a physical-culture expert or the proprietor of a health institute or gymnasium has earned an excellent livelihood from the fact that these men take up exercise and try to prove to themselves that they are better than they really are. The wise man will realize that aging is a natural process and that the conditions that come with advancing years must be treated with respect. If the thyroid gland, the sex glands, and the pituitary are less efficient, the deficiency will be reflected in the body generally. A doctor can prescribe glandular substances to overcome such deficiencies in part.

Hardening of the arteries and high blood pressure are two of the most important symptoms. Many years ago a wise physician said that a man is as old as his arteries. Incidentally, men are more frequently affected with hardening of the arteries than women.

Arthritis is another condition especially frequent in people after the age of forty and which cripples and disables a good many older people.

Medicine can do a great deal for these disturbances if they are brought soon enough to medical attention. But man is not immortal and the wise man will recognize the aging process and conduct himself accordingly.

EYES OF THE AGED—The aging process is continuous from the time of birth to the time of death. Some human beings age more slowly than others.

Many of these changes in the vision of older people are associated with changes in the circulation, including hardening of the arteries. The eyelids of old people develop wrinkles.

Old people seem to cry easily and sometimes suffer from an overflow of tears. This is often due to relaxation of the tissues of the eye, which do not hold the material as do the elastic tissues of the young. Surgeons have developed technics for maintaining the normal relationships between the tissues, overcoming this overflow of tears when it becomes a nuisance.

Elderly people often complain of heaviness of the eyelids and inability to raise them, especially in the morning. The weakness may be due to a gradual disappearance of the elastic tissue from the eyelids.

In the old person the pupil of the eye becomes smaller and less movable, and the color of the eye becomes lighter. The lens of the eye grows and increases in weight throughout life. Sometimes a ring seems to form around the colored center of the eye. This is called an "arcus senilis" and is characteristic of aging.

Cataract is typical of the aged, and the exact cause is not known. The decision as to whether or not a cataract is to be removed by surgical operation depends on many factors having to do with the patient's physical and mental condition as well as the actual condition of the eye.

Old people need much higher intensities of light than young persons. In fact, improvement of the light often decreases the need for stronger eyeglasses.

WHAT OLD PEOPLE REMEMBER—With the improvement in health our life expectancy at birth has gradually risen. The ancient Greeks apparently lived to an average age of just under thirty years. In 1900 the average age at death in the United States was forty-five. Now we have raised the average life expectancy at birth to almost seventy years and for white girl babies to more than 70 years.

Our mental activities are dependent to some extent on our physical condition. The more any mental activity is dependent on some physical activity of the body, the more that activity is likely to decline with age.

From birth to fifteen years the growth of the human being is rapid. At around twenty-five years of age the human physique reaches its maximum in strength and skill. Most human beings descend slowly from this level until the age of forty-five, when the momentum of decline increases. Then at about fifty-five years of age the rate of decline again increases until the age of seventy.

Intelligence, which is the effective organization of mental abilities for a certain purpose, matures quickly, so that by sixteen years of age the intelligence of the human being is about at its peak. It remains on this level until the early twenties. From twenty years on, the intelligence decreases. By the age of fifty-five many human beings have receded to the fourteen-year-old level. Not all of the factors involved in intelligence are lost at the same rate. The voice and the hearing remain efficient until well along in life. The reaction time is, however, likely to decrease more rapidly.

Memory reaches its peak in the late teens and early twenties and declines rapidly with age. The inability to remember recent events is always a telltale sign of senescence. Old people remember happenings of their childhood and forget what happened yesterday. With senescence they become careless of accuracy, but some youngsters never learn accuracy.

LEARNING AND OLD AGE—"Never too old to learn" is a trite phrase; also "some people never learn." The ability to learn reaches its maximum in the late teens and early twenties and then declines slowly. One psychologist found that there is a 1 per cent loss in learning ability every year from the age of twenty-five on.

Few people develop new interests after fifty. Most people tend to dislike change as they approach old age. The interests of people after middle age are reflected in the physical condition of their bodies. As people get older they enjoy sedentary pursuits and dislike strenuous physical or mental activities. Television has proved to be a wonderful medium of interest and enjoyment particularly for old people.

As people get older their love of amusement declines in the majority of instances in favor of distinctly cultural pursuits. Older men are likely to prefer forms of amusement and relaxation which they can do alone rather than the gregarious types of amusement which interest younger men. Of course there are exceptions to every rule, and some older people possess the ability to renew their minds continually. Thus many old people find their chief delight in reading history and biography.

The world tends to reject the older individual and to make less opportunity for him to take up new jobs or new interests. The man who takes up a new job or profession or returns to school at sixty-five or seventy is rare.

Some men who take up amateur gardening or collection hobbies exhibit surprising skill. Wars give the old people opportunities far beyond those of peacetime.

The suggestion has been made that our recreation experts and our adult education groups ought to plan particularly for the special needs, interests, and abilities of men and women who are more than sixty years old. The mental stimulation which they would receive in such courses would not only help them to live longer and more healthfully but would also be exceedingly productive for the world as a whole.

SEPTICEMIA Whenever infection invades the blood, the condition is called septicemia. Such infection is always accompanied by chills, profuse sweating, and prostration. The appearance of these symptoms indicates that the doctor should be called immediately because every moment counts in controlling the spread of such an infection.

SEPTIC SORE THROAT A germ called the *Streptococcus hemolyticus,* which is one of the many different forms of this organism, is responsible for a condition called septic sore throat. Of all the sore throats, septic sore throat is the worst. Usually the condition begins with a severe chill and a rapidly developing fever which may reach as high as 105 degrees Fahrenheit. Occasionally, however, the infection takes place more slowly, with some sore throat, headache, and slight fever for a day or two, intensifying as the disease progresses. Soon the swelling in the throat makes swallowing difficult. The head and neck are held stiffly because movement is painful. As the infection extends downward, the voice becomes hoarse, coughing occurs, and there may even be shortness of breath.

When the doctor looks at the throat, he discovers that it is dark red and that there are patches of grayish material. This inflammation may extend even to the point of ulceration. Because of the extent of the infection the glands in the side of the neck become greatly enlarged and this type of inflammation may go on to the formation of abscesses.

The number of fatalities from septic

sore throat is not exceedingly great because the location of the infection makes it possible for the doctor to attend to it promptly. However, many instances occur in which the infection may extend to the heart, causing heart disease, or to the abdominal cavity, causing peritonitis, or indeed to any other portion of the body.

Fortunately we now have a remedy which is practically specific in the control of septic sore throat. The various sulfonamide drugs are known to have a definite effect on the streptococci and particularly on the *Streptococcus hemolyticus*. Therefore the doctor gives large doses of this drug at once and continues until the infection is under control. Anyone with septic sore throat should go to bed immediately.

As an aid to causing the infection to break up, hot wet packs are applied to the neck. Little is gained, however, by using gargles or sprays or washes of any kind applied to the surface of the throat.

In severe cases when the obstruction in the throat becomes so bad as to interfere seriously with breathing, the administration of oxygen may be used. Naturally any secondary infections such as abscesses or inflammations elsewhere in the body are given immediate attention.

SHINGLES An important fact about the occurrence of shingles, or herpes zoster, is the appearance of the blisters in groups along the course of one or more of the nerves of sensation in the skin of the body. The condition is thus quite definitely a nervous disease as well as a skin disease. Shingles usually are found in people whose nervous resistance has been lowered by overwork, disease, or some long-continued toxic action on the human body. The blisters are usually preceded by pain of a neuralgic character in the region of the body that is affected and the disappearance of the blisters is not infrequently followed by burning, tingling, or other irritation.

Sometimes one crop of blisters will persist for a week or ten days, then dry up, form crusts, and disappear. Shortly thereafter a new crop of blisters will appear at the same place or near by. The blisters vary in size from a pinhead to that of a small pea. The walls are thick but they will break eventually. Then a fine fluid appears and dries. If, however, there has been secondary infection of the blisters, they will be filled with a white puslike material.

Young people usually get over the shingles in short order but when they appear in old people they are painful and are quite frequently followed by repeated attacks of nerve pain in the region affected.

In most cases the shingles appear on the sides of the chest, the back, or above the eye. They may appear in the groin and actually, of course, on any portion of the surface of the body.

There are all sorts of superstitions about shingles, one of which is that when shingles occur on both sides of the body and meet in the center the condition will be fatal. This, of course, is ridiculous.

In persistent cases of shingles the specialist in diseases of the skin is sometimes able to prevent recurrences by the use of the X ray, ultraviolet ray, and by various other measures applied directly to the area concerned. A real advance in the control of shingles has been the use of ACTH or Cortisone. In some cases antihistamines have helped.

SHOCK The condition called shock has been in the past one of the most difficult emergencies that confronts a physician. Loss of blood is one of the most serious effects of a wound. Many physicians are convinced that the cause of shock is in most instances loss of blood. Therefore the modern treatment of shock places emphasis on maintaining the blood supply through the use of blood plasma. The first change that occurs in shock is dilation of the blood vessels on the surface of the body. In connection with the dilation of these blood vessels, perspiration occurs and the skin is relatively warm. The blood pressure becomes low and the pulse feeble and slow.

The first step in aiding the person in shock is to place him with the head low because a loss of blood from the brain may result in a failure of that tissue to function. The patient in shock must be kept comfortably warm. Pain is relieved by sedative drugs because it is known that pain may be a contributing factor to the intensity of shock.

Following initial shock from a wound or an injury there develops a condition called secondary shock due to the damage of the tissues. This may come on an hour or more after an injury. People with secondary shock are pale, weak, or exhausted. They may complain of thirst if they are conscious; the perspiration is cold and clammy; the pulse is rapid and thready; the breathing rapid and shallow; the blood pressure low; and the superficial blood vessels are collapsed. This type of shock is seen particularly after severe burns or as a late manifestation following a surgical operation. Fortunately the condition is preventable to a large extent, so that in modern surgery continuous transfusion of blood or of plasma may be a feature of the operative procedure and thus greatly lessen the incidence of shock.

SHOULDER The shoulder is a joint in which several bones, ligaments, and muscles are involved. This joint has the greatest range of motion of any joint in the body. For that very reason the shoulder is injured most easily. If the shoulder joint gets stiff and painful, you may as well quit work, for any further effort will merely make it worse.

Scientific authorities believe that the shoulder evolved from a walking joint like that possessed by animals which walk on four legs and changed to a weight-carrying joint. Therefore the shoulder has lost much of its stability, strength, and durability.

The shoulder joint may, like any other joint in the body, become infected or injured in various ways. One of the most frequent injuries is a torn tendon,

which gives rise to what is called a stiff, painful shoulder. Such a tendon may tear due to dislocation of the shoulder or to a fall or to an unusual strain such as occurs when one is trying to tie a rope or pull a chain hoist. A middle-aged woman slipped on an oiled floor and in trying to save her balance threw her arm up so high that she tore a tendon in the shoulder.

Fractures of any of the bones involved in the shoulder joint demand surgical attention. Dislocations also demand setting of the bones in the proper position and frequently bandaging, often the use of a cast.

There are also bursas in the region of the shoulder joint which may become inflamed and thus produce inability to move the joint properly.

Whenever there is serious pain in the shoulder joint after a sprain, a severe infection, or the tearing of a ligament, it is desirable that there be no excessive motion. The position of greatest comfort is to have the arm carried in a sling, which permits the arm to be supported and to be held rather close to the side. Often this treatment in itself is sufficient to prevent any further difficulties.

In other forms of injury to the joint it is desirable that the arm be held in a position away from the body or in the abduction position. In order to secure this position it may be necessary to put a splint and a plaster cast on the body.

Heat, massage, and early active exercise, which will utilize not only the shoulder joint but the other joints in that vicinity, as soon as possible after the splint and the plaster cast have been removed are important in preventing loss of function.

A rather common disability is a recurrent dislocation of the shoulder joint. Apparently this is controllable only by surgical operation, with subsequent use of a plaster cast and still later suitable exercise of the joint.

SINUSES The sinuses are cavities in the bones of the head which connect with the inside of the nose by means of small openings. The sinus in the cheekbone is called the antrum, the one above the eyes is the frontal sinus, and deeper behind the nose is the ethmoid sinus.

Infectious germs gain access to the sinuses and infect the membranes which line their walls. If the opening of the sinus into the nose becomes blocked, the presence of infectious material causes headache and pain, and the absorption of infectious material leads to fever. An ordinary cold will clear up in three to five days, but if the sinuses become infected, the symptoms will last for weeks and weeks. Eventually such conditions become chronic, and there is an exacerbation which is like the original infection.

When a patient with an infection of the sinuses comes to the doctor, the doctor usually cleans the nose, shrinks the membranes by applying adrenalin or epinephrine, and then studies the openings from the sinuses into the nose to see whether or not infectious material is coming out. The sinuses are also studied by use of the X ray and by transillumination. Any blocking of the sinuses is shown by a shadow. It is also possible, when the physician believes there are growths like polyps or tumors in the sinuses, to inject an opaque substance into the sinuses and then to make an X-ray picture.

The presence of infection may be controlled with drugs given by mouth, materials applied directly to the nose by washing out the sinuses, and sometimes by surgical procedures. Modern developments in drug treatment, including the sulfonamides and penicillin, are known to be especially valuable in some of the infections that attack the sinuses.

Some of the recent studies on infections of the sinuses have shown that nutritional deficiencies are sometimes related to persistent infections of the sinuses. This applies particularly to deficiencies of vitamin A, since this vitamin is associated with the proper development of mucous membranes. Some have insisted that an excess of starch in the diet is responsible for sinus infec-

tions, and others say that calcium is an important factor. All of this merely means that the nutrition of the patient needs to be properly controlled in order that he may receive all of the essential substances.

People with infections of the sinuses should avoid swimming, diving, and strenuous outdoor exercises. Sometimes they find relief where the climate is hot and dry.

SKIN The skin is living tissue, not just an envelope on the outside of the body. The skin of a grown person weighs about 6 pounds and if spread out flat on the ground would cover an area of about 16 to 20 square feet. The skin on the palms of the hands, the soles of the feet, the shoulders, and the back of the neck is the thickest skin of the body, varying from .02 of an inch to .16 of an inch in thickness.

Externally the skin is full of furrows which are formed by the attachment of the skin to the structures underneath and by the movement of the skin. These furrows are constant for each person. Between the furrows are ridges which are dotted with numerous depressions that are openings of the pores which release sweat through the skin.

Doctors view the skin as being made of three layers—an outer layer, which is called the cuticle; the next layer, which is the true skin; and finally, the lowest layer where the blood vessels, lymph vessels, and similar structures necessary for the health and life of the skin are located. Here also are some of the glands and the beginnings of the hair follicles. The blood vessels are extremely important to the skin because the skin receives one third of all of the blood that circulates in order to nourish it.

The skin is constantly rejuvenating itself until old age comes on. The outermost layers are detached as the lower layers produce new cells. Billions of new cells are made every day and billions of dead horny cells are shed by the body. There are thirty layers of cells constantly being added to from below and shed from above.

One of the functions of the skin is the evaporation of heat from the body so as to maintain a constant temperature. The amount of heat radiated depends on the climate in which one lives. The skin keeps the body from drying up through evaporation of fluid. Other glands in the skin secrete an oil or grease which maintains the skin in a flexible condition. On the palms of the hand there are more than 5000 sweat glands for each square inch of surface.

The skin is an organ of the body just as are the liver, the heart, and the lungs. When the flow of blood to the skin is hindered for any reason, the skin hardens, thickens, and loses its normal appearance. In old age when the circulation to the skin is lessened, the skin loses its youthful appearance. Wrinkles form and the color of the skin also changes.

The color of the skin is dependent to some extent on the effects of sunlight. In most people the pigment or color of the skin depends on inheritance and, finally, on the amount of blood that circulates through the skin.

Many people believe that it is possible to feed the skin or cause it to fill out by the use of oils, creams, pastes, ointments, or similar preparations which are rubbed on or into the skin. There is no way to feed the skin by anything put on the surface. Fatty substances and ointments placed on the skin are not absorbed but if they are rubbed hard enough they may be pushed into the glands, from which they are taken up by the blood. Thus some substances rubbed on the skin are picked up by the blood.

With a reasonable amount of cleanliness the skin gets along quite well. The skin of a baby requires more attention than that of an adult since it becomes more easily irritated by rubbing between the folds of the skin or by the constant contact with secretions of the body. If the skin is kept clean, it will seldom become irritated except through rubbing or from exposure to irritating substances.

Any inflammation of the skin is called dermatitis. Ninety-five per cent of people who come to doctors with disturbances of the skin have simple inflammations that are due to some external cause such as an irritating chemical or an infection.

The amount of attention given to the skin depends on the kind of skin it is. An oily skin may require more cleaning and a different type of cleaning than a skin that tends to be dry. The skin of a baby is often benefited by being oiled, since the oil serves as a protection. People with oily skins need to bathe more frequently than those with dry skins. People with dry skins may require added oil.

The face is usually adapted by years of exposure to sunlight, fresh air, and the elements to get along satisfactorily merely with simple cleansing. This means washing two or three times a day either with water alone or with soap and water. The face may be washed more frequently, however, if it needs it. Generally it is satisfactory to wash the face frequently with plain water during the day and then to give it a thorough washing with warm water and soap before going to bed at night.

Men who shave frequently put plenty of soap and water on the face during the shaving process. Women often like to steam the skin by covering it with hot towels and thereafter softening it by rubbing in cold creams. The application of any cream to the face should usually be preceded by thorough washing with warm water and soap.

For a skin that is especially dry, the use of a toilet powder aids in preventing damage. The daily use of creams with powder on top will incline, however, to clog the pores of the skin. Secondary infection then may seriously damage the skin.

Nowadays there is a great tendency to expose the skin to tanning by the sun. Most specialists are convinced that excessive exposure to the sun will damage the texture of the skin and, in older people, perhaps set up processes which, in the long run, are quite harmful.

In many of the deficiency diseases,

such as pellagra, changes in the skin are prominent. We know that the vitamins have a definite relationship to the skin. There are six conditions affecting the skin which are also definitely related to vitamin deficiencies. Practically all the vitamins have been offered at one time or another for specific effects for ordinary acne with pimples and blackheads. Actually, however, the use of the vitamins for the control of pimples and blackheads has not been proved to be especially beneficial. In some instances improved activity of the bowels brought about by the taking of yeast or the vitamin B complex has been found to be of some help to the skin. This, however, is not a specific vitamin action.

A deficiency of vitamin B_2 (called riboflavin) has been definitely related to the appearance of blisters and cracking at the corner of the mouth. If it can be shown in such a case that there is a deficiency of riboflavin in the diet or if it can be shown that the riboflavin is not absorbed, the use of the riboflavin may be helpful. There are, however, many cases of blistering and cracking at the corner of the mouth in which the giving of extra riboflavin does not bring about a cure.

It has been well established that a deficiency of vitamin C will produce scurvy with hemorrhages in the gums and in the skin. The claim has been made that excessively large doses of vitamin D will help patients with psoriasis. However, careful testing of great numbers of patients indicates that there are many in whom this form of treatment has not been helpful. A well-established deficiency of vitamin A will be associated with a dryness of the skin and hair. However, the taking of excessive doses of vitamin A does not seem to benefit most people who complain of excessive dryness of the skin and hair.

This all adds up to the explanation that the human body is a highly complex mechanism and that many different factors may be involved in the conditions described, so that the mere addition of one vitamin or of several vitamins may not bring about improvement.

Many people feel that all of their skin troubles are due to something that they ate. There is hardly a skin disease that has not at one time or another been treated by a diet of one kind or another. In the majority of instances, however, attempts to control a skin disease by diet alone are not satisfactory. An examination of the books on nutrition shows that there is no single diet that is specific for any single inflammation of the skin. This does not mean that dieting is without value; it means rather that many diseases of the skin that are said to be due to foods are not related to food at all. The skin diseases that with certainty are related to diet are those like urticaria and forms of eczema, which represent a sensitivity of the body to certain proteins.

All sorts of diets have been tried for pimples and blackheads including diets without meat, diets without sugar, and diets without fats. At present most specialists agree that a low fat diet is useful because there is an overactivity of the glands in the skin that secrete oils. Such a diet is said to be helpful, but, again, there are many of these cases in which the adoption of a low fat diet is not necessarily associated with a cure. Here again the constitution of the body and particularly its glandular mechanism is such that the condition cannot be controlled by diet alone. One fact is certain: the skin, like every other tissue of the body, needs to be nourished by proper amounts of all of the essential substances. A well-balanced diet is helpful in every disease.

THE SKIN IN WINTER—In winter the cold slows down the circulation of blood in the skin and as a result there is a lessened amount of secretion of oil from the skin. This failure to keep the skin well lubricated results in dryness, irritation, and cracking. Incidentally, the extreme dry heat of most modern apartments and homes merely intensifies the exposure of the skin to dry heat.

Next most serious are the sudden changes of temperature that are inevitable when you leave your home or your office to go outdoors and submit yourself to cold and wind. People who have skin diseases such as psoriasis, eczema, inflammations of the skin, and chilblains discover frequently that the skin gets much worse during the winter. People who work a great deal with the hands are more likely to have cracked and chapped skin and to become secondarily infected. The modern habit of girls of going out in cold weather without stockings has been reported to bring about inflammations and difficulties with the skin in winter.

Fortunately there are available today a great variety of treatments for chapping of the skin and for the lack of a sufficient amount of lubrication. Any of the widely advertised hand lotions will be useful if properly used during the winter months.

Certainly the ears, the cheeks, and the nose should be protected against frostbite. The wearing of babushkas or scarfs is a great help in this direction. When the hands are washed in winter, they should be thoroughly dried and treated with a suitable hand lotion or with a powder.

One must be sure that clothing is warm but not so tight as to restrict the circulation of the blood. This is an added factor of danger to the skin in winter.

SLEEP Sancho Panza, who accompanied Don Quixote on his travels, is famous for one of his most simple sayings: "God bless the man who first invented sleep." Most people know that sleep is necessary for health. People differ in sleep requirements. One investigator deprived himself for 115 hours, but all of the evidence shows that the longer a person goes without sleep the less he is able to carry on any kind of important activity and the less reliable to accept any kind of responsibility.

Fortunately sleep is rest, no matter whether it is taken in large or small doses. If one has difficulty in getting enough sleep at night, a nap of even just a few minutes is helpful. The difficulty with naps is that they tend to become prolonged. A number of people have invented technics for controlling the length of a nap. One New York captain

of industry always took his nap with a bunch of keys in his hand. When his sleep became sufficiently sound, relaxation of the hand resulted in dropping the keys; the keys would jangle, and he would wake up.

An important journalist takes his nap immediately after lunch each day in a barbershop. He has become accustomed to fall asleep the moment he gets into the chair for his shave, and he awakens when the shave is completed.

A number of people insist that they cannot sleep at night if they sleep at all during the day. However, the physiologists say there is no essential or inherent inappropriateness in reversing the time of sleep. Night watchmen, newspaper workers, railroad men, factory men on night shifts, and a great many others became accustomed during the period of accelerated war industry to sleeping in the day and working at night. Just as soon as daytime sleep became sufficiently established as a habit, they obtained adequate rest from their sleep during this period.

Some people find it especially difficult to sleep while traveling. For a long time there was a superstition that one sleeps better with the head toward the north. Others insist that they sleep better with the head toward the east. It should not make the slightest difference whether you sleep with your head toward the north, south, east, or west, provided you do not have in your mind the continual question of whether the position in which you lie is the most healthful one. In most European countries passengers always ride sidewise in sleeping cars, and in many of our modern American sleeping cars the sidewise position has been adopted.

Much of the ability to sleep while riding in trains depends on the ventilation, which has been continuously improved, on the comfort of the mattress, the number of pillows, and a good many other small factors which do or do not duplicate the sleeping conditions at home. One may become a nuisance to the porter by insisting on a duplication of home habits of sleep as much as possible when traveling, but, nuisance or not, it is well to attempt such duplication if sleep is to be sound and comfortable.

How Long Can You Go without Sleep?—The first experimental study of the ability of human beings to get along without sleep was made by two investigators in 1896. They kept three young men awake for from 88 to 90 hours and reported that there was no significant change except a decrease in reaction time, slower motor performance, failures to memorize, and a slight loss of ability to perceive.

Since that time studies have been made on other people who have gone without sleep for periods like 65 hours. Not long ago some experts at the University of Chicago tested thirty-five students who were willing to try the experiment. They found that sleepiness comes in waves, with the greatest difficulty from three to six in the morning. When sleepiness occurs, there is increased difficulty in writing, reading, and studying. The eyes feel and become tired. Sometimes one begins to see double. The effect on the emotions is to make the individual resentful and irritable.

Dr. Kleitman, who made these studies, concluded that the effects of loss of sleep are to produce a general disturbance of the body and that greatly increased amounts of effort are demanded for any performance when there is loss of sleep for periods longer than 24 hours.

Investigators at the University of Georgia have studied the effects of loss of sleep for 100 consecutive hours, utilizing a number of volunteers. They found, too, that sleepiness comes in waves and that people who have been going without sleep feel quite wide-awake sometime after breakfast and early in the evening.

After 48 hours without sleep it is difficult to read. Eventually one finds it difficult to maintain balance and may stagger. Some people suffer severe headaches. Many people see flashes of light. Some who go without sleep have the feeling of a band pressing on the head.

The longer one goes without sleep the less becomes the ability to be certain as to one's location or destination when walking.

The irritability of one man who tried to do without sleep became so great that he reported that he felt like fighting all the time. A girl who took part in the experiment began hearing voices which sounded far away. Another girl constantly counted the people to see if everybody was there and found one missing all the time; this person was herself.

Especially interesting also was the report as to how long it takes to recover after one goes 100 hours without sleep. Some made up their sleep with about half the sleep that they had lost. One man reported that he did not feel recovered until he had had extra sleep for two weeks. The smallest and least athletic man recovered in 57 per cent of the time lost, but the most powerful made recovery in 86 per cent of the lost time. The women came through the experiment as well as or better than the men. The smaller and lighter individual suffered the least; the stronger and more athletic men suffered the most.

Everyone likes to have a good night's sleep.

Inadequate feeding, colic, hunger, thirst, temperature of the room, lights, and noise are likely to interfere with a baby's sleep. If these obstacles are eliminated, it will be found that babies like to sleep. Many authorities hold that babies cannot get too much sleep. Yet even among babies there are variations.

Doctors agree that methods of putting children to sleep artificially by means of monotonous sensations are not desirable. This includes rocking of babies in cradles or in the arms, and singing of monotonous lullabies. The latter method is in the nature of hypnotism.

Investigators have found that young children will get enough sleep almost regardless of direction by their parents. Over a long period of time each child finds the normal amount of sleep that he needs, provided of course he is a healthful child.

Authorities are convinced that it does not make much difference what hour a child goes to bed, except that he must get enough sleep. One expert feels that children are put to bed early in the evening not for their own benefit but for the parents to be able to arrange their evening as freely as possible. Thus the baby is put to bed early more to get him out of the way than to give him enough sleep.

Another expert insists that children ought to go to bed later in the winter so they will not wake up in the dark. These views may be revolutionary, but there seems to be a certain amount of truth behind them.

There is a great deal of agitation about the problem of a daytime nap for older children. This is another factor that cannot be regulated by any sort of an absolute law.

Some experts recommend one to two hours a day in bed for children from the ages of six to thirteen. Afternoon naps should be encouraged until they seem to delay the onset of sleep in the evening.

Anything that causes a child to remain awake after going to bed is undesirable. It is a bad habit to put a child to bed and then to have him play, read, look at pictures, or do anything else that keeps him from associating going to bed with going to sleep. This may set up habits which persist in later life and which may bring about insomnia in the adult.

Experts who have studied sleep in children claim that heavy evening meals have a disturbing effect on children as have mental work and exciting games in the evening, certain types of motion pictures, and serious emotional states.

The question as to how long an adult ought to sleep has never been satisfactorily answered, and probably never will be, because of the differences in human beings.

It is hard to study the matter because many people get enough sleep and complain that they do not rest; others do not get enough sleep and say nothing about it. Some people sleep too long.

Experts say that oversleeping is just as bad as overeating.

The mental aspects of sleep have been insufficiently studied. Some people have a good night's sleep and still wake up moody and mean. Others will sleep only five or six hours and awaken in the best of spirits, quite refreshed.

There has been some study of the optimum time for going to bed. One expert says that an hour before midnight is worth two after midnight.

Another expert says that there are two types of sleepers. One is tired in the evening, quickly falls asleep, soon reaches the greatest depth of sleep, and wakes up refreshed and well rested. The other is alert in the evening, does not fall asleep easily, reaches the greatest depth of sleep during the early hours of the morning, and wakes up feeling tired.

Some people have two phases of sleep. They awaken from a first phase but are not quite rested. After lying awake for a brief time they fall asleep again and awaken shortly quite refreshed.

Any effort that upsets the routine of daily life may bring about a restless night. The eating of foods to which people are sensitive or which they find difficult to digest may result in restless sleep. Authorities have found that an empty stomach is irritable and that any light snack taken around bedtime tends to enhance restful sleep. Yet some people are restless if they eat or drink anything at all before going to bed.

City dwellers take great pains in purchasing sleeping equipment. It is possible not only to get mattresses which are especially designed for good sleep, but also eyeshades to keep out the light, ear stops to keep out noise, and many special kinds of pillows.

A large portion of mankind sleeps on bedsprings on the ground, sometimes only on mats, sometimes on the bare floor or soil.

These people seem, once they have established the habit, to sleep as well as those who use a hard mattress, a soft mattress, a spring mattress, or a solid mattress.

Specialists in orthopedic surgery say

certain forms of mattress prevent spinal curves by placing stress on the bones of the spine.

The argument has been made that a sag in the middle of the bed is bad for good sleep. A cat sleeps curled up, the Japanese sleep on the ground and do not make it conform to the curves of their bodies, and sailors who sleep in sagging hammocks sleep quite soundly.

The sagging of a mattress and bedsprings may discourage frequent changes in position of the sleeper once he has become used to that particular mattress and spring. Most of these matters seem to be questions of individual likes and dislikes.

This is true also of bedcovers. Some people sleep better on cool nights with a full covering of quilts and blankets. Others sleep better when they use no covers. There are some people who cannot sleep well unless they wear gowns or pajamas; others insist the only way they can sleep well is "in the raw."

A few sleepers insist the only way to sleep comfortably is with the face and stomach down. Others never feel well unless they are lying on their backs.

Before there was suitable indoor heating, it was customary to use a bed warmer. Some people prefer an ice-cold bed. They say they fall asleep quicker as they must lie still in order to warm up the part of the bed with which they are in contact.

As early as 1834 an expert found that a person changes his sleeping positions frequently during the night. With the development of the motion picture and suitable timing devices, studies have been made which establish definitely the fact that no normal person sleeps "like a log," but that all of us change our positions frequently during sleeping hours.

If we remain too long in one position, there is likely to be a feeling of discomfort and stiffness which disturbs sleep. This happens particularly with people who are exceedingly tired when they go to bed or with people who have taken enough alcoholic liquor to make them semiconscious.

It is desirable to have the air in the room sufficiently cool because too much warmth and humidity interfere with sleep. It is well to have the air mildly in motion, but a draft will interfere with sleep.

A question of more importance is whether everyone should sleep alone or whether the bed should be shared by two people. Apparently some people sleep better double and others single. This indicates that habits are of the utmost importance in relationship to sound sleep.

Some people insist that exercise before going to bed makes them rest better. Some practice breathing exercises before an open window, others practice complete relaxation. These factors again indicate that there is no absolute rule for every person and that the establishment of a good routine is of the utmost importance.

The psychology of falling asleep has brought on a number of formulas like the counting of sheep. Other rituals suggested include the repetition of prayers, the naming of large numbers of animals or objects in certain classifications (i.e., everything made of wood, every animal that walks on four feet), or any other routine and monotonous task.

One psychologist suggests that all one has to do is to paint a large imaginary figure 3 on an imaginary wall by means of an imaginary brush and a can of imaginary white paint. He says that anybody who has painted three of these 3s will shortly find it impossible to stay awake. You can easily imagine why.

Practically all that has been really learned about the hygiene of sleep is that the adaptation of the body to a regular rhythm of sleeping and wakefulness in the 24-hour cycle of day and night is an individual affair; that it depends on the mind to a large extent for its establishment and maintenance; and that the development of regular habits with respect to the activities of the waking hours, as well as those of sleep, is most significant in falling asleep promptly and in sleeping restfully.

Sleep, as a factor in the development of the child, was given special consideration in a recent survey of the growth and development of the child, made under the auspices of the White House Conference on Child Health and Protection.

Even though numerous physiologists throughout the world have studied the phenomena of sleep, it has not been possible to determine satisfactorily just why we go to sleep, why we remain asleep, or why we awaken. There are numerous theories, however, all of which have a fair amount of reason behind them.

Most of these theories are based on the idea that fatigue gradually develops in the body due to action of the nerves and muscles and that as a result chemical changes occur which lead to the development of sleep. During sleep the reverse process goes on and when fatigue is overcome the body awakens.

However, it must be pointed out that the hours of waking and of sleeping are usually rhythmical and associated in periodicity with the movements of the planet on which we live.

There is usually a drop in the blood pressure during sleep. The sleep becomes more intense during the first hour and then gradually lessens. Young children tend to sleep more quietly than older children, but there are also differences in the sexes, the time of the year, and other factors.

In one series of scientific investigations it was found that there was a slight tendency to sleep less at night among children who had taken a long nap during the day, but at the same time that children who took no nap at all or who took only a nap for a few minutes had a definite reduction in the total number of hours of sleep in the 24 hours; that is to say, sleeping at night does not compensate for the loss of the nap during the day.

Up to four years of age a nap taken in the daytime rarely interferes with sleep at night. However, after four years of age children as a rule should not be allowed to sleep more than one and a half hours during the day because this will tend to interfere with going to sleep at night.

The authorities believe that children up to the seventh or eighth year should sleep 12 hours daily and at the sixteenth year 9 hours.

If good sleeping habits are established early in life, they tend to persist. It is recognized, however, that there is considerable individual variation in requirements of sleep and that there is not yet sufficient scientific knowledge to make absolute rules.

Newborn babies sleep most of the time except as the demands of nature serve to stimulate and awaken them. The desire for food, pain in the digestive tract, sudden noises or flashes of light, or sudden changes in the temperature of the body will awaken the baby.

If, therefore, the child is kept warm, is placed in the crib in such a manner as to avoid muscular activity, if the stomach is kept free from discomfort by proper feeding, if the clothing is not too tight and the room not too warm, the child will probably sleep well. However, children can be taught to disregard slight noises, slight changes in lighting, the position of the bed, and similar external factors to which it is possible to become accustomed.

The one interference that is serious is irregularity in the hour of going to sleep. The child is therefore best put to bed at a regular hour and if left alone will probably go to sleep by himself.

Psychologists recommend that the attitude of children toward sleep should always be pleasant. They should not be punished just at bedtime.

There must be no possible suggestion that will induce fear connected with the dark or with being left alone. Adults should not discuss before children their own difficulties in sleeping. Too much excitement just before bedtime is likely to make sleep difficult.

For this reason it is extremely unfortunate that many modern radio programs planned for children are exciting mystery stories or detective stories full of warfare, shooting, explosions, and murders rather than the type of material that will lead to a rested mind.

Authorities suggest that the infant, from birth on, be accustomed to sleep in a room by himself. But he should not be so secluded as to have artificial conditions develop which are not likely to be followed later in life; by this is meant complete absence of all noise or the daily activities of life.

SLEEP OF THE CHILD—People spend approximately a third of their time in sleeping, which naturally results in sleep being one of the most important and interesting subjects for human discussion. A research was devoted to the sleep habits of preschool children. In this study 29 boys and 29 girls were included and the investigators made a most meticulous record of their daily lives including eating, speaking, eliminating, learning, which are quite normal in human conduct, and also thumb and finger sucking, nail biting, nose picking, handling of the sex organs, patterns of sleep, the duration of sleep, restlessness and similar characteristics. Specific inquiries were made as to anxiety, fears, and dreams. This was not the first research done on the subject of sleep, since it has interested the medical profession for many years.

Children two or three years old sleep about twelve and a half hours out of twenty-four and those three to five years old sleep from eleven to twelve hours. However, as great variations were found as to the amount of sleep required by different boys and girls as can be found among adults. Some parents have rigid standards about hours of sleep and even try to force children to sleep by threatening not to love them any more. Some parents give children candy to get them to sleep. Obviously these are also abnormal reactions.

Among the children studied, some had their own rooms and slept alone, some slept in a room with a nurse, some slept with another child in the room, frequently a baby, and one child slept in a room with his mother, who happened to be a divorcee. Frequently the presence of another person in the room makes a great deal of difference in falling asleep and in the duration of sleep. Children vary greatly in the length of time required to fall asleep. Some fall asleep immediately and others take anywhere from a few minutes to half an hour to fall asleep. One child slept usually ten hours but took two hours to fall asleep. Many children are restless during sleep, moving around in the bed, removing the covers, getting up, crying, and in some instances almost invariably going to the bed of the mother. Early attitudes toward parents are observed in that some boys consistently went to the mother's bed while one girl consistently went to her father's bed during periods of restlessness. One boy went to a doll's bed or a nurse's bed when his sister did not let him sleep in her bed.

Parents develop all sorts of patterns toward getting the child to go to sleep. Some play with the child, others tell stories, and some cuddle and rock the child to sleep. Some children reported that they were being spanked and being locked in their rooms and told to go to sleep. The majority of children sleep face down or on their backs. Children who suck their thumbs are usually those who sleep face down. Most school children, even including those who sucked their thumbs, sleep on their side. Among the children who were restless at night, one third were also bed-wetters. Out of the whole study comes the conclusion that most parents are too rigid about children's sleep and will do much better by less strictness. Many a sleep problem was developed by parents putting too much attention on the number of hours of sleep that had to be obtained daily at all costs. When the means selected by parents to force children to sleep are wrong, the child tends to develop methods of deceiving the parents and that may give him a sense of guilt. When a child develops an elaborate ritual about going to sleep, the pattern is usually developed to overcome a sense of anxiety.

SLEEP PRODUCERS—Among the greatest blessings of mankind are those drugs and preparations which either completely remove consciousness from the human being or temporarily inhibit it so that the human being becomes insensible to pain or to outside stimuli. The ancient Arabs and Egyptians were familiar with the drugs that would produce sleep or temporary unconsciousness. Only with the coming of modern centuries, however, have we been able to develop a great variety of such drugs and preparations, so that they vary in their strength from those which act for a few moments only and which produce slight degrees of insensibility to those which may produce complete unconsciousness for long periods of time.

All such drugs are poisons if taken in large quantities. They should, therefore, be used with the utmost caution, preferably never except under the advice of a physician. In many places druggists are not permitted to sell such preparations to anyone without a doctor's prescription. If they have been prescribed by the doctor for use according to his directions, they should always be kept safely so as to avoid any possibility of error in their use.

BROMIDES—Among the older sleep producers are the bromides, which are now available in many forms. They are used chiefly to quiet the spasms and convulsions associated with epilepsy, but the dose and intervals of taking them must always be regulated by the doctor. Bromides used to be the chief ingredients of patent medicines sold for epilepsy. Today most patent medicines sold for epilepsy contain some derivative of barbituric acid. These vary in their strength or toxicity and poisoning character.

NOT TO BE KEPT IN FAMILY MEDICINE CHEST!—The narcotic preparations should never be used by anyone without a doctor's prescription. Any drug that has to be administered with a hypodermic syringe should not be kept in the average family medicine chest. There are some persons with diabetes who have been taught by the doctors to inject themselves with insulin. Even these people should always keep their syringe outfits separate from the family medicine chest.

SLEEPLESSNESS See *Insomnia.*

SMALLPOX Most of the civilized countries of the world now control smallpox by isolation, quarantine, and vaccination. In the United States we still have more smallpox than any other civilized country in the world except British India. In thirteen of our states, with a population of more than 42,-000,000, vaccination is compulsory. In these thirteen states there are each year about 230 cases of smallpox or 1 case for every 200,000 people. In fourteen states every town is permitted to decide for itself whether or not its citizens ought to be vaccinated against smallpox. In these fourteen states the population reaches more than 38,000,000 people, and in these states there are more than 1300 cases of smallpox every year, or 7 cases of smallpox for every 200,000 people. Now there are still twenty-two other states, including the District of Columbia, in which vaccination is not compulsory in any form. In these states there are 44,000,000 people who have more than 6000 cases of smallpox every year. They have 28 cases for every 200,000 people.

Smallpox is a foul disease. Once it was so frequent that the rare person in any community was the one without scars on his face from this disease. Now it is rare to see a person with scars of smallpox. They are a manifestation of ignorance or stupidity either on the part of the person concerned or on the part of those responsible for him.

In the typical case of smallpox chills, high temperature, vomiting, aches, and pains begin ten to fourteen days after exposure. The characteristic eruption appears about fourteen days after exposure. It consists of blisters which become filled with pus. In some cases the infection is so severe that hemorrhages occur.

How pitiful that there should still be instances in which this condition is permitted to occur to a child who is unable to protect himself. Practically every school in the United States that is conducted along scientific lines now requires that a child bring with him on his first day of school a certificate that he has had a recent and satisfactory vaccination against smallpox. Vaccination against smallpox is as safe a procedure as is known to medicine. Complications are rare when the vaccination is properly performed. The protection is so certain that neglect of this scientific procedure represents the height of foolhardiness.

While this procedure brings about immunity in the vast majority of cases, there are a few instances in which repeated vaccination may be necessary to build up immunity. This means not only that a person should be vaccinated at certain definite periods of life but also that he should be revaccinated whenever there is the possibility of being brought into contact with smallpox. The fact that smallpox is now so rare has made many people neglectful or evasive of vaccination.

The recent experiences in Great Britain, where there were outbreaks of smallpox both in civil communities and in troops, indicate the desirability of keeping the danger constantly in mind. Indeed one British physician says that the situation there in relation to smallpox is like the situation that existed in foreign affairs among the democratic nations in 1933 when the prophets kept on saying that there was danger ahead and that we ought to be preparing whereas the stupid and the conscientious objectors kept on insisting on "peace in our time."

SMELL   Odors are sometimes pleasant and sometimes disagreeable. Usually the sense of pleasure is associated with some previous experience; likewise the sense of displeasure. The smell of roses is more pleasant than that of asafetida. One man who smelled camphor immediately associated it with the door of the wardrobe and was then reminded that he had been placed in a closet in which were clothes that had been treated with camphor as a moth preventive over thirty years previously. A girl who smelled cedarwood oil associated it with a summer evening on the Norwegian coast and with the cigar box in which her mother had kept the family funds. A woman who smelled cedarwood oil thought about spring cleaning and the use of the mop. A Scotchman who smelled asafetida thought of a streetcar in Edinburgh and it was discovered that these cars were formerly lighted by acetylene gas which gave off a similar odor.

The odors of the human body vary with different races, although some people insist that the odor is wholly a matter of cleanliness. An ethnologist has said that Indians smell of acetylene, Australians of phosphorus; the Chinese are said to have a musty odor and the Negro an odor slightly suggesting ammonia.

Once doctors thought that certain diseases had a definite smell associated with them, particularly diphtheria and diabetes. It is now recognized that the odor of diphtheria is the odor of infection in the throat which has injured the tissues. The odor of diabetes is the sweet acetone odor associated with acidosis.

In some people the sense of smell is greatly deficient; in others it is exceedingly sensitive. Usually the sense of sight dominates by far the sense of smell, so that even when the sense of smell is wholly lost, life is not greatly affected except by such pleasures as come from perfumes.

In testing sensitivity to smell, certain well-defined odors are used. An extremely sensitive person can detect camphor in a solution of 1:400,000; musk in a solution of 1:30,000,000; and vanilla in a concentration of 1:10,000,000. Apparently the strongest odor is that of the substance called mercaptan. This can be detected when 1/23,000,000th of a milligram is present in a quart of water.

SNEEZING   A sneeze is elicited by irritation of the mucous membrane of the nose. The impulses responsible for a sneeze are set up by the irritation of the nerve endings of the trigeminal nerves and probably also by the stimulation of the nerves that are concerned with detecting odors. A sneeze usually begins, as does a cough, with the taking of a deep breath and the violent expulsion of the air. The deeper the breath taken the longer and louder will be the sneeze.

Experts, using flash photography, have studied the effects of the sneeze on contamination of the surrounding air. When you sneeze, most of the droplets that are expelled come from the mouth but there is also a large discharge of material from the nose. The material carried from the nose is carried forward horizontally by the blast from the mouth. The size of the droplets varies greatly. When the mouth is open, the droplets are larger; when the sneezing is done with the mouth closed or partially closed, the droplets are smaller.

A British bacteriologist exposed some culture plates before a healthy sneezer at a distance of three feet from the nose. Then the germs deposited on the culture plate were counted after they had grown. The investigators counted 19,000 different colonies, which would mean that a least 19,000 different droplets must have been projected at least three feet.

The droplets with the germs that they carry will hang in the air for some time. After a man sneezed in a dry, dust-free room, some plates were put out twenty minutes later. Some 493 germ colonies grew on these plates.

Since it is known that coughs and sneezes spread diseases, various means have been sought to control such contamination. The wearing of a gauze mask helps but the mask becomes messy after there have been many sneezes through it. A large handkerchief would prevent the escape of droplets almost entirely but the bits of flimsy linen used by most women permit droplets to escape around it. Masks of cellulose acetate which are used sometimes now in surgeries apparently trap everything but they are often warm and uncomfortable. The placing of a hand to the mouth and nose will deflect the spray but it contaminates the hand, after which everything in the neighborhood of the hand may become contaminated. One Britisher suggested that the best way to sneeze is from a short distance directly into a coal fire or a grate fire.

During the great influenza epidemic of 1918 the wearing of gauze masks was popular. It was then found that a thin gauze mask is an inefficient filter. A six-layer gauze mask will filter away 97 per cent of the germs. Laundering tends to destroy the ability of the mask as a filter of germs.

SNORING Somehow the habit of snoring in sleep is usually greeted with a good deal of ridicule and embarrassment. Whenever the question arises in any home, the father and mother will affirm positively that each of them individually never snores, yet each is likely to affirm with equal glee that the other snores to the high heavens.

Old people are likely to say—with a good deal of irritation over the accusation—that they not only do not snore but never did snore. Now practically everyone under certain circumstances may snore, because the conditions that cause snoring may occur at one time or another in every person.

The actual noises made by the snorer are due to intermittent passage of air at places in the nose and throat where there may be partial obstruction to the passage. What are the conditions that may bring about such obstruction?

First, there may occur during sleep a partial relaxation of the muscles holding the vocal cords, so that they fall more or less closely together and thus interfere with the passage of air.

Second, when a person in deep sleep or one who is unconscious lies on his back, the tongue may fall back and partially close the opening through which the air passes.

Third, when a person lies on his back, the muscles controlling the soft palate may fail to hold it, so that it falls against the hard palate and obstructs the passage of air up through the nose.

Fourth, because of irritation or inflammation mucus may collect in the nose or in the passages behind the nose.

Fifth, the muscles associated with the throat and nose may be abnormally tense and thus create interference to the passing of air.

Sixth, if the nose is blocked and the lips are held rather close to the air, a whistling sound occurs as the air passes out.

Many people can produce snoring sounds during their waking hours by trying any or all of the muscle arrangements that have been mentioned. This, however, is not an especially desirable performance because snoring sounds are seldom pleasant.

It is interesting to realize that snoring seldom disturbs the soundness of the sleep of the snorer himself. Even though he is sensitive to noise while asleep, his own noises do not wake him up.

The most that we can do to prevent snoring is to make sure there are no obstructions in the nose and throat. Then snoring is less liable to occur if the person goes to sleep and stays asleep on either the side or the abdomen instead of on the back.

SODIUM BICARBONATE The common name for this drug is baking soda. Its chief uses are to overcome excess acidity of the juices of the stomach and excess acidity of the body generally. In cases of acidosis large doses of baking soda are usually given by mouth. The drug is also used occasionally as a mild alkaline wash. Baking soda baths are sometimes used to overcome itching.

SOMNAMBULISM This term comes from two Greek words meaning sleep and walk. Therefore any person who habitually walks in his sleep is known as a somnambulist. There are many different causes for this condition. In practically every instance, however, the condition is due to stimulation of the brain by thoughts that are carried over from the waking period into the sleeping state. Proper mental hygiene and attention to the stimuli which may disturb sleep are helpful in the control of this condition.

SPASMS A spasm is any sudden contraction of a muscle that occurs without any desire or wish on the part of the person affected. Almost anybody can at one cime or another have a muscle spasm. Sudden chilling of the body after swimming may bring about spasm of the muscles. Whenever the circulation of the blood in any part of the body is greatly diminished, sudden involuntary contractions of the muscles may occur. Of this type is the muscle spasm of the calf of the leg that is called intermittent claudication. This may be so severe as to bring about pain and inability to walk. If the person will rest for a few minutes or more, he finds that he is able to walk again. The spasm of the muscle relaxes and the circulation improves.

Difficulties in the nervous system, as for instance the death of a nerve cell in the interior portion of the spinal cord, may result in paralysis of the muscles with spasm of the opposing muscles.

Spasms are not to be confused with what are called tics. Tics occur as a result of habit. Among the most common of all spasms are those that affect the face. This is particularly due to the fact that the muscles of the face are easily movable. They are affected easily by many different emotions or activities. Spasms of the face may be sudden and pass so quickly that they go unnoticed. Sometimes they affect only the little muscles around the eye. Sometimes when the eye becomes especially tired the eyelids will develop a spasm or twitching which is known as blepharospasm.

The habit spasms of children are not to be confused with chorea, or St. Vitus' dance, which is a rheumatic disorder. The movements of habit spasms differ from those of chorea by being quicker and always being repeated in the same way. The movements of chorea are irregular and variable.

Whenever a spasm of the muscle occurs, it needs investigation with a view to removing the cause. If the cause is in a condition affecting the nerves, medical or surgical treatment may be required. In some instances the only way to stop a spasm is to inject various substances around the nerves of the area involved.

Sometimes the spasms in children occur in association with distress, such as fear of punishment. These children do well with encouragement and pleasantness. Constant faultfinding makes them worse.

SPEECH About the most exciting time in an average family is the moment when the new baby begins to talk. In the first few months of life babies make sounds which have little significance to those who hear them but which must be a source of satisfaction to the baby; otherwise the baby would not spend so much time working at it.

The first sounds that a baby makes are variations of the sounds of *a* and *u*. Then the consonants *m*, *p*, and *b* are added to these vowels. These are the

sounds that can be made with the lips closed. After the baby is three months old he will combine these sounds so that *umm, da, ma* and *goo* are formed. When he puts two *da's* together, the father is flattered. When he puts two *wah's* together, the mother insists that the baby wants water. Soon the baby begins to see that there is value in the sounds he makes. People bring things. Then the baby imitates adult sounds and thus learns to speak. As soon as possible the baby makes noises that sound like words and people begin praising and encouraging him. This causes the baby to try to imitate himself and he becomes proud of his ability. This encouragement also helps him to speak.

A baby can probably understand a number of words before he can say any of them. A bright baby will speak his first word about the time he is eight or nine months old. Almost any baby can be expected to say something about the time he reaches the tenth or twelfth month. Some babies know one or two

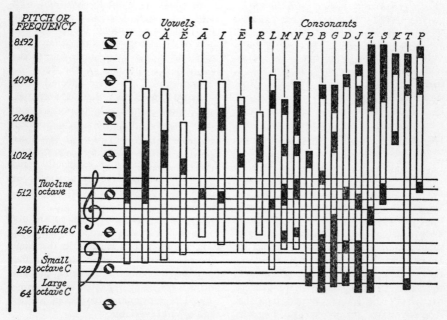

Musical scale indicating pitch or wave frequency of various sounds used in speaking

words by the time they are a year old. The ability to combine words in phrases and sentences comes usually between the time the child is one and a half to two years old. The vocabulary grows almost daily. By the time the child is seven years old, he is probably familiar with about 3000 words. However, the number of words that a child can use varies with his intelligence. In general smart children talk earlier and dull children talk later than the average. The development of speech is one of the methods that experts use for measuring intelligence.

Speech is the chief characteristic by which we distinguish men from animals. Twenty-five or thirty years ago the country was well covered with elocution teachers. Many little boys and girls were taught to recite poetry with gestures. Nowadays less attention is paid to such recitation and much more attention is paid to simple talking for purposes of living.

Children learn speech largely through imitation. Many a child is ruined as to his speech habits by the bad speaking habits of his older brothers and sisters, his mother and father, and his playmates. When children enter kindergarten, the teachers classify them according to their ability to express themselves. Statistics show that about 10 per cent of people have speech defects. At least 1,500,000 children stutter and stammer. Many others just have bad speaking habits.

One writer has coined the phrase "lip laziness" to describe people who do not trouble to talk correctly. The ability to speak distinctly requires a certain amount of attention to the formation of sounds exactly as ability to swing a baseball bat or a golf club requires mental and physical co-ordination.

When young children are learning to speak, they may be made to realize the importance of speaking correctly by suitable rewards for correct speech. The words used by a small child are not nearly so important as the manner in which the words are spoken. Children who live in homes in which the parents speak distinctly and use correct words will, if they have ordinary intelligence, learn to use the same words in the same way.

Here are seven rules which parents should follow in developing habits of good speech in their children.

1. Do not correct the child's pronunciation or enunciation. Applaud that which is right. Do not stress that which is wrong.

2. Do not imitate the child's baby talk. When you say "dravy" for "gravy" and "wed" for "red," simply because the baby talks that way, you confirm him in his difficulty. But do not correct him too severely. If you keep on talking English, he will talk it as soon as he can.

3. Never talk down to babies and little children.

4. Do not nag, coax, or raise your voice in an effort to get the baby to talk. Speech will come naturally.

5. If the baby's uncle and aunt stammer, or if you stammer yourself, give the baby a chance to learn how to talk from someone else. Children will imitate.

6. Give the child a chance to talk, and listen to him when he talks. This will encourage him.

7. Tell the child to listen. Do not ignore him, but include him whenever possible in the conversation.

SPINA BIFIDA In 1 out of every 1000 childbirths the infant comes into the world not quite properly grown together, at least as far as the lower portion of the spine is concerned. In most instances the difficulty is simply a failure of the coverings of the spinal cord to grow together. In some instances, however, one or more of the bones of the spine may be lacking. In such instances there may be a hernia or projection of the coverings of the spinal cord to the exterior. This makes a large sac or balloon filled with fluid. The condition is serious because it exposes a part of the nervous system directly to the exterior.

Occasionally a failure of the spinal

tissues to grow together properly is associated with a collection of fluid inside the skull and enlargement of the bones of the skull occurs to make room for the fluid. This condition is called hydrocephalus, meaning water on the brain. Such people have tiny bodies and large heads.

If nothing is done for a child with spina bifida, there occurs such pressure and stretching of the nerves of the spinal cord that they do not function satisfactorily. If the condition is in the lower part of the spine and damage to that part of the spine occurs, the child will suffer with paralysis, including inability to control the motions of the bowels and bladder. There may be ulcers on the legs due to the fact that certain portions of the skin do not have a satisfactory nerve supply.

Certainly a child with this deformity should be taken to a doctor as soon as possible, so that the doctor may study the condition to see what is the most that can be done. In some instances a simple surgical operation to eliminate the protrusion of the coverings of the spinal cord and to repair the sac will yield a satisfactory result. This type of surgery is called reconstructive or plastic surgery. At least one half of the babies born with this deformity can be helped by surgery. Everything possible should be done to see that help is given to them early, since cure is much more likely when help is given early.

SPINAL CURVATURE   The spine sometimes curves to one side or another. To this the scientific name of scoliosis is given. This may be a symptom or a sequel to many different diseases but often seems to be a condition of the spine itself. Occasionally it results from an insufficiency of the muscles and ligaments that hold the bones in place. Sometimes it occurs from the permanent adoption of a faulty posture. In still other instances the bones themselves are at fault and a breakdown in the structure of a bone allows other tissues to collapse.

In the early stages of twisting of the spine due to bad posture there will not be found any definite changes in the tissues of the spine. If, however, the condition is not corrected, such changes do occur, and when the tissues have changed, the condition is more or less permanent.

Naturally, with the twisting of the spine, changes in the position of the organs occur. The lung may be compressed more on one side than on another. Often there is an absence of important symptoms except for the appearance, so that a child with a twisted spine is first brought to the doctor because of the bad posture. Eventually pain will develop because of pressure of the ribs on the thighbone or pressure on various nerves. In such cases it is customary to examine the child and to make certain of the alignment of the spine. The child should be examined with the body fully exposed. The outline of the back is examined both with the child trying to stand erect and with relaxation in the habitual position. Sometimes a plumb line is used to find out just how straight the spine really is.

Every parent should watch carefully the postural development of a child, and everything possible should be done to avoid faulty attitudes. Sometimes gymnastic treatment and exercise will correct bad posture and encourage the strength of the muscles necessary to hold the spine in proper position. In serious cases an orthopedic surgeon gives help by the use of braces and supports, sometimes even by a plaster cast. However, it is considered to be unwise to use spinal supports until everything possible has been accomplished by suitable exercises and training.

SPINAL FRACTURE   A broken back used to be considered about as serious an injury as could occur to a human being. In those days the only way to be certain that anyone had a broken back was the presence of paralysis of certain portions of the body due to injury to the nervous system. Now, with the discovery of the X ray and with improvements in the use of the X ray, breaks in the bones of the spine are detected much more frequently.

Most injuries to the spine occur when people fall from a height, in traffic accidents, in being thrown from a horse, or in sudden pressures resulting from lifting or straining.

Fractures of the spine may occur in the upper portion of the spine called the neck or the cervical region, in the middle, or at the bottom. Most of the serious breaks occur in the neck region. A broken neck is much more serious than a break in the spine lower down. Sometimes a serious injury to the spinal cord will occur when the bones of the spine are twisted away from each other without actually breaking a portion of one of the bones.

The most serious results follow when there is a break directly into the spinal cord with hemorrhage into the spinal cord or tearing of the spinal cord itself.

Sometimes following an injury to the back there is loss of sensation below the level at which the injury occurred and loss of control of the ordinary actions of the bowel and the urinary bladder. The appearance of these symptoms is a clear indication of a serious condition demanding immediate medical attention.

The doctor will suggest first of all that anyone with an injury to the spine should be moved only when lying on a flat board and with the minimum amount of manipulation. If the injury is in the region of the neck, some technic should be found to hold the neck absolutely still. Usually an injury to the spine that is serious will bring on shock. This means again that the patient must lie with the head down and with sufficient warmth to maintain the circulation of the body.

As soon as the condition of the patient permits, the diagnosis of fractures of the spine should be verified by the use of the X ray in order to determine how much damage has occurred. Then a surgeon or orthopedic surgeon will get the bones in proper position and provide supports and braces to hold the tissues in proper position until there has been healing and as much recovery as possible.

During the period of recovery it may be necessary to aid the action of the bowels and the urinary bladder until the person is recovered.

When there has been injury to the spine or any other portion of the nervous system, a specialist in conditions affecting the nervous system will have to make a complete study to determine the extent of the damage that has been done and the possibilities for bringing about a full recovery through specialized treatment.

Curvature of the spine sometimes results from tuberculous infection of the bones so that they fall together. In the worst cases of curvature of the spine the difficulty may be due to disease. The earliest possible application of modern methods is necessary in such cases to prevent serious deformity.

SPINE The spinal cord is one of the most remarkable mechanisms of the human body. It is strong enough to support many hundreds of pounds; at the same time it is pliant and elastic. The muscles and tendons attached to the bones away from the spine help to move it in every direction.

Between each two of the bones of the spine there is a soft cushion which is known as the intervertebral disk. This serves like a ball bearing and a shock absorber. Shock between the bones of the spine that occurs when walking or sitting down is absorbed by this cushion. Its presence permits the bones of the spine to rotate more easily one on the other.

In the middle of this intervertebral disk is a soft material called nucleus pulposus. A sudden shock such as occurs when an airplane comes down or in a traffic accident, may cause the whole intervertebral disk to be pinched or pushed out of place. Occasionally it will break the nucleus pulposus and permit loss of fluid.

Only recently has the importance of this tissue come to be realized. Squeezing or dislocation of the intervertebral disk may produce constant and long-continued pain in the back. A new disease called "jeep disease" is simply an injury to the intervertebral disk which was common during World War II among drivers of jeeps and tanks and which occurred as they bounced over ditches and foxholes.

Exercises that involve sudden strains on the spine, such as football, soccer, baseball, and cricket, are sometimes productive of injury to the disk. Even organized gymnastics, or what the British call "organized jerks," may, if taken too precipitously or with too much force, injure the delicate tissues of the spine. These movements are especially dangerous for people with long legs and short arms who have a special problem of balance.

The presence of an injury to an intervertebral disk cannot be detected simply by running the fingers up and down the spine or by asking questions. The doctor is aided in determining such injury by taking an X-ray picture, often first injecting into the area concerned a substance which makes the position of the bones and soft tissues of the spine quite clear. This type of study, combined with application of the knowledge that the doctor has of the structure of the spine, will give him the necessary information to determine whether or not the condition can be corrected by braces and supports or whether or not a surgical operation is required.

SPLEEN In the abdomen on the left side there is a large pulpy organ known as the spleen. From the earliest times the spleen has been associated with emotions of anger. From this came the phrase "to vent one's spleen."

Even today all of the functions of the human body are not clearly understood. Contraction of the spleen occurs with the forcing of blood out of the spleen into the circulation. This has given rise to the concept that the function of the spleen is to maintain a proper amount of blood in the blood vessels, thus keep-

ing up the blood pressure through controlling the volume of the blood.

For some time it has been thought that the spleen is concerned not only with the breaking down and disposal of worn-out blood cells but also with the production of new blood cells.

Some of the studies of the spleen have been made by a very interesting process. Using an animal for the experiment, the doctor puts a celluloid window in the wall of the body and watches directly the function of the organ. It is also possible to transplant an organ outside the abdominal cavity and thus observe its action. The spleen itself is insensitive to pain.

When an animal exercises severely, the spleen contracts due to the discharge of blood into the circulation. Also when an animal exercises severely, the kidney may be deprived of blood to the extent of being actually injured. Injury to the kidney has been known to accompany severe and excessive exercise. Thus the spleen is helpful in putting more blood into the circulation and preventing damage to the vital organs, like the kidney.

Some truth must lie in the idea that the spleen is associated with emotions. The famous physiologist, Dr. Joseph Barcroft, made some tests on a dog which had developed the habit of chasing any cat in the neighborhood. If this dog lay on a table and a duster was placed in front of its nose, the spleen remain unaltered. If that duster were removed and another which had been in a basket with a cat was held in front of the dog's nose, the spleen would contract, even though none of the muscles of the dog moved. The noise of a cat mewing in another room caused the spleen of the dog to contract.

These observations help to explain why a person gets pale when he gets angry and how he can get so mad that he will faint away.

SPLENIC DISEASE The spleen is one of the large organs of the body least understood by medical science. It lies in the abdomen on the left side under the ribs. It seems to be concerned in the formation of blood cells, perhaps also in their destruction. In certain diseases the spleen enlarges greatly. Like other tissues of the body, it may be subjected to injuries such as occur in motor accidents, gunshot wounds, or falls. The spleen is likely to become much enlarged in leukemia, in which there are a tremendous number of white blood cells in the circulation.

Among unusual conditions affecting this organ are the appearance of accessory spleens scattered through the abdomen. Sometimes the spleen becomes detached or the tissues which hold it in place become relaxed, so that the spleen will move from the position it ordinarily occupies. It then is called a floating or wandering spleen, a condition which occurs far more often in women than in men.

When the spleen is ruptured or broken, as occurs in a road accident, the bleeding is usually severe because of the extensive amount of blood going through this organ. A rupture of the spleen is followed by an intense hemorrhage into the abdomen.

The spleen is often found enlarged in malaria and in blood diseases of various kinds. It is particularly large in a condition called Banti's disease, when the tremendous enlargement of the spleen is associated with severe anemia.

In certain diseases surgical removal of the spleen is considered to be especially helpful, for instance in severe cases of purpura hemorrhagica, a condition in which the blood does not clot easily. The spleen may also be removed because of the presence of tumors. Removal of the spleen has not been considered especially desirable in Banti's disease.

The spleen is not necessary to life as is the liver.

SPRAINS Among the most common injuries which affect human beings are sprains, particularly of the ankles and the wrists. A sudden movement or a fall will stretch or overstretch a ligament so that it tears. Fluid or blood

then gets into a joint. Sometimes a sprain is so severe that a bone is broken. For this reason every serious sprain should be subjected to an X-ray picture. The opening of the football season and the coming of winter produce a sudden increase in the number of sprains, particularly of the ankles.

Ordinarily a simple sprain is treated by rest, elevation of the leg and ankle, and the application of an ice bag. The doctor can immobilize the joint with strapping—use adhesive—or even with a plaster cast. Modern treatment, however, calls for movement of the joint. Since this is likely to produce pain, the physician in some instances injects an anesthetic substance into the injured area and permits the patient to use the foot or the hand.

After a joint has been fixed in one position for a considerable length of time and particularly if there has been much inflammation and swelling, it is difficult to move the joint. In such cases movement is not attempted rapidly but slowly; massage is used to aid softening of the tissues and relaxation of the stiffness. Heat should not be applied to a sprained ankle until the danger of congestion and hemorrhage has been controlled. The value of heat is greatest in the final stages when repair has begun in order to encourage circulation and absorption of excess fluid.

SPRUE Among the tropical conditions which affected a good many of our soldiers in the war was one called sprue. In this condition diarrhea, loss of weight, and inflammation of the mouth are the chief symptoms. Often the condition is mistaken for food poisoning. The tongue becomes red and sore, the abdomen is suddenly swollen with gas, and there may be repeated cramps.

The word "sprue" comes from a Dutch word that is used to describe an inflammation of the mouth. The disease was known more than two thousand years ago. The exact cause of sprue is not now known but the generally accepted view is that sprue follows some nutritional deficiency. This impression is confirmed by the fact that proper feeding with certain materials brings about improvement. The symptoms of sprue are like those of pellagra and pernicious anemia, in both of which the addition of certain substances to the diet brings about improvement. Incidentally the existence of sprue is associated with the growth of a yeastlike fungus called the monilia, but the evidence that the monilia is the cause of the sprue is not generally accepted.

Because there are many types of infection in tropical areas associated with dysentery, inflammation, and even bleeding from the bowel, a correct diagnosis of sprue is most important. The doctor, therefore, must get a careful record of the diet and of the action of the bowel. The failure of appetite in these patients makes it more likely that they will have an inadequate diet. Often patients with sprue lose one third to one half their normal weight.

The material from the bowel in a case of sprue has a large excess of fat. Apparently the difficulty is the inability of the body to take up this material. Until recently sprue was treated with a great variety of special diets. Then it was found that liver treatment is just as effective in sprue as it is in pernicious anemia. When the treatment with liver is begun early, the results are brilliant. In far-advanced cases the damage to the tissues of the body has been so great that complete recovery is impossible. Because of the nature of the disease the feeding of liver alone never gets as good a result as injection of liver into the body by the veins or the blood. During the course of treatment the diet is also modified to cut down the fats and to provide extra protein and extra vitamins. Often these patients improve tremendously merely with a high-protein and high-vitamin diet.

SQUINT See discussion of *Cross-Eyes* under *Eye*.

STAMMERING See *Stuttering and Stammering*.

STERILITY The future of any nation depends on the continued growth of its population. When people do not have children, nations must seek elsewhere for their population. An example is the way in which Germany imported workers because her men were all engaged in war. Fortunately the desire to have children is a natural human desire. Unfortunately some people who want children, who are even anxious to have them, do not do so because physical conditions prevent.

People who have many children are called fertile. Sterility is the opposite of fertility and it means inability to have children. Either the woman or the man may be responsible. In many cases the responsibility is shared by both. Some people make up their minds early in their married life that they do not want children and take steps to prevent childbirth. Experts say that at least 10 per cent of marriages in Great Britain and in the United States are completely sterile. This means that there is nothing that can be done that will cause these people to have children.

Many people are not absolutely sterile but merely relatively sterile—that is to say, they are sterile under the conditions of the marriage but might not be sterile under some other conditions.

Once, when we knew far less about childbirth than we know now, it was taken for granted that failure to have children meant that the woman was responsible. Nowadays we realize that investigations of childless marriages involve exhaustive examination of both husband and wife before it may be determined which is responsible and to what extent.

From the point of view of the woman who is sterile, the doctor determines whether or not the ovaries produce and give off eggs capable of being fertilized. He must find out whether or not such eggs pass down through the tubes into the uterus in which the child develops before birth. He must know whether or not it is possible for the male cells to reach the female cell in the uterus. He must know whether or not the lining of the uterus is capable of forming tissues that are necessary for the development of the child.

From the point of view of the man, the doctor must find out whether or not the male sex glands produce the fertilizing element in sufficient amount and with sufficient strength or life to travel the necessary distance to reach the female cell.

If any of these prerequisites fall short of perfection, the result is a definite lessening of the possibility that a child may be conceived or developed.

The most recently accumulated figures show that the man is responsible wholly or in part for from 30 to 40 per cent of all cases in which a family does not have children. The first step in sterility studies should always be an investigation of the husband. In case a complete absence of the fertilizing element is demonstrated, there is no further need to examine the wife. In many instances the number of male elements is small and the product is weak. Frequently several examinations are necessary because these qualifications differ from time to time.

When a man and woman marry and live an apparently normal sex life and still fail to have children, physical conditions are usually responsible for the failure. When such people consult the doctor to determine what is wrong, they must realize that conditions affecting the man are just as likely to be responsible as conditions affecting his wife. Since the child is formed by the union of a cell from the man with a cell from the woman, the study must include an actual investigation of the ability of the man and of the woman to provide the necessary cells.

Furthermore, there must be certainty that the cells of the father can travel the necessary route to join the cell from the mother in the organ in which the child is carried after conception. The physician must make certain that the cell from the mother developed by the ovary can travel successfully down the tube into the uterus. The male cells undergo greater risk of damage or de-struction in their route to join the female cell than does the ovum of the mother in passing from the ovary to the uterus. The normal male can provide each time from 3,000,000 to 4,000,000 cells; yet only one of these is neccessary to fertilize the female cell. The destruction of the male cells or damage to them en route by secretions or other materials on the path that they follow may be responsible for failure of the woman to conceive.

Obviously, if the number of male cells deposited is less than it should be, or if the cells are without the necessary vitality to travel their course, the chance of conception is greatly lessened.

Another factor of importance is the time when the female cell reaches the uterus in relationship to the time when the male cells start their journey. There are about two weeks between the periodical functions of the woman when impregnation of an ovum by a sperm cell is exceedingly unlikely.

The term "sterility" usually means that a woman has not given birth to a child after living with her husband for three years, during which time no efforts have been made to interfere with conception. This does not mean, however, that the woman cannot become pregnant. Some women become pregnant ten years after marriage, while others may never be able to become pregnant.

If the tubes which carry the egg cell from the ovary to the uterus are permanently blocked as the result of abnormal construction or disease, the woman cannot possibly become pregnant. There may have been infections early in life which injured the organs involved in this procedure. For instance, mumps is known to affect the organs involved in the production of the sex cells. Experiments with animals have indicated that diets seriously deficient in certain necessary vitamins may damage the reproductive function. Indeed, even serious mental or emotional disturbances may affect the physical relationships to such an extent as to make conception unlikely. If, therefore, any couple is disturbed about failure to have children, a complete physical examination of both the prospective father and mother is necessary in order to determine the responsibility for the failure. The examination may include a study of the cells developed by the father, the use of modern methods to determine whether or not the tubes of the mother are open, and finally a complete record of the sex life of the people concerned.

Unfortunately the tubes of the woman, once sealed by serious disease, are not likely to be capable of repair by surgical procedures, or by blowing of air through the tubes or other technics which physicians use.

STOMACH ULCERS The stresses and exigencies of war resulted everywhere in an increase in the incidence of ulcers of the stomach and duodenum. The duodenum, the portion of the intestines which comes immediately after the stomach, was called that by the ancients because it was about twelve fingers long.

Ulcers of the duodenum have been described as the commonest disease of the upper part of the intestinal system and the condition is found four times as often in men as in women. Also ulcers are found ten times as often in the duodenum as they are in the stomach. Occurring usually in people who live under high tension, the condition has often been called "nervous indigestion."

Simply because we are not certain of any one cause of ulcers of the stomach or duodenum, we are likely to assign any one of a number of causes. Apparently they are more prevalent in certain families, but this can be related to the fact that a nervous constitution occurs also in certain families.

Undoubtedly there are physical causes as well as mental, but apparently the physical causes become operative under certain mental conditions. When there are stock-market crashes, when there are wars, when there are constant bickerings and arguments in the family, ulcers appear.

There has been a tendency to associate the presence of ulcers with an increased amount of acid in the stomach. The excess acid is responsible for the continuation of the symptoms. It has been customary to treat the condition largely with a view to combating the excess acidity. An ulcer of the stomach or of the intestines is like an ulcer elsewhere in the body: when it heals, there is a tendency to form a scar.

Because of the increased emphasis on psychological relationship in ulcers, modern treatment calls for mental rest and special attention to decreasing the worry or strain from which the patients suffer. Many men with ulcers improve when they take a vacation. It has been observed that when patients travel long distances to get some kind of treatment they sometimes arrive at their destination with the beginning of healing already in progress.

Apparently the continuation of the stress and strain will be reflected in the nervous system. The drugs used are antacids, antispasmodics like atropine, banthine, or prantal which block the nerve impulses, and sedatives. In severe uncontrollable cases surgical treatment prevents perforation and leads to more permanent results.

The big problem for the doctor is to correct the excess acidity by the provision of a proper diet and proper drugs. Diets have to be calculated for the individual patient, and they must take into account the necessity for vitamins and mineral salts in order to maintain general health as well as the treatment of the ulcer.

In the hygiene of the person with ulcers, authorities recommend discontinuation of smoking and of the use of alcohol and of excessive exercise. In occasional instances change of occupation and of residence seem to make the difference between health and continued disease.

STROKE See *Apoplexy.*

STRABISMUS Another word for *Cross-Eyes.* See under *Eye.*

STUTTERING AND STAMMERING

Modern views of stuttering point to the concept that it is a nervous condition based on some mental conflict. The stutterer has a tenseness and spasm of the muscles involved in speaking. He is unable to co-ordinate them properly. Back of his failure to co-ordinate is a state of the nervous system involving some mental conflict. History shows that stutterers are in good company. Among the great names in history of people who stuttered are Aristotle, Aesop, Demosthenes, Virgil, Charles Lamb, Erasmus, Darwin, Moses, Mendelssohn, and several of the kings of England and France.

Although stuttering may be largely mental in causation, physical factors are sometimes associated and may act to aggravate the stuttering. The doctor therefore makes certain that adenoids, abnormal length of uvula, abnormal size of the tongue, and improper development of the mouth are not present. Such defects are not, however, found with great frequency as the primary cause of stuttering.

The stutterer usually has most trouble with p, b, m, and w, which are the sounds made by the lips. The stutterer does not, however, always stutter on the same sound. His emotional status at the time of speaking may be a factor in determining the particular word or phrase that is associated with stuttering.

Often children who stutter develop behavior changes due to a lack of confidence with the fear of appearing ridiculous. Some children who stutter are even considered to be mentally retarded because of their speech defect.

Because stuttering is primarily a mental affliction, treatment directed to the mental conflict is of the greatest importance. When the nature of the conflict is discovered and revealed to the stutterer, self-confidence returns and there may be a readjustment toward life in general.

Since all people who have difficulty in speaking display disturbances of the normal rhythm of breathing and speaking, training is useful in developing the power of speech. This has been observed through the fact that many people get along without stammering when they whisper or sing or recite poetry or speak to a large audience but have difficulty under other conditions. Musicians who stutter sometimes become blocked in playing certain notes. This means that they stutter in their thinking as well as in their speech.

The re-education of the person who stutters requires training in relaxation, in breathing, in vocal gymnastics, and in phonetics. Such training is, of course, combined with proper mental study designed to release the block that occurs in the mind. The first task is to break down the spasm of the unco-ordinated muscles and liberate the imprisoned voice. This requires teaching in the relaxation of the muscles. The stutterer must be made to forget his problem by exercises in relaxing the muscles of the body, the head, the tongue, the throat, and the vocal cords. Excess effort toward speaking brings about wrong action of the diaphragm. The stutterer tries to talk while he is inhaling. This, of course, is difficult if not impossible. Therefore exercises are given in proper breathing and in control of breathing in relationship to speech.

Because of the difficulty in speaking stutterers form bad speech habits that need correction. These habits affect particularly the articulation of certain sounds. It becomes necessary to teach them how to articulate the sounds with which they have trouble.

Dr. John A. Glassburg has described a routine of approach to speech which is useful.

1. Before you speak, think, inhale, and visualize the words.

2. When you speak, never go back, never repeat; lengthen your vowel sounds.

3. Always speak quietly, slowly, and calmly.

There is a good deal of trouble trying to distinguish between stuttering and stammering. Some people say that stuttering is reduplication of sound and stammering is hesitation in speaking. Some define stuttering as difficult speech and stammering as incorrect speech. This merely confuses a condition which has been considerably confused for a variety of reasons. For all practical purposes the average person may consider stuttering and stammering as the same kind of difficulty.

STYES See discussion under *Eye*.

SUICIDE Every year about 20,000 people in the United States kill themselves. Suicide is not, therefore, an exceedingly prominent cause of death. Nevertheless, suicides are always attracting attention because of the natural drama associated with them.

Why do three and a half times as many men as women attempt suicide? Why is the tendency to commit suicide greater among older than among young people? It seems that suicide results chiefly from the discouragement and hopelessness of later years of life. During war the suicide rate always drops.

People differ as to the methods by which they commit suicide. The agents most frequently used are firearms and poisons, which account altogether for about one half of all suicides. Then there are asphyxiation and hanging. These four technics account for 83 per cent of all suicides.

People who commit suicide represent a group who are easily upset emotionally. They break down under strains which other people manage to surmount. Sometimes the strain arises from economic conditions, sometimes because of trouble with friends and relatives.

The psychologists are convinced that there is a steady progression of the tendency to self-destruction long before the self-destruction is finally consummated. Obviously, therefore, there is time when such a tendency is discovered to undertake corrective action with a view to overcoming the desire.

The ability to adjust oneself emotionally to one's surroundings is perhaps most important to the prevention of suicides. The conditions that influence people, such as poverty, unemployment, ill-health, mental abnormality, physical suffering or handicaps, may lead people to thoughts of self-destruction. Loss of honor and prestige, disappointment in love, failure in achieving one's ambitions, or any other failure in adequacy may result in thoughts of suicide.

Obviously the way to prevent suicide is to develop a proper attitude toward life in the young. This is the responsibility of the entire community as well as of the home. Young people must be given a proper mental and emotional outlook. They must learn to act properly toward the difficult situations that invariably arise in the human life.

SUN- AND HEAT STROKE (See also *Heat Sickness*) Sunstroke, as the term is popularly understood, is not the result of the light of the sun, but of the infrared, or heat, rays. The same symptoms may occur as the result of exposure to heat and humidity in a laundry, a steel mill, a fireroom, a deep metal mine, or any other industry. Among the more severe manifestations are symptoms of complete exhaustion and the occurrence of heat cramps.

When heat stroke occurs, the temperature-regulating mechanism of the human body is thrown out of order. Usually there are premonitory symptoms such as headache, dizziness, and nausea, but sometimes the worker goes on without paying much attention to the minor symptoms, to be stricken as by a flash of lightning, and to die suddenly before anything worth while can be done to save his life.

Among the symptoms of exhaustion are physical weakness, profuse perspiration, a moderate amount of fever, although sometimes the temperature may be lower than normal, and sometimes severe cramping pains in the abdomen or in the arms and legs. In the more severe cases the patient promptly becomes unconscious, his pulse gets very rapid, his breathing gets deep, and the pupils of the eye dilate.

Usually if the person afflicted lives through the second day of his attack he gets better, so that the most important measures are those taken promptly to meet the emergency and to permit the patient to survive the first shock.

In the case of heat exhaustion the first thing to do is to get the person into a cool place and absolutely at rest, flat on his back. If the temperature is high, sponging with cool water will help to control it. It may be necessary to give stimulation such as can be had from stronger drugs or from coffee in order to help the patient over the acute stage of the condition.

In the case of heat stroke with the more severe symptoms prompt action is even more necessary than in heat exhaustion. In such cases the body may be washed in ice water; cold sprays and injections of cold water may be used to bring the fever down rapidly.

The effects of the stroke on the heart should be watched by a physician who may remain constantly in attendance until the heart action is satisfactory. He can give supportive drugs that will control the heart and this may make the difference between life and death. Sometimes congestion may be great and it may be necessary for the doctor to permit some blood to flow from the veins in order to relieve the congestion.

Many industrial plants and many golf clubs are now providing their employees and their patrons with little tablets made of common table salt. Special dispensers have been developed which are placed beside the drinking-water fountain. In the industrial plants the employees are encouraged to take one of these tablets every time they take a drink of water. It has been found by actual studies that this helps to eliminate the occurrence of heat stroke or heat exhaustion.

The human body is unable to adjust itself satisfactorily to high temperatures for a long time. The workers who are most likely to develop heat stroke or heat cramps are miners, firemen, laundry workers, and kitchen workers, but many a golfer who tries to play thirty-six holes of golf in a day may collapse halfway around because he failed to realize that the human body needs help in such a situation.

Some years ago a study was made of the miners in Boulder City, Nevada. It was found that heat cramps which occurred in these miners were associated with disturbances which resulted from a lack of salt in the body. A British investigator named Haldane found that miners at work may lose as much as five and a half pounds in an hour. A person in a Turkish bath may lose two pounds in an hour.

When large amounts of salt solution are taken into the body, the effects of heat cramps and heat stroke disappear. The blood of a person suffering from heat stroke is found to contain less salt than normally.

In some industries all of the drinking water is modified by the addition of salt. This serves to protect even those workers who will not realize the importance of taking a salt tablet at fairly frequent intervals. In Great Britain miners are supplied with salted beer and are told that the food which they take daily should be salted liberally.

Our number of cases of sunstroke, heat stroke, and heat exhaustion is relatively slight for the year as a whole, but in the summer the number of cases rises quite definitely. The number of deaths from heat stroke vary, of course, with the severity of the temperature during the summer, but it has reached as high as 4000 in one year.

SUNBURN As with every other disease, the doctors have coined a special name for ordinary sunburn. It is known as erythema solare, which merely means that it is an inflammation caused by the sun. The same term can, of course, be used to apply to an inflammation of the skin caused by ultra-violet rays from other sources.

The inflammation that develops varies from a slight flush to the severe burn that results in blistering and loss of skin. Immediately after burning there may be a sensation of heat which is followed in a few days or a week by itching and by peeling of the skin. Usually if the person protects the skin and avoids further sunburn, healing occurs promptly. Sunburns seldom produce scars unless there is a secondary infection of the damaged area.

If the sunburned area is very extensive, the effects of absorption of the material that has been damaged may be shown by dizziness, headache, fever, vomiting, and other symptoms of a constitutional disturbance.

Most people have at one time or another suffered the effects of sunburn and know just about what to do. The application of ordinary cold cream or any similar medication will stop the sensation of burning and dryness that results from the exposure of nerve endings. In the very severe cases it is necessary, however, to apply treatment exactly as if the surface of the body were burned by any other burning agent.

The dangers from sunlight are chiefly the effects of the ultraviolet rays. These are the short rays rather than the longer heat rays.

When doctors use sunlight in the treatment of disease, as, for example, tuberculosis, they carefully regulate the dosage of the rays that are given and also gradually accustom the person concerned to the sunlight. It is customary to apply the sun bath in a succession of short periods, particularly at the beginning, because these brief and repeated exposures to the sun enable us to escape any inflammation of the skin and the subsequent blisters, burning, and nervous reactions which result in loss of sleep.

Certain skins are much more delicate than others. Blonds, particularly with thin skins, react so quickly that even a short exposure may bring about a reaction to the heat and even the symptoms of sunstroke. The skin of the infant is much more delicate than that of the adult and will burn and become inflamed much more promptly.

A person of intelligence can determine for himself how much sunlight he ought to have, but the infant is certainly not able to settle such a question for himself.

SWEAT See *Perspiration*.

SWIMMING POOLS Hot weather means to the doctor an increasing number of infected ears and noses because people are careless about the places where they swim and bathe.

There are in the United States at least 6000 indoor swimming pools. No one knows how many beaches there are along the shores of lakes, rivers, and oceans. Great numbers of golf clubs have added swimming pools as a special accessory for summer enjoyment. In 1900 there were said to be only 67 swimming pools in the United States.

The chief diseases that are transmitted through swimming pools are inflammation of the eye, boils and other infections in the ear, chronic inflammation of the nose and the sinuses, sore throat, various infections of the skin (including particularly the so-called athlete's foot), and, finally, infection of the bowels with dysentery. All swimmers who enter public swimming pools should be free from visible infections or acute disease at the time they enter the pool. Most managers now require a shower bath before each person enters the pool. This means at least one shower bath for every forty bathers and adequate comfort facilities for men and women as an accessory.

Drinking water near swimming pools must be controlled. The common use of drinking cups, towels, combs, hairbrushes, and other toilet articles should be strictly prohibited.

Most American swimming pools provide for the use of chlorine in the water as a means of keeping it pure, although the ultraviolet ray has also been developed as a useful technic for this purpose. Regular draining of the pool and the removal of sediment and infectious material also help to maintain sanitation. If a swimming pool is submitted to proper sanitation, there is less likelihood of infection for a swimmer unless he happens to come in contact with a heavy dose of germs from some person who should not be using the pool.

Few cases of infection develop from swimming in the ocean or in rivers or lakes where the people are not packed together. On crowded beaches, where there is hardly room to move the arms, people are constantly exposed to the excretions and secretions of their neighbors. This kind of crowding must bear the burden for infection of the respiratory tract and for dysentery.

Another important measure for use around swimming pools to prevent infection of the feet is to insist on a protected walk next to the pool to be used only by bathers who have previously had a shower and thus have cleansed their feet. This protected walk should be forbidden to visitors who are walking in their shoes and who thus carry infectious organisms and put them down where they come in contact with the naked feet of the bather. Such surface contamination may also be washed into the pool.

Scientific health standards demand that the germs in swimming pools be counted at fairly frequent intervals in relation to the total amount of water used. Large city engineering departments have facilities for conducting such studies.

SYMPATHETIC NERVOUS SYSTEM

Many functions carried on by the human body go on without any conscious activity by the brain. For instance the glands regularly secrete the glandular substances necessary to life. The blood is formed in the appropriate tissues. Associated with many of these necessary activities is the function of the sympathetic nervous system, also called the autonomic nervous system.

The nerve tissues of the autonomic nervous system go to practically all of the important organs of the body, to the sweat glands in the skin and the salivary glands. The nerves of the autonomic nervous system run alongside the spinal cord. Some of them are associated with important nerves affecting the eyes and ears. Certain drugs are known to influence particularly the sympathetic nervous system, although of course they do not affect that system alone but are likely to affect other portions of the body as well.

The blood supply to any part of the body can be increased by interrupting the sympathetic nerves that go to that part. This can be done by a surgical operation. It sometimes becomes necessary to undertake procedures of this kind in certain diseases. Nothing is to be gained by trying a procedure of this sort when the walls of the blood vessels are permanently hardened so that they cannot carry a greater blood supply.

One of the operations on the sympathetic nervous system that is sometimes used is the operation for high blood pressure, the idea being to increase the flow of blood into the abdominal area and the lower limbs and thus to decrease the pressure. Many cases are reported now in which this operation has been useful.

Occasionally interruption or treatment applied to the sympathetic nervous system has been used in conditions affecting the heart, like angina pectoris, or in severe pain involving the uterus. Operations have been done even to aid the activities of the bowel and the bladder and to control serious disturbances of the sweat glands.

In certain conditions that seem to be almost wholly emotional, the manifestations appear through activities of the sympathetic nervous system. This occurs, for instance, in shell shock, nervous breakdown, and in other conditions of the type called psychosomatic.

SYNDROME

Whenever a number of symptoms occur together regularly, the group of symptoms is called a syndrome. There are a wide variety of diseases that are known as syndromes, most of them named after the physician who first observed the occurrence of the symptoms as a group. Among the best known of these conditions, for example, is the Cushing syndrome, which is a series of symptoms due to certain tumors of the brain; the Christian syndrome, which is associated with the condition called diabetes insipidus.

SYNOVITIS The membranes which line the joints are known as synovial membranes. The fluid in a joint is known as synovial fluid. Inflammation of these membranes is known as synovitis.

SYPHILIS The word "syphilis," coined in 1530 by an Italian physician, has attained recognition.

Known to the world for many centuries, this disease gradually has developed increasing prevalence and prominence simply because one of its methods of transmission made its discussion taboo.

If syphilis were transmitted by a fly or mosquito, we could long since have stamped it out. It happens, however, to be spread in the vast majority of cases by contact between human beings, and by a form of contact which itself has been taboo as a subject for general discussion.

Through years of research the medical profession learned that the disease is caused in every case by an organism known as *Spirochaeta pallida*. Literally this means "pale coil of hair." It refers to a germ which appears under the microscope as a spiral germ of pallid coloring. One of these germs is about as long as an ordinary red blood cell.

IMITATES OTHER DISEASES—Were it not for the fact that this germ is susceptible to sunlight and air, and also to fairly mild antiseptics, syphilis might long since have destroyed human life upon this earth.

When the germ gets into the body, it multiplies quickly and gradually invades every organ and tissue. Some germs are limited largely to the lungs, others to the throat, and still others to the intestines, but the syphilis germ attacks any kind of tissue, and it has been said that because of this syphilis can imitate every other disease.

One of the most famous physicians, Sir William Osler, once said: "Know

syphilis in all its manifestations and relations and all other things clinical will be added unto you."

IT CAN BE CURED—Until 1903 it was thought that syphilis occurred only in human beings. In that year it was first transmitted to monkeys, and since that time it occasionally has been transmitted to rabbits and white mice. Transmission of the disease to these animals has enabled us to study it on a larger scale and as a result has made it possible for us to say that syphilis can be cured.

Cure means not only elimination of the first lesion that the disease causes on the skin, but even the elimination of the organisms and their poisons from the entire body.

Clearing the germ from the body also halts secondary eruption on the skin, damage to internal tissues, and the germ's invasion of the brain. When syphilis attacks the brain, there results the condition called general paralysis of the insane and locomotor ataxia.

DEVELOPING TREATMENTS—The advance against syphilis has depended largely on certain epoch-making, world-famous discoveries. When the organism that causes the disease was discovered by Schaudinn in 1905, a great step forward was taken.

Wassermann's description of the test by which infection can be determined was another tremendous advance.

The final, most significant advance was the development of the product called 606, salvarsan, or arsphenamine, by Paul Ehrlich. This was important not only for its own value but also as a stimulus to subsequent discoveries which have led to the development of other drugs of great importance in the treatment of this disease.

Especially significant have been the new developments in relationship to the use of mercury, the determination of the germ of syphilis in the brain, and the development of bismuth and heat treatment and of penicillin in most recent years.

Syphilis can be transmitted from parents to their children. In these cases the germ that causes the disease passes from the mother to the child and infects the organs of the baby.

Usually the tissues that connect the mother to the baby act as a filter and keep back the germs of most diseases, including those of tuberculosis, but the germs of syphilis seem to be able to find their way through.

BIRTH TOLL IS GREAT—After a baby has been infected, he may die, and syphilis is recognized today as one of the important causes of premature birth of dead babies and stillbirths.

It is also recognized that babies born either prematurely or at the right time may be so enfeebled by syphilis that they will die while they are very young.

Moreover, if these enfeebled babies survive the first few months of life, they may later develop sores that leave ugly scars, deformed bones, bad teeth, blindness, deafness, paralysis, or even mental disturbances, as a result of the syphilis that has been transmitted to them.

It has been estimated that three out of every one hundred babies born have syphilis which they acquired in the period before they were born, and it has been stated that out of all of the babies who die before they are twelve months old 40 per cent die before they reach the age of one month, with syphilis outstanding as the cause of such early deaths.

EARLY TREATMENT BEST—The saddest fact in relationship to this misfortune is that this is all preventable but that modern social organization and science have not yet found the way to make prevention the practice.

Most important step in this prevention is the examination of every prospective mother, including the making of a Wassermann test. If the mother is found to be infected, arrangements must be made immediately for her to take treatment of the most active kind in order to prevent the birth of an infected child.

The best time to cure the disease is before the baby is born. If the mother begins treatment during the first three months of her expectant period, infec-

tion of the baby can be prevented. Treatment will drive the germs out of her blood so that they cannot travel from her circulation into that of the baby. But even if the treatment is not started until the fourth or fifth month, she still may have a healthy baby.

If treatment of the mother has been insufficient or if she has had no treatment before the birth of the child, then the immediate treatment of the baby after his arrival is of the utmost importance. This can be arranged without much difficulty because of new methods of administering the necessary drugs and other treatments important in controlling this disease.

It is commonly estimated that from 8 to 10 per cent of the American people have syphilis. That means that from 10,000,000 to 12,000,000 are infected.

It has been estimated that 21,000,000 working days are lost by infected men. Allowing for this at the rate of $4 per day, there is an immediate loss of $84,-000,000. This does not take into account time lost by women. It has been estimated that the annual bill for treatment of syphilis in New York State is more than $23,000,000.

The amount of infection seems to vary according to the status of society and the occupations of those who are concerned. Women of the "red-light" districts are said to be infected invariably sooner or later.

Among criminals in penitentiaries as many as 20 to 40 per cent have been found infected. Among men of better families the amount of infection seems to vary from 2 to 10 per cent.

ACTIVE DEATH CAUSE—The number of people who die from syphilis is not definitely known, because there is a disinclination to report syphilis as the main cause of death, and also because it is covered up by other more important causes.

If it is remembered, however, that syphilis is the real cause of death in all cases of general paralysis and locomotor ataxia, in many cases of epilepsy, and in a considerable number of other diseases, the importance of the condition as a cause of death is more easily estimated.

Life insurance companies are not likely to be willing to insure people who have syphilis. The sickness and death rates of those who have had the disease are likely to be higher than those for other people in the community.

If insurance companies do accept for insurance those who have had syphilis, they are likely to want a higher rate. Some companies will, however, insure people who have had a thorough course of treatment and who have been without symptoms for some three to five years.

MARRIAGE PRECAUTIONS—In many states syphilis is a bar to marriage. Twenty-two states demand a physician's certificate or a statement or affidavit from one or both candidates that they are free from venereal disease.

In Michigan and Oklahoma marriage by a person with venereal disease is expressly stated to be a felony. In Utah a marriage under such circumstances may by annulled.

Doctors everywhere warn people in the early stages of syphilis against marriage, and in every instance when syphilis has not been cured it is the duty of the doctor to warn the prospective partner against marriage until cure has been accomplished.

No one can possibly estimate the cost in money represented by the damage that syphilis does to human health and life. The amount is so tremendous that the figures stagger the imagination.

There are some records of syphilis infection by accident when a person with a sore on his finger has come in contact with syphilitic material on the body of another person.

There are records of infection from kissing, and babies have been infected from wet nurses. These secondary types of infection are, however, so unusual in comparison with the ordinary methods of spread of infection that this fact should not frighten anyone into a constant fear of this disease.

In the vast majority of cases syphilis is transmitted from one human to another during sex relationship.

Hotel beds, public lavatories, bathtubs, doorknobs, books, dishes used in restaurants, and similar materials are not easily infected. It is necessary for the germ to get into the body through a sore or through an easily infected spot if it is to invade the body generally.

USUAL SYMPTOMS—As has already been said, the organism that causes syphilis is killed by drying and is susceptible to soap and water. Thorough washing is an important factor in preventing the spread of the infection.

The first sign of the disease usually is a sore at the point where the germ has entered the tissue. The doctor who finds this sore will make his diagnosis by studying the material from the sore under the microscope, either fresh or after staining.

He also takes some blood from the veins and tests this blood with what is known as the Wassermann test or with the Kahn test. These tests determine usually at a fairly early stage whether or not a person has been infected with syphilis.

If the disease is not promptly treated, it will spread to the interior of the body, ultimately causing eruption on the skin, and all of the other serious conditions that have been mentioned.

MAY BE OTHER CAUSES—There are a few simple facts that everyone ought to know about syphilis:

This disease does not cause pimples.

It does not cause itching conditions of the skin.

It may cause ulcers of the legs, but more frequently these are due to varicose veins.

It may be responsible for failure to produce children, but there are also other conditions which may produce such failures.

It is not a form of blood poisoning. Testing of the blood will show whether or not the patient has syphilis.

It is not responsible for the vast majority of cases of baldness, but some cases of loss of hair not only of the head but of the entire body may be due to syphilis.

It has not been established in any way

that syphilis is the cause of cancer or that these two conditions are in any way related.

BASIC RULES—There are a few simple instructions which were widely circulated during World War II to all soldiers who were found to be infected with this disease:

If you have any sore on your genitals, no matter how small, or if you think you have syphilis, consult your physician.

Do not under any conditions rely on the "blood medicines" that promise to eradicate syphilis, and do not be caught by advertising doctors—quacks—who try to get your money by promising to cure you quickly.

Do not let druggists prescribe for you; they are not qualified to treat syphilis.

Do not hesitate to tell your doctor or dentist of your disease. Later in life, if you get sick at any time, you should tell your doctor that you have had syphilis, since this fact may furnish a clue to treatment on which your cure depends.

Live temperately and sensibly. Do not go to extreme in any direction in your habits of life.

Try to get a reasonable amount of sleep—eight hours is the amount needed by the average person. And as a safeguard to others, sleep alone.

Take good care of your teeth. Brush them two or three times a day. If they are not in good condition, have them attended to by a dentist. But when you go to him, tell him that you have syphilis.

DON'T SPREAD TROUBLE—Do not have sexual intercourse until you are told by your physician that you are no longer contagious. It will interfere with the cure of the disease, and it is criminal, for it is likely to give the disease to your wife.

You must not marry until you have the doctor's consent, which cannot be properly given until at least two years have passed after cure seems complete. If you do, you run the risk of infecting your wife and your children with syphilis.

Early in the course of syphilis, while it is contagious, the greatest danger of infecting other people is by the mouth. Because of this danger do not kiss anybody. Particularly do not endanger children by kissing them.

Do not allow anything that has come in contact with your lips or that has been in your mouth to be left around so that anybody can use it before it has been cleaned. This applies to cups, glasses, knives, forks, spoons, pipes, cigars, toothpicks, and all such things. It is better to use your own towels, brushes, comb, razor, soap, et cetera, though these are much less likely to be contaminated than objects that go in your mouth.

If you have any open sores—you will not have any after the first week or two, if you are treated—everything that comes in contact with them should be destroyed or disinfected.

As a result of the examination of 10,000,000 men in World War II, it has been found that the incidence of syphilis varies in different parts of the United States.

Early in the war men with a positive Wassermann test were eliminated from military service. Later it was decided to take these men into the service and to treat them. As a result syphilis is now being brought much more definitely under control.

In the modern treatment of syphilis, technics have been developed for shortening the period of treatment. These include an intensive treatment, occupying ten weeks, using principally the arsenical drugs; also a five-day treatment carried on in the hospital, in which the patient is given intensive, continuous treatment with drugs put directly into the veins. Sometimes there is combined with this a long period of heat treatment, using special devices known as hypertherms that have been developed for the purpose.

More recently syphilis is being treated with penicillin and other antibiotics. By giving penicillin either continuously over a period of five days or by repeated intramuscular injections one may stop the progress of the disease and change a positive Wassermann test to a negative Wassermann test inside of a week. The percentage of relapses with this treatment is relatively slight, being certainly well under 4 per cent of all the cases. The method has been found useful not only in the treatment of early syphilis but in halting the progress of syphilis of the nervous system.

Because of the great success of these methods of treatment many authorities now predict that syphilis may be completely eliminated from the United States within the next generation.

TABES See *Locomotor Ataxia.*

TACHYPHAGIA The word "tachyphage" is another one of those long medical words composed of two Greek words: "tachy," meaning rapid; and "phage," meaning to eat. A tachyphage is a rapid eater, and the United States is full of them. A tachyphage is likely to wake up in the morning with a tight feeling in the abdomen at the thought of the day that is before him. He lies in bed too long thinking about his troubles, skips his bath, rushes through his dressing, grabs a glass of orange juice and a cup of coffee and runs for the train chewing on a piece of toast. Then he is troubled with discomfort in his abdomen most of the morning. At noon he bolts his luncheon, eating it off the corner of a desk or speeding through service at a luncheon club so that there will be time for the speaker. He gets home just in time to bolt his dinner so that he can be off to a movie or a bridge game.

Sooner or later the constant discomfort in his interior gives him an anxious look. He begins to think that he has hyperacidity or a gastric ulcer—and maybe he has. Thereafter he takes large quantities of baking soda an hour or two after each meal.

Most of the trouble is due to the fact that he eats too rapidly. Because of his mental state he has trouble in digesting what he eats. The chief step in his cure is the establishment of regular hours for his meals, insistence on spending enough time to eat the meal slowly, and, finally, the avoidance of all business discussions and telephone conversations or other anxieties during the meal.

The woman worker is no advance on the big businessman when it comes to being a tachyphage. She gulps her lunch, including a sandwich and a cup of coffee, with possibly also a piece of pie, in five or ten minutes and spends the remaining time in gossip or shopping. Such a luncheon is of little use either for nutrition or the satisfaction of hunger. Therefore it is supplemented all day long with candy, soda-fountain drinks, and similar items.

Not long ago a number of the New York literati formed a Three-Hours-for-Lunch Club. That was probably a reaction against the establishment of tachyphagia as a universal American disease.

TALIPES (See also discussion under *Clubfoot*) Talipes is a deformity of the foot in which it is twisted out of shape or position. The common name for this condition is clubfoot. The condition has been classified according to the direction in which the foot is twisted. Sometimes when the foot stands on the toe the condition is called talipes equinus because it is like the foot of a horse. If it is twisted to the side, it is called talipes valgus. These conditions can be controlled by care given exceedingly early in life by an orthopedic surgeon.

TANTALUM This new metallic element has been found to be non-corrosive and malleable and is, therefore, used not only as a plate to replace areas lost from the skull by injury but also for the making of sutures to sew together damaged tissues.

TATTOOING With every outbreak of war and recruitment of men into military service tattooing becomes prominent. Then when the war ends, great numbers of men and even some women begin asking specialists in diseases of the skin how to get rid of the pictures.

In the process of tattooing mineral and vegetable substances are introduced into the skin by means of needles. Primitive savages pigmented the skin and tattooed the body largely in connection with religious worship. Soldiers and sailors apparently indulge in tattooing as a form of obtaining a permanent souvenir of some country that they have visited or some person whom they want to remember. Sometimes it is difficult to explain just why anyone has himself tattooed. One soldier had a tombstone in black tattooed on his forearm and below this in red letters "To the Memory of My Mother." A sailor from Liverpool had sixteen girls' names tattooed on his back. Fifteen out of thirty men with tattoo pictures had mermaids as the perdominating figure in their personal art galleries.

Tattooing of the skin sometimes occurs accidentally, as in the case of powder stains, in which particles of powder are deposited in the skin. Miners sometimes have permanent discoloration due to the imbedding of coal dust in scratches. Other metals which have been deposited in the skin with the effect of tattooing are silver and iron.

In the tattooing process the moistening is sometimes accomplished by the saliva of the tattooer. By this technic various diseases, including tuberculosis, erysipelas, bacterial infections, and even venereal diseases have been transmitted from the tattooer to the subject. Occasionally tattooing sets up reactions in the skin which result in the development of tumors.

Among the methods known for removing tattoo is the peeling of the skin by the use of caustic substances. This is quite dangerous, and even specialists in diseases of the skin dislike to attempt its use. It is, of course, possible to cut away entirely the tattooed area if it is not too large and to take care of the defect that is thus developed by grafting new skin from another portion of the body. A new successful method involves sterilizing the area with antiseptics, then sandpapering the tattooed skin off its base, controlling the bleeding and encouraging healing.

TEETH (See also *Dentifrices*) Thousands of years ago men, without the advantages that we possess today, recognized the importance of teeth. Human beings who have to get along without knives and forks—for instance, the Eskimos—learn to use the jaws and teeth in a manner in which civilized men never have used them. Eskimos will bite through bone and tear tough meats with their teeth.

The ancient Egyptians, Greeks, and Romans used abrasives to keep their teeth clean. They made gold supports to hold loose teeth in the mouth and even tried to replace lost teeth with teeth taken from sheep or calves. They endeavored to make their teeth more beautiful by inserting diamonds and other ornaments. There are still people who decorate their mouths in this manner, but most of us prefer porcelain or similar material, which gives the teeth as normal an appearance as possible.

The famous artist Leonardo da Vinci was among the first to recognize that the teeth in a normal mouth are of different shapes and different sizes in order to perform special functions. In the normal mouth there are thirty-two permanent teeth. These permanent teeth are preceded by baby teeth which must also be protected if the permanent teeth are to come in properly.

Until modern dentistry was developed in the United States, the care of the teeth was a side line for blacksmiths and goldsmiths. Decayed teeth were pulled and false teeth were made of gold, bone, and ivory. They were not the same size and shape as natural teeth.

The teeth George Washington wore were held in his mouth by spiral springs which often jammed and would not work. Washington's teeth were made about 1790. Ten years later a Frenchman in Philadelphia discovered how to keep false teeth in the mouth without springs.

About that time also the celebrated physician, Benjamin Rush, one of the signers of the Declaration of Independence, pointed out that infected teeth could bring about diseases in other parts of the body.

The first school of dentistry was established in Baltimore in 1840. Other dental schools were established promptly thereafter. Today dentistry in the United States leads all the world.

There is no known diet that alone will insure good teeth. A diet that contains the right proteins, carbohydrates, fats, mineral salts, and vitamins is a good diet for the teeth as well as for the rest of the body. However, teeth need minerals, like calcium and phosphorus, and these are found to best advantage in milk and milk products. If, however, you happen to be sensitive to milk, or if the milk acts unfavorably for your digestion, remember that other foods also provide these minerals.

These minerals are found in the leafy green vegetables. Moreover, the whole-grain cereals and the flesh of fish are also rich in phosphorus. In order that the calcium and phosphorus may be usable by the body for the production of sound teeth and bones, it is desirable that we take regularly enough vitamins A, C, and D. The use of the right amounts of cod-liver oil or halibut-liver oil helps to supply vitamins A and D.

The ultraviolet rays of the sun help the body to make vitamin D. The juice of tomatoes, oranges, and grapefruit and other citrus fruits provide plenty of vitamin C.

The dentist says give your teeth plenty of chewing exercise. If you eat the foods that require chewing, you are more likely to get the chewing exercise than you are if you try to get along with soft foods only. People who live largely on a liquid diet fail to remember that chewing is important for the preservation of their teeth.

In the first place the mouth provides saliva which contains a ferment capable of digesting sugars and starches. In the second place chewing benefits the teeth, the jaws, the nasal and breathing passages, as well as the stomach. The jaws should be well developed not only because we have learned to admire a well-developed jaw, but also because a well-developed jaw gives the teeth plenty of room. When the mouth is not well developed, the teeth become crowded together and get out of line. That makes

chewing more difficult—in short, a vicious circle.

Chewing can be performed not only by chewing gum, which exercises the teeth and jaws and helps to keep the teeth clean, but also by chewing fruits and vegetables with fiber, such, for instance, as carrots, apples, the hearts of cabbage and celery.

Your dentist says, "Keep your teeth clean." This can be made a habit. The dentist says, "Brush your teeth the way they grow." Since the upper teeth grow down, brush them down, and brush the lower teeth upward, and do not forget the surface between the teeth. Brush all the teeth—not just the front ones.

Once you form the habit of brushing your teeth, at least morning and evening if not after each meal, you will learn to relish the sensation of clean teeth.

Your dentist may not say that you ought to see him three times a year, but the facts are that small cavities appear in the teeth and persist and grow larger if they are not promptly cared for. It is, therefore, to your advantage to have your dentist look your teeth over three times a year.

Remember these four rules:

1. Eat the right food.
2. Give your teeth plenty of chewing exercise.
3. Brush your teeth at least twice a day.
4. See your dentist for an examination and cleaning of the teeth three times a year.

TEMPERATURE, BODY The ordinary fever thermometer has a red arrow at 98.6 degrees Fahrenheit, which is supposed to be the normal body temperature.

The human being is built with a thermostat device that controls his temperature. He is kept at the normal temperature by a regulating device in the body which gets rid of excess heat or produces extra heat if it is needed. When we perspire, water evaporates from the skin, and the temperature of the body is lowered. When we shiver or move our muscles, heat is produced and the temperature of the body is raised.

The sensation of heat or cold is not due to a change in the temperature of the body but to a change in the temperature of the skin. When the skin feels cold, a message is sent to the brain; the brain turns loose the mechanisms that arrange for the temperature to be raised or lowered as needed. In the brain there is a little mechanism that works just like the thermometer that turns the oil heater on and off in your home. About four o'clock in the morning your body temperature as recorded by a thermometer in the mouth is likely to be 97.3 degrees Fahrenheit. About four o'clock in the afternoon it will probably be recorded as 99.1 degrees Fahrenheit.

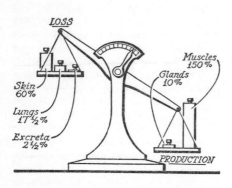

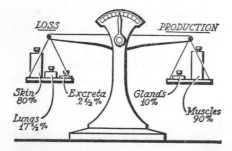

When the body's chemistry operates normally, the heat produced by muscles and by glands is lost by way of the skin, the lungs, and the excreta. When there is fever, the loss is unable to keep up with the production

If you are sick with a fever, the temperature may move up to 104 degrees or even higher. In severe infections at the time of death the fever may reach as high as 107 to 109 degrees. The average fever thermometer has a top of around 110 degrees. Above that temperature human beings usually die. Above 110 degrees conditions occur which affect the cells of the body generally and which are incompatible with life.

Cases are recorded of people who died of heat stroke and who had temperatures over 110 degrees. In one group of 14 cases 6 died and the remainder recovered.

When people report temperatures over 110 degrees lasting beyond a momentary or brief rise, it may be taken for granted that somebody is malingering or manipulating the thermometer.

Repeatedly it has been said that chilling of the human body is bad for health. Some people are much more susceptible to chilling than others. In general it is believed that chilling is more serious for a person with chronic infections of the nose and throat than for a person who is in excellent health. Some people are so sensitive to chilling that they suffer even after having a haircut, after washing the hair, from the coolness of the evening air or any other chilling process. Their response to the chilling is congestion in the nose and sinuses, and the appearance of a condition like a cold. Investigations have shown that people can be especially sensitive to either heat or cold and respond with symptoms of the type described.

TENIA (See discussion under *Worms*) Tapeworm.

TESTICLES See discussion under *Orchitis.*

TETANUS People used to think that tetanus or lockjaw was caused by scratching oneself with a rusty nail. This belief still prevails among many people, although the germ that causes lockjaw was isolated in 1886. The disease was known more than two thousand years ago and was described by Hippocrates.

The poison that is produced by the germ of tetanus is one of the most powerful poisons known. When the germ gets into the body, it sets up inflammation of nerve tissues. These germs have a special predilection for nerves. Some types of wounds are, therefore, more likely to be associated with tetanus than others. Most important are deep, penetrating, lacerating or crushing wounds which contain particles of foreign material. The soil of many areas contains the tetanus germ. The germs of tetanus seem to live preferably in the intestinal tract of cattle, horses, and man. In this way soil is contaminated. The germs live much better in the absence of oxygen; in deep wounds, therefore, they multiply more rapidly than in shallow wounds.

Tetanus begins about seven days after a wound which permits the germs to get into the tissues. The first signs are a sense of drawing pain in the wound with a twitching of muscles near by. Also there is irritability, headache, chills, and fever. Then comes the stiffness of the muscles of the jaw and neck which gives this disease its name. Serious spasms and convulsions ensue. In some cases there may be from three to forty spasms in an hour. All of the muscles of the body may be involved, including those of the bowels and of the bladder.

Even with the best of treatment patients with lockjaw may die because of the poisonous nature of the secretions of this organism. Fortunately medicine now has a preventive of tetanus so efficient that we are able to say that there was not one death from tetanus in the armed forces in World War II.

For the prevention of tetanus people who have been wounded, particularly when the wound is contaminated, should receive immediately an injection under the skin of the specific antitoxin against tetanus. Another injection may be given one week later. The physician who treats the case will open the wound widely, remove any clothing, soil, or other visible contamination that may be present, and treat the wound with appropriate anti-

septic substances. Under the best of treatment it is possible to save the lives of one half to two thirds of the people who are infected.

THERMOMETER The thermometer is used in medicine to ascertain the temperature of the human body. The temperature is usually reported in terms of Fahrenheit, which makes the normal temperature 98.6 degrees when taken with the thermometer in the mouth, a degree higher when the temperature is taken inside the rectum, and a degree lower when the temperature is taken under the arm. Temperatures are also sometimes reported in centigrade according to the decimal system. In the decimal system 37 degrees corresponds to 98.6 degrees Fahrenheit as a normal temperature. A good thermometer registers the temperature in two or three minutes. Even if the thermometer is marked one minute, it is well to leave it in place two or three minutes for an accurate recording.

THROAT There are general inflammations of the throat associated with redness, swelling, and excessive discharge of mucus due to many different causes. Most common, of course, is exposure to cold, an extension of inflammation from the tonsils, the adenoids, or the nose.

Excessive use of tobacco, excessive exposure to dust, smoke, irritating fumes, and sudden changes in temperature, excessive dryness, and similar atmospheric conditions may cause irritation of the throat.

People who are sensitive to certain food substances sometimes react with blisters on the tissues of the throat, which become secondarily infected and produce irritations and inflammation.

There may be severe pain associated with swelling and inflammation of the throat, including pain in the ears because of blocking of the tubes which lead from the nose to the ears; there may also be a sense of fullness or obstruction, with much hawking and spitting.

The first thing to know about any inflammation of the throat is its cause. If the condition happens to be due to diphtheria, prompt action is necessary, including the giving of diphtheria antitoxin. If, however, it is due to some other type of germ, other methods of treatment are employed.

The pain of an inflamed throat is best relieved by use of an ice bag filled with cracked ice. Most doctors are now convinced that gargles seldom go deep enough in the throat in sufficient quantity or strength to permit them to have much effect in killing germs or in curing disease.

To have a definite effect from any antiseptic in the throat, it is necessary to apply it directly to the infected or inflamed part. This is best done by spreading material with a cotton swab or by using an atomizer properly. In order to get the antiseptic into the back of the throat, it may be necessary to hold the tongue or to use a tongue depressor.

The primary purpose of a mouth wash or throat wash is to clean and soothe. A good cleansing mouth wash is merely salt solution made by adding a fourth of a teaspoon of salt to a half glass of warm water. If there is much mucus, the addition of a quarter of a teaspoon of bicarbonate of soda or ordinary baking soda may be beneficial.

THROMBO-ANGIITIS OBLITERANS See *Buerger's Disease*.

THROMBOPHLEBITIS See discussion under *Phlebitis*.

THROMBOSIS The formation of a clot in a blood vessel is called thrombosis. Clots form in all sorts of places and the thrombosis may be described in relationship to the place where it is formed. In various types of inflammation of the blood vessels, thrombi may form. When a portion of the thrombus breaks away and floats in the blood stream, the condition is called embolism.

THRUSH Children become infected by various fungi which attack the tissues of the mouth. This condition is called thrush.

THYMUS GLAND The thymus gland lies in the chest in front of the windpipe, between the lungs and above the heart. Its nature is not yet fully understood.

During the first period of growth the thymus gland and a small gland in the brain called the pineal gland are greatly concerned. The thymus gland is large during the first eight or nine months of life, after which it gradually gets smaller and finally disappears. If it fails to get smaller and continues to send its secretion in large amounts into the body, changes may occur that are serious for life and health. If, however, the thymus gland fails to act during the early years of life, the results are also serious.

If the gland becomes quite large, its situation is such that it may cause difficulty in breathing and in the circulation of the blood in infants. In the condition called status lymphaticus sudden death sometimes occurs, apparently due to the enlargement of the thymus gland. If a physician finds the condition of enlargement on examination, he may wish to expose the gland to the X ray and in that way bring about a reduction in its size.

If the thymus gland continues to secrete beyond the time when it should have stopped, the skin of the person concerned becomes soft, smooth, and velvety. In fact the skin develops a "peaches and cream" complexion. When a boy with this condition becomes a man, he may find that it is unnecessary for him to shave or perhaps he will have to shave only once a week. Persons with persistent thymus glands appear younger than they are; the hair over the body is scanty, and the teeth rather a bluish-white in color. Moreover, they may have a low blood pressure and be easily fatigued.

If, however, the thymus gland discontinues to function too soon, the person concerned seems to grow old a little too soon. Such people are short in stature, the body hair develops early and is thick, and the blood pressure is usually too high.

Recently investigators have been injecting animals with thymus extract. They find that there is marked precocity in the offspring of the animals in the second generation. In the second generation the young animals show increased growth and development. The young of the third generation also grow and develop physically, sexually, and psychically at an unbelievable rate. They do not, however, become giants because the rapid rate of growth decreases from the second month on.

Some investigators believe that the thymus may control to some extent the mental make-up as well, namely, that those in whom thymus action persists remain childlike, self-centered, and simple in their mental processes and initiative, whereas those in whom the thymus disappears too soon become easily aroused to anger and are resentful. While they seem quite advanced when young, they never seem to mature completely.

It should be emphasized that work on the thymus gland is still in an exceedingly early experimental stage. The thymus gland seems to influence to some extent the growth of the skeleton. It seems to be concerned with calcium utilization by the body and also with the development of the sex glands.

THYROID (See also *Goiter*) The gland in the throat in front of the windpipe which secretes an internal secretion called thyroxin. Simple enlargement of the thyroid is goiter; excessive action is hyperthyroidism, also called Basedow's disease, Graves' disease, or exophthalmic goiter.

TIC Any spasmodic movement or twitching, particularly of the face, is called a tic. People can develop tics as a habit, under which circumstances they are called habit spasms. Most serious of all tics is an actual neuralgia involving the facial nerves called tic douloureux. This condition is treated usually with certain drugs which are known to have an effect in many cases. Occasionally, however, all drug treatments fail, so that the condition has to be treated by injection of a substance that will paralyze the nerve or by surgical operation on the nerve or the ganglion cell.

TOBACCO Today the American people spend more for tobacco than for education, religion, or health. The smoking of tobacco is a social habit which has become so firmly established in the American system of living that it represents a fixed charge on the expenditures of every family. The consumption of tobacco has gradually risen as our habits have changed.

Since 1905 the public taste has shifted largely from cigars to cigarettes. The consumption of large cigars dropped from 8,500,000,000 in 1920 to 5,500,-000,000 in 1952. In the same period of time the consumption of cigarettes increased from 50,409,000,000 to over 400,000,000,000 cigarettes.

During this period of time doctors and psychologists have been seriously concerned with the study of the effects of tobacco consumption on the nation's health and welfare. The psychologists particularly have been concerned with the question as to why people smoke. A serious scientific questionnaire showed that sociability, relaxation, and steadying of the nerves are among the most significant of the reasons given. Less significant were the effects of smoking on hunger and the pleasures associated with the sight of the smoke, the feel of the cigarette, and the social charm associated with the habit.

From the point of view of the effects of tobacco on the body, the smoking of nicotine affects the nervous system and the blood vessels. Most serious of the effects of tobacco are its effects on the circulation of the blood. Thus the smoking of tobacco is definitely related to the increase in the condition called Buerger's disease or thrombo-angiitis obliterans. Especially important is the possible relationship of excessive cigarette smoking to cancer of the lung.

Secondary effects on the digestion and on the throat and lungs have also been established. These vary, however, in different people, depending on the amount of tobacco smoking that is done. Among the symptoms credited to excess smoking are irregular neuralgias, vague gastrointestinal discomfort, headache, insomnia, disturbances of the bowels, palpitation of the heart, and diseases of the circulation of the blood.

However, the records of thousands of persons who have smoked considerably over long periods of time indicate that, on the whole, the habit of smoking is not nearly so harmful as the sound of this list of symptoms would indicate. There is a tendency for the individual smoker to establish a certain amount of tolerance to the use of tobacco.

TONGUE Doctors of a previous generation always looked first at the patient's tongue. A tongue that is dry, dark, and furred indicates disease. A tongue that is moist and clean reflects a normal condition.

A healthy tongue can be moved quickly or slowly in all directions. Various diseases modify the movements of the tongue. In people who have overactivity of the thyroid gland, the tongue moves quickly and snappily; those who have underactivity of the gland are likely to have a sluggish tongue. People who are weak or exhausted and those in a stupor or in a coma will put the tongue out just a little and leave it out until they are told to put it back.

Paralysis that affects only one side of the tongue results in having the healthy side push the tongue toward the paralyzed side. This sign is seen especially in people who have had a hemorrhage into the brain or who have lost the function of one side of the brain from some other cause.

Among the most common of the peculiar sensations that disturb many people is a burning feeling in the tongue. The tongue, like all of the other tissues of the human body, is connected with the nervous system. A burning sensation in the tongue is reflected through its nerves. Many investigations have been made of this symptom. Sometimes the tongue is inflamed by coming into contact with the edges of rough teeth or by the wearing of unsatisfactory false teeth. In some cases of pellagra or pernicious anemia there are burning sensations in the tongue. The symptom is also found occasionally associated with difficulties of the digestive system. When, therefore, a patient complains of a burning sensation in the tongue, the physician will want to make a complete examination, including particularly a study of the digestive system and of the blood.

In a few instances burning and even ulcers of the tongue have been found to be due to the fact that metals of different electric potentials are used to fill the teeth on opposite sides of the mouth. There are, of course, instances in which the tongue is itself infected by germs, also cases in which the tongue may be subject to cancer or other specific diseases.

Sometimes the surface of the tongue, instead of being smooth, becomes marked by deep furrows and elevations. As a result, it looks like a relief map. This condition is called geographic tongue. Sometimes the condition can be improved by the use of mouth washes, mild antiseptics, and the adoption of a diet that is rich in vitamins and antianemic substances like iron and liver. The exact cause of geographic tongue has not been definitely determined.

TONSILS Why do we have tonsils? Apparently they serve some purpose in taking care of infectious germs that come into the throat. They respond to infection with swelling and inflammation associated with pain, soreness, difficulty in swallowing, swelling of the glands in the throat, fever, a rapid pulse, and illness generally.

The list of diseases that have been attributed to infection through germs of one kind or another attacking the tonsils is like the index of a medical book. Definite relationships have been traced between infection of the tonsils and infections of the ears, eyes, diseases of the skin, the heart, and the joints. In cases in which there is such inflammation or infection it has been found that removal of the tonsils has a good effect on the general health. Moreover, there are subsequently fewer disturbances of the throat and of the nose and chest.

The child who breathes constantly through the mouth because of the presence of tonsils or adenoids will be found after their removal to breathe through the nose. This has an excellent effect not only on the child's frame of mind but also in aiding sleep and improving the child's appearance.

An enlarged tonsil is not necessarily an infected tonsil. Enlargement may, however, be the result of repeated infections which subsequently heal.

Many hundreds of thousands, if not millions, of people have had their tonsils removed, and it is now possible for the doctors to draw some positive conclusions as to the desirability of removal of the tonsils in certain instances. The modern operation for the removal of the tonsils has been so well perfected that complications are exceedingly rare, and an occasional fatality even rarer. When the operation for the removal of the tonsils is properly performed, preferably in a hospital, with the anesthetic either general or local properly controlled, the operation is likely to be completely successful.

In very old people or in instances of heart disease or in other cases when the taking of an anesthetic is not possible, tonsils are sometimes treated with the X ray. The X ray is also used occasionally to treat fragments of tissue that may be left after removal of the tonsils. The experts consider this technic as suitable only in exceptional cases rather than as a routine.

TORTICOLLIS When a person's neck appears to be twisted, so that the head leans or is tilted toward one shoulder or the other, the condition is called wry neck, twisted neck, or torticollis.

There are various causes for this condition. Sometimes an accident of birth is responsible. Many people tilt their heads to one side as a habit. In cases of wry neck that have lasted a long time, the tissue on the short side of the neck becomes shortened to accommodate itself to the twisting. The face as well as the skull may become deformed, giving it a slanting appearance. There may even be twisting of the spine to compensate for the twisting of the head.

In the ordinary case of wry neck the application of heat and the use of drugs to overcome the pain will frequently bring about relief. In every such instance, however, the doctor must make a thorough search to find out whether or not there are infections elsewhere in the body, since failure to overcome sources of infection may bring about repeated instances of twisting of the neck.

Occasionally wry neck occurs as the result of a nervous or mental disturbance associated occasionally with overwork or mental strain. This is called a functional nervous disorder and is treated by mental methods.

Wry neck sometimes occurs as a result of infection of the lymph glands in the neck. In still other cases it may be associated with damage to the spine or the spinal cord.

In the difficult chronic case of wry neck a surgical operation may be desirable to prevent secondary deformities such as those that have been mentioned. In this operation ligaments are cut and occasionally muscles are operated on to permit placing of the head in proper alignment to the neck. By the use of suitable braces or casts the head is held in this position until complete recovery has occurred. Regular exercises and massage are useful in the postoperative period to bring about better results.

TRACHEA The scientific name for the windpipe is the trachea. It is often involved in infections of the throat and the bronchial tubes. Any virus or germ that can produce inflammation of the respiratory tract can also cause the lining of the trachea to become infected. It is possible for the experts to see the lining of the trachea by the use of the bronchoscope.

In World War I there were many instances of severe inflammation of the lining of the trachea due to mustard gas poisoning. When the lining of the trachea becomes inflamed, the most typical symptom is the cough. These coughs are non-productive, hacking, and metallic. They tend to be worse after the person goes to bed and during the night. An acute inflammation of the trachea is accompanied by rawness, tightness, and discomfort, sometimes even pain, in the lower part of the neck and behind the upper part of the breastbone, or sternum. As the inflammation goes on, there is mucus and finally a good deal of sputum and mucus may be expectorated. If the infection is purulent, as with the staphylococcus or streptococcus, the material coughed up will be a mixture of mucus and pus.

These conditions can be helped by the usual treatment that is given to other inflammations of the respiratory tract. That means going to bed for a few days, applying warmth, and producing rest by the use of appropriate remedies which the doctor prescribes. Often inhalations of warm vapor treated with medicated oils help to bring relief.

In some instances the acute inflammation of the trachea becomes chronic. In such cases the cough is irritating and frequent. When these symptoms are present, it becomes necessary for the doctor to make certain that the patient does not have tuberculosis or any other condition affecting the lungs. In such cases it is customary to prohibit smoking. Often residence in a warm, dry climate is advisable. The use of anti-infectious remedies such as the sulfonamides and penicillin are important in eliminating infection.

TRACHOMA One of the most widespread diseases of the world is an inflammation of the eyes called trachoma, now believed to be due to a specific virus. The condition is so common in Egypt, Palestine, and India, except among the upper classes, that it is almost a universal disease.

The infection is carried by the transfer of the secretions from the eyes through the use of the hands, towels, handkerchiefs, pillows, or even by sneezing. It has been thought indeed that in some areas the infection is carried by flies.

In this condition the eye becomes inflamed and red; then blisters and crusts form. The scarring and injury may change the shape of the eyelids. If the infection of the cornea of the eye becomes sufficiently severe, the eyesight may be destroyed.

This infection should be avoided with every possible effort. People who are in an area where trachoma is common should be exceedingly careful about the use of common towels and about rubbing the eyes with the hands.

The modern treatment of trachoma, using the sulfonamide drugs and aureomycin has been helpful in stopping the progress of the disease.

In treating the symptoms of trachoma, including the inflammation and the secretion, attempts are made to check and remove the granules and to overcome the enlargement of the tissues of the conjunctiva. This is accomplished by the application of caustic substances like sulfate of copper or nitrate of silver and by mechanical and surgical methods such as scraping or cutting away the excess material. This demands the utmost judgment and care on the part of the physician, since overirritation demands soothing treatment, so that there is no routine. Each patient must be treated according to the condition that exists at the time he is examined. It becomes necessary to keep the eyes clean for some time by the frequent use of solutions of salt or alkaline washes or other preparations which the physician may prescribe.

In the United States at least 10 per cent of the entire Indian population are said to be affected. Since the development of new methods of treatment, the condition is gradually being eliminated even from our Indian tribes.

TRENCH MOUTH See *Vincent's Angina.*

TRICHINOSIS When the Jewish leaders prohibited the eating of pork around 1500 B.C., they probably did so because there had been trouble with infected pork. The infection that usually occurs is trichinosis, first recognized as a disease around 1822. The organism that causes trichinosis was not demonstrated, however, until 1835. This is a small, round worm, scarcely visible to the naked eye, quite slender and tapering. The organism multiplies freely in the intestines. After development it passes by way of the blood to the muscles, where it lives and causes pain and other serious symptoms. Occasionally considerable numbers of people are infected by eating pork that has been improperly inspected, insufficiently cooked, and improperly handled.

The United States Department of Agriculture requires storage of pork at a temperature of 5 degrees Fahrenheit or below for twenty days before it is used. This will destroy all the trichina organisms. Occasionally, however, meat of animals killed for home consumption is not properly controlled; then the people who eat the meat get the symptoms of trichinosis. A temperature of 137 degrees Fahrenheit for a sufficient period of time will destroy the organisms of trichinosis; therefore proper cooking of pork will help to prevent an outbreak.

In a typical case the symptoms begin with headache, chills, and a general feeling of illness. Then the eyes become swollen and painful. There may be sore throat and a general soreness of the muscles. Fever appears. Examination of the blood reveals the presence of great numbers of white blood cells and especially an increase of one type of white blood cell known as eosinophiles.

There is not much to be done in the way of specific treatment of the disease. After a while the tissues of the body surround the organisms and encapsulate them.

The way to avoid this disease is to make sure that all pork products are properly inspected, properly stored, and properly cooked. At the same time there must be a campaign of education as to the feeding of swine. Swine which are fed on garbage are infested with trichinae from three to five times as often as swine that are fed on grain. In some instances the infection gets into the hogs from the eating of rats. The feeding of garbage to swine may seem economical, but if it is to result in any considerable number of cases of trichinosis, it will prove far more costly than will the feeding of suitable material free from the possibility of infection.

TUBERCULOSIS Tuberculosis has destroyed more human beings than any other disease. Today it is still seventh in the list of causes of death. It destroys life mostly in early and middle adult ages, at the time when people are most productive economically and most useful. It kills more men than women proportionately and attacks colored people much more seriously than it does the white race. Some 80,000 people die each year from this infection.

In 1910, 136 out of every 100,000 people in our country died from tuberculosis. In 1932 it was 56.4. Today the rate is near to 20. Nevertheless, our present death rate means that between 7,000,000 and 8,000,000 people now living in the United States will die eventually of tuberculosis unless some new discovery or wider use of present methods materially controls the condition.

The discovery of new drugs like streptomycin, paramino salicylic acid, and isoniazid has stimulated research. New methods are now being intensively studied. Combinations of various new remedies are so effective in treatment that many people are now treated while ambulatory instead of being placed in sanatoriums.

Tuberculosis is a germ disease. It is not an inherited disease. Usually it attacks children through contact of the child with some older person who has the disease or with an animal suffering from the disease or with food products or other materials contaminated by the germ. Sometimes the disease attacks not in childhood but later along in life. Modern methods of diagnosis reveal that the tendency is more and more for protection of the child against the disease until a later period in his life.

We now have tests which show whether or not a child has been or is infected with the germs of tuberculosis. These tests can be applied to large groups of children to determine the extent of infection. In some areas every child is examined by these methods. England has just arranged for their use on a large scale.

People seldom suspected tuberculosis in previous times until severe coughs with expectoration began with loss of weight and night sweats. With modern methods the disease is detected long before any such serious signs are present. The use of the X ray shows promptly changes which occur in the lung. The use of the tuberculin tests can demonstrate the presence of the disease. Many people now arrange to have their family doctor use such technics at regular intervals to find out whether or not children are in danger.

In the tuberculin test a small amount of material called tuberculin is applied to the skin or in some cases injected between the layers of the skin. If the skin reacts positively to this material, the significance is that the tissues have been sensitized to the material of the germ of tuberculosis. A positive tuberculin test means that the tubercle germs have entered the body and that somewhere in the body there is infection.

There may, of course, be cases in which the reactions are doubtful and other cases in which other possible evidence of tuberculosis cannot be found by any of the well-accepted measures. In most instances this should indicate, however, either the necessity for further testing or the necessity for continued watchfulness and further study to determine the point at which the infection is localized.

Not always will a person who has a positive tuberculin test become severely sick with this disease. Approximately 20 per cent of those who react positively to this test do present manifestations of the disease at some subsequent time.

We do not, however, have any certain way of knowing which of those who react positively will fall into the 80 per cent of those who are going to be safe and which will fall into the 20 per cent of those who are going to be severely infected. The safe measure is, therefore, to examine carefully at regular intervals those who react positively to the tuberculin test.

CAUSE—Tuberculosis is caused by a germ, first described by the bacteriologist Robert Koch. There are different kinds of tubercle germs—those which affect human beings primarily, those which affect cattle, those which affect birds, and those which affect cold-blooded animals like the frog and the turtle. The ones which affect cattle are most like those which affect man, but the human type is more dangerous to a human being than it is to domestic animals, and the cattle type is more dangerous to domestic animals than it is to man.

The cattle type may, however, infect human beings, especially children. Indeed the bovine, or cattle, form of tuberculosis is known to be largely responsible for tuberculosis of the bones, joints, and lymph glands of children who have been in the past infected by drinking milk from cows infected with bovine tuberculosis.

As a result of the recognition of this menace to health milk supplies are controlled by submitting cattle to the tuberculin test and by eliminating from the herds of cows those which are found to have the disease. In the United States we have cut down the incidence of tuberculosis in cattle to the vanishing point. There are still countries in the world, however, including England, where tuberculosis, particularly of bones, joints, and glands, has not been well controlled. In the United States tuberculosis of the glands of the abdomen is exceedingly uncommon and, when it does occur, is mild. In other countries in which control of tuberculous cattle has not been so efficient, such tuberculosis continues to appear. In most instances tuberculosis of the glands of the abdomen is due to the swallowing of germs which have been coughed up from the lungs or to milk products containing the germs of tuberculosis.

One of the saddest forms of tuberculosis is that which causes a crippling of the spine. This condition is called Pott's disease after a British physician named Pott who first described it. When one of the bones of the spine becomes involved, the central portion of the bone is broken down and softened so that the muscles pull the bones together and produce the buckling of the spine which is characteristic of Pott's disease. Tuberculosis may also affect the hip joint or other joint or other bones, producing crippling injuries which are easily recognizable. Tuberculosis may affect the glands, the covering of the brain, the spinal fluid, the eye, and many other tissues as well as the lung. In each instance it is necessary for the doctor to make a suitable diagnosis and then to treat the condition according to the portion of the body that is concerned. It is quite possible for a person to have not only tuberculosis of the lung but at the same time some of the other forms of the disease that have been mentioned.

At one time it was thought necessary for every child to have tuberculosis in order to develop resistance against the disease. We now recognize that this was a view like the old belief that every child ought to be exposed to measles so as to have the disease and get it over with.

There now is in Britain a definite increase in bone and joint tuberculosis among children. Be sure that children get grade A pasteurized milk; that is insurance against milk as a source of tuberculosis.

PREVENTION—The truly extensive knowledge of tuberculosis which we now have should make its complete prevention an ultimate possibility. The disease cannot be stamped out overnight, but persistence can control it, as some states and cities already are proving. The first step is elimination of the exposure of young children to infection from adults with whom they come in contact. Today we are crowded together beyond anything that occurred in the past. The home has largely disappeared in our great cities. We have tremendous apartment houses, tenements, and barracks. These apartments are occupied by from three to a hundred families, where the children come in contact not only with their own parents and relatives but with vast numbers of other children and other families. A child of an earlier day played in his own back yard until the age of six. Today the child goes early to nursery school or plays about with others while his mother is at work. Then he goes to kindergarten and afterward to assemble with other children in public schools. Human beings are crowded together in streetcars, busses, and elevators, and assemble in crowds of thousands in motion picture houses and in crowds of tens of hundreds of thousands at various public events. It is not possible for any person living in a modern city to avoid contact with other human beings.

We know that the people of many portions of the world did not have tuberculosis until it was brought to them by civilized human beings. We know, moreover, that the first infection coming into a population which has not been previously subjected to tuberculosis is far more destructive than an infection coming into a community in which there has always been tuberculosis.

The attack on tuberculosis must be not only a medical but also an economic attack. This is a disease associated with bad hygiene. It multiplies when there is an insufficient amount of food, rest, sunlight, and fresh air. It can be shown that a sudden drop in wages or financial depression will result in an increase of tuberculosis.

When the germ of tuberculosis gets into the body either by direct inhalation of germs or by inhaling dust containing the germs or by any of the other methods that have been mentioned, it tends to localize and to set up an infection. The infection may be a sudden, severe one or a slower and more chronic infection. It seems likely that sometimes a child is lightly infected with the disease, recovering quite promptly, but that it is thereafter sensitive to a new infection with the same organism.

The germs which establish themselves in the body form lesions or spots of infection which are typical of tuberculosis. These areas may become secondarily infected with other organisms which, of course, change the general picture of the disease.

SYMPTOMS—The symptoms by which most people know tuberculosis include the cough, which is an indication of an infection of the lung, whether by tuberculosis or by some other germ. Any cough that lasts for three or four weeks is always suspect of the possibility that it presents a disease of the lungs. With the cough there is frequently expectoration. There is also in certain cases enough destruction of lung tissue so that the person with tuberculosis may expectorate some blood. Also there may be pouring out of fluid into the walls of the chest—an example of the attempts of the body to control the infection.

Because of the manner in which the disease attacks the human body, the person with tuberculosis is generally rather sick and complains of loss of strength and loss of weight. There may also be a slight afternoon rise of temperature or fever and associated with that an increase in the rate of the pulse. The night sweats are commonly found in the presence of tuberculosis, but they may be caused by many other conditions as well. When a physician finds symptoms and signs of this character in a patient, he then extends his examination promptly to take advantage of modern methods of diagnosis. Chief among these methods of examination is the use of the X ray. The X-ray pictures will show in many instances the extent of involvement of the lung. The doctor will also put to use all of the older systems of examination which have been proved valuable by many years of experience. These include a general examination of the chest to determine any changes that have taken place in its shape or its contour and

also in its movements. The doctor puts his hands on the chest to find out whether or not there are spasms of the muscles or vibrations associated with the passing of air into the lung or out of it. He thumps the chest in order to find out by the sounds whether or not there is dullness, tympanic response, or increased resonance.

These and other signs indicate to the doctor the nature of the changes in the tissue of the lung. Next he listens with his stethoscope, because the various sounds made by the air passing into the lung indicate the presence of interference with the passing of the air, the presence of fluid, the presence of solid tissue, or other changes.

The sputum of the patient is examined for the presence of the germs of tuberculosis, and if these are found present by suitable straining methods, the evidence is well-nigh unimpeachable. The absence of the germs does not, however, exclude the disease because in the earlier stages of the disease they may be absent in as many as 35 per cent of cases.

The hope of successful treatment in this disease depends largely on the recognition of the disease at the earliest possible moment. Hence, whenever there is any question of tuberculosis, those concerned should have everything in the way of diagnostic aid that modern medicine can offer to prove the presence or absence of this disease.

TREATMENT—Once the doctor has determined the extent of the tuberculosis, the age of the infections, the portions of tissue involved, and other important factors, it is necessary for him to decide what to do about treatment and also to decide what to tell the patient about his future. The future of the patient depends on the extent of the disease at the time treatment is begun, the character of the disease—namely, whether it is a rapidly progressive or slowly progressive type—the extent to which other organs have been involved by complications, and the general condition of the body so far as relates to its nutrition and general existence.

Much depends on the amount of response that the patient may make to the proper treatment. If he responds favorably and promptly, he is much more likely to do well than if it is difficult to get any change. The age of the patient is also of great importance.

Generally speaking, the more advanced the disease happens to be at the time when the diagnosis is made, the poorer is the likelihood of recovery. In cases of tuberculosis that are far advanced recovery in more than 10 to 20 per cent of the cases is unlikely. Tuberculosis is more quickly fatal and more serious in the extremely young than in those who are older. Where living conditions are exceedingly bad, the likelihood of recovery is not so great. The temperament of the patient and his attitude toward the disease are important factors, because a patient without hope and without anxiety to recover will not give to his doctor or his nurse the kind of co-operation that is necessary in this disease. If the patient happens to have diabetes, heart disease, or some kidney disturbance in addition to tuberculosis, his chance of recovery is less.

Nowadays cases of tuberculosis are classified as minimal, moderately advanced, or far advanced. Another classification describes the cases as apparently cured, arrested, apparently arrested, quiescent, improved, or unimproved. A decision as to the exact status of the case rests in every instance on a complete study of the condition, using all of the best available modern methods of physical and laboratory examination.

One of the first measures to be considered formerly was a change of climate. Nowadays it is believed quite possible to get a suitable climate anywhere in the world. The only advantage in traveling to hunt a cure is the advantage that accrues from a change of surroundings.

In general it is well established that open air is helpful to the tuberculous and that it is most effective when the temperature of the air is cool and bracing. One authority points out that the favorable effect of rest in the open air on the toxic symptoms of tuberculosis is often striking. This measure of treatment may be begun promptly and developed until it becomes a habit. The patient can be out of doors during all of the daytime and in many cases sleep out of doors as well, although outdoor sleeping is not essential if plenty of air is available by use of screened porches or open windows. In general cold air seems to be helpful, but if the circulation of the blood is not good and the reaction to cold air is insufficient, exposure to cold air need not be a routine. In any type of outdoor life exposure to dust, wind, rain, and fog is undesirable. Heat or cold in great excess are dangerous to health. In general warm, moist climates are believed to have a depressing effect, and cool, dry climates to be stimulating. There is really no one best climate for all who are tuberculous. Proper treatment under scientific conditions is more important than climate alone.

New remedies such as streptomycin and neomycin and para-aminosalicylic acid have revolutionized the treatment of tuberculosis. They are used particularly for tuberculosis in the young, tuberculous meningitis, and tuberculosis of the larynx.

CLIMATE AND TUBERCULOSIS—There was a time when everyone who had tuberculosis immediately began traveling. Not long ago the United States Government, through the United States Public Health Service, protested against the shipping of patients to certain states when such patients did not have the means for the necessities of life after they arrived at the new location. The minimum costs of care approximate twenty-five to fifty dollars a week. Unless an invalid is able to provide from twelve to eighteen hundred dollars a year for his care, he cannot do himself much good by moving to another state in which neither his citizenship nor his residency is established. When the burden of providing for himself in a strange town is added to the burdens of the disease from which he suffers, the invalid loads himself with a handicap so great that it may mean the difference between life and death.

After a consideration of all of the various factors involved in the climatic factors of tuberculosis, Dr. James Alexander Miller summarizes the situation with ten aphorisms which follow:

1. The regimen of regulated rest and exercise, proper food, and open-air life is the fundamental essential in the treatment of tuberculosis. Suitable climatic environment makes this open-air life more easy, enjoyable, and beneficial.

2. When these essentials are assured, a change of climate is of definite value in a considerable number, probably the majority of cases, but with the proper regimen many cases will do well in any climate.

3. Any change of climate involving the fatigue of travel is contraindicated in acute cases with fever or hemorrhage, or in very far advanced and markedly debilitated cases. Absolute bed rest is the one essential here.

4. No patient should be sent away in search of climate who cannot afford to stay the reasonably-to-be-expected time and to have the necessary food, lodging, and care.

5. Competent medical advice and supervision are essential.

6. One of the most valuable assets of change is the education of the patient. This may, of course, be obtained in a suitable environment without reference to climate, as in a sanatorium near home.

7. Selection of a suitable locality is an individual problem for every patient, depending upon his temperament, tastes, and individual reaction to environment, as well as the character of his disease. The advising physician should have an appreciation of these as well as a knowledge of the particular environment to which the patient is being sent. Contentment and reasonable comfort are essential.

8. There is no universally ideal climate. For each patient there may well be a most favorable environment, if we are wise enough to find it.

9. There is a reasonable amount of evidence that certain medical types of cases are more favorably influenced by certain conditions of climate, everything else being equal. For example reasonably cold, dry, variable climate, such as is found in the mountains, for young or vigorous constitutions which will react well. Dry, sunny climates for laryngeal cases and those with marked catarrhal secretions. Equable mild climates at low altitudes for the elderly and those of nervous temperaments, as well as for those with arteriosclerosis, weak hearts, or marked tendency to dyspnea.

10. Successful selection of climate and environment for cases of tuberculosis requires wide knowledge of human nature, of places, and of the disease. This can only be acquired by patience, skill, and experience.

ARTIFICIAL PNEUMOTHORAX—Among the many ways in which the lung of the person with tuberculosis may be rested, that which has received the greatest consideration in recent years is the so-called application of pneumothorax, sometimes called collapse treatment. There are many different ways by which a lung may be collapsed so that the tissues may be quiet and out of use until they have opportunity to recover. The purpose of collapse is not only to give rest to the lung but also to hinder the spread of the disease from one portion of the lung to another.

The first of the procedures is known as artificial pneumothorax, and it seems to be applicable in anywhere from one fourth to one half of all cases, preferably those in which only one lung or a portion of one lung is involved rather than a considerable amount of both lungs. This method is not suitable to patients who have large amounts of fluid in the chest or those in whom there has been a great deal of pleurisy with attachment of the lung to the chest wall.

In brief the method of treatment involves the insertion of a needle into the chest cavity and the passing of air into the cavity from without in sufficient amounts to compress the lung tissue and to stop its motion. Some investigators have suggested the injection of mineral oil into the chest cavity instead of air, but this procedure has not been widely adopted.

It is also possible to put the lung at rest by cutting the nerve which goes to the diaphragm. Elimination of movement of the muscles of the diaphragm and of the chest on the side concerned causes the diaphragm to be rested and thus to diminish the amount of work in the chest cavity.

Another method is wholly surgical and is seldom used until after pneumothorax has been tried and failed or else has been found to be impossible to apply. In this method, known as thoracoplasty, there is an actual operation on the chest wall involving the removal of portions of the ribs, thus bringing about collapse and complete rest of the lung tissue.

In many instances the method of artificial pneumothorax fails because it is not applied soon enough. When the method of treatment is applied soon enough and in the proper manner, patients who would in previous years have been compelled to remain constantly in the sanatorium are actually given opportunity to go about their work. It cannot be expected, however, from this or any other method of treatment that the patient will recover immediately. In many instances the pneumothorax must be kept up for one, two, or three years before signs of healing appear as shown by the use of the X ray and other modern methods of investigation.

TULAREMIA   Almost twenty years have passed since Dr. Edward Francis of the United States Public Health Service announced the discovery of a disease infecting human beings who had been in contact with diseased rabbits. Rarely the condition is carried to a human being by a tick. By far the most common source of infection is an infection of the hands of a person who has dressed the flesh of a diseased rabbit for cooking purposes. The rabbit meat thoroughly cooked is harmless as a food, since a temperature of 130 degrees Fahrenheit will kill the germ of tularemia.

When tularemia appears on the body, there is usually an ulcer at the point where the germs entered through the skin. The ulcer usually appears several days after the exposure to the infected rabbit. Following the appearance of the ulcer, there develop aching of the muscles and joints, weakness, chills, and fever, which may last for several weeks.

Tularemia, or rabbit fever, gets its name from Tulare County, California. Some years ago the wild game in Tulare County were found to be dying by the thousands because of a plaguelike condition that was spreading among them. The germ isolated was the germ of tularemia.

Chiefly it is the wild rabbit that is infected, although the past twenty years have brought to light cases of infection in almost every other type of small wild animal, including muskrats, opossums, and water rats, also squirrels, cats, and sheep.

During the year 1938, 545 cases of tularemia were found in a survey of twenty large cities with a total population of 20,000,000 people.

Men who hunt rabbits should be warned of the danger of bringing home for cooking any rabbit that can be knocked over with a stick. A healthy rabbit is one that can run like a "scared rabbit" when the hunter approaches. The animal that can be knocked down is one that is likely to be infected with tularemia or some other disease.

People who handle rabbits for any purpose ought to wear rubber gloves. If they do not, they should wash their hands thoroughly in some mild antiseptic solution and most thoroughly with soap and water after they have finished the handling of the rabbits. Never let a scratch, a cut, or a sore come in contact with the flesh of the rabbit or with the dish or pan in which rabbit meat has been kept. Wrapping paper which has contained the bodies of dead rabbits should be burned. The attention of the doctor should be called to every cut or sore just as soon as there is the slightest evidence of swelling or secondary infection.

TUMORS A word describing any overgrowth of tissue. See discussion under *Cancer*.

TYPHOID FEVER Once typhoid fever was first in the subjects seriously discussed in textbooks of medicine. Today it has been relegated to a less important position because modern sanitary methods have practically eliminated the danger of typhoid fever in a modern community.

If the case rates and death rates that prevailed in Chicago in 1880 existed today, there would be 60,000 cases of typhoid fever and approximately 6000 deaths from that disease every year. Instead Chicago has seldom had as many as 200 cases with 10 deaths in any one year.

Typhoid fever is an acute infection caused by a germ known as the typhoid bacillus. The germ can be found in the blood of a person seriously sick with the disease, and in 80 per cent of cases the typhoid germ is found in the material that is passed by the bowels. The germ of typhoid fever is spread by means of the excretions of the body, by contaminated food and clothing, and by water and milk which contain the germs. The primary menace in typhoid fever today is the typhoid carrier, the person who has had the disease and recovered but who still continues to give off the germs.

Typhoid fever follows a long and serious course once a person becomes infected. From three to twenty-one days after the infection, which is known as the incubation period, the germs develop in the body and liberate their poisons. Typhoid fever begins with the usual symptoms of infection, such as headache, pains all over the body, the feeling of exhaustion, chills, and fever. Frequently there is nosebleed, and almost invariably there is serious disturbance of the bowels due to the fact that the typhoid germs produce ulcers

in the bowels. As the disease goes on, the infected person becomes sicker and sicker; clots may form in the blood vessels; rose spots appear on the skin at the end of the first week or beginning of the second week. Because of the damage to the bowels, there is formation of gas with bloating and sometimes severe hemorrhages from the bowels. Occasionally the infection also attacks the nervous system, producing pains and even delirium.

The doctor who examines the patient with typhoid fever makes his diagnosis from the history of the case, the nature of the symptoms, and also by careful studies of the blood. A blood test called the Widal test is a means of determining with reasonable certainty that the condition is typhoid fever.

A person who has typhoid fever must be kept alone and preferably cared for by an experienced nurse. The room should be screened if the illness occurs during the summer when flies are common.

Because the person with typhoid is likely to remain in bed for a long time, he should have a firm mattress, and arrangements must be made to change the bed linen any time it is soiled. The patient must be bathed at least once a day and kept clean in order to prevent secondary infections. It is also important that the mouth be rinsed each time after food is taken.

There was a time when it was thought advisable to starve typhoid patients. It is now known that the condition is so serious as to break down the nutrition of the patient, so that present methods involve the giving of a diet of from 3000 to 3500 calories. Then the patient will not lose weight during the course of the illness.

It is well established that a vaccine made of the killed germs of typhoid fever is of value in preventing the disease. It is customary to give three injections of the vaccine at ten-day intervals, although the intervals between injections may be shortened. Obviously such vaccines should be given by a physician or a trained nurse. Only rarely indeed are there reactions of a serious character.

It is probable that persistent attention to water supplies and disposal of sewage, pasteurization of milk, education of the public in hygiene, and the control of typhoid carriers will eventually eliminate typhoid fever entirely throughout the civilized world.

In typhoid fever chloromycetin or chloramphenicol is effective.

TYPHUS Typhus fever is one of the most important of all epidemics in the world today. An epidemic of this disease, which has in the past been called hospital fever, spotted fever, jail fever, camp fever, and ship fever, is devastating.

We know that the condition is spread by the body louse and that a similar condition is spread by the rat flea. There are other diseases like typhus— perhaps different forms of the same disease—that are spread by various insects in different parts of the world.

A Chicago physician named Howard Taylor Ricketts proved that the Mexican form of typhus fever called tabardillo is spread by the body louse. This disease has been named in his honor Rickettsia.

Usually typhus appears about twelve days after a person has been bitten by an infected louse. Prostration is one of the first symptoms. About five days after the first signs of illness a dark red, mottling eruption occurs, later changing to blood spots. In the form of typhus that occurs in civilian life away from war fronts, the condition begins like any other infectious disease with rapidly increasing fever. The eruption takes place on the fifth or sixth day. Then there may be a crisis with recovery or perhaps death.

The prevention of typhus fever involves measures associated with the elimination of lice and fleas. In time of war all of the clothing of our soldiers is sterilized in special delousing apparatus. One of the greatest discoveries of World War II has been the development of extracts of pyrethrum with which the underwear of soldiers may be treated

so that a louse cannot live in contact with the underwear as long as six weeks after the underwear is first sprayed or dipped in the solution.

Another great development is DDT powder. By the liberal use of this powder the spread of typhus fever was stopped in Naples immediately after the American troops captured that city. The DDT powder is freely sprinkled in the clothing, particularly in the seams. The body lice cannot live in contact with this powder.

Finally, vaccines have been developed which are made by preparing emulsions of Rickettsia organisms. All of the American soldiers going into typhus-infested areas are given immunity against the disease with the vaccine.

By the use of all of these measures our troops were kept relatively free from typhus throughout the war.

There is always some typhus in various portions of the United States, and our health authorities are constantly on the watch for it. We have every reason to believe that the spread of the disease in this country can be halted by the methods known to modern medical science.

ULCERS Any open sore, other than a wound, is called an ulcer. The term is applied to a loss of substance inside the body. Ulcers may occur from infection, from injury to the blood supply, from damage to nerves, and from a wide variety of other causes. The occurrence of an ulcer is an indication for a physician to find out exactly what caused the ulcer. The method of treatment is definitely related to the cause.

UMBILICUS See *Navel, Diseases of.*

UNDULANT FEVER Among the other names common for the condition called undulant fever are brucellosis, Malta fever, Mediterranean fever, abortus fever, and melitensis fever. These names represent the history of the condition and the investigator who first determined its cause.

Undulant fever has existed in the

Mediterranean region from early times. It was first definitely studied on the island of Malta. A British physician named Bruce first isolated the causative germ. Then a similar organism was found to be responsible for contagious abortion in cattle.

The disease occurs as a natural disease of goats, sheep, and cattle and is commonly contracted in man by consumption of infected milk or milk products such as butter, cheese, and ice cream. Occasionally it may result from direct contact with infected animals. It may also spread through contamination of soil and water. Instances are known in which an infection has followed puncture of the skin by a contaminated needle, and it is conceivable that the condition may at times be carried by biting insects.

Somewhere from twelve days to three weeks after the person has been exposed to the condition the fever begins. It is of an undulating type, climbing like a stepladder with morning remissions of one degree. Then, having reached a level of 102 or 103 degrees, the fever will remain raised for a few days and gradually fall by a stepladder descent. Successive waves of fever and intermissions may go on in this way for weeks or months. With the fever come headache, disturbance of the bowels, principally constipation, and occasionally the cloudiness and dulling of the intellect which accompany continued fever. There are cases in which the fever is continuous. Instances also occur in which undulant fever is a very severe disease, rising to a sudden high temperature and not infrequently causing death.

Because of the nature of this disease it has at times been confused with typhoid fever, tuberculosis, malaria, and a variety of tropical diseases.

Before 1927 undulant fever was regarded in the United States as a medical curiosity. Now cases have been recorded in every state. In the Southwest the condition has been called goat fever, Texas fever, and Rio Grande fever.

Methods have now been developed for testing the blood of people who are believed to have this condition, using a test similar to that used for typhoid fever. These tests, carried out now by our state medical laboratories, aid the physician in confirming the diagnosis.

For many years little could be done for the person with undulant fever. Now, however, vaccines have been developed, made from the killed organisms, which seem to be helpful in some cases. The injection of foreign protein substances causes a fever reaction in the body, which helps in some cases. In some instances the sulfonamide drugs have been useful, particularly when combined with treatments in the hypertherm, or heat cabinet. Combinations of streptomycin and sulfonamides have been found effective in undulant fever.

UREMIA If both kidneys are removed, the person concerned, or the animal concerned, will die in a few days because poisons formed in the body are not eliminated. This condition is called uremia. It begins with drowsiness, promptly followed by convulsions. Most cases of uremia occur as complications of inflammation of the kidney. Uremia may occur from conditions lower down in the urinary tract which block the flow of urine from the body.

One of the first signs likely to attract attention is severe headache. The headache may precede all other symptoms by weeks. If the headache is associated with constant nausea, occasional vomiting, and a good deal of restlessness and disturbance of sleep, the physician will probably suspect uremia. An immediate examination of the urine will help to determine whether or not satisfactory excretion is taking place.

As the materials that are toxic accumulate in the body, shortness of breath develops. Sometimes the shortness of breath resulting from this type of poisoning is difficult to differentiate from the shortage of breath due to weakness of the heart. Heart weakness is not uncommon in late forms of kidney disease.

Doctors recognize various forms of uremia associated with different types of inflammation of the kidney. When the uremia is due to a retention of the toxic products in the body, the patient may become drowsy and apathetic and then pass into a quiet unconsciousness during which he may die. In other forms there may be a vast accumulation of fluid in the body. The patient gradually becomes short of breath due to pressure on the lung, and he also becomes increasingly sluggish in his thought and speech.

In children particularly, when inflammation of the kidney associated with acute infection occurs, the swelling of the face and of the tissues may appear suddenly and be followed almost immediately by a severe convulsion. These convulsions may come on so rapidly and continue so persistently that death follows. Therefore physicians are particularly watchful for the changes in the urine associated with conditions like scarlet fever, severe sore throats, inflammation of the tonsils, and pneumonia.

Whenever a patient shows signs of uremia, quick action is imperative. Everything necessary must be done to help out the action of the heart. Sometimes if the pressure on the brain and the spinal fluid is too great, the patient is helped by withdrawing some of the spinal fluid after puncture of the spine.

Headache, which is a warning symptom, should not be treated with sedative or hypnotic drugs. The patient should go at once to bed, and the diet should be kept under suitable control, the urine being examined regularly to determine the extent to which the kidneys are functioning. After the diagnosis is made, suitable drugs may be prescribed for the control of the headache in patients with chronic inflammation of the kidney.

URETER The ureter is the tube that passes from the kidney to the bladder. It may be blocked by a stone; it may become twisted; it may become infected. Specialists in conditions affecting the urinary tract are known as urologists. Any serious condition affecting the ureter demands that kind of specialistic care. One of the first steps is to take an X-ray picture after injecting a substance which will cause the ureter to be visible.

URTICARIA See *Hives*.

UTERUS (See also *Hysterectomy, Pregnancy,* and *Prenatal Care*) This is the scientific name for the womb, the organ which carries the child previous to childbirth. The uterus is a muscular organ which has a lining of tissue from which the menstrual fluid comes each month. Like any other tissue of the body, the uterus may be infected so that its lining is seriously inflamed. An inflammation of the lining of the uterus is called endometritis. The opening of the uterus into the vagina is called the cervix. It is possible for the cervix to become infected by various germs. The cervix may also be injured during childbirth. An examination of the cervix and of the uterus at least once each year after the age of forty is recommended to every woman as a preventive against cancer.

Sometimes an irritation of the wall of the uterus results in damage to the tissues so that it becomes necessary to dilate the cervix and by means of the curette to scrape the lining of the uterus. The tissue thus removed is examined under the microscope for the presence of cancer or determination as to the nature of the disturbance in the tissues. The process of dilating and scraping, or curetting, is called dilation and curettage and is commonly spoken of around the hospitals as the "D & C" procedure.

UVULA From the middle of the palate there hangs down into the throat a small fleshy mass which is known as the uvula. Rarely it becomes infected; otherwise it is best let alone. Seldom is it necessary to clip, cut, or treat it in any way.

VACCINATION See *Diphtheria, Immunization, Smallpox, Tetanus,* etc.

VAGINA The canal which in the woman extends from the outer sex organs to the uterus is known as the vagina. The outer organs are called scientifically the vulva.

VARICELLA See *Chicken Pox.*

VARICOSE VEINS Once human beings were so modest that it was undesirable even to mention varicose veins. Now comedians crack jokes about them on the radio.

Most of the veins of the body are provided with valves which keep the column of blood going back to the heart from settling back in the veins. When the valves break down, the veins dilate. Such dilated veins are called varicose veins. When the veins dilate, they project above the skin in lumpy masses. If they get blocked, clots may form in the veins. Occasionally these become secondarily infected.

The veins of the legs are first affected, for the simple reason that the power of gravity has a stronger influence on the veins of the leg than on those higher up in the body. Varicosity of the veins around the bottom of the bowel produces hemorrhoids. Women who are pregnant are likely to develop varicose veins because of the blocking of the return flow of blood through the veins.

In the prevention of varicose veins the mechanism of causation must be kept in mind. If the veins have been blocked because of the wearing of tight belts or tight garters, discontinuance of such garments is indicated. After the birth of a child the pressure on the circulation is relieved, but the valves may be broken down, and they do not again recover. Excess weight may interfere with the action of the circulation and also with exercise. Hence fat people tend to have varicose veins more easily than thin ones.

Among the methods used to control varicose veins are the wearing of elastic bandages or stockings, removal of the varicose veins by surgery, and obliteration of the veins by the injection of caustic substances. If the procedure that brought about the varicose veins still operates, new veins will become varicose as older ones are blocked. In severe cases the physician may tie off a large blood vessel high up on the thigh so as to prevent the secondary effects that have been mentioned.

Ordinarily the injection method of treating small varicose veins is simple. The doctor, having located the extent of the dilated portion of the vein, frees the blood vessel of blood and then injects into it a substance which causes irritation of the walls of the blood vessel so that the walls will grow together. A variety of solutions are used for this purpose, the doctor determining in each instance the one which he prefers to use for the individual patient.

VENTILATION While most people worry most about ventilation in hot weather because it is hard to keep cool, the real problems of ventilation are those of the winter. In summer you can always get fresh air by opening the windows; in winter a cold, drafty room is uncomfortable. A hot, dry room may be even more uncomfortable.

Most American homes are too hot and too dry in winter. The windows are closed, the steam heat is left at capacity, and people forget that air requires a certain amount of moisture to be comfortable for men and safe for furniture. If the air is too dry, it will pick up water wherever it can. Therefore the skin of the body, the membranes of the nose and throat become dry. The furniture becomes dry and brittle and cracks at night. The groaning and crackling of the furniture which is warping and pulling apart interfere with sleep.

Nowadays many types of air moisteners are available. However, many of the devices that evaporate fluid rapidly cause a sensation of dampness. The valves on radiators that are supposed to release moisture keep up a hissing noise and occasionally drop water on the floor, so that you have a choice between crackling furniture or hissing radiators. Pans of water placed over radiators help to put a certain amount of water into the air, but the water evaporates rapidly, and most people forget to keep the pans full. Among the efficient humidifiers are those with troughs of water and belts of cloth that pass through the water, a fan that blows the water, and a motor that operates the fan. This is a lot of machinery for a very simple purpose.

Experts in ventilation of the home are now agreed that the proper use of a barometer is the first important step. This will show the extent to which the air contains moisture. Careful use of the doors and windows, coupled with the cracks in the ordinary residence, will provide for circulation of fresh air. Good ventilation provides for the prevention of smoke, dust, and gases in the air. A comfortable house temperature in summer varies from 70 to 85 degrees Fahrenheit. The best temperature of the air in winter is from 65 to 68 degrees, with sufficient water vapor in the air to produce a relative humidity of from 30 to 60 per cent.

VERTIGO See *Dizziness.*

VINCENT'S ANGINA During World War I many of our soldiers suffered with a condition that was called trench mouth. In this ailment sores and ulcers occur on the lining of the cheeks and gums, sometimes also on the tonsils and in the back of the throat. The ulcers may become so large as to incapacitate the person who is infected. The gums become acutely inflamed and bleed easily.

Trench mouth is not, however, purely a war condition. A French physician named Vincent found that it was due to an infectious organism which has been called Vincent's organism.

The person who has Vincent's infection may spread it to other people by kissing, by contaminating eating utensils or drinking cups. Cases have been reported in which the disease has been spread by improper sterilizing of dental instruments.

The prevention of Vincent's infec-

tion demands constant watchfulness of the condition of the mouth, teeth, and gums. Persistent bleeding of the gums or the appearance of an unpleasant odor or the occurrence of ulcers in the mouth demands that the patient consult a competent dentist or physician at once. Control of this infection is much easier in the early stages than at a time when the condition has become chronic.

Vincent's infection occurs most frequently in those with bad teeth and with mouths that have been badly cared for. Regular, competent attention to the teeth and gums helps to prevent the spread of such infection. The removal of deposits around the teeth and proper attention to the cavities and crevices make it difficult for the germs to grow and persist around the teeth and in the gums.

Such conditions as scurvy, diabetes, lead or bismuth poisoning, and syphilis may produce damage to the mouth and gums and ulcers, to which Vincent's infection may be secondary. It is important, therefore, that in each instance the physician determine exactly what is wrong.

In the modern treatment of Vincent's infection drugs like hydrogen peroxide are used to remove the dead tissue and infected material. The drug called sodium perborate is believed to have a definite effect in destroying the germs of Vincent's disease. These drugs must be used with great care because they may cause chemical burns of tender gums and of the lining of the cheeks.

It is known that the sulfonamide preparations are sometimes helpful. Materials constantly in contact with the teeth and gums have been developed, including solutions and the incorporation of the sulfonamides in chewing gum. The dentist or the physician who treats Vincent's infection may apply the drugs directly to the infected area and may by such technics keep the materials closely in contact with the area in which the germs are found. In some instances the use of arsenical preparations injected directly into the veins has been helpful.

Often Vincent's infection is a persistent condition, difficult to cure and demanding attention over long periods of time.

VITAMINS VITAMIN A—A characteristic disease of the eyes, usually called xerophthalmia, results from a deficiency of vitamin A; one of the first signs of its absence is a condition called night blindness; a deficiency of this vitamin sometimes results in a condition of the skin which is called hyperkeratosis, meaning a thickening or hardening. There has been a tremendous amount of experimentation with vitamin A, with a view to proving that it has many other virtues. The Council on Pharmacy and Chemistry of the American Medical Association does not permit the claim that the giving of extra vitamin A to drivers of automobiles will diminish accidents from driving at night in any considerable number of people. Neither does the Council accept the view that the taking of extra amounts of vitamin A is of any value in preventing colds, influenza, or other respiratory infections. Neither is there proof that the taking of a sufficient amount

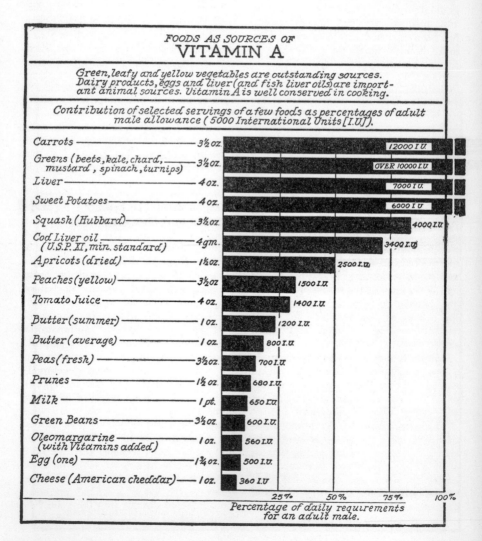

FOODS AS SOURCES OF
VITAMIN A

Green, leafy and yellow vegetables are outstanding sources. Dairy products, eggs and liver (and fish liver oils) are important animal sources. Vitamin A is well conserved in cooking.

Contribution of selected servings of a few foods as percentages of adult male allowance (5000 International Units [I.U.]).

Food	Serving	I.U.
Carrots	3½ oz.	12000 I.U.
Greens (beets, kale, chard, mustard, spinach, turnips)	3½ oz.	OVER 10000 I.U.
Liver	4 oz.	7000 I.U.
Sweet Potatoes	4 oz.	6000 I.U.
Squash (Hubbard)	3½ oz.	4000 I.U.
Cod Liver oil (U.S.P. XI, min. standard)	4 gm.	3400 I.U.
Apricots (dried)	1½ oz.	2500 I.U.
Peaches (yellow)	3½ oz.	1500 I.U.
Tomato Juice	4 oz.	1400 I.U.
Butter (summer)	1 oz.	1200 I.U.
Butter (average)	1 oz.	800 I.U.
Peas (fresh)	3½ oz.	700 I.U.
Prunes	1½ oz.	680 I.U.
Milk	1 pt.	650 I.U.
Green Beans	3½ oz.	600 I.U.
Oleomargarine (with Vitamins added)	1 oz.	560 I.U.
Egg (one)	1¾ oz.	500 I.U.
Cheese (American cheddar)	1 oz.	360 I.U.

25%　　50%　　75%　　100%

Percentage of daily requirements for an adult male.

of vitamin A or vitamin A in excess will prevent the formation of kidney stones in man. There does not seem to be any proof that vitamin A, either in normal amounts or in excess amounts, will help excessive action of the thyroid gland, anemia, degenerative conditions of the nervous system, sunburn, or ulcerations of the skin.

Vitamin A has fortunately gotten by without having affixed to it a popular promotional name. There was for a while an attempt to call it the anti-infective vitamin, but science caught up with promotion, and that name has gradually disappeared from both public and medical writing. Oleomargarine has been enriched with this vitamin to make it more nearly resemble the virtues of butter.

Vitamin B Complex—Vitamin B complex is the name for a group of substances which have been shown to be a part of what was once known as vitamin B. The list includes thiamine, riboflavin, nicotinic acid, pantothenic acid, pyridoxine, and most of the other substances which have been found to have some relation to nutrition of animals, but apparently little, if any, importance in human nutrition.

Thiamine—The name "thiamine" for the vitamin once called B₁ was selected by Dr. R. R. Williams, who showed the chemical character of the substance. This factor was first isolated in 1927, but long before thiamine was isolated it was known that polished rice produced beriberi and that unpolished rice prevented that condition. Fortu-

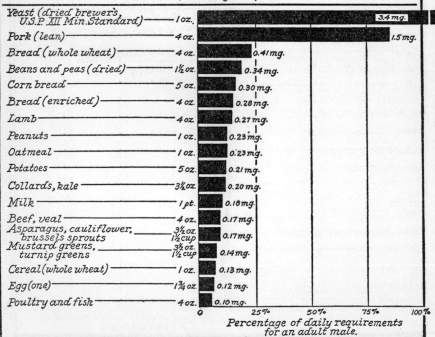

FOODS AS SOURCES OF
THIAMINE (Vitamin B₁)

Except for pork, common foods supply only small amounts of thiamine, the best sources being nutritionally unimpaired cereals and meats; some thiamine may be lost in cooking, either through destruction by heat or extraction by water. . .

Contribution of selected servings of a few foods as percentages of adult male allowance (1.8 milligrams)

Food	Serving	mg
Yeast (dried brewer's, U.S.P. XII Min. Standard)	1 oz.	3.4 mg.
Pork (lean)	4 oz.	1.5 mg.
Bread (whole wheat)	4 oz.	0.41 mg.
Beans and peas (dried)	1½ oz.	0.34 mg.
Corn bread	5 oz.	0.30 mg.
Bread (enriched)	4 oz.	0.28 mg.
Lamb	4 oz.	0.27 mg.
Peanuts	1 oz.	0.23 mg.
Oatmeal	1 oz.	0.23 mg.
Potatoes	5 oz.	0.21 mg.
Collards, kale	3½ oz.	0.20 mg.
Milk	1 pt.	0.18 mg.
Beef, veal	4 oz.	0.17 mg.
Asparagus, cauliflower, brussels sprouts	3½ oz. 1½ cup	0.17 mg.
Mustard greens, turnip greens	3½ oz. 1½ cup	0.14 mg.
Cereal (whole wheat)	1 oz.	0.13 mg.
Egg (one)	1¾ oz.	0.12 mg.
Poultry and fish	4 oz.	0.10 mg.

0   25%   50%   75%   100%

Percentage of daily requirements for an adult male.

nately there is not much beriberi in the United States. However, thiamine is also of value in correcting and preventing the loss of appetite that is apparent in many digestive conditions.

There seem to be conditions in which vitamins, although taken into the body, are not properly absorbed. For instance when there is constant vomiting, when patients have to be fed with tubes, when there is a paralysis of the muscles associated with swallowing, when there is excessive alcoholism, it may be necessary to give thiamine in amounts beyond those ordinarily taken, and perhaps even by direct injection into the body.

In animals disturbances of the heart and blood vessels are sometimes associated with lack of this vitamin. But few conditions, apparently, exist in human beings in which there is waterlogging

of the system associated with lack of thiamine. We know that excessive action of the thyroid gland or fever or vigorous muscle activities use up more thiamine than is ordinarily available, and that people with these conditions need extra amounts of the vitamin.

RIBOFLAVIN—Another portion of the vitamin B complex is riboflavin. When it is absent, characteristic disturbances appear on the tongue, the lips, and the face. These conditions differ from those that affect the same tissues in pellagra. Sometimes itching, burning, and a sensation of roughness of the eyes are associated with lack of riboflavin. But actually these conditions are so difficult to diagnose that the doctor tries to make certain first that the riboflavin in the diet is inadequate before he recommends extra riboflavin.

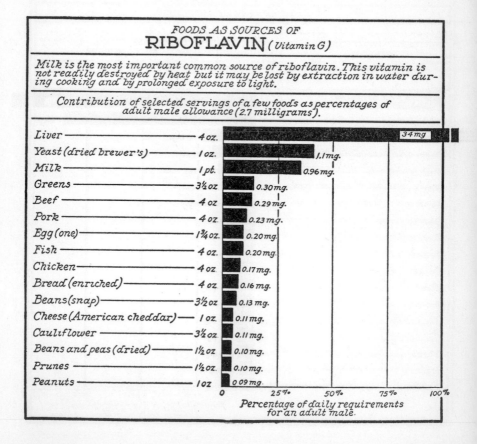

FOODS AS SOURCES OF
RIBOFLAVIN *(Vitamin G)*

Milk is the most important common source of riboflavin. This vitamin is not readily destroyed by heat but it may be lost by extraction in water during cooking and by prolonged exposure to light.

Contribution of selected servings of a few foods as percentages of adult male allowance (2.7 milligrams).

Food	Serving	Amount
Liver	4 oz.	34 mg.
Yeast (dried brewer's)	1 oz.	1.1 mg.
Milk	1 pt.	0.96 mg.
Greens	3½ oz.	0.30 mg.
Beef	4 oz.	0.29 mg.
Pork	4 oz.	0.23 mg.
Egg (one)	1¾ oz.	0.20 mg.
Fish	4 oz.	0.20 mg.
Chicken	4 oz.	0.17 mg.
Bread (enriched)	4 oz.	0.16 mg.
Beans (snap)	3½ oz.	0.13 mg.
Cheese (American cheddar)	1 oz.	0.11 mg.
Cauliflower	3½ oz.	0.11 mg.
Beans and peas (dried)	1½ oz.	0.10 mg.
Prunes	1½ oz.	0.10 mg.
Peanuts	1 oz.	0.09 mg.

0   25%   50%   75%   100%
Percentage of daily requirements for an adult male.

Nicotinic Acid or Nicotinamide— The discovery that another portion of the vitamin B complex known as nicotinic acid or nicotinamide is specific in the treatment of pellagra is one of the greatest discoveries of modern medical science. When pellagra is present, the use of this substance will lead to the disappearance of the symptoms related to the skin, the digestion, and the nervous system. However, there does not seem to be much good evidence that extra amounts of nicotinic acid are good for the wide variety of conditions in which they have been tried and recommended.

Vitamin C—Vitamin C is the antiscurvy vitamin. This has been established experimentally and proved on patients. However, a tremendous number of articles have been published about the use of vitamin C in a great many other conditions.

Apparently there are people who do not have outright scurvy, but something resembling scurvy. There are evidences that dental caries, pyorrhea, certain infections of the gums, loss of appetite, anemia, undernutrition, and infection are sometimes found along with insufficient amounts of ascorbic acid. However, again it would be desirable to prove always that there is a deficiency of this vitamin taken into the body and properly utilized, rather than to begin the treatment of such a wide variety of conditions by assuming in advance that the deficiency of the vitamin was responsible and that the giving of large amounts of ascorbic acid or orange juice or tomato juice would bring about a cure.

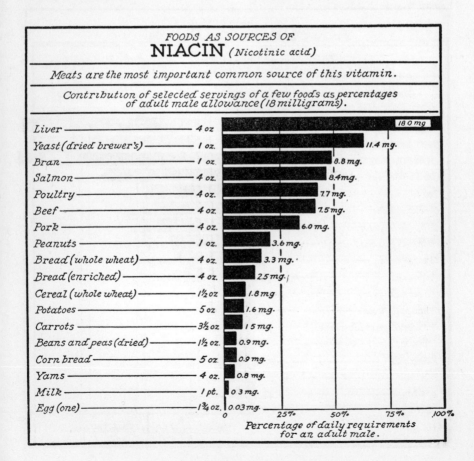

FOODS AS SOURCES OF
NIACIN *(Nicotinic acid)*

Meats are the most important common source of this vitamin.

Contribution of selected servings of a few foods as percentages of adult male allowance (18 milligrams).

Food	Serving	Value
Liver	4 oz	18.0 mg.
Yeast (dried brewer's)	1 oz.	11.4 mg.
Bran	1 oz.	8.8 mg.
Salmon	4 oz.	8.4 mg.
Poultry	4 oz.	7.7 mg.
Beef	4 oz.	7.5 mg.
Pork	4 oz.	6.0 mg.
Peanuts	1 oz.	3.6 mg.
Bread (whole wheat)	4 oz.	3.3 mg.
Bread (enriched)	4 oz.	2.5 mg.
Cereal (whole wheat)	1½ oz	1.8 mg
Potatoes	5 oz	1.6 mg.
Carrots	3½ oz	1.5 mg.
Beans and peas (dried)	1½ oz.	0.9 mg.
Corn bread	5 oz	0.9 mg.
Yams	4 oz.	0.8 mg.
Milk	1 pt.	0.3 mg.
Egg (one)	1¾ oz.	0.03 mg.

Percentage of daily requirements for an adult male.

VITAMIN D—Vitamin D is known in many forms, of which at least two are definitely related to proper use of calcium and phosphorus by the human body. Reports have appeared claiming improvement in chronic arthritis and in some allergic conditions by use of massive doses of vitamin D. The statement has been made that massive doses of this vitamin will improve psoriasis. The Council on Pharmacy and Chemistry of the American Medical Association has held, however, that there is not sufficient evidence to prove either of these claims, although the Council does not discourage further experimentation.

VITAMIN E—For years it has been known that vitamin E must be included in the diet of the rat if there are to be little rats. In other words, this is the anti-sterility vitamin, as the imaginative boys of the press describe it. But the Council on Pharmacy and Chemistry, which talks very concretely on these subjects, simply says that vitamin E is of no value in the treatment of sterility. There are indications that it may be of value in case of habitual abortion, but further studies are necessary to clarify the picture.

VITAMIN B₁₂—This substance has cobalt as a chief chemical ingredient. The product is known also as Cyanocobalamin. This has blood-stimulating activity like that of the anti-anemia factor of liver. Therefore, it is used especially in pernicious anemia. The drug is used also

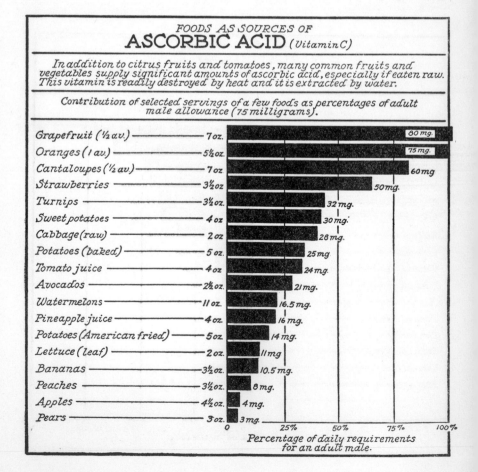

FOODS AS SOURCES OF
ASCORBIC ACID (Vitamin C)

In addition to citrus fruits and tomatoes, many common fruits and vegetables supply significant amounts of ascorbic acid, especially if eaten raw. This vitamin is readily destroyed by heat and it is extracted by water.

Contribution of selected servings of a few foods as percentages of adult male allowance (75 milligrams).

Food	Serving	Amount
Grapefruit (½ av.)	7 oz.	80 mg.
Oranges (1 av.)	5½ oz.	75 mg.
Cantaloupes (½ av.)	7 oz.	60 mg
Strawberries	3½ oz.	50 mg.
Turnips	3½ oz.	32 mg.
Sweet potatoes	4 oz.	30 mg.
Cabbage (raw)	2 oz.	28 mg.
Potatoes (baked)	5 oz.	25 mg
Tomato juice	4 oz.	24 mg.
Avocados	2½ oz.	21 mg.
Watermelons	11 oz.	16.5 mg.
Pineapple juice	4 oz.	16 mg.
Potatoes (American fried)	5 oz.	14 mg.
Lettuce (leaf)	2 oz.	11 mg
Bananas	3½ oz.	10.5 mg.
Peaches	3½ oz.	8 mg.
Apples	4½ oz.	4 mg.
Pears	3 oz.	3 mg.

0   25%   50%   75%   100%

Percentage of daily requirements for an adult male.

in sprue and in anemias resulting from vitamin B₁₂ deficiency. Combined with material from the wall of the stomach, the mixture is effective in anemias with neurologic complications. These substances can be taken by mouth.

VITAMIN K—Vitamin K represents again one of the greatest discoveries of medical science. It is the anti-hemorrhagic vitamin. It is useful in obstructive jaundice, in hemorrhagic states associated with certain intestinal diseases, and in some hemorrhagic conditions of the newborn. The evidence is accepted that the mother should have some of this vitamin before childbirth and that the infant should have a normal amount of prothrombin in his blood at the time of birth.

VITILIGO In vitiligo the pigment in the skin entirely disappears from some spots on the skin, so that these appear quite white in contrast with the rest of the skin. Because of the absence of any pigment mechanism in these portions of the skin they are much more prominent when the rest of the skin is tanned or sunburned. The cause for the absence of pigment from some portions of the skin is not known.

When vitiligo occurs in Negroes, as it sometimes does, they appear to be turning white, and there are cases on record in which most of the pigment has disappeared from the skin of a colored person. Some of these also have been exhibited in museums and side shows.

Recently a drug called ammoidin was found in Egypt which seems to be able to control vitiligo. The drug is painted on the area involved and is also prescribed to be taken internally.

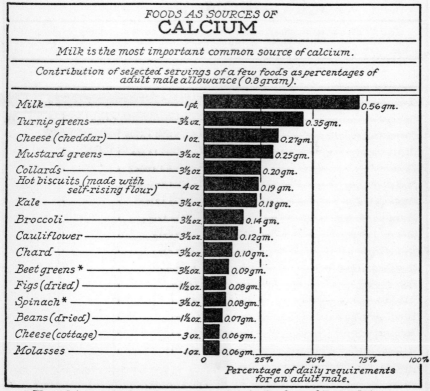

FOODS AS SOURCES OF
CALCIUM

Milk is the most important common source of calcium.

Contribution of selected servings of a few foods as percentages of adult male allowance (0.8 gram).

Food	Serving	Calcium
Milk	1 pt.	0.56 gm.
Turnip greens	3½ oz.	0.35 gm.
Cheese (cheddar)	1 oz.	0.27 gm.
Mustard greens	3½ oz.	0.25 gm.
Collards	3½ oz.	0.20 gm.
Hot biscuits (made with self-rising flour)	4 oz.	0.19 gm.
Kale	3½ oz.	0.18 gm.
Broccoli	3½ oz.	0.14 gm.
Cauliflower	3½ oz.	0.12 gm.
Chard	3½ oz.	0.10 gm.
Beet greens *	3½ oz.	0.09 gm.
Figs (dried)	1½ oz.	0.08 gm.
Spinach *	3½ oz.	0.08 gm.
Beans (dried)	1½ oz.	0.07 gm.
Cheese (cottage)	3 oz.	0.06 gm.
Molasses	1 oz.	0.06 gm.

0   25%   50%   75%   100%

Percentage of daily requirements for an adult male.

* The calcium in beet greens and spinach is in the form of the oxalate which is not assimilated by the body.

It has been suggested that those who are exceedingly sensitive have their skin painted with some of the cosmetic preparations now available so that the white spots will not appear so prominently.

VOCAL CORDS See *Laryngitis, Larynx.*

VOICE See *Laryngitis, Larynx,* and *Speech.*

VOMITING Two of the most common symptoms of all sorts of disease are nausea and vomiting. They occur not only in infections and disturbances affecting the nervous system, in diabetes and in kidney disease, but often from purely mental causes.

The doctor does not treat nausea and vomiting as if they were diseases. He controls them as symptoms and then endeavors to determine exactly what may be the underlying condition responsible. If a person vomits, something has happened to cause the stomach to wish to be emptied. Not much is to be gained, therefore, by pouring a lot of things into the stomach. There are, of course, instances in which the vomiting occurs because of irritation by poisons. In this event the drinking of a great deal of fluid, which is promptly vomited back, serves to wash out the stomach.

In the average case of vomiting the doctor is likely to recommend, first of all, that the patient take no food for at least twenty-four hours. It is necessary,

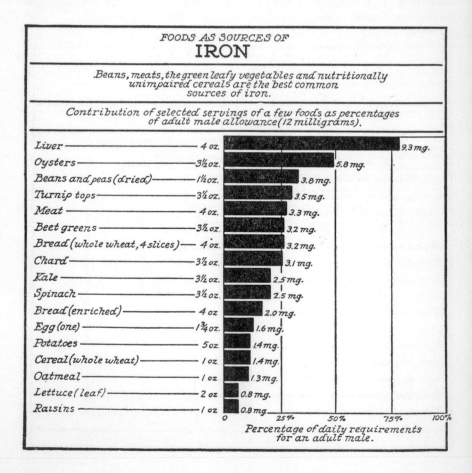

FOODS AS SOURCES OF
IRON

Beans, meats, the green leafy vegetables and nutritionally unimpaired cereals are the best common sources of iron.

Contribution of selected servings of a few foods as percentages of adult male allowance (12 milligrams).

Food	Serving	Iron
Liver	4 oz.	9.3 mg.
Oysters	3½ oz.	5.8 mg.
Beans and peas (dried)	1½ oz.	3.8 mg.
Turnip tops	3½ oz.	3.5 mg.
Meat	4 oz.	3.3 mg.
Beet greens	3½ oz.	3.2 mg.
Bread (whole wheat, 4 slices)	4 oz.	3.2 mg.
Chard	3½ oz.	3.1 mg.
Kale	3½ oz.	2.5 mg.
Spinach	3½ oz.	2.5 mg.
Bread (enriched)	4 oz	2.0 mg.
Egg (one)	1¾ oz.	1.6 mg.
Potatoes	5 oz.	1.4 mg.
Cereal (whole wheat)	1 oz	1.4 mg.
Oatmeal	1 oz	1.3 mg.
Lettuce (leaf)	2 oz	0.8 mg.
Raisins	1 oz	0.8 mg.

Percentage of daily requirements for an adult male.

however, to keep the body supplied with fluid, since vomiting serves to diminish the fluids in the body. The loss of fluid may, in itself, produce serious symptoms. If the fluid cannot be kept in the stomach, the doctor may recommend the injection of fluid into the body by other means.

The mechanism of vomiting has been studied under the X ray. First the valve at the bottom of the stomach through which the food passes from the stomach to the bowels closes. Next come a series of waves in the wall of the stomach which do not pass downward, as is the case ordinarily, but upward in a reverse order. As these waves continue, the person affected begins to breathe deeply; then there is a powerful contraction of the diaphragm and of the abdomen, so that the contents of the stomach are forced, as by an explosion, up the esophagus, into the mouth and out. Sometimes this takes place so rapidly that the material is evacuated through the nose, if the passage from the throat to the nose is not closed.

The initiation of the vomiting of seasickness probably takes place in the organs of the body that have to do with maintaining its balance.

A severe pain associated with conditions affecting the heart may produce reflex vomiting. The severe pain associated with a violent blow on the abdomen may cause vomiting. The sight of an unpleasant or revolting object, a fetid smell, or even an unpleasant sound or an insulting word may be followed by vomiting.

Often there is a feeling of dizziness preceding the vomiting, which itself is a part of the accumulated nerve impulses that bring about the emptying of the stomach.

WARTS When warts are studied scientifically, they are found to be growths of the skin. Many doctors believe that they are infections. They appear to be slightly contagious. In fact inoculation of material from warts has been followed by the growth of new warts.

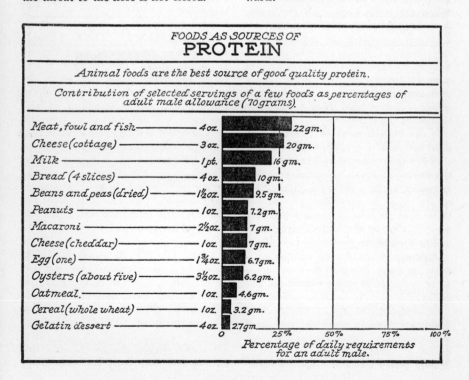

FOODS AS SOURCES OF
PROTEIN

Animal foods are the best source of good quality protein.

Contribution of selected servings of a few foods as percentages of adult male allowance (70 grams).

Meat, fowl and fish	4 oz.	22 gm.
Cheese (cottage)	3 oz.	20 gm.
Milk	1 pt.	16 gm.
Bread (4 slices)	4 oz.	10 gm.
Beans and peas (dried)	1½ oz.	9.5 gm.
Peanuts	1 oz.	7.2 gm.
Macaroni	2½ oz.	7 gm.
Cheese (cheddar)	1 oz.	7 gm.
Egg (one)	1¾ oz.	6.7 gm.
Oysters (about five)	3½ oz.	6.2 gm.
Oatmeal	1 oz.	4.6 gm.
Cereal (whole wheat)	1 oz.	3.2 gm.
Gelatin dessert	4 oz.	2.7 gm.

0   25%   50%   75%   100%

Percentage of daily requirements for an adult male.

Warts seldom produce any symptoms except when they are on the soles of the feet, in which case, of course, they may become painful.

It has been found that picking of warts and spreading of the blood or material from the wart over the adjacent skin may result in multiplication of the warts in the same person by autoinoculation. It is better, therefore, not to attempt to treat them unscientifically.

When a specialist in diseases of the skin is called upon to treat warts, he applies any one of a number of treatments, including injections of bismuth directly into the wart, destruction of the warts by strong chemicals, freezing with carbon dioxide snow, electric desiccation of the wart, and surgical removal if the warts are large or multiple in any one spot.

Radium and X rays are also used for warts and in some instances seem to work most satisfactorily. This method is used especially when there are many warts around the fingernails. When the warts appear on the scalp, it is customary to treat them first by softening them with the application of various acids and then to make the final removal by freezing with carbon dioxide snow or by the electric needle. However, none of these materials or methods should ever be used except by those trained in the technic.

Warts on the soles of the feet are most resistant to treatment. Frequently they are best removed by surgery. After the horny material has been properly cut away, caustics are used on the base of the wart to prevent regrowth. In these cases also the X ray is frequently used to destroy the wart-bearing area and to prevent the growth of new warts.

Although warts disappear spontaneously in many cases, it does not seem to be desirable to wait too long for this to occur.

In addition to the common wart there are similar growths associated with venereal infections. These are called venereal warts. They develop around places where the mucous membranes join the skin. They are usually aggregate collections of overgrowths like warts. Because of irritation, friction, heat, moisture, and a large supply of blood they grow luxuriantly and spread rapidly. Such warts demand special treatment because of their nature. Most important, however, is the application of treatment as promptly as possible in order that the condition may be fully controlled before it has spread too widely.

Old people have a special form of wart known as senile wart. These also demand prompt attention because continued irritation may cause them to develop the malignant growth that is characteristic of cancer. It is best in such instances to have each wart removed as it develops and to have a careful study made of the tissues under the microscope to make certain that cancerous changes have not occurred. Such warts develop most often on the body rather than on the hands or the exposed skin. As far as is known, this type of wart never disappears spontaneously.

WASSERMANN TEST People with syphilis are usually submitted to an examination of the blood by a test called the Wassermann test which determines the presence or absence of the disease. Various modifications of this test have been discovered, most prominent of which is the so-called Kahn test, also the Eagle and the Hinton tests. Such tests are necessary at the earliest possible moment to determine whether or not the disease is present and at fairly frequent intervals throughout the course of the disease to determine the extent of improvement.

WEIGHT, OVER- AND UNDER- People get fat because they eat too much. After a good many years of study experts have come to the conclusion that the only source of fat for the human being is food. As pointed out by Dr. Edward H. Rynearson, there are many people who by the inherited structure of their body are more likely to be fat than other people. Exceedingly few people are fat because one of their glands of internal secretion fails to work.

A great many people are fat for psychologic reasons. For instance there are children who eat as a means of escape from personal distresses. There are people who eat as a habit to pass time just as there are others who smoke as a habit to pass time. However, none of these modifications of the situation in any way alters the statement that the only source of fat in the human body is the food taken into the body. Therefore the only successful way to cut down on the fat is to restrict the total amount of food taken into the body. This was called by Professor Lafayette B. Mendel "physiologic bookkeeping."

The proteins taken into the human body are necessary to repair the cells and to correct new tissue. Vitamins and minerals also act in the essential metabolism of the human body. The fat taken into the body need only be sufficient to carry the essential fatty acid and the fat-soluble vitamins and to make it unnecessary to eat too large a total amount of food. All the rest of the calories necessary for maintenance of weight and for the energy of the body can be taken in the form of carbohydrates or sugars. In fact the highly refined grains and sugars are the cheapest sources of calories. They need to be supplemented always, however, by the protective elements such as the essential amino acids, the vitamins, and the minerals.

People who are underweight have much less trouble than those who are overweight because they can be comforted by the fact that life insurance statistics indicate that they are likely to live long and have, in general, better health than the people who are overweight. However, people who are thin because of illness or who suffer from lack of appetite and inability to eat represent a problem for both the psychologist and the nutrition expert. Just as the person who is overweight can im-

prove his condition by physiologic bookkeeping, so also can the one who is underweight produce a gain if he will decrease expenditure of energy and increase the intake of calories.

As to those people who prefer to put all the blame for overweight or underweight on the glands, Dr. Rynearson says, "The race horse and the draft horse are not 'endocrine problems.' They are the result of intentional breeding, feeding, and training. No one in his right mind would attempt to convert a draft horse into a race horse, but by diet alone he can convert a fat draft horse into one of normal size."

WEN   The wen is scientifically known as a sebaceous cyst. It is due to the fact that the sebum or material excreted from these glands in the skin does not get out because of some obstruction; therefore, a black plug of sebum will be found choking the outlet to the gland.

The material is dammed back and sooner or later is reacted on by itself and by the material from the blood so that the semisolid mass becomes semifluid. The material is likely to have a rancid odor.

If the wen does not become infected, it can go on swelling as long as the release of the material is prevented. Such bumps have been known to grow as large as a golf ball or even larger before the person concerned consulted a doctor and had the material let out.

Because of the inflammation that may set in, the skin over the bump may become adherent to the wen. Moreover, the clothing rubbing against a bump of this kind will irritate it.

Should these cysts become infected, they are a much more serious matter. Frequently the bumps on the scalp will be multiple and if they are allowed to grow too large, it may be necessary to remove a considerable amount of skin to get all of the material out.

When the wen becomes infected, merely cutting the opening in order to cause the material inside to flow out will not cure the wen. The difficulty is in the structure of the tissues; the lining of the cyst continues to secrete the sebaceous material, which again hardens and begins to collect.

The permanent cure, therefore, involves a complete surgical dissection which will take away the lining walls of the cyst and thus prevent a repetition of the swelling.

WHOOPING COUGH Doctors call whooping cough pertussis. They prefer pertussis because not every patient with whooping cough whoops. The disease got its name because it is characterized by a series of repeated, spasmodic coughs which cause the patient to get out of breath. As a result he is forced to draw air into his lungs, and the sound of this forced inspiration is the whoop.

Whooping cough has been known to the medical profession for a great many years. The earliest reference to it appeared in medical literature as far back as 1540. In those early days the condition was called quintana.

Often vomiting follows the coughing spell, and this was noted as far back as 1578.

Many people consider whooping cough a trivial disease of childhood. It is, nevertheless, one of the most serious conditions that affect mankind, causing more deaths than measles. Most of the deaths from whooping cough are associated with secondary conditions like bronchopneumonia or infection of the intestinal tract, and thus they are not always reported as whooping cough.

The number of days lost from school by children with whooping cough is greater than that for any two other infectious diseases. Most of the cases of whooping cough occur in children under five years of age, but it may affect people of any age and is more serious in the very young and in the very old than in those of intermediate ages.

For years there has been an argument as to the cause of whooping cough, but now bacteriologists are convinced that the disease is caused by a germ to which the name *Hemophilus pertussis* is given. It is found almost invariably in the throat during the early stages of the disease. It is seldom found in people who have not been exposed to whooping cough. Inoculation of the germ into animals will produce infection. Conceivably the case of whooping cough is complicated early by the invasion of other germs. This happens to be the case also with the common cold, in which infection with a virus is associated with secondary infections.

The modern technic for establishing with certainty the existence of whooping cough is to have the child cough on a plate which contains a substance on which the germs grow easily. The plate test is now used to prove, first, that the child has the disease, and, second, that the child is free from the germs and recovered from the disease. This is particularly important because it prevents wider dissemination of the disease from healthy carriers.

The first stage of whooping cough is a period of about ten days, in which the symptoms are like those of a person catching cold. This is the incubation period. After five or six days, however, the cough usually gets worse instead of better. Then come the typical seizures of whooping. This introduces the second stage of whooping cough. If the coughing spells are severe, the face becomes deep red or purple; the veins of the face and scalp swell, and the eyes fill with tears. Very young children vomit immediately after a spell of coughing, particularly when the coughing follows the taking of food.

Since the cough is provoked by exposure to cold, tobacco, or overexercise, much can be accomplished by keeping the child quietly at rest during the severe period of the disease.

The doctor diagnoses whooping cough not only by the typical coughing spells but also by changes in the blood. The white blood cells increase in number, particularly one form known as the lymphocytes, which are cells with a single nucleus, or central body, when seen under the microscope. The cough is so characteristic in whooping cough that special studies are seldom necessary to establish with certainty the nature of the disease.

For the prevention of whooping cough children with this condition should never be allowed to attend school. Tiny babies particularly must be guarded against contact with those who have the disease. Since the child should be kept closely confined for periods of nearly six weeks or even two or three months, other children in the family for whom exposure would be dangerous may, when possible, be sent away from the house. If the child is permitted to play outdoors during the time of gradual recovery, arrangements should be made to guard carefully against contact with other children.

I have heard children with whooping cough contaminating the air of motion picture houses, trains, busses, streetcars, and even churches. Parents ought to be more careful about the danger the child with whooping cough presents to other children. In some communities it has been suggested that the child who is recovering from whooping cough ought to wear a red band with the words "Whooping Cough" prominently displayed.

For the prevention of whooping cough all sorts of methods have been tried, such as those that have proved efficient in other diseases. Children may be inoculated with the blood of people who have recently recovered from whooping cough. They may be injected with vaccines made from germs that have been isolated, permitted to grow, and then suitably killed. These vaccines are believed to be useful in shortening the attack of whooping cough and making it milder. They are used also now in the treatment of whooping cough. Their development has taken more than thirty years; they were first prepared in 1914. Gradually they have been improved, tested in epidemics, and studied as to dosage and duration of efficiency. Furthermore, technics have been developed by which the efficiency of the vaccine can be tested. The vaccines now available have been proved to be useful and to provide considerable protection. They are given preferably after the child is six months of age. It is now accepted that they reduce the total number of cases of infection and greatly minimize the severity of the disease when infection does occur.

Parents can be of great help to the child with whooping cough. On the first appearance of the symptoms the child should be put to bed and isolated from members of the family who have not had the disease. In bad weather the child should be kept away from drafts and should be protected suitably with light but warm bed clothing. Since there may by considerable strain on the muscles of the abdomen during coughing, a binder such as is worn by babies may be wrapped around the abdomen to support the muscles.

Due to persistent vomiting, children with whooping cough may become undernourished and particularly short of fluids. The diet is watched closely. Preferably small amounts of food are given at frequent intervals. Food should be chosen by the doctor especially for its nutritious and easily digestible qualities. By all means make certain that the child gets and retains enough water in the body. Large amounts of food must be avoided because they cause irritation and more vomiting. The best time to give a small amount of food is ten or fifteen minutes after a coughing spell. Among the foods particularly recommended are small amounts of meat, carefully chopped or sieved, and vegetable soup properly prepared. Foods to be avoided in whooping cough include excess of bread, starchy foods, sweet pastries, and potatoes. Dry and crumbly foods like crackers and nuts should be avoided. Particularly helpful are drinks of fresh fruit juices.

The doctor can do a great deal toward diminishing the severity of coughing spells by the prescription of drugs which lessen the severity of the cough. These drugs are potent and cannot be given without a doctor's prescription. The doctor will prescribe those that are just up to the strength of the child concerned. For many years it has been known that inhalations of steam with various soothing oils may be useful in lessening the severity of coughing spasms.

An interesting observation is the fact that children sometimes imitate the coughing of others. Even a small baby will soon learn that a handsome demonstration during a spell of coughing brings presents, sympathy, and attention which otherwise he might not receive. The wrong mental attitude, therefore, may make a serious invalid out of what might otherwise be rather a mild attack of whooping cough. Children need to be encouraged to control coughing as much as possible.

Most dangerous of all the complications of whooping cough is secondary pneumonia. The child with a combination of whooping cough and pneumonia is probably best cared for in a hospital.

WOMB See *Uterus*.

WORMS A recent survey showed in certain Southern areas that from 50 to 60 per cent of the children had intestinal worms at one time or another. A survey made of children in Washington, D.C., revealed pinworms in from 35 to 65 per cent in various groups of children.

Apparently the worms may often be present in the bowels without causing much in the way of serious symptoms. In other instances they produce all sorts of disturbances.

By far the most common and most widely distributed of all of the worms that live on man is the pinworm, which is also called the seat worm or the threadworm. This worm is exclusively a human parasite. It is a small white worm about ⅛ to ½ inch long. When the eggs are taken into the human body, they hatch in the small intestine, where the worms mature and mate. The males are then passed out of the body, while the females move on to the large bowel and develop the eggs. As the worms are passed out of the bowel, the eggs are discharged. The entire life cycle is a matter of about two months.

The eggs of the pinworm may lodge in the area around the opening of the bowel, may get onto the sleeping garments or bedclothes. By scratching they get under the fingernails of the infected child and again contaminate his food, so that reinfection and dissemination go on constantly.

The most disturbing symptom from pinworm infestation is the itching which is associated with the presence of the female worms and their eggs at the lower end of the bowel. Scratching sometimes leads to secondary infection. Occasionally in girls the worms migrate to the genital area. Occasionally the trouble with the worms may be sufficient to interfere with eating, so there is loss of weight and some anemia.

In the control of pinworms the utmost care is required in maintaining cleanliness of the parts affected. There must be daily bathing. All infected members of the family should be treated at the same time. The doctor can prescribe suitable antiseptic ointments for application to the area involved.

All of the drugs that are taken for the control of this infection are of such character that they should be used only when prescribed by the doctor and in the amounts prescribed in each case. The dosage necessary for a child is quite different from that for an adult. In the treatment of the condition enemas of suitable amounts of hexylresorcinol are used. Reports are also made of the use internally of a dye substance called gentian violet. Here again the exact amount and the manner in which the drug is to be taken must be left to the doctor.

ROUNDWORMS—The roundworm is known as the *Ascaris lumbricoides*. This is exceeded in its frequency of infection in the human being only by the pinworm. In the Appalachian Mountain area investigators found over 40 per cent of infection with the roundworm among preschool and early school age children in rural and mining camp districts. Similar rates have been reported from the Gulf and Atlantic coasts. Infestation with this type of worm is much less common in the Northern states; a small survey made near Detroit showed only 2 per cent of children infected.

The roundworm is a large white worm which lives normally in the small bowel of the human being. The female is 10 to 15 inches long and is about as thick as a lead pencil. The male is 6 to 8 inches long and is more slender. They hold themselves in the bowel by a sort of springlike pressure with the two ends of the worm held against the intestinal wall. Throughout life the female worm discharges about 200,000 eggs each day. These develop to an infective stage on the surface of the soil in from two weeks to a month. They may survive for many months in a moist, shaded soil.

Infection is acquired only when the eggs are taken into the body of the human being. They hatch in the small intestine. The larvae then penetrate the intestinal wall and are carried to the liver and from the liver to the lungs. In the lungs they are coughed up and swallowed again and then develop to maturity in the intestine. The development of this worm in the body of human beings requires a month to six weeks, and it may live for six months thereafter.

This worm does not cause much in the way of serious symptoms in the human being except that sensitivities have been noted which produce some of the symptoms of allergy. Under various conditions like fever or when people are being treated with drugs the worms may wander from where they are and have sometimes shown up in the nose and mouth or even in the tube that passes from behind the nose to the ears. When the worms wander into a tube like the one that carries the bile or into the appendix, they can obstruct the passage of fluid and do serious harm. Obviously, therefore, anybody who has these worms ought to get rid of them. Fortunately such drugs as hexylresorcinol have been found especially effective against this worm. It is given to a patient after a minimum of twelve hours' starvation. It should be taken only when prescribed by the doctor and in the manner which the doctor prescribes. After the drug has been given, the person must abstain completely from food of any kind for at least five hours. Less disturbance follows if semifluid foods only are taken for the next five hours. Twenty-four hours after the drug has been given, a saline cathartic is taken so as to wash all of the material out of the bowel. Usually one treatment with the drug, properly given, will rid the patient of worms.

HOOKWORMS—The parasite that causes hookworm disease in the United States is known as *Necator americanus*.

The story of the way in which the hookworm infects the human being is one of the fascinating stories in medicine. A female hookworm can lay from 6000 to 15,000 eggs a day. When the skin of man is exposed to infected soil in which the hookworm eggs have been deposited, the larva of the hookworm penetrates the skin, enters a blood vessel, and is carried to the lungs, where it breaks out into one of the open spaces in the lungs. The worm then makes its way up the bronchial tubes into the throat, where it is swallowed. Next it passes to the small intestines, where it develops into an adult worm. It takes about six weeks for this program from the time when the larva penetrates the skin until the eggs appear in the human excretions.

A human hookworm is something less than ½ inch long, and the females are a little larger than the males. The worm has teeth by which it attaches itself to the wall of the bowels, and the worms secrete a toxic fluid which causes dilatation and rupture of the small blood vessels and prevents coagulation of the blood. The worms feed mainly on blood.

From this description of the hookworm it is easy to understand the harm it does. First, when it penetrates the skin, it produces conditions that are called "ground itch." Second, when it passes through the lungs, it may produce an inflammation. Third, when it gets into the intestines, it causes anemia through loss of blood, weakness of the muscles, and a distaste for work. As a result of the long-continued, mild anemia a person with hookworm disease has a face that is dull, hair that is dry and lusterless, and usually an inordinate appetite. If the condition is not corrected, the anemia may become so severe as to cause permanent invalidism or death.

A doctor can easily establish a diagnosis of hookworm by examining the material excreted from the bowel. The eggs of the worm will be found through such studies. Fortunately we know today many different ways to eliminate hookworms from the bowel, including a variety of remedies like hexylresorcinol, oil of chenopodium, and tetrachlorethylene. All these remedies are poisonous and should be given only by the doctor according to the prescribed method. There are, however, several things that the average person can do when he lives in an area where hookworm is prevalent. First, he should wear shoes and, second, he should provide for sanitary disposal of material excreted from the bowel. Since the larva of the hookworm cannot climb up a vertical surface to any height, the use of places of disposal that are sufficiently deep in the ground will control the dissemination of the hookworm from infected excretions.

Notwithstanding all that has been learned, hookworm is still an important public health problem in many parts of the world and in certain portions of the southern United States.

TAPEWORMS—Among the worms that live in the human intestine the tapeworms are among the most frequent and perhaps also among the most interesting. The quacks who used to go about in buggies carried with them huge glass jars displaying tapeworms and peddled their worm medicine on the basis that one look at the worm in the jar would bring the customers around.

Although there are thirty or forty different species of tapeworms that can get into the human intestine, six of them, known as the beef tapeworm, pork tapeworm, fish tapeworm, dwarf tapeworm, rat tapeworm, and dog tapeworm are the most common.

A complete beef tapeworm will measure 1 to 15 feet long and contain as many as 2000 parts. Cattle pick up the eggs when grazing on moist pasture land that has been contaminated with human sewage. The meat of the cattle is infected, and when man consumes this infected meat, inadequately cooked, he can acquire the infection. This is especially frequent when people eat raw beef.

The pork tapeworm seldom reaches 10 feet long and has about 1000 parts. Hogs that feed on human sewage become infected, and then human beings become infected from eating insufficiently cooked pork.

The fish tapeworm occurs wherever human excrement is discharged into bodies of fresh water. The swimming embryos are eaten by water fleas; the fresh-water fish eat the fleas; the human beings eat the infected raw fish. Occasionally the water fleas are eaten by little fish, which are eaten by bigger fish, which in turn are eaten by human beings. This condition was formerly frequent chiefly in Europe, but immigration from the Scandinavian areas and Poland has brought the infection to the United States.

The dwarf tapeworm is less than 1 inch long and is correspondingly small in its other dimensions. Infection with this worm is more frequent in children than in adults. Usually this infection is passed from one person to another through the eating of food contaminated by human excrement.

The rat and dog tapeworm are relatively uncommon in the human being, although cases are known.

The damage done by a tapeworm to a human being depends on the size of the worm, the kind of worm, and similar factors. Often the existence of the tapeworm is marked by toxic diarrhea and false hunger pains, frequently by the appearance of secondary anemia, loss of appetite, and loss of weight. The diagnosis is made certain by examining the excrement and finding the parts of the tapeworm or eggs in it.

Many different substances have been used to get rid of these worms. The doctor will starve the patient for a while and then give him a large dose of salts. The next day the patient takes medicine as prescribed by the doctor, and after waiting another day, during which the patient takes nothing but water, he gets another dose of salts. This succeeds in destroying the worms and getting them out of the body. Several different medicines are known which doctors can use and which are effective against the tapeworm.

WORRY See discussion under *Hygiene*.

WOUNDS A wound is any injury that breaks the skin or the underlying tissues. Wounds are classified according to the way in which they occur and according to the type of the wound. Wounds may be made by a razor blade, a knife, a bullet, a pin, or a burn. The wound may be clean-cut, lacerated, punctured, or due to a breaking force.

The chief danger arising from a wound is the danger of secondary infection. Hemorrhage or bleeding may be dangerous if large in amount or persistent. Hence the treatment given to wounds is designed first to control the bleeding; second to prevent infection. The control of bleeding is usually accomplished by putting a gauze compress over the wound. It should be made of sterile gauze. Under circumstances in which a first-aid pack is not available and bleeding is serious, a recently laundered handkerchief may be used. It is especially advisable, however, for people who are hunting, fishing, or touring in motorcars or in areas far removed from access to medical care to carry a first-aid cabinet with proper amounts of sterilized bandages.

The antiseptics commonly applied to wounds include iodine, boric acid, hydrogen peroxide, mercurochrome, tinctures of metaphen and merthiolate, and many others. Soap and water also act to destroy germs. Since many of the antiseptic substances are poisonous, it is a good rule never to put anything on or in a wound unless you have used it before and know exactly what you are doing. If you are not positive, it is much better to cover the wound with a clean dressing and wait for the doctor. In the case of a small wound, thorough washing with soap and boiled water is helpful.

Following any injury, the injured place may heal slowly or may become reddened, hot, and painful. Large red streaks may appear running up the arm or leg or away from the wound. There may be swelling, pain, chills, and fever. This means that infection has occurred and that a physician should be called immediately to take care of the condition; otherwise death may ensue.

Whenever a wound is seriously contaminated with clothing, soil, or similar materials, the doctor must also take into consideration the possibility of tetanus, or lockjaw, and advise the use of the anti-tetanus serum.

WRY NECK See *Torticollis*.

XANTHOMA Certain tumors develop a yellow color. The word "xanthoma" means yellow tumor. Quite often flat plaques of a yellow color appear on the skin due to deposit of fatty substances. These are called xanthomas. It is quite possible for these benign tumors to become mixed with malignant tumors, giving rise to such conditions as xanthosarcoma and xanthocarcinoma.

XERODERMA This is a skin disease in which there is marked roughness or drying of the skin and in which there may be discoloration. The term merely means dry skin. The prefix "xero-" refers to dryness.

X RAY The discovery of the X ray was first announced in December 1895. Since that time the X ray has become one of the greatest aids of the medical profession.

One of the chief uses of the X ray continues to be for the diagnosis of broken bones. Nowadays pictures are made from different angles so that the exact relationship of the broken bones to the tissues may be determined.

An X ray of the skull shows the presence of disease of the bone, sometimes the presence of a tumor or changes in the blood vessels in the brain.

Once an X ray could be used only to show tissues like the bones. Nowadays, by the use of accessory materials, it is possible to visualize various organs and tissues. These materials include various dye substances which may be taken into the body and which localize in certain organs and tissues. Then by the use of the X ray these tissues and organs are made visible. One dye substance is used in taking X rays of the gall bladder; others are used for the kidney and the urinary bladder; still others for the female genital system or the spinal column. A substance called lipiodol may be injected into the lungs or sinuses and thus make them visible.

By the use of the X ray the exact size of the heart may be determined. The ability of the bowels to carry food forward may be studied and the outlines visualized.

The X ray is used also in the treatment of disease, particularly in the treatment of tumors, conditions affecting the skin, inflammations of various kinds such as bursitis, and, in fact, for a wide variety of purposes.

Since the X ray was described by Wilhelm Konrad von Roentgen, innumerable improvements have been made. Portable apparatus is now available that can be taken directly to the patient's bedside. In our armed forces there is portable X-ray equipment together with portable darkrooms for developing the plates, so that complete X-ray equipment is set up close to the front within twelve minutes after the arrival of the trucks that carry the boxes.

One of the most important developments in the use of the X ray has been the taking of a 4×5 chest film of every man in the armed forces as a means of ruling out the presence of tuberculosis.

YAWS Tropical disease which is contagious and in which there are raspberrylike growths on the face, the hands, the feet, and the genital organs is called yaws. It is also called frambesia. Occasionally it has been called leishmaniasis. While the condition is not seen frequently in the United States, it is likely to be seen more frequently when great numbers of soldiers have returned from tropical areas.

YELLOW FEVER In 1918 the eminent Japanese investigator Noguchi found what he believed to be the causative organism of yellow fever. The disease had previously been shown to be definitely related to a mosquito of a particular type. As a result of this investigation yellow fever has been eliminated from the United States; Havana, Rio de Janeiro, and Panama have been made safe places in which to live.

However, there seems to be plenty of evidence to show that yellow fever is capable of infecting the monkey, and that it can be found among monkeys in the jungles of South America. For that very reason cases occasionally break out in various parts of Brazil and even in Rio de Janeiro.

While studies were going on in Brazil, it was found that the organism discovered by Noguchi was not the organism of yellow fever, but rather the organism which causes infectious jaundice. Noguchi himself died of yellow fever in Africa, but even before his death he had become convinced that the cause of yellow fever was not the spirochete which he discovered but a virus—a toxic agent so small that it can pass through a clay filter.

In 1930 investigators at Harvard University developed a serum that would act against the yellow fever virus; still later, workers in the Rockefeller Foundation were able to prepare a vaccine against this condition. In the making of the vaccine against yellow fever they plant the virus on chicken embryos —the same type of procedure that is used for the making of vaccine against influenza. Today vaccination against yellow fever is a well-recognized public health measure. Almost 2,000,000 people have been vaccinated against this disease in Brazil.

It does not seem possible that the disease can be eradicated as long as there are jungles in which animals may be infected and in which mosquitoes may propagate, to infect human beings.

It takes six days for yellow fever to develop after a person is bitten by an infected mosquito. As part of the procedure which is used to keep yellow fever out of the United States airplanes are regularly inspected when they come from South America or other infected parts of the world. Fumigation is used to kill any mosquitoes that are present; passengers are examined and questioned as to whether or not they have been in contact with possible sources of yellow fever. The crews which fly the airplanes to South America and Africa have been vaccinated against yellow fever. With these precautions this menacing disease has been kept out of our own borders.

ZINC The uses of zinc in medicine are chiefly as a component of zinc chloride and zinc oxide and similar combinations used in the treatment of conditions affecting the skin. These drugs are combined with ointments and dusting powders.

ZYGOMA A portion of the temple bone in the head is called the zygoma. It is occasionally involved in fractures of the skull.

ZYME Zyme is a short word taken from the Greek which means ferment. Enzymes are ferments which develop inside the body. Many different forms of ferments are used in medicine.

INDEX

Afterbirth, 11; immune globulin obtained from, 310
Agalactia, 11
Agar, 11
Age, old. *See* Senescence
Agglutinin and agglutinogen, 70
Agranulocytosis. *See* Granulocytosis
Ague, 11
Ainhum (tropical disease), 11
Air conditioning, 11–13
Airsickness. *See* Seasickness
Airsickness remedy: dramamine, 183
Air swallowing, 112, 115, 148, 151
Albinos, 13–14. *See also* Vitiligo
Albuminuria, 14; in eclampsia, 88; in nephritis, 330. *See also* Kidneys
Alcohol, 14–16; asthmatic attack from excess use, 43; biliousness from, 57–58; in diabetes, 173; in gastritis, 231; in gout, 238; heatstroke promoted by, 254; injection for neuralgia, 334; longevity, effect on, 304–5; during nursing, 109; during pregnancy, 376; in stomach ulcer, 431
Alcoholism, 14–16; alcoholic coma, 153–54; delirium tremens, 167–68; offspring, effect on, 259; symptoms produced by excess of insulin in blood, 347; thiamine (vitamin) deficiency in, 58
Aldosterone, 8
Alexia, 16
Alimentation, 16
Alkalies, poisoning from, 361
Alkalinity: acetic acid as alkalizing agent, 4; and acidosis, 4–5; sodium bicarbonate as alkalizing agent, 274
Alkalosis, 16; and acidosis, 4–5
Allergy, 16–17; and asthma, 41–43; bronchitis, allergy patients prone to, 79–80; dust as causative factor, 183–84; in eclampsia, 187–88; in eczema, 188–89; in hay fever, 244–45; headache caused by, 245; histamine in, 54; in hives, 262; location of body regions affected by, *illus.*, 16; throat, in food allergy, 445
Aloes, 17
Alopecia (baldness). *See* Hair
Altitude sickness, 17–18; and seasickness, 403–4
Aluminum, 18
Amaurosis, 18–19
Amblyopia, 19
Amebiasis, 19, 185–86
Amenorrhea, 19. *See also* Menstruation
Amino acids, 19; in deficiency diseases, 167
Aminophylline (drugs), 19
Aminopterin (drug), in leukemia, 299. *See also* Cancer
Aminopyrine, 186, 239, 246
Ammonia, 19
Ammonia, aromatic spirits of, 314
Amnesia, 19; and memory, 316
"Amog" (amuck), 19
Amphetamine, 57

Amyl nitrite (drug). *See* Angina pectoris
Amyotrophic lateral sclerosis, 19–20; vitamin E not a remedy, 468–69
Anacidity. *See* Achylia
Analgesia, 20. *See also* Anesthetics
Anaphylaxis. *See* Allergy
Ancylostomiasis (hookworm disease), 477–78
Anemia, 20–22; and anemia, pernicious, 22–23; chlorosis, of adolescents, 10, 21; eyes, changes from, 204; gastritis as a cause, 232; hookworm disease as a cause, 477–78; iron in treatment, 290; in kala azar, 294; and leukemia, 299; spleen, enlargement of (Banti's disease), as a cause, 428; ulcerative colitis as a cause, 153
Anemia, cerebral. *See* Brain concussion
Anemia, pernicious, 22–23; folic acid and vitamin B12, in treatment, 23; iron in treatment, 23; liver extracts in treatment, 303
Anesthesia, 24–25, *illus.*, 24; analgesia, 20; cocaine, 145; chloroform, 24; cyclopropane, 163; liver, damage from, 303
Aneurism, 25, *illus.*, 25
Angina, Vincent's. *See* Vincent's angina
Angina pectoris, 25–27; aminophylline, in relief of, 19; pain characteristically brief, 26; oxygen, in relief of, 344
Animals as carriers of disease: asthmatic symptoms caused by animals, 43; cats, 93–95; cattle, 452–53, 478; dogs, 93–95, 387–88, 478; fish, 478; hogs, 451, 478; insects, 285–86; parrots, 382; rabbits, 457–58; rats, 388–89, 389–90, 478; snails, 58. *See also* Carriers of disease; Insect pests
Aniseikonia, 28
Ankle, sprained, 28; do not apply heat, 428
Ankylosis, 190–91
Anopheles (mosquito), 307–8, *illus.*, 307
Anorexia, 28
Anosmia. *See* Odors
Antabuse (drug). *See* Alcohol
Anthrax, 28–29
Antibiotics. (*References to antibiotics are too numerous to be cited. Mention of their use will be found under many infectious diseases.*)
Antifebrin (drug). *See* Acetanilid
Antihistaminic drugs: in allergy, 17; in asthma, 42; benadryl, 54, 57, 148, 262; in colds, 147; dramamine, 183, 404; in hives, 262; in itching, 290; pyribenzamine, 54, 148, 262; in shingles, 408
Antiseptics: acriflavine and proflavine, 6; cuts and bruises, children, 137; germicides, 233; hexylresorcinol, 476; hydrogen peroxide, 463; iodine, 289–90; in medicine chest, 314; sodium perborate, 463. *See also* Disinfection
Antitoxins, 29–30, 180, 401, 445
Antrum, 30, *illus.*, 30; other sinuses, 409–10

Happiness, 321; and hypochondriasis, 269–70; and melancholia, 315–16

Harelip, 142, 301

Haverhill fever. *See* Ratbite fever

Hay fever, 244–45; and allergy, 16–17; benadryl, in relief of, 57

Headache, 245–46; in uremia, 461

Headache powders. *See* Sedatives

Head banging and head rolling, 246–47

Health, 264–69; noise, a health hazard, 335; relation to climate, 142–43

Hearing: adenoids, impairment by, 9; babies, hearing of, 103; deafness, 163–66; hearing aids, 165; mechanism of, 163–66; noise, excessive, damages, 165, 278, 335–36; operation to restore, 166; and otosclerosis, 342–43. *See also* Ear

Heart, 247–53, *illus.*, 66, 248, 375; altitude, effect of, 143; angina pectoris, condition in, 25–27; bee venom, harmful to, 54; blocking of (coronary thrombosis), 248–49, 252–53; blood pressure, high, effect of, 67; and cyanosis, 162–63; delirium tremens, collapse of heart in, 168; digitalis, as stimulant, 177; electrocardiograph, 192; endocarditis, 251–52; fibrillation, 222; function of, 25–27; in obesity, 338; in old age, 249; pericarditis, 351; pulse, 383; rheumatic fever, 250, 392–96; weakness of, in uremia, 460

Heart block, 253

Heat cramp and exhaustion. *See* Sun- and heat stroke

Heat sickness, 253–54; and sun- and heat stroke, 278, 433–34

Heat treatment: in acne, 6; ankle, sprained, not good for, 428; in arthritis, 39; in Bell's palsy, 57; infrared rays, 255; in joint disturbances, 292; in paresis, 349; for septic sore throat, 408; in tonsillitis, 134; for torticollis (wry neck), 449. *See also* Fever treatment

Height, 254–55; in acromegaly, 6–7; in infantilism, 287; lilliputians, 4. *See also* Growth

Heliotherapy, 255, 434–35

Hemarthrosis. *See* Joint disturbances

Hematuria, 255–56

Hemoglobin, 65, 256; in anemia, 20–21; in carbon monoxide poisoning, 92; hemoglobin test, 21–22; hemoglobinuria, 256; in high altitude, 17

Hemophilia, 256

Hemorrhage, 21, 256–57; anemia, caused by, 20–22; apoplexy, brain hemorrhage in, 31; in arteriosclerosis, 36; brain concussion, 75–76; ergot, checks hemorrhage, 199; hoarseness, from hemorrhagic diseases, 296; metrorrhagia, 322; from perforation of stomach ulcer, 274; prothrombin, anti-hemorrhagic vitamin, 469; shock, 408; tourniquet, 257, 314; tourniquet, complications from use of, 230–31; wounds, 479

Hemorrhoids, 257–59

Hemosmia. *See* Odor

Heparin (drug): in treatment of embolism, 193; in treatment of endocarditis, 252

Hepatic duct, *illus.*, 229, 277

Hepatitis infections, 259. *See also* Biliousness

Heredity, 259, 378; adoption calls for investigation of, 10–11; albinos, 10–11; in alcoholism, 14, 259; allergy, 16–17; arteriosclerosis, 35–36; ataxia, 44; baldness, 240; blood pressure, high, 66; cancer, 89; chorea, 140; color of eyes, 204; cross-eyes, 211–12; deaf-mutism, 164; deafness, 164; diabetes, 171; fertility, 219–20; hemophilia, 256; longevity, 304–5; multiple births, 61; obesity, 473; otosclerosis, 164; Rh factor, 71; stomach ulcers, 431; syphilis, 438–39; youthfulness into old age, 405

Hermaphroditism, 259–60

Hernia, 260; diaphragmatic, 175–76, 260; ruptures in babies, 133–34; spina bifida, 424–25

Herpes simplex, 91, 260–61

Herpes zoster. *See* Shingles

Hexylresorcinol, in treatment of worm disease, 476

Hiccups, 261–62; and diaphragm, 175–76

High blood pressure. *See* Blood pressure, high

Hinton test. *See* Wassermann test

Histamine, in bee venom, 54; chills caused by secretion of, 68; in hives, 262

Hives, 262

Hoarseness, 262–63; in cancer, 87; and coughing, 159–61; in laryngitis, 296–97; in septic sore throat, 407–8

Hodgkin's disease, 263–64

Home remedies. *See* Medicine chest

Homosexuality, 264

Hookworm disease, 477–78

Hormones, 264; adrenocorticotropic hormone, in treatment of arthritis, 40; estrogens, 201; growth hormone, 254, 355; male sex hormone, in development of musculature, 322; menopause, caused by hormone deficiency, 318–19; ovary, hormone from, 343; pituitary gland, 355–57; replacement in hormone deficiency, 316

Horseshoe kidney. *See* Kidneys

Hospital fever. *See* Typhus

Hot flashes. *See* Menopause

Housemaid's knee. *See* Bursitis

Humerus, *illus.*, 191

Hunger. *See* Appetite

Hydrarthrosis, intermittent. *See* Joint disturbances

Hydrocephalus. *See* Spina bifida

Hydrochloric acid: achlorhydria, 4; in indigestion, 273–74; salt, in formation of, 399; sodium bicarbonate, to offset excess of, 274

Hydrophobia. *See* Rabies

Hygiene, personal, in health, 264–69;

"Naphtha jag," 364
Naps, 414–15, 417–18
Narcolepsy, 327–28
Narcotic addiction, 45, 328
Nausea. *See* Vomiting
Navel, diseases of, 133–34, 328–29
Nearsightedness, 28, 203–4, 206–7, *illus.*, 28
Neck, broken, 329–30, 425–26; twisted (wry), 449
Neo-antergan, 17, 54
Neomycin, 455
Nephritis, 330–32
Nephrosis. *See* Edema
Nervous breakdown, 332–33; and mental depression, 319–20; and mental hygiene, 321
Nervous system, 436; and brain, 74–75; calcium, function of, in, 85; and cerebrospinal fluid, 245, 355; and pain, 345–46; spinal cord, 426; vitamin E, in treatment of disorders of, 468–69
Nervous system, diseases and disorders of: aeroneurosis, 18; alcoholism, 14–16; allergy, 16–17; amyotrophic lateral sclerosis, 19–20; anemia, pernicious, involvement in, 22–23; anosmia, 340; ataxia, 44; Bell's palsy, 56–57; beriberi, 57–58; brain concussion, 75–76; in brain tumor, 76–77; bulimia, 327–28; in carbon disulfide poisoning, 91–92; chorea, 140–41; dysphagia, 200; in electrical injuries, 191–92; and emotions, 193–94; encephalitis, 195–96; epilepsy, 197–98; in exhaustion, 201–2; hyposmia, 340; hysteria, 270–71; infantile paralysis, 279–84; insomnia, 286–87; locomotor ataxia, 303–4; meningitis, 317–18; in menopause, 318–19; multiple sclerosis, 324–25; narcolepsy, 327–28; in neck, broken, 329–30; nervous breakdown, 332–33; neuralgia, 333–34; neuritis, 334; neurosis, 334; night terrors, 334–35; nystagmus, 338; oxygen, lack of, as cause, 18; paralysis agitans, 347–48; paresis, 349–50; psychogenic pain, 345–46; in rabies, 387–88; and sciatic neuritis, 402; in scleroderma, 402; in seasickness, 403–4; shingles, 408; sleeping sickness (encephalitis), 195–96; somnambulism, 422; spasms, 422; in spinal fracture, 425–26; stomach ulcers, relation to, 431; stuttering and stammering, 432–33; tetanus, involvement in, 444–45; tic, 447; tobacco, effect of, 447–48; in torticollis, 449; tumor (glioma), 235. *See also* Mental diseases and disorders
Nettle rash. *See* Hives
Neuralgia, 333–34, 447; and Bell's palsy, 56–57; dental, 333; tic douloureux (facial), 334
Neuritis, 334; in beriberi, 58; and sciatic neuritis, 401–2
Neurosis, 334; and nervous breakdown, 332–33

"New Skin." *See* Collodion
Niacin (nicotinamide, nicotine acid), 467; food sources of, *chart,* 467; in pellagra, treatment of, 350
Night air. *See* Air conditioning
Night blindness (xerophthalmia), 167, 464
Night sweats. *See* Bronchiectasis
Night terrors, 334–35
Nitrogen balance. *See* Amino acids
Nitroglycerine. *See* Angina pectoris
Nitrous oxide oxygen gas. *See* Anesthesia
Noise, 335–36; and deafness, 163–66; decibels, for measuring volume of, 166–67; as a health hazard, 278–79
Nose, 336–38; olfactory sense, 340; and smells, 420; and sneezing, 420–21
Nose, diseases and disorders of: adenoids, 8–9, 133–35; atrophic rhinitis, 344; catarrh, 96; congestion, relieved by benzedrine, 57; foreign bodies in, 135–37, 226, 336–37; and hay fever, 244–45; mastoiditis from bad habits in nose blowing, 309; odors, 339–40; ozena, 344; rhinitis, 396; rhinophyma, 396
Nosebleed, 17–18, 198, 257, 336; in psittacosis, 382
Nucleus pulposus, 180, 426
Nursing, 108–12. *See also* Babies, breast feeding; Breast feeding
Nursing care (of the sick): in apoplexy, 31; in bed sores, 53; in bronchitis, 80; in chicken pox, 100; of children, 129–38; in chorea, 140–41; convalescence, 157–58, 251, 395–96; in coughing, 160; in croup, 161; in diphtheria, 180; disinfection, 180–81; fever, 220–22; hygiene of the sickroom, 131–32; in infantile paralysis, 282–83; in laryngitis, 296–97; in measles, 310–11; in rheumatic fever, 251, 395–96; in scarlet fever, 401; in typhoid fever, 458; in whooping cough, 475–76. *See also* Diets, special; First aid; Quarantine and isolation
Nutrition: amino acids, 19; in arctic climates, 34–35; boils, indicate poor nutritional states, 72; calories, 86; marasmus, 309; obesity, 338–39, 472–73; skin indicates nutritional state, 410–12; undernourishment in obesity, 68; vitamins, 464–69. *See also* Deficiency diseases
Nymphomania, 338
Nystagmus, 338

Obesity, 338–39; and blood pressure, high, 67–68; chafing caused by, 98; diabetes, associated with, 172; glands, not often caused by, 473; and hemorrhoids, 258; overeating, 338–39, 381, 472–73; undernourishment in, 68; varicose veins more frequent in, 462
Occupational diseases. *See* Industrial health
Odors, 71, 339–40, 420. *See also* Breath odor

Roughage, 155–56; bran, 156; in colitis, 150–51; excess may bring on diarrhea, 177
Roundworms, 476–77
Rubella. *See* Measles, German
Rupture. *See* Hernia

Sacroiliac joint, 402
Sacrum, 399
Sadism, 399
"Safe" period, 156–57, 373
St. Vitus dance. *See* Chorea
Salicylic acid, 36; in arthritis treatment, 39; in corn removers, 218; in dandruff treatments, 163; in gout, 237–38; home supplies, 313; para-aminosalicylic acid, in treatment of tuberculosis, 456; in rheumatic fever, 394; in ringworm treatments, 397
Saliva, 399
Salk vaccine, 272
Salmonella (bacteria). *See* Food poisoning
Salpingitis, 215, 399
Salt, 399; blood pressure, low, helped by, 68; in hot weather (salt tablets), 253–54, 434; iodized, for prevention of goiter, 235, 378–79; kidney disease calls for minimum in diet, 332; pneumonia patient needs much, 359
Salts of gold, in treatment of arthritis, 39
Salvarsan (606), 349–50, 437
Sanitation (public hygiene), 268–69; quarantine, 389–90; rat control, 389–90; summer camps, children, 127–28; swimming pools, 435–36. *See also* Carriers of disease; Infection; Milk; Quarantine and isolation
Sarcoma, 89, 399
Scabies. *See* Insect pests
Scarlatina. *See* Scarlet fever
Scarlet fever, 131, 400–1; and antitoxin, 29–30, 271–72; mastoiditis from, 309–10
Scarring: from burns, 84; from chicken pox, 100; in esophagus, 200, 364–65; keloid, 294–95; from smallpox, 419
Schlatter's disease. *See* Joint disturbances
Sciatica, 402. *See also* Sciatic neuritis
Sciatic neuritis, 401–2; and neuritis, 334
Scleroderma, 402
Sclerosis, 402
Sclerotic, *illus.*, 203
Scoliosis. *See* Spinal curvature
Scrofula. *See* Cures
Scurvy. *See* Vitamin C
Seasickness, 403–4; and altitude sickness, 17–18; treatment with dramamine, 183, 404
Seat worm, 476
Sebaceous cyst. *See* Wen
Sebaceous gland, *illus.*, 5
Seborrhea, 404–5. *See also* Dandruff
Seborrheic dermatitis. *See* Dandruff
Sedatives (pain killers): acetanilid, dangers of, 222, 313, 362; aconite, poisoning from, 6; aminopyrine (amido-

pyrine), dangers from, 186, 239, 246; habit formation, 186, 313, 319; in medicine chest, 313; pryamidon, dangers from, 186, 246, 300, 362. *See also* Salicylic acid
Semicircular canals, 182–83, 403, *illus.*, 187
Semilunar cartilage. *See* Joint disturbances
Seminal ducts, *illus.*, 374
Seminal vesicle, 374, 381
Senescence, 405–7. *See also* Old age
Senile wart. *See* Warts
Senility. *See* Senescence
Sepsis. *See* Abscess
Septicemia, 407
Septic sore throat, 353, 407–8, 445–46; associated with rheumatic fever, 393
Sertane, 39
Serums. *See* Measles; Pneumonia
Setting-up exercises, 201, 222, 268–69
Seven-year itch (scabies). *See* Insect pests
Sex function, 146; in acromegaly, disturbed, 6–7; aphrodisiac, 30; cantharides, 91; conception, 373; contraception, 156–57; fertility, 219–20; and hysterectomy, 270; in infantilism, disturbed, 284; libido, 300; and menopause, 318–19; menstruation, 319; orgasm, 341; puberty (sex maturity), 9–10, 219–20, 319; pituitary gland, role of, 355–57; and sterility, 429–31
Sex function, abnormal: exhibitionism, 202; hermaphroditism, 259–60; homosexuality and lesbianism, 264; nymphomania, 338; sadism, 399
Sex glands and organs, *illus.*, 373, 374, 375, 381; acne, relation to, 5; arthritis, relation to, 38; backache, from pulling by female organs, 49; circumcision, 141; Fallopian tubes, 215; damage to, from gonorrhea, 237, 341; hormone, male, in relief of cancer, 90; hormone, male, in building of musculature, 322; hymen, 269; ovary, 270, 343; penis, 351; pineal gland, relation to, 355; pituitary gland, relation to, 355–57; prostate, 381–82; testicles, *illus.*, 374, 381; uterus, 461; vagina, 462. *See also* Breast; Breast feeding
Sex glands and organs, disorders of: abortion, spontaneous, 3; acromegaly, 6–7; cancer, 87–88; endometritis, 196; epididymitis, 197; in eunuchs, 201; gleet, 235; gonorrhea, 236–37; gynecomastia, 239; hermaphroditism, 259–60; in infantilism, 284; leukorrhea, 300; mastitis, 309; metritis, 322; mumps, impairment by, 325–26; orchitis, 341; sterility, 429–31
Shaving, 239, 314, 411
Shell shock. *See* Hysteria
Shingles, 408
Ship fever. *See* Typhus
Shock, 408–9; in Addison's disease, 8; danger of, from burns, 83